Handbook of Medical Informatics

Handbook of Medical Informatics

J.H. van Bemmel
M.A. Musen

Editors

J.C. Helder

Managing editor

Houten/Diegem   1997

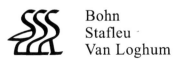
Bohn
Stafleu
Van Loghum

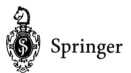
Springer

ISBN 90 313 2294 6 (Bohn Stafleu Van Loghum edition)
ISBN 3-450-63351-0 (Springer-Verlag edition)

This book will be distributed by Bohn Stafleu Van Loghum in The Netherlands and Belgium, by Springer-Verlag in the rest of the world.

Eerste druk, 1997
Eerste druk, tweede oplage 2000

Bohn Stafleu Van Loghum
De Molen 77, 3995 AW Houten, The Netherlands
Kouterveld 2, B-1831 Diegem, Belgium

Springer-Verlag
Tiergartenstrasse 17, D-69121 Heidelberg, Germany

Preface

Developments in medical informatics are progressing at great speed. As a consequence, there is a need for a broad overview of the field, recognizing that current students in medicine and health care will be the clinical professionals of the next millennium. By then, computers will be in widespread use for the support of patient care, the assessment of the quality of care, and the enhancement of decision making, management, planning, and medical research.

Medical informatics has both an applied and a theoretical dimension. These two aspects of the discipline have expanded dramatically during the last decade, and will continue to do so in the years to come. We are witnessing a radical change as technologies that primarily support administrative processes are augmented with systems that address the core of medicine: patient care in both the ambulatory and in-patient setting, disease prevention and health promotion, rehabilitation, and home care. Computer-based patient records and electronic communication will be the most visible developments in the years ahead.

The field of medical informatics is too extensive to be covered by only a small number of experts. Therefore, this *Handbook of Medical Informatics* has been written by a host of renowned international authorities in medical and health informatics (see the Table of Contents and the List of Authors).

The development of the Handbook has been the work of the two editors, one from Europe and one from the United States, assisted by a managing editor. The editors took much care that the Handbook would not be merely a collection of separate chapters, but rather would offer a consistent and structured overview of the field. They are aware that there is still considerable room for improvement and that certain elements of medical informatics are not fully covered, such as modeling and simulation. These shortcomings will be addressed in future editions and by the provision of material for advanced studies on the World Wide Web site associated with this Handbook (see below). Whereas this Handbook provides a comprehensive survey of current work performed to develop information technology for the clinical workplace, we recognize that the exciting and rapidly expanding discipline of bioinformatics is beyond our scope. Although many of the basic methods described in this Handbook are also applicable to work in computational biology, students will want to consult other sources for specific discussions of topics in bioinformatics.

Purpose

The purpose of the Handbook is to provide a systematic overview of medical informatics for medical students and nursing students, for physicians, nurses, and other health care professionals, and for students in other areas, such as informatics and computer science. There are three main reasons that we developed the Handbook:

1. Informatics is becoming part of the curriculum in an increasing number of universities and institutions for the higher education of health care professionals worldwide. The Handbook may serve as an introduction to the field for these students.

2. Health care workers are frequently confronted with information systems for the support of patient care, the assessment of the quality of care, research, or management and planning. For these professionals, the Handbook can serve as an orientation to the rapidly developing field of computers in health care.
3. Expanding numbers of graduate students are turning to medical informatics as a discipline for study and investigation. The more advanced chapters of this Handbook provide comprehensive overviews of topics in medical informatics that should be of value to specialists in the field.

Organization

The Handbook has been organized systematically. The 37 chapters are grouped into three main clusters that are subdivided into nine parts:

The first cluster deals with *data*:

I. The transformation from data into information.
II. The processing and storage of data in computers.
III. The acquisition of data from patients.

The second cluster describes the different types of *systems* in medicine and health care:

IV. Patient-centered information systems.
V. Systems for knowledge and decision support.
VI. Systems that are used to support institutions such as hospitals.

The third cluster pertains to *methodological* aspects of medical informatics and is intended to be used for more advanced or specialized education. The third cluster contains:

VII. The methodology for information processing (an extension of Parts II-V).
VIII. The methodology for information systems (an extension of Part VI).
IX. Medical informatics as a profession and academic discipline.

The Handbook contains only a few references to the literature, given at the end of most chapters. An extensive list of further literature for advanced study can be obtained from the Handbook's Web site (see below). This list will be continuously updated.
The editors invite readers, teachers, and students to send comments and feedback (suggestions, remarks, corrections, exercises, demonstrations, questions and answers, and so forth) to further improve and expand future editions of the Handbook and to be included immediately on the Web site (see the section below on Electronic Support for the Handbook).

The Editors,
Jan H. van Bemmel, Rotterdam, The Netherlands
Mark A. Musen, Stanford, California, USA

Electronic Support of the Handbook

Because medical informatics is a rapidly developing discipline, not all aspects of the field, let alone the most recent advances, could be contained in this Handbook. Therefore, the Handbook contains *links* to the Handbook's Web site, and from this Web site one can further branch to other Web sites around the world. The Web site contains the following sections:

1. An extensive *glossary* on terminology;
2. An electronic version of parts of the *Handbook*;
3. Electronic versions of *figures* and *tables* in the Handbook;
4. Questions and answers (*Q&A*);
5. References to the *literature*;
6. Published *articles*;
7. Interactive *exercises*;
8. Multimedia *demonstrations*; and
9. Short *videos.*
10. Pointers to *Web sites* worldwide;

(Some parts of the Web site are under continuous development, and certain parts of the Web site are only accessible by using a password that can be obtained on request from the editors.)

The blue-colored words (the *hyperlinks*) in the printed Handbook refer both to the glossary at the end of the Handbook and to the glossary on the Web site. Many hyperlinked words also refer to the 10 sections on the Web site listed above. Experts in the field and all readers and students are encouraged to contribute to the material on the Web site. The editorial board of the Handbook (composed of a selection of authors) will evaluate the quality of the proposed material.

> The Web site can be reached at the following addresses:
>
> http://www.mieur.nl/mihandbook
> and
> http://www.mihandbook.stanford.edu

Acknowledgments

The editors are most grateful to our authors for providing valuable text material, figures, and tables and for making helpful suggestions.

They are also most indebted to the managing editor, Dr. Jan C. Helder, for his careful reading of all material, for his many suggestions, and especially for the composition of the glossary and the insertion of hyperlinks into the glossary for access to additional information on the World Wide Web. Much work was done to generate the figures and the final text by our colleagues Peter C.G.M. Sollet and Sandra C. ten Bergen, who also made many suggestions regarding the layout and the language used. The editors are also very much indebted to Michael K. Hayes, Washington, DC, for carefully copyediting the Handbook.

Many thanks are also forwarded to Joop S. Duisterhout and Bob J.A. Schijvenaars, who have laid the foundation for the Handbook's Web site. Bob Schijvenaars also generated some of the complex figures on biosignal analysis. The editors are grateful to several colleagues elsewhere for providing illustrations for the Handbook.

Our publishers (Bohn, Stafleu and Van Loghum, and Springer Verlag) gave much help and encouragement to start the comprehensive endeavor of developing this text.

Finally, the editors were much stimulated by the extremely helpful feedback from many students and colleagues worldwide who commented on the preliminary version of this Handbook that appeared in 1996 and of which the present Handbook is the result. The present, color version would not have been realized without the help of the following colleagues:

J.E.C.M. Aarts, Polytechnic Eindhoven, The Netherlands;
H. Abdeslami, Erasmus University Rotterdam, The Netherlands;
P.W. Achterberg, RIVM, Bilthoven, The Netherlands;
H. Ahlfeldt, Linköping University, Sweden;
D. Assanelli, University Hospital Brescia, Italy;
N.C. Black, University of Ulster, Newtownabbey, United Kingdom;
H.M. Bos-Menting, Polytechnic The Hague, The Netherlands;
S. Cerutti, Polytechnic University of Milan, Milan, Italy;
J.J. Cimino, Columbia Presbyterian Medical Center, New York, United States;
E. Contini, Data and Telematics Services, Torino, Italy;
J. de Vries, University of Groningen, The Netherlands;
O. Ferrer-Roca, University La Laguna, Tenerife, Spain;
P. Ferrer-Salvans, University de Bellvitge, Barcelona, Spain;
M. Fieschi, University of Marseille, France;
G. Gell, University of Graz, Austria;
J.L. Grashuis, Erasmus University Rotterdam, The Netherlands;
R.A. Greenes, Harvard Medical School, Boston, United States;
F. Grémy, Montpellier, France;
J.B. Grimson, Trinity College, Dublin, Ireland;
T. Groth, University of Uppsala, Sweden;
A. Hasman, Maastricht University, The Netherlands
M.G.M. Hunink, University of Groningen, The Netherlands;
M.G. Kahn, Washington University, St. Louis, United States;
J.A. Kors, Erasmus University Rotterdam, The Netherlands;
P. Le Beux, University of Rennes, France;
N. Maglaveras, Aristotle University, Thessaloniki, Greece;
P. McCullagh, University of Ulster, Newtownabbey, United Kingdom;
K. McGlade, Queen's University, Belfast, United Kingdom;
G.I. Mihalas, University of Medicine and Pharmacy, Timisoara, Romania;

R.A. Miller, Vanderbilt University, Nashville, United States;
J.R. Möhr, University of Victoria, Canada;
P.W. Moorman, Erasmus University Rotterdam, The Netherlands;
J.A. Newell, Stratford-upon-Avon, United Kingdom;
T. Olhede, Swedish Institute for Health Services Development, Stockholm, Sweden;
V. Olchanski, Medical College of Virginia, United States;
M.H. Overmars, University of Utrecht, The Netherlands;
V. Rajkovic, University of Ljubljana, Slovenia;
J.H.C. Reiber, University of Leiden, The Netherlands;
F.H. Roger France, Catholic University of Louvain, Brussels, Belgium;
J.R. Scherrer, University of Geneva, Switzerland;
R.J.A. Schijvenaars, Erasmus University Rotterdam, The Netherlands;
M.A. Shifrin, Burdenko Neurosurgical Insititute, Moscow, Russia;
P. Spijns, University of Gent, Belgium;
W.W. Stead, Vanderbilt University, Nashville, United States;
M. Stefanelli, University of Pavia, Italy;
T. Stijnen, Erasmus University Rotterdam, The Netherlands;
C.A. Swenne, University of Leiden, The Netherlands;
T. Takahashi, Kyoto University, Kyoto, Japan;
B. van den Bosch, University Hospital Leuven, Belgium;
A.A.F. van der Maas, Catholic University Nijmegen, The Netherlands;
H.S. Verbrugh, Erasmus University Rotterdam, The Netherlands;
M.A. Viergever, University of Utrecht, The Netherlands;
J.E. Vos, University of Groningen. The Netherlands;
O.B. Wigertz, Linköping University, Sweden;
B. Zupan, University of Ljubljana, Slovenia;
J. Zvárová, Charles University, Prague, Czech Republic;
Chr. Zywietz, Medizinische Hochschule, Hannover, Germany.

How to Use this Handbook

This Handbook is intended for a wide readership. In fact, the Handbook offers only a first introduction to medical informatics, but even within the Handbook the depth of discussion in the different chapters varies. The following matrix may offer help in studying the different chapters. The various shades of grey indicate chapters that are strongly recommended, recommended, or optional for studying, depending on the reader's background.

Part	Chapter No.	Chapter Title	Students Medicine	Students Health Sciences	Professionals Health Care	Professionals Medical Informatics
I	1	Introduction and Overview				
	2	Information and Communication				
II	3	Data Processing				
	4	Database Management				
	5	Telecommunication, Networking, and Integration				
III	6	Coding and Classification				
	7	The Patient Record				
	8	Biosignal Analysis				
	9	Medical Imaging				
	10	Image Processing and Analysis				
IV	11	Primary Care				
	12	Clinical Departmental Systems				
	13	Clinical Support Systems				
	14	Nursing Information Systems				

▶

| Part | Chapter No. | Chapter Title | Students | | Professionals | |
			Medicine	Health Sciences	Health Care	Medical Informatics
V	15	Methods for Decision Support	■	■	■	■
	16	Clinical Decision-Support Systems	■	■	■	■
	17	Strategies for Medical Knowledge Acquisition	▨	▨	▨	■
	18	Predictive Tools for Clinical Decision Support	■	▨	■	▨
VI	19	Health Care Modeling		■	■	■
	20	HIS: Clinical Use	■	■	■	■
	21	HIS: Technical Choices	■	■	■	■
	22	Health Information Resources		■	■	■
VII	23	Logical Operations	■	■		■
	24	Biostatistical Methods	■	■		■
	25	Biosignal Processing Methods	■	■		■
	26	Advances in Image Processing	■	■		■
	27	Pattern Recognition	■	■		■
	28	Modeling for Decision Support	■	■		■
	29	Structuring the CPR	■		■	■
	30	Evaluation of Information Systems	■	■	■	■
VIII	31	Human-Computer Interaction in Health Care	▨	▨	▨	■
	32	Costs and Benefits of Information Systems	▨	▨	▨	■
	33	Security in Medical Information Systems	■	■	■	▨
	34	Standards in Health Care				■
	35	Project Management			▨	■
IX	36	Education and Training				■
	37	International Developments				■

■ Strongly recommended
▨ Recommended
☐ Optional

Table of Contents

PART I: Data and Information

PART II: Data in Computers

TC

PART III: Data from Patients

TC

Chapter 8: Biosignal Analysis 117

Chapter 9: Medical Imaging 127

PART IV: Patient-Centered Information Systems

TC

PART V: Medical Knowledge and Decision Support

TC

PART VI: Institutional Information Systems

TC

TC

PART VII: Methodology for Information Processing

TC

TC

PART VIII: Methodology for Information Systems

TC

TC

TC

PART IX: Medical Informatics as a Profession

Table of Contents

TC

Table of Authors

TA

TA

TA

What is Medical Informatics?

Medical informatics is located at the intersection of information technology and the different disciplines of medicine and health care. In this Handbook, we shall also use the term *health informatics* without entering into a fundamental discussion of the possible differences between medical informatics and health informatics (see Panel 1 for some other names of the field).

Medical informatics has both distinctly applied features and more fundamental characteristics. Just as medicine itself is multidisciplinary, so is medical informatics. The main reason for this convergence of disciplines is that, in principle, medical informatics deals with the whole field of medicine and health care. Blois[1] summarized the heterogeneity of medical science quite eloquently and related the multi-disciplinary nature of medicine directly to the basis of medical informatics:

It is sometimes asserted that medical science is no different than any other science. I would strongly disagree with this view; medical science (human biology) in its describing, reasoning, explaining, and predicting, necessarily draws upon a number of lower-level sciences, while physics, for example, does not. This obvious state of affairs (that medicine rests upon a hierarchy of natural sciences) has profound consequences. Because medicine derives its experimental content from a set of sciences (including both "hard" and "soft" sciences), the processing of the

observational data of medicine faces a number of problems. This is one of the reasons why there is a "medical' information science, and why there is not a "physics" information science.

The health care process is very different from medical science. The former is more related to the art of medicine, whereas the latter is closely connected to the 'academic aspects and the basic disciplines of medicine. A synonym for *art* is, for instance, *skill*. Science is related to *knowledge*, as expressed by Webster's Dictionary:

Science is accumulated and accepted knowledge that has been systematized and formulated with reference to the discovery of general truths or the operation of general laws.

Specialization can be accomplished in both art and science. The more specialized one's health care (the art of practicing health care), the more detailed must be one's medical knowledge (the science of medicine). What is the origin and the nature of the scientific knowledge that lies at the root of health care? How and where is that knowledge acquired? The latter appears to happen in two different locations:

1. in the medical research laboratory and
2. in clinical practice.

From the foregoing we may conclude the following: Scientific research in medical informatics is multi-disciplinary because

---

1   Blois MS. Information and Medicine: The Nature of Medical Descriptions. *Berkeley, CA: Univ of California Press, 1984.*

PANEL 1

What's in a Name?

The term *medical informatics* dates from the second half of the 1970s and was borrowed from the French expression *informatique médicale*. Before that time, other names were used (and are sometimes still in use), such as *medical computer science, medical information science, computers in medicine, health informatics*, and more specialized terms such as *nursing informatics, dental informatics*, and so on. These terms have their parallels with similar ones in areas outside health care, such as *computer science, information processing*, and *informatics*, and in specialized areas, for instance: *computational physics, computational linguistics*, or *artificial intelligence*. In informatics as such, one may discern three different layers of research: fundamental computer science, applications-oriented informatics, and applied informatics. Research for the realization of medical information systems mainly belongs to the third category.

The more usable and more comprehensive the software tools that come out of research in computer science, the better medical informatics can direct its efforts on applications-oriented projects where specific knowledge is required in the specialized area.

- we deal with medicine and health care as a whole, and
- it is done by investigators who come from different scientific disciplines.

Research in medical informatics aims not only at the incorporation of

- knowledge from the natural sciences, but also of
- special knowledge or clinical experience.

Finally, research in medical informatics must deal with the normative aspects of our knowledge.

It is appropriate to ask whether medical informatics has a research domain of its own and a specific methodology or whether it borrows its methods from other disciplines and just applies these methods to medicine and health care. Is medical informatics, for instance, different from statistics or epidemiology? Are the methods of medical informatics different from those of computer science or physics? Furthermore, if in medical informatics we deal with the whole of medicine and health care, in what respect are its methods different from those that are used in medicine and health care? In addition, how should we

reckon with ethical aspects in applying the results from medical informatics research?

We may state that if medical informatics is a science, then some of the following properties should be applicable:

- It contains a *domain* where a *theory* is developed.
- It is not merely *applied* science.
- It is not solely determined by *technology*.
- *Models* are developed to illustrate and prove theories.
- Problems are solved in a methodical way, following scientific principles of *abstraction and generalization*.

The *domain* of medical informatics is determined by the intersection of the terms "medicine" and "informatics" (or "health" and "information") (see also Panel 2 for two definitions). The first term indicates the area of research, the second one its methodology. Medical informatics has both applied and theoretical aspects; models are developed both in applications and in theoretical activities. As in all science, in medical informatics research we strive for the collection of generally applicable knowledge, so that we may use it within a particular domain: health care.

> ## PANEL 2
>
> ## Definitions of Medical Informatics
>
> Several definitions of medical informatics (medical information science, health informatics) have been given. Some of these take into account both the scientific and the applied sides of the field; other definitions are more pragmatic. We cite only two definitions:
>
> *Medical information science is the science of using system-analytic tools . . . to develop procedures (algorithms) for management, process control, decision making and scientific analysis of medical knowledge.*[2]
>
> *Medical Informatics comprises the theoretical and practical aspects of information processing and communication, based on knowledge and experience derived from processes in medicine and health care.*[3]
>
> ---
>
> [2] *Shortliffe EH. The science of biomedical computing. Med Inform 1984;9:185-93.*
> [3] *Van Bemmel JH. The structure of medical informatics. Med Inform 1984;9:175-80.*

In summary:

In medical informatics we develop and assess methods and systems for the acquisition, processing, and interpretation of patient data with the help of knowledge that is obtained in scientific research.

Computers are the vehicles used to realize these goals. In medical informatics, we deal with the entire domain of medicine and health care, from computer-based patient records to image processing and from primary care practices to hospitals and regions of health care. Some areas of the field are relatively fundamental; others have an applied character. The challenge in developing methods and systems in medical informatics is that once the systems have been made operational for one medical specialty, they can also be transferred to some other specialty.

As much as possible, this Handbook attempts to stress the general methodology behind all methods and applications. Examples of this cross-fertilization are methods for image processing in cardiology, pathology, and radiology; the common structure of computer-based records in internal medicine, primary care, and pediatrics; or the way that medical knowledge can be structured and documented in surgery, obstetrics or oncology.

In Chapter 1 we cluster the field of medical informatics into six *levels of complexity*. This clustering shows a strong resemblance to the diagnostic-therapeutic cycle, which we also discuss in Chapter 1.

Related to the two types of knowledge, medical treatment consists of indisputable *conclusions* on the one hand and responsible *decisions* on the other. The conclusions are, within the domain and the limitations of scientific a prioris, absolute and objective in nature. At the same time, they are of limited scope, since they are based on the application of scientific research. Although the final diagnostic decision is based on such conclusions, it is still oriented toward the individual patient and his or her personal circumstances and expectations. The final decision is, for all that, not absolute, but is made in freedom and under the responsibility of the treating clinician (and, it is hoped, in agreement with the patient). The decision also takes into account those aspects of patient care that cannot be formalized. Therefore, the final decision regarding the therapy to be selected requires experience and insight, but it also has ethical and legal aspects and foremost should be a wise decision. These last qualities are unsuitable for formalization, let alone fit for delegation to a computer.

In conclusion:

- Medical informatics is both an *Art* and a *Science*.
  - *Science*: where methods are conceived and experimentally validated by means of computer models and formalisms.
  - *Art*: where computer processing systems are built and assessed.

- Research in medical informatics is multidisciplinary and follows scientific methods; applications have a technological foundation.
- Research and applications in medical informatics should take into account the responsibilities of investigators and users.

Data and Information

Authors of Part I

Chapter 1: Introduction and Overview
J.H. van Bemmel, Erasmus University Rotterdam

Chapter 2: Information and Communication
J.H. van Bemmel, J.S. Duisterhout, Erasmus University Rotterdam

1 Introduction and Overview

1 Introduction

The purpose of this introductory chapter is to present an overview of computer support in medicine and health care as reflected in the *collection* and interpretation of *data*, in decision making, and in subsequent actions. This and the following chapters review different aspects of computer support and provide many examples.

Conscious thinking and reasoning characteristically precedes most human activity. This applies to daily pursuits as well as to scientific activities. Patient care and medical research are examples of areas in which human reasoning is pivotal. Such thinking essentially entails the interpretation of real-world observations or *data* with the help of *knowledge* that is provided by experts. In principle, both data and knowledge can be stored in *computers*. This is why human reasoning can now be assisted by computers.

If computers are able to assist human reasoning, it is important to know the strong points and the limitations of computers in general and in health care in particular. Therefore, we want to investigate where and how human thinking can be supported by computers in patient care and related activities, such as medical research or management and planning in health care. It is also important to investigate to what degree computers might help in *decision making* and how the latter is related to the clinician's responsibility for patients.

Information plays a key role when interpreting data and making decisions. It is therefore essential to know what information is and to understand the difference between data, information, and knowledge. In this and the following chapters we will discuss how reliable data can be acquired, in what way information is derived from the data, and what type of knowledge is necessary for interpreting the data and how this knowledge can be stored in computers. Figure 1.1 shows that the patient or some (biological) process generates *data* that are observed by the clinician. From those data, by a process of interpretation or reasoning, *information* is derived, and this information guides the clinician in taking further action. In Fig. 1.1 the arrow labeled "information" indicates the first *feedback* loop to the clinician. By carefully studying many such interpretation processes in medicine or by collecting interpreted data from many patients, inductive reasoning may lead to new insights and new *knowledge*. This knowledge is then added to the body of knowledge in medicine and, in turn, is used to interpret other data. Computers may help in the collection and the interpretation of the data and in the derivation of new knowledge. As indicated above, both data and knowledge can be stored in computers, and computer programs can be developed for the *acquisition* and the interpretation of the *data*.

The bird's eye view of computer applications in health care, as presented in section 4 of this chapter will show that there are many possibilities, but also fundamental limitations, in the use of computers in medicine, the more so if they are used for direct patient care. This introductory chapter intends to offer a handle that can be used to order and structure computer applications

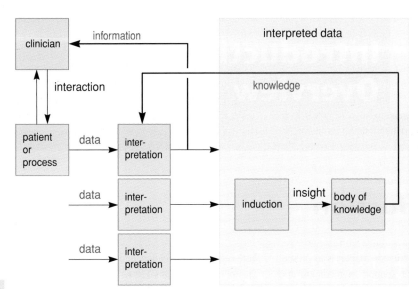

Figure 1.1
A patient or a biological process generates data that are observed by the clinician. Information is derived from the data by interpretation, which is fed back to the clinician. By inductive reasoning with the interpreted data, collected from many similar patients or processes, new knowledge is obtained, which is added to the body of knowledge in medicine. This knowledge is used for the interpretation of other data.

with respect to the strong and weak aspects of using computers in health care. This structure will be presented in the form of a scheme of levels of complexity or levels of dependence on human involvement, with the user being the physician, the nurse, or some other health care provider, or the medical researcher.

2 Diagnostic-Therapeutic Cycle

In almost all human activities we can discern three stages (Table 1.1):

1. observation,
2. reasoning,
3. action.

These stages in human activity play a role not only in daily life, but also in patient care, management, and research. For instance, if we find ourselves in a dangerous or unpleasant situation, we observe the facts and the circumstances, make a plan to get away from the problem and, if possible, carry out our plan to improve the situation. On the battlefield, for instance, generals collect data on the military situation, design a strategic plan, and carry it out. Beforehand, they may even simulate the battlefield situation and the plan on a computer. The same three stages can also be seen in scientific research (Table 1.1). The investigator collects the observations (measurements or data), arrives at a conclusion in view of hypotheses and, on the basis of his theoretical knowledge and reasoning, comes to an interpretation and rejects or revises the theory, and, finally, plans new investigations or experiments to widen his or her knowledge.

Also in health care the same three stages can be seen in the so-called diagnostic-therapeutic cycle (Fig. 1.2):

1. observation,
2. *diagnosis*,
3. *therapy*.

A patient tells his or her history, the clinician collects the data (e.g., during a physical examination, by laboratory tests or radiology), comes to a conclusion and possibly even a diagnosis, and prescribes a therapy or carries out some other treatment. In health care, in contrast to scientific research, we are not confronted with the issue of solving an abstract, general problem, but are confronted with solving the problems of individual patients. These problems can only partly be generalized. For solving patient-related problems, the clinician must use as much as possible methods that were assessed in scientific research but must always address the specific problems of the individual patient in the real, nonabstracted world. Often, therefore, patient-related problems cannot be solved in a way that abstracts from how patients function in society.

In practice, the three stages of human activity are often cycled iteratively, because it may appear that hypotheses have to be refined or altered. Where and when, precisely, during the process of making a diagnosis or carrying out research the creative spark to obtain insight in the human brain jumps is generally a mystery. This is particularly true for research, including medical research.

After this more or less philosophical introduction it must be stressed that this book is not a course in computer programming, but deals with the use of computers for solving problems dealing with data, information and knowledge in health care. These problems are related to both scientific issues and patient-related prob-lems. The medical sciences are not different from other disciplines when using computers for scientific research. The use of computers for solving patient-related problems, however, is different from the use of computers in most other areas. For that reason, we first discuss the three stages in the diagnostic-therapeutic cycle (Fig. 1.2). It is a brief description of common clinical practice, in which care providers are dealing with data, information and knowledge.

2.1 Observation

In the observation stage we deal with the acquisition of data, preferably, only data that provide relevant information (other aspects about the difference between data and information will be dealt with in Chapter 2). In short, with information we can diminish the uncertainty that exists about a patient's disease. In many cases this uncertainty can be decreased by data from the patient history (the **anamnesis**); in other cases physiological or biochemical data must be collected from the patient (e.g., by a physical examination), from an analysis of blood samples, or the recording of biological signals (**biosignals**) such as electrocardiograms (**ECGs**) or **spirograms**.

In collecting data, we are often faced with sometimes considerable anomalies in the data, such as incom-

1

Areas of human activity				Table 1.1
Stage	General	Scientific research	Health care	Computer processing
1	Observation	Measurement	Patient data collection	Data entry
2	Reasoning	Theory	Diagnosis	Data processing
3	Action	Experiment	Therapy	Output generation

Table 1.1
Three Stages of Human Activities: Observation, Thinking or Reasoning, and Action, for Different Areas.

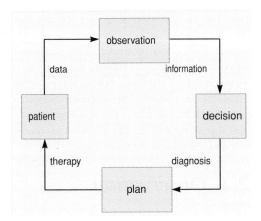

Figure 1.2
Diagnostic-therapeutic cycle. In this cycle information circles around from observed data, via interpreted data, to data that are used for the therapy. The cycle can be circled only once, e.g., during patient consultation, or many times, e.g., when a patient is monitored in an intensive care unit.

1

ischemic heart diseases: the patient history, the *exercise ECG, coronary angiography,* and *echocardiography*). Sometimes we have so many data at our disposal that we can speak of data **redundancy**. In fact, while cycling the diagnostic-therapeutic cycle, during each pass the clinician attempts to decrease the uncertainty about the patient's disease or the actual state of the disease process. For that reason, the first stage in this cycle is always the patient history, if one is available, and then less expensive procedures (e.g., a physical examination or a laboratory test) generally precede the more expensive and invasive ones (e.g., a magnetic resonance imaging (**MRI**) scan or a cardiac **catheterization**). By using data in different ways and using different methods, in most circumstances a complete view of the patient's condition is obtained. It is the task of medical informatics to support the clinician in obtaining the necessary data and providing decision-support methods so that the diagnostic-therapeutic cycle can be traversed in an efficient manner while maintaining quality of care and decreasing inconvenience for the patient as much as possible.

plete or incorrect answers from the patient, noise on biosignals, or errors in biochemical analyses (see also Chapter 2). In many cases we may not be able to obtain the data in which we are interested because the organ or process of interest cannot be reached by noninvasive procedures. Only in certain circumstances the physician may decide to invade the body and collect data by carrying out an exploratory examination, for instance, with a *catheter*, an *endoscope*, or a *laparoscope* or by obtaining a specimen by performing a *biopsy*. In some diseases, the process in which we are interested is unstable or nonstationary, that is, the disease process is in a dynamic state and the process parameters are continuously changing. This occurs, for instance, in patients with runs of extrasystoles, patients in shock, or patients with epileptic seizures.

It is a challenge for medical informatics to assist in interpreting the data that are acquired from patients. Section 4 of this chapter and the following chapters give numerous examples of the use of computers to derive parameters that are of importance for diagnosis and therapy.

Patient data that are derived in completely different ways often supplement and reinforce each other so that a more reliable diagnosis can be reached (e.g., in

2.2 Diagnosis

Part V (Chapters 15-18) returns to the relationship between computers and making a diagnosis. Therefore, only some preliminary remarks that fit into the introductory character of this first chapter are made here. Human thinking (by the treating clinician) precedes the diagnosis. For that reason the computer can be of great support in the diagnostic stage as well. However, this concerns only that part of the diagnosis that can be structured, generalized, and made objective, in other words, the part that is based on scientific and well-structured methods. A clinician is often not aware of what he does not know; computer-generated lists may prompt him to suggestions he was not aware of. The computer may help, for instance, to find the necessary background information from the literature.

A clinician bears responsibility for the patient and, consequently, for the diagnosis, when using computer support, but computers will never be allowed to take over the human responsibility of making a diagnosis.

The objective and scientifically based part of the diagnosis, however, may be left to the computer. Those elements of the diagnosis that deal with unique and individual problems of the patient cannot and should not be handed over to a machine. For instance, a diagnosis always has, to some degree, subjective aspects that may never be generalized and transferred to a computer. At first sight it seems that the practical experience of clinicians in making diagnoses and treating patients is highly subjective and cannot be transferred to a computer. This is only partly true, as will be seen later (see Chapter 15), because even clinical knowledge and experience stored in human brains can be structured and made operational in a computer (e.g., documented in a *knowledge base*), although only partially and only to a certain degree.

2.3 Therapy

The clinical knowledge and experience required in the therapeutic stage are different from those required in the diagnostic stage; a therapy is characterized by the practical aspects of human activity, which is less governed by theoretical reflections than by decision making. The therapeutic stage is therefore dependent on the outcome of the preceding stage, the diagnosis and implicitly the prognosis (i.e., the most probable future patient outcome) predicted by *decision analysis* (see Chapter 18).

Often, the therapy is given by a physician or a nurse other than the clinician who made the diagnosis. Examples of therapies often given by other care providers are surgery and radiotherapy. It is inconceivable that the surgical or exploratory activities of clinicians will ever be completely taken over by computers or robots. However, the preparation for and the monitoring of the therapy can be supported by computers. Examples of the latter are the administration of drugs (their amount, possible *drug-drug interaction* or *contraindications*), the *monitoring* of severely ill patients, or radiotherapy.

Although these latter examples are directly related to patient care, the computer can also be used to analyze large collections of data derived from many patients to draw conclusions by induction (see Fig. 1.1). This type of analysis, sometimes also referred to as *data mining* (see Chapter 22), is seen in *epidemiology*, health services research, decision analysis, and medical research in general. Computers are also indispensable for the assessment of different therapies, for which in many instances *controlled trials* or intervention studies must be carried out.

3 Information Processing

In anticipation of Chapter 3, where we shall discuss the structure of an information processing system, we want to show the parallels and differences between information processing by humans and machine. In information processing by a computer we also observe the same three stages that we discerned earlier (see Table 1.1):

1. measuring and data entry,
2. data processing,
3. output generation.

Essentially, we can only speak of *information* processing if a human is involved in one way or the other.

Computers, as we shall see, do not process information but merely process *data*. Only a human being is able to interpret the data so that they become information. There is a parallel between computer-assisted data entry and observation with the human senses (see also Chapter 2). Computer processing, too, has some parallels with thought processes in the human brain, but as mentioned earlier, this concerns only that part of the processing that can be structured and generalized. In patient care, computers cannot and should not *replace* thought processes in the human brain but should *amplify* the brain's capabilities. A computer can extend the brain's memory, increase its data processing capabilities, and improve the accuracy and consistency of our data processing. Similar to the way that the human senses are amplified by a microscope or a stethoscope, the human brain can be amplified by a computer.

In the framework of information processing by computer, humans have a very specific role in that a human takes the initiative, prepares the processing, and interprets the results. In developing or using information processing systems, one should ensure that the human responsibility is left intact and prevent a situation in which the human merely becomes a replaceable part of the information processing system, who is called for only when human activity is cheaper, but who is replaced as soon as the computer offers a better alternative. This is even more applicable to health care, in which not only economical aspects, but also ethical issues apply. Particularly when computers are applied in health care, in which human beings are both the subjects (physicians and nurses) and the objects (patients) of information processes, we should be careful to have the right balance between human and machine.

3.1 Support of Human Thinking

Developments in informatics and computer technology follow each other at very rapid speed. Who could have imagined only a few decades ago (it was the time of the ENIAC, the first calculator built with electronic tubes, with about 1,000 operations per second) that there would be pocket-sized computers able to perform a 100 million or even 1 billion operations per second? A computer from the early 1950s that at that time cost about $1 million would now cost, with comparable functionality, on the order of $25 or less.

Through the accomplishments of informatics and telematics, our time is rapidly and dramatically changing to an information age. The *Internet* and the *World Wide Web* are well-known terms, and increasing percentages of people own a personal computer (*PC*). In fact, we do not know what information really is or what substance it consists of! (Chapter 2 discusses in some detail the different aspects of information.) Do we really understand the essence of gravity or electri-

city? We have no idea what an electron or a neutrino really is. In science we build theories that are valid until they are falsified or until somebody develops some other theory that shapes a better model of the world in which we live.

In a similar way, a clinician also often does not fully understand the disease itself, its nature or its origin, although genetics is broadening the horizon of our knowledge to a far greater distance. Physicians often do not quite understand how they arrived at the proper insight that put them on the right track to finding the correct diagnosis (Chapter 15 discusses this issue in greater depth). However, is a chess grand master, having played many games, really able to describe how he came to the insight of what his best next move would be? (see also Panel 15.1.) In the same way, clinicians come to such insight, on the basis of knowledge and experience, and also in health care we successfully apply models and theories for the benefit of patient care, even when they are not fully understood. Modern health care would be nonexistent without such models and theories, which are the results of medical research. Both in science and in health care, our thinking (stage two of human activity) and action (stage three) are dominated by man-made rules or laws that have been discovered and theories that have been developed in the course of scientific research. A computer may support us in structuring and ordering the world in which we live, both in science and in society at large. Thus, in our research and in virtually all areas of modern society computers have become indispensable.

In medical informatics we also attempt to formulate rules, discover laws, or structure models that provide a better insight into information processes. Such models are made operational using computers with the intention of applying them to patient care. There is, however, a danger that must be pointed out and that applies to the use of models in general. It is tempting to view the real world from the perspective of our models. In doing so, we reshape the world around us, reduce it, and put it in the harness of our own, limited view of the world. If we put on a pair of red glasses we should not be surprised that the world is red and no longer colorful. If our computer models contain knowledge related to only a limited number of diseases, we should not be surprised that the true disease

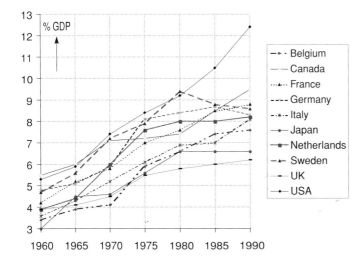

a Source: OECD, 1995

Figure 1.3
Costs of health care in different countries as a function of time and related to the GDP.[a] Health care costs tend to increase as a function of higher demands (e.g., a growing population of elderly people) and a larger spectrum of diagnostic and therapeutic possibilities. Information systems may assist with controlling the costs of health care while maintaining a high quality.

will never be diagnosed. When applying the results of research to the real world, we should be aware of both the possibilities and the limitations of the underlying models. This book also intends to make users of computers in health care aware of these limitations.

3.2 Developments in Health Care

The introduction of computers in health care goes in parallel with a growing concern that the costs of health care are increasing too quickly or have already surpassed a level that is acceptable to society. Figure 1.3 outlines the costs of health care as a function of gross domestic product (GDP) in some countries. In Western countries this ranges from about 6% to more than 12% of GDP.

It is no surprise that much is expected from using computers to control and stabilize the costs of health care. One of the proposed measures is the reinforcement of primary care in combination with providing physicians and nurses with computers. This would involve a shift from hospital care to primary care and home care. This implies collaboration between care providers supported by computer-based **shared care** and electronic interchange of patient data, computer-supported teleconsulting by experts and decision-support systems, and the introduction of **protocols** and **managed care**

(see Chapters 5 and 11). All this results in new responsibilities for clinicians and changes in the tasks of different care providers. It also means increased responsibilities for patients themselves, who could have a greater role in self-care if they were supported by computers.

The data in computer-based patient records are increasingly used to evaluate the provision of care and for medical audits. In all possible future scenarios of health care, information streams will only increase; hopefully for the benefit of patients and healthy people. This information stream is wide and shallow in primary care, but it is much wider and deeper in hospital-based care. Patient data will also increasingly be used for management and planning in health care organizations and national institutions and to support the assessment of quality of care. At all levels of health care, from individual patient care to health care management, decision makers are interested in patient data or aggregations of patient data.

3.3 Parallels

As we already observed, information processing and computers have penetrated our entire society. No wonder that in health care, too, changes similar to those in society as a whole have taken place. Indeed, we can observe many parallels between computers in

1

Computer Applications			
Level	Society	Health Care	
1	Use of the Internet	Health-care communication	
2	Airline booking	Hospital registration	
3	Satellite pictures	X-ray imaging	
4	Process control	Patient monitoring	
5	Computer-assisted design	Radiotherapy planning	
6	Model of traffic flow	Model of the blood circulation	

Table 1.2
Parallels Between Computer Applications in Society and Health Care.[a]

[a] Many applications seen in other areas have their counterpart in health care, such as booking a flight and patient registration in a hospital, the control of an industrial process and patient monitoring, or the processing of satellite images or X-ray images. The levels of the six examples refer to the same levels mentioned in Fig. 1.4.

society and computers in health care, and we may even wonder why we need to develop information systems especially for health care and why we need a separate profession called *medical informatics*. We will come back to this issue in section 4, but first we list in Table 1.2 examples of computer applications in health care and society, to show the many parallels in processing methodology and information systems. From the examples in Table 1.2 we see the correspondence between computer applications in different areas. At first sight, these examples look somewhat arbitrary; any structure about information processing in the different areas does not become apparent. Yet, it appears from this enumeration that in some application areas the computer is used for pure administrative goals (booking of seats on airplanes or registration for a hospital bed), in others it is used for the analysis of data (industrial or hospital laboratories), and in yet others it is used for the support of decisions, either in management or in health care. In the next section we bring some further structure to these different applications, and it will appear that differences in the nature of the computer applications are reflected in their complexity and dependence on human involvement.

4 Systematization of Computer Applications

At first sight the applications of computers in health care look very extensive and the field of medical informatics does not seem to be structured or orderly. After a superficial acquaintance with medical informatics, not only may the newcomer have this impression, but sometimes even the insider may have the same impression. Systematization of the applications in medical informatics is not easy and is not self-evident. Systematization is of importance, however, for different reasons. First, it is of great use in education. Second, it may provide to students a better understanding of the possibilities and limitations of certain computer applications in health care, and, third, structuring of the field might help to advance its scientific basis. For instance, it might be of great help to understand why progress in certain applications is lagging behind expectations, or it might give insight how to better balance the involvement of humans and computers in certain application areas.

The systematization that we want to discuss intends to address all three areas. It will appear that the limitations of computers in health care and their dependence on human interaction is more fundamental than was thought at first sight. In addition, although the field of medical informatics is very wide, we will show that it is possible to bring structure in all applications so that we can gain more insight into what to expect, even when new generations of information systems are developed. Structuring of the field will also be useful for gaining insight into the coherence between the different chapters of this book.

In discussing our systematization, we want to make use of the scheme depicted in Fig. 1.4, which offers a model with six levels for the structuring of applications of computers in health care. It will appear that we are less dependent on human involvement in information processing if we are better able to generalize our application, which applies especially to the lower levels of our scheme. However, in direct patient care we rarely deal with a generalized problem; rather, we deal with an individual patient. This structuring is also of importance for all other applications in society: when we can systematize and structure a problem in the form of a model, computers are better suitable for offering help. However, the solution of unique problems and situations, not covered by a model, can hardly ever be assisted by computers, independent of human involvement. An airplane can be flown by computers, but in situations that are not foreseen, human interaction is required. Cars can completely be manufactured by robots, but the ingenuity of engineers is required to develop a new prototype. Administrative processes such as those used in banking can be almost fully automated, but a high-level corporate decision should be taken by the board of directors after carefully balancing pros and cons. Successful application of computers is only possible when a proper systems analysis precedes systems development and programming. In

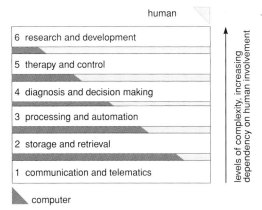

Figure 1.4
A model for structuring computer applications in health care by a scheme of levels of complexity or dependence on human involvement. The model can be seen as a building with six floors or levels. Each level contains different types of computer applications with, from bottom to top, an increasing complexity and a growing human involvement (see text).

that respect, in health care as well, some computer applications are better suitable for systematization and generalization than other ones.

For the reasons mentioned above, the scheme in Fig. 1.4 has been designed in such a way that it expresses at higher levels an increasing complexity of computer applications in health care and an increasing dependence on human interaction. We shall discuss these levels of complexity in the following paragraphs and, while doing so, give concrete examples in health care. The scheme in Fig. 1.4 can be imagined as a building with six floors or levels. On each floor we see different types of computer applications that, from bottom to top, increase in complexity and require increased human involvement. At the lower levels in the building, computer applications can be better structured and controlled and they can more often operate without human interaction. For that reason we have given the wall of the building two different colors: the triangle at the lower left represents a decreasing degree of automation, and the triangle at the upper right represents a steadily growing human involvement. It is not possible to reach some higher level without passing slowly or quickly through all lower levels. Furthermore, the results that are obtained on the highest level influence the applications at all lower levels.

On the ground floor we enter and leave the building; here the main usage of computers is *communication* and *telematics*. In principle, time here is real time. On the second level, time is frozen, that is, data do not leave the building immediately but are stored in computer memories. However, in principle, the data are left untouched; that is, they are not processed, transformed, or interpreted. On the third level not only is time (temporarily) frozen but the data are also changed by processing. This is the level where automated data processing takes place. The results of such processing are either stored on the second level or presented to the fourth level, where the (processed) data are interpreted. Human involvement and, possibly, the human-machine interaction are far greater here than on the levels below. The results of the interpretation are used on the fifth level to assist in therapy or to control processes. On the sixth level, human involvement is greatest: it is the level where new discoveries are made during research and development. The results of this are used at all lower levels. The first two levels deal mainly with the first stage of the diagnostic-therapeutic cycle, the observation and data acquisition phase. Levels 3 and 4 deal primarily with the second stage, where the diagnosis is made. Level 5 is most related to the third stage of the diagnostic-therapeutic cycle, therapy.

The following sections discuss the activities that take place on all floors and give illustrations of some representative applications.

Level 1:

Communication and Telematics

One of the best-structured applications is one in which a computer is used for *data acquisition* and data transmission. This frequently involves some *decoding* or coding process that transforms the data into a standardized form and sometimes into an *encrypted* format. Computers are increasingly used for data transfer and communication, also called *tele-*

matics. In case of transmission, the data are first stored on some temporary storage medium before being transmitted. The following are some examples of applications on this level.

- The visualization of biological signals such as an ECG or an arterial blood pressure tracing on a computer screen during intensive patient care. The data are usually derived from the patient by *electrodes* or *transducers*, amplified, *digitized*, entered into a computer in the intensive care unit, and presented on a display terminal, laser printer, or plotter.

- A *local area network* in a clinical department that interconnects personal computers or a network of *workstations* in a hospital that are used to transfer the results of biochemical analysis from the laboratory to clinical departments or to transmit orders of clinicians for drugs to the hospital pharmacy.

- The electronic interchange of patient data between computer-based patient records in a region where primary care physicians are collaborating in *shared care*, or the electronic transfer of referral letters and discharge reports between general practitioners and hospitals.

- The transmission of radiological images from a district hospital to a university hospital for teleconsulting or the transmission of *ECGs* from remote places to a department of cardiology for computer interpretation.

- Using the *Internet* and the *World Wide Web* it is possible to transmit data from one location to the other.

When developing such applications, we seldom meet fundamental problems of a technical nature (except for speed in data interchange) or are hampered by limitations caused by information technology; most of the remaining problems are caused by the very nature of problems in health care. On the ground level of the scheme in Fig. 1.4, data enter the building of information processing and are coded, transmitted, decoded, and presented to the user or to another processing system. In general, the use of computers for telematics in health care is not very different from other application areas elsewhere in society.

Level 2:

Storage and Retrieval

The applications in the preceding section are now extended with the possibilities that computers offer for storage and retrieval of data in databases. With the present-day computers and PCs, it is possible to store an extremely large amount of data at a cheap price, and these data can be retrieved quickly. Combined with the applications in level 1, the storage capacity for data is virtually infinite. Medical databases can grow very large, and a capacity of more than 100 *gigabytes*[1] or even more than a *terabyte* (see Chapter 3 for the size of computer memories) in hospital information systems is certainly no exception, especially when patient data are continuously updated. Hospitals may have a hospital database containing data for more than 1 million patients. The storage of medical images requires a huge capacity; for that purpose industry has developed efficient storage media that can contain many thousands of images (after data compression: see Chapters 13 and 34). There are now industrial standards to transport these images efficiently from one place to another. Examples of applications on level 2 include the following:

- *Databases* of patient data are in use in hospitals, clinical departments, and primary care practices and are used for statistical purposes. In *ancillary departments* databases are also used to control the stock of goods necessary to run an institution.
- Several institutions serve health care by providing central databases and systems where knowledge is stored. This knowledge can be borrowed for the benefit of patient care or research. Examples are *MEDLINE* of the National Library of Medicine (*NLM*) in the United States, national databases of drugs, or international databases for the storage of diagnostic codes, such as the International Classification of Diseases (*ICD*) or the Systematized Nomenclature of Human and Veterinary Medicine (*SNOMED* International).

---

[1] *kilo: 10^3, mega: 10^6, giga: 10^9, tera: 10^{12}.*

- Now that medical imaging systems increasingly deliver pictures in digital form and computer memories are becoming steadily larger and have lower prices, picture archiving systems (*PACS*) are now also more affordable, and PACS have begun to be implemented in departments of radiology.
- In several countries, national databases are constructed for management and planning or, increasingly, for the quality assessment of care or postmarketing surveillance of drugs.

Computer applications on this level are not essentially different from the ones we see in industry, banking, or trade and transportation. All areas of society use database management systems and standards for the coding and compact storage of data, signals, and images. Health care is no exception in this respect. The main difference between applications in health care and those in society is the wide variety of different data that are stored, from purely financial items to radiological pictures, and the large number of potential users of these data. The complexity of the applications on this level therefore consists of the *semantic* interconnection of these data and the wide variety of different goals that are to be served with these data. This is also reflected in the way that the databases are constructed (see Chapter 4 for a more detailed description).

Level 3:

Processing and Automation

A more complex use of computers concerns its more "intelligent" applications in areas such as laboratory automation or processing of biological signals. Here also most of the processing can be done without much human interaction, although in all applications on this level only those problems that can be standardized can be solved, for example, if they are repetitious. For the design of systems on this level, much more knowledge that is specific to health care is required. Use is also made of the systems available on the lower two levels, that is, data input and output, and data storage and retrieval. Some examples of applications on this level are given below.

1

- The analysis of samples of blood or urine in the clinical laboratory, which is fully automated for the majority of all blood and urine tests (see Chapter 13). Analysis equipment is usually equipped with computers so that the results (data) can immediately be transferred to laboratory computers for further processing, including quality control and report generation.
- The processing of biological signals acquired during surgery, in intensive care, or during diagnostic function analysis. Examples are estimations of **ST depression**s in ECGs during physical exercise or the computation of frequency spectra of **electroencephalogram**s (see Chapters 7 and 25). In most instances there is a tight coupling between measuring devices and the computers that process the data.
- The computation of the radiation dosage and different plans for radiotherapy is another example of computer support that serves patient care (see Chapter 12, Section 10). In such cases the physician is responsible for the choice of the plan that should be applied, and in this respect, computing on this level is preparatory for the two levels higher up in our scheme.
- Medical imaging is another area that belongs on this level, where applications are seen in radiology (X-ray images, **computer tomography**, **magnetic resonance images**, and **positron emission tomography**), **nuclear medicine**, and **ultrasound** (see Chapter 9). Without computers, in view of the enormous computational load, medical imaging would be nonexistent.

The complexity of computer processing and of the mathematical, physical, and biochemical problems involved is much higher on this level than on the two lower levels. Insight is necessary into the underlying physiological and pathophysiological processes of organs and organ systems to arrive at solutions for the problems concerned. Dependence on people is higher because most applications are specifically developed for health care applications, in contrast to most software at the two lower levels. Level 3 of our scheme is closely connected to the first stage of the diagnostic-therapeutic cycle, the observation stage.

Level 4:
Diagnosis and Decision Making

A preeminently human occupation is the recognition of visual images and situations, which allow people to prepare for subsequent decision making and plan further actions. Recognition can be done only if enough knowledge and experience are available in human brains and computers and if the data are accurate and reliable enough for recognition, that is, are complete and not blurred. The ultimate challenge in this area is how to formalize medical knowledge in such a way that it can be used for decision support. The methods on this level are related to pattern recognition and heuristic reasoning techniques (see Chapter 15). The following are examples of applications on this level:

- The diagnostic interpretation of ECGs by computer is an illustration of systems operational on this level (Chapters 8, 12 and 13). ECG interpretation is one of the most successful applications of computers for medical decision support, and it runs almost fully automatically, without human intervention. The final ECG **classification**, however, falls under the responsibility of the treating physician, who should acknowledge the computer classification by his or her signature.
- Many **decision-support systems** have been developed to assist the clinician in arriving at a correct diagnosis. One of the early systems is a method for the differential diagnosis of abdominal pain (see Chapter 16). On the basis of the signs and symptoms entered by the clinician, the computer lists the different possible diseases as a function of probability, but here also, the physician must make the final decision.

On this level, we may encounter in health care almost insurmountable difficulties when using computers in a fully automatic fashion. The reason is that on this level we are involved with typical human pursuits such as making a diagnosis for an individual patient. If computers should serve us on this level, then one cannot avoid the design of formal decision-making criteria and models for medical decision making. In pattern recognition, image processing, and decision making there is therefore only limited room for completely automated systems. Most of the time we see computer-assisted diagnostic systems rather than systems that operate independently of humans. The systems on level 4 concern the second stage of the diagnostic-therapeutic cycle, the diagnosis.

Level 5:
Treatment and Control

The final goal of all information processing is, of course, the achievement of concrete results that can lead to some action, such as a treatment or increased insight. In health care we find on this level only a few computer applications that have a direct effect on patient care. The injection of a drug or surgery will always primarily remain a human activity. Full automation of process control, including the last stage, the action, is much more common in industrial processes that deal with technological problems. Yet, also in patient care we can give examples of situations in which computers play a pivotal role on this level and in which the results of decision making are the input to the last stage of the diagnostic-therapeutic cycle, the treatment:

- During intensive care of patients, the *fluid balance* must be carefully monitored. Researchers have developed computer *algorithms* that control the automatic administration of infusion on the basis of fluids given or withdrawn, (e.g., by drains). Automatic *feedback* has also been realized for anti-coagulation therapy or for the administration of insulin. Infusion algorithms can be better developed if, for instance, they are based on a *pharmacokinetic* model.
- In *radiotherapy*, the radiation equipment is often automatically adjusted and calibrated on the basis of output from computer models and radiation plans, such as the ones computed under level 3.
- The prescription of drugs is assessed by integrating patient data from computer-based records with decision models that check the possible existence of *drug-drug interactions* or *contraindications*.

Protocols are successfully applied for the treatment of chronic diseases, such as hypertension or diabetes.

- Data in *computer-based patient records*, if they are coded, can also be used for decision support. Examples are decision-support systems that are integrated with computer-based patient records and that generate comments on the clinician's choice of therapy. This type of decision-support system is usually called a *critiquing system*. A more extensive discussion of critiquing systems can be found in Chapter 16.
- On-demand pacemakers trigger patients' hearts only when an implanted special-purpose computer (integrated on a chip) detects too low a voltage or an irregular heart beat.

On this level, there is much human involvement and the therapeutic and control processes are complex. This level is primarily related to the third stage of the diagnostic-therapeutic cycle, the therapy, that is, the feedback after the decision-making stage to the patient or the process. The more the process can be structured and formalized, which is particularly the case when we deal with sheer physical or biochemical processes, the better automatic feedback can be realized.

Level 6:
Research and Development

We have covered all possible computer applications in health care in the five levels discussed above and have accounted for all three stages of the diagnostic-therapeutic cycle. However, there is one human activity in medicine that has not yet been accounted for and that belongs to the most creative occupations of humans: scientific research and its complement, the development of new methods during research and development. In medical informatics there is also a great need for basic and applied research and the development of methods that are based on such research. As mentioned earlier, a computer program is only successful when we are dealing with a problem that can be structured and a model that can be generalized. This is exactly the object of research in medical informatics, in which we investigate processes to be able to describe them

1

formally, to develop and assess models and algorithms, and to develop processing systems. In this respect medical informatics is both an experimental and an applied science that uses the formalisms from, for instance, mathematics and physics and the tools from informatics. When such models cannot be defined, no computer programs can be designed. Such models are required for the electronic interchange of medical data (level 1), departmental information systems or computer-based patient records (level 2), the three-dimensional reconstruction (*3-D reconstruction*) of medical images (level 3), the interpretation of *ECG*s or the differential diagnosis of abdominal pain (level 4), or therapeutic support by critiquing systems (level 5). Examples of activities on level 6 are as follows:

- Development and validation of different models underlying computer-based patient records and models that support sharing of patient data.
- The use of computers for the analysis of data acquired in epidemiological studies, for example, by using *database management systems*, statistical methods, *spreadsheet*s, and graphical presentation software.
- Computer models for the electric *depolarization* of the cardiac muscle. Such models may give more insight into the functioning of the heart and lay the foundation for a better interpretation of ECGs.
- Models for the investigation of nervous or hormonal control systems of the circulation. Only by use of such models can different control systems and their interconnection be studied. Computer models ena-

ble verification of hypotheses and preparation of protocols for in vivo experiments.
- The development and assessment of models for image, signal, and *pattern recognition* with the help of databases of well-documented patient material.
- The use of *virtual-reality* models in surgery, for training (comparable to flight simulators) or to assist surgeons in so-called minimal invasive surgery.

Research and development for the realization of systems on all five levels is done on level 6. Here, in fact, human ingenuity and creativity reach their climax. Here, interaction between computers and people is the most intense in the sense that the computer truly "amplifies" the human brain with respect to data storage (memory), speed (retrieval and computations), and accuracy. Computer models may assist with the verification of theoretical assumptions, and prototypes may help in the assessment of ideas for the development of information processing systems. In experiments with patient databases, hypotheses can be tested and models can be validated.

Especially on this level, it should continuously be kept in mind that all models are abstractions of the real world and are valid only within the framework of the assumptions and a priori notions that we have defined ourselves. Before the resulting systems on the sixth level are allowed to be introduced on one of the lower levels, they should be thoroughly assessed and their possibilities and limitations should be carefully documented. A model and its resulting system should not be used outside the definition domain that was defined on level 6.

5 Concluding Remarks

In the next chapters we shall discuss many applications, some of which were briefly mentioned in this introductory chapter.

When studying this book, the reader should be aware of the sometimes principal limitations of systems on the different levels. These limitations might bear a more or less permanent character, independent of technical possibilities. It is one of the chal-

lenges in medical informatics to continuously gain more insight into all processes so that models can be defined and refined and systems can be designed and improved. At the same time it should be clear that most systems in practice have subsystems on different levels.

The scheme with levels of complexity therefore has particularly an educational character.

Key References

Blois MS. *Information and Medicine: The Nature of Medical Descriptions.* Berkeley CA: Univ of California Press, 1984.

Blum BI. *Information Systems for Patient Care.* New York: Springer Verlag, 1986.

Shortliffe EH, Perreault LE, eds. *Medical Informatics: Computer Applications in Health Care.* Reading MA: Addison-Wesley., 1990.

Van Bemmel JH, McCray AT, eds. *IMIA Yearbooks of Medical Informatics.* Stuttgart/New York: Schattauer Verlag, 1992 and following years (see Chapter 37).

See the Web site for further literature references.

1

2 Information and Communication

1 Introduction

The era we are living in is often referred to as "the age of communication." Within a short period of time, portable radio, satellite television, cellular telephones, multimedia personal computers (*PCs*), and *Internet* have all become familiar terms. The purpose of all these media is to transmit messages from one party to the other. Technically, the way that these messages are communicated can differ from medium to medium (e.g., one-way or bidirectional). In some instances the sender and the receiver are integrated in one device; in other instances the transmission channels and devices are separate.

Most often, the people who send or receive messages are only interested in the message itself and not in the carrier of the message or the route that the carrier has to take to reach the receiver with a message. For instance, for an intercontinental telephone conversation it does not matter whether the signal that carries the message is transmitted via satellite or by submarine cable. The receiver may notice the difference between the two, however, by a longer delay for the satellite

connection and the receiver may experience an echo. When low noise and optimal data protection are required, a cable connection is preferable.

As stated, most of the time the receiver is interested in the *message*, not the *medium*. In some instances, however, our interest may lie in the medium through which the message passes before it arrives at the receiver's end and not in the message as such. Later on in this chapter we give some examples of this in the medical area. Before doing so, we first want to sketch the general situation of a sender, a receiver, and a transmission channel, a situation that is relevant to the communications between a patient and a physician or a nurse, and for the exchange of patient data, medical images, or biological signals. In addition to what has been remarked in Chapter 1 on Level 1, dealing with data acquisition and transmission, it should be realized that all data in health care have a source or sender (usually the patient) and a receiver (the care provider). Without transmission the data would not reach the receiver and could not be interpreted.

2 Sender, Channel, and Receiver

Between any sender **S** and a receiver **R** there is always a transmission channel **T** through which the message must pass (Fig. 2.1). This channel can be long or short, and it may cause some delay or it may be instantaneous, as in the example of the submarine cable or the

satellite transmission. Part of the transmission channel is the transducer, which picks up the message and generally transforms it into an electric signal suitable for further processing.

Even in cases where we may assume that the transmit-

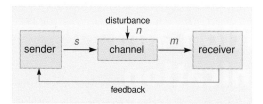

Figure 2.1
Sender, receiver, and transmission channel. The sender transmits the signal s, and in the transmission channel the noise n is superimposed on s, so that at the receiver's site the mixture m = s + n is received. On the way from the sender to the receiver, the information entropy therefore tends to increase. The only way to maintain a low entropy is by keeping the disturbance low and by adding intelligence to both the sender and the receiver. One way of adding intelligence to the communication system is by incorporating feedback from the receiver to the sender.

ted message has a well-known structure and a clear meaning, the message may become distorted during transmission (see Fig. 2.1). The message or the signal s may be corrupted by some disturbance or noise n, resulting in the mixture m, consisting of signal plus noise. Disturbance may be caused by:

- the sender,
- the transmission channel, or
- the receiver itself.

If the message is distorted, the receiver tries to extract the correct message s from the mixture m (e.g., by requesting that the sender repeats the message).
In this chapter we assume, for simplicity's sake, that the disturbance is additive, that is, the mixture m is the sum of signal s plus **noise n**:

$$m = s + n.$$

Examples of superimposed disturbance are environmental noise, for example, from the clinician's room or the street, corrupting the speech sounds during a conversation between a patient and a clinician or the noise generated by active muscles, for example, during patient movements, superimposed on a recorded electrocardiogram.

In general, the variables m, s, and n are time-varying signals. Furthermore, they may be either analog or digital variables, and they may consist of several parallel components, such as a 3-channel *electrocardiogram* or a 16-channel *electroencephalogram*. In some instances, s can also be a time-varying image, for example, an echocardiographic movie recorded during examination of the heart or the vessels.
If we generalize the different situations in which a sender **S**, a channel **T**, and a receiver **R** are involved, we can discern five different configurations of **S**, **R**, and **T**, which are described in the following sections.

1. S → R
This is a situation of one-way transmission, in which both the sender and the receiver are known and in which the receiver is interested in the message itself and not necessarily in the transmission channel. An example is the auscultation of the heart (**S** is the heart; s is the audible sound generated by the closure of the heart valves and cardiac murmurs, for instance, caused by a turbulent or regurgitating blood flow; n could be respiration or noise in the room; **R** is the stethoscope or microphone plus the ears of the examining clinician; and **T** is the chest and the air between the heart and the transducer).
Another example is the registration of an *EEG* (**S** is the *depolarizing* neurons in the *cortex*; s is the weighted sum of depolarization waves of groups of neurons; n is the electric disturbance from the environment, active muscles, and even the ECG; **R** is electrodes, amplifiers, and recording equipment; and **T** is the tissue, skin, and electrode gel between the skin and the electrodes).

2. S ↔ R
This is a configuration of bidirectional communication. Here, too, the sender and the receiver are known, and the receiver is only interested in the message transmitted by the sender. An example is a conversation between a patient and a clinician, such as during history taking (**S** is the patient listening to and answering the questions of the clinician; s is speech; n is noise from outside resulting in words that are misunderstood; **R** is the clinician who both listens and asks questions; and **T** is the channel between voices and the ears of both patient and clinician, see also Example 4 below). A further example is the response

of a nerve or muscle cell after administering an electric stimulus from an electrode (**S** is the cell or muscle sensing the stimulus and generating the response; *s* is the electric nerve cell or muscle response; *n* is the disturbance from adjacent cells or muscle bundles; **R** is the microelectrode administering the stimulus and receiving the response; and **T** is the channel between cell or muscle and the tip of the electrode).

3. S = R

In this situation, the sender and the receiver are one device. In typical situations, we are not interested in the message as such but in the channel between the signal that was transmitted and received by the combined sender-receiver. An example is *ultrasound* that is generated by an array of *piezoelectric* crystals (e.g., by a so-called sector scanner) and the echoes that are received from tissue boundaries (**S** is the crystals that radiate ultrasound into surrounding tissues; *s* is the ultrasonic wave of several megahertz generated by the crystals (see also Chapter 9 for a discussion on ultrasound for medical imaging); *n* is distorting reflections received from other tissues or caused by tissue inhomogeneities; **R** is the same receiving crystals that generated the ultrasonic wave but that is now receiving the echoes; and **T** is the channel between the crystals via tissue and back to the same crystals).

4. S → ?

This is an academic situation in which the receiver is not present, does not pay attention, or has no correct transducer. This happens, for instance, under circumstances in which symptoms are not picked up by the clinician or are only occurring randomly or in which the disease is asymptomatic (e.g., in case the heart generates *extrasystoles* that are not detected).

5. ? → R

This is a typical situation in medicine in which symptoms are detected, but in which the cause of the symptoms is still unknown. For instance, deviating values may be seen in blood chemistry without the possibility of tracing the organ that causes the deviation.

In medicine, numerous examples that are comparable to one of these five situations can be given. We pre-

sent some examples in which communication between the sender and the receiver in one of the situations sketched above is most essential in medicine. In fact, health care would be nonexistent without data that are transmitted from the sender (the patient or an organ) to the receiver. It is the task of the receiver to ask for the most relevant data that are to be used for the diagnosis or to monitor the course of the disease. In discussing the examples below it will become apparent that we are not always able to shape ideal circumstances for communication. Sometimes, we are not certain that the organ sends enough signals and symptoms that are relevant to the diagnosis of the disease. Furthermore, we often cannot approach the organ closely enough to pick up the message. In the following are some examples of communication that can occur in health care and where different types of information are acquired and processed by computers.

Example 1:

Ultrasound

Ultrasound is used for diagnostic purposes in many areas of health care such as neurology, cardiology, internal medicine, and obstetrics (see also Chapter 9). Ultrasound is a signal or wave front *s* with a frequency of 1, 2, or even 8 MHz, depending on the desired resolution. The ultrasonic wave is radiated toward the organ of interest or, in the case of obstetrics, to the entire fetus or part of it (e.g., the fetal heart or skull). The echoes that are received are the mixture of signal and noise, in which the original signal *s* has been transformed to a signal s^* by the tissues through which *s* has passed. The receiving transducer detects only reflected signals. In this case **S** = **R**. The message that is carried by s^* is information about the structure of the tissue, encoded as a delay and, partly, a lower amplitude of the wave. The echoes that are presented as a signal or, most often, as a picture can, for instance, give information about the position of the fetus, a tumor in the esophagus, or asymmetry in brain tissue (e.g., asymmetry caused by internal bleeding). Increasingly, ultrasonic signals are digitized and processed by a computer to obtain a better presentation of the images or to compute parameters, such as the speed of blood flow.

2

Example 2:

Imaging

Imaging is an area in health care that is of great importance for making a diagnosis. In Chapters 9, 10, and 26 special attention is paid to this area. Here we discuss an example from cardiology. When we are interested in the filling of the ventricles with blood as a function of time, a **radiopaque fluid** is injected in the veins and is transported to the heart by the blood. X rays are the signal s that is used to offer information on the size of the ventricles. The X rays are radiated toward the chest and pass through it, and the received signal s^* gives information about the density of the tissues in between the X-ray tube (**S**) and the sensing device **R**, which can be a photographic emulsion or a **photonmultiplier**. Apparently, the tissue and the body fluids have distorted (weakened) the original signal s, and this is exactly the information in which we are interested. Superimposed on s^*, however, are also effects from tissues other than only the heart, such as the lungs and the ribs, causing the mixture m from which s^* should be extracted. After receiving the signal (i.e., the transmitted picture) processing can be applied to measure the area of the ventricles or, in the case of two simultaneous orthogonal or nonparallel pictures, to estimate the ventricular volume as a function of time. In this case the cardiac output can, in principle, be measured as a function of time.

Example 3:

Wireless Transmission

In some instances it might be of interest to fix a wireless transmitter on the body (e.g., in the case of **Holter** monitoring; see Chapter 12) to implant a **transducer** or even a **transmitter** in the body (e.g., to measure intracranial pressure). The transmitter **S** then sends the signal s to some receiver **R** not too far remote from the body. Radio transmission is used to avoid wires that would hamper the natural protrusion of the micro-transmitter.

In all three of these examples, both the sender and the receiver were man-made and so were the signals generated by the user. In the first example, **S** and **R** are identical; in the second example, **S** (the X-ray tube) and **R** (the camera) are physically opposite and mechanically coupled; in the third example, the connection between sender and receiver is looser.

The next few examples deal with other types of communication in which the patient or organs function as sender or receiver. We shall specifically point to the disturbance generated in the transmission channel.

Example 4:

Transmission by Natural Language

During patient history taking, the message s is carried by natural language (i.e., it is spoken). It should be noted that an experienced clinician also acquires information from nonverbal messages, such as from body language. The receiver, that is, the clinician, has enough expertise to extract the message from the mixture m. In this case, however, the disturbance is not merely the added noise from the environment but is also the fact that the true meaning of the message is hidden in the natural language. In other words, to comprehend the message, the receiver must immediately interpret the message so that a meaningful feedback can be given to the patient. The mere superposition of s and n no longer applies here; the message also has no truly physical or quantitative value, but is carried by natural language. Only by interpretation and coding is the true message filtered out of the mixture of words. If clinicians have not been properly trained, they will be unable to find a meaningful message in the medium, the language. This is the reason why natural language interpretation by computers is extremely difficult and, perhaps, never fully attainable.

In some applications an artificial situation is created in which the patient is still the sender **S**, but the receiver **R** is a computer that is equipped with a program that generates (sends) questions to be answered by the patient in a structured manner (e.g., in a multiple-choice mode). In some cases it is useful to let the human interview be preceded by a structured patient-computer interview (for a more extensive description of the pros and cons of computer-supported data entry, see Chapter 7).

Example 5:

Biosignals

Every living cell, organ, or organism generates signals for internal communication or to make itself known to the outside world. In general, we may express this situation as a biological process that generates some output, and in some circumstances we might even be interested in offering this process an input signal to examine its response, as we have seen in the example above of the cell that was stimulated with an electrode.

Such biological signals can have a different nature:

- electrochemical, for example, the depolarization of a cell, which is the result of flows of ions, that pass the cell membrane, such as Ca^{++}, Na^+, or Cl^-;
- mechanical, for example, the respiration, set in motion by thoracic muscles and resulting in air-flows and pressures;
- biochemical, for example, blood gas values such as PO_2 or PCO_2;
- hormonal, for example, the release of **oxytocin** during labor.

In most instances we deal with transmission situations 1 or 5 indicated above. The received signal s is sometimes very distorted by the transmission channel in the body if s must pass different tissues on its way to the transducer. An example of a signal s that passes many tissue layers before it reaches the transducer is the fetal ECG (see Fig. 2.2). In the first three months of pregnancy this signal is too weak to be detected, and during labor it is much distorted by the uterine and abdominal muscles. On top of the fetal signal, the maternal ECG (which can be considerably larger in voltage than the fetal ECG) is also superimposed. The intervals between fetal heart beats can reveal information about possible fetal distress during birth.

There are many other examples of situations in which information is transmitted from the sender to the receiver by means of temperatures, mass, electric current, hormones, biochemical parameters, **DNA**, and so forth, but the examples given thus far are sufficient to provide a representative picture of the role of patient data in making a diagnosis.

In general, we may conclude that from the viewpoint of

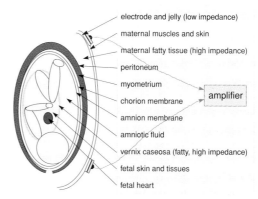

Figure 2.2

Different tissue and fluid layers between fetal heart and abdominal electrode when recording the fetal ECG. This physically small sender (the fetal heart) and the transmission channel (the many layers with different electric impedances) cause the fetal ECG to be rather small compared to an adult ECG. The maternal ECG is usually seen superimposed on the fetal ECG, together with disturbances from active muscles (electromyogram) and external sources (e.g., power line disturbance).

2

information and communication, patients and organs can be considered as time-varying *processes* that generate signals s that are of interest for determining or monitoring the state of the process. Unfortunately, the signals are often distorted or the processes cannot be approached closely enough to be able to record the signals with a high enough fidelity. In some circumstances, as we shall see, we are able to improve the situation in which communication takes place, for example, by removing sources that cause disturbances or by bringing our transducers much closer to the process of interest. The most important factor, however, is that the receiver be tuned to the sender and able to pick up the correct message. This deals not only with technical tuning, but also with the ability to understand the message, as seen in the example of natural language. In the latter case, the receiver should be properly trained (in a way, also tuned) and have enough prior knowledge to understand the message and to ask the right questions. This knowledge is of a nonphysical nature and cannot easily be made operational on a computer unless both the sender and the receiver are forced into a structured environment, as discussed in the example of the computerized patient interview, which may hamper, however, a spontaneous and more human communication.

3 Perception and Transducers

As discussed in Section 2, all communication situations suppose a sender, a receiver, and a transmission channel. This also applies to information processing in living organisms, in which messages are generated, transported by the nervous or the hormonal system, and transported to a sensing organ. The organism as a whole communicates with the outside world by using physical or chemical carriers (voice, gesture, and scent) and the five senses as receivers.

For the reasons just given, we briefly summarize some aspects of human information processing, which are also of interest to understanding the limitations of human information processing in health care. The most important senses for the acquisition of information from the outside world are our eyes and ears. The human eye is able to receive 3 million bits per second via the retina (the *bit* being the smallest unit of information; see Chapter 3). The retina has about 100 million rods and 10 million pyramids. This enables us, in principle, to discern at daytime more than 400,000 separate picture points (not to be confused with the picture elements or pixels of digital images, see

---

Table 2.1
The Human Senses and Their Information Processing Capacity [a] (adapted from **Steinbuch**[b]).

	Senses					
	Sight	*Hearing*	*Sense of Touch*	*Sense of Heat*	*Sense of Smell*	*Sense of Taste*
Stimulus	Electro-magnetic (3,800-7,600 Å)	Mechanic	Mechanic deformation of the skin	Temperature differences in place and time	Chemical substances	Chemical substances
Location	Retina	Basilar membrane	Epidermis	Epidermis	Nasal cavity	Tongue, palate
Number of receptors	1×10^7 pyramids (day, color) 1×10^8 rods (twilight) 4×10^5 picture points discernible	Hair cells: $1\text{-}3 \times 10^4$	Pressure: 5×10^5 pain: 3×10^5	heat: 1×10^4 cold: 3×10^5	1×10^7	1×10^7
Number of nerve bundles to central nervous system	$(1 \text{ to } 2) \times 10^6$	$(1 \text{ to } 2) \times 10^4$	1×10^4	1×10^4	2×10^3	2×10^3
Information capacity (bits)	3×10^6	$2\text{-}5 \times 10^4$	2×10^5	2×10^3	10 to 100	10

[a] The number of sensors and the parallel information processing capacity of the human senses is most impressive, especially if one realizes the small size (10^{-2} to 10^{-5} mm³) of all processing elements (neurons). It should also be realized that the structure and the processing of information in the human brain is radically different from that in a digital computer (and the mechanism is largely unknown).

[b] Steinbuch K. *Mensch und Automat*. Berlin: Springer Verlag, 1954.

Chapter 9). This human ability to acquire pictures is impressive if we realize that most television cameras have a much lower resolution. A high-resolution computer screen may have 1,620 x 1,280 image points (around 2,000,000 pixels) which is five times the resolution of the eye (personal computer screens usually have 640 x 480, 1024 x 768 or more pixel points). Table 2.1, after Steinbuch, illustrates the information acquisition and processing capacity of our senses.

The most impressive difference between information processing by computers and human beings is that the human brain, starting with the retina from which more than 1 million nerves lead to the cortex, is able to accomplish *parallel* information processing, whereas most computers do it serially, albeit at an extremely high speed. Only for very advanced computational work, such as in science and technology, do we see parallel computing (e.g., with more than 50,000 *parallel processors*). It is tempting to compare a neuron with the most elementary unit of information storage in a computer, in which only one bit can be stored. How the brain stores and processes information is, however, still a mystery, despite basic research in neurophysiology, cognitive psychology, and brain research in general.

It can be stated, however, that the differences between the human brain and a computer are fundamental, and go far beyond expressing information in just bits and in number of operations per second. If, however, we would like to express the storage capacity of the brain in bits, then it can be estimated that this is on the order of 1 million bits per cm^3, giving the entire brain on the order of 10^{12} bits (1 million megabits) of storage capacity, with more than 1.5×10^{10} neurons being involved. One of the devices used to store the largest amount of data with the highest density is the *compact disk*, which can easily store more than 5×10^9 bits. This is still far less than what the brain may contain in less

space. We underline, however, that the brain stores its information in a fundamentally different way that is at the same time less accurate (i.e., nonnumeric) and more global. For further discussion on some differences between brains and computers, see Chapter 15.

In many instances, our senses are not able to pick up the information that is of interest for diagnostic purposes. We have already seen several examples: ultrasound of several MHz, which falls far above the range of acoustic signals that we are able to hear (say, from about 40 to about 8,000 *Hz* or, at a young age, even 16,000 Hz) or electromagnetic waves such as X rays or infrared light, which are outside the spectrum of visible light that we are able to see. Moreover, we have no senses for electric currents (except that they may stimulate nerves and muscles, such as during *cardiac defibrillation*) or for magnetic fields, and the way that we sense temperature or pressure is very crude and not reliable enough to be used to acquire information, except that we may feel someone's forehead and conclude that the person has a high fever.

In all such cases we make use of *transducers* that transform a mechanical or biochemical variable into an electric one. In this respect, we have already discussed use of the piezoelectric crystal for ultrasound, the microelectrode for the detection of weak ionic currents across cell membranes, a microphone for the detection of cardiac sounds, or a photonmultiplier for the detection of X rays. However, the *data* that arrive at our senses do not all contain *information*. Information is only contained if the message can be interpreted by the receiver or, as we have seen, if the receiver is tuned to the sender and has enough knowledge. Obtaining the knowledge necessary for the interpretation is one of the fields of interest in medical informatics research (taking place on level 6, as discussed in Chapter 1).

The next section will discuss in more depth the differences between data and information.

2

4 Aspects of Information

It is impossible to define exactly what information is. (Neither can we precisely say what energy or gravity is.) Such questions belong to the limits of our scientific

knowledge. Although scientific research implies shifting the horizon and the limits of our knowledge, there always remain first or last questions: the former being the a priori notions of science and the latter being related to the limits of our present knowledge. In the natural sciences, however, we trust that we live in an orderly world and that the laws that we discover are valid, independent of place and time, without being able to scientifically prove the existence of the reality in which we live, let alone its origin and meaning.

We approach scientific problems dealing with information the same way that we approach problems dealing with energy or gravity (from experiments we know they exist, but we cannot prove their existence from first principles); in our scientific research we try to formulate the rules that govern the informational aspects of reality. Although we have no true idea of what information is (an ontological issue that is philosophical in nature), we are nevertheless able to investigate the structure of information.

Information can exist only if there is a carrier for the information. (There are also other examples in which a phenomenon only exists by the grace of something else. For instance, in physics Albert Einstein showed us that space exists only if matter is present.) Information science is the science that makes use of symbols and their combination or, in general, language. Natural language is the way in which we express ourselves most directly; by a computer language we express ourselves in a structured way. A message, expressed by any language, can only be interpreted by living creatures, from cells to humans.

Information has three different aspects that are directly related to the three stages of human activity discussed in Chapter 1, and particularly to the three stages of the diagnostic-therapeutic cycle (observation, diagnosis, and therapy): *syntactic*, *semantic*, and **pragmatic** aspects.

4.1 Syntactic Aspect

The syntactic aspect of information concerns the grammar or syntax for the description, storage, or transmission of messages. In fact, the syntax describes the rules of conduct for the information carriers, such as a set of codes or symbols, the letters of some alphabet, the way that words must be spelled in a language, the way that musical notes must be composed, the frequency spectrum and amplitude range for certain biosignals, and so forth. The rules of conduct are agreements and definitions made by people or are implicitly defined by the processes that we

study. The syntactic aspect of information is strongly related to the carrier of the information, that is, the specific language or the type of image or biosignal. The purely syntactic aspect of information can best be called **data**. Data do not necessarily have to be interpreted by the receiver. Many observations in health care are just data. Only after human interpretation, do the data acquire meaning, which is the next aspect of information.

4.2 Semantic Aspect

The semantic aspect of information pertains to the meaning of the message. When dealing with the semantic aspect we are not interested in the way that we have received the information or in the syntax as such, but only in its significance for interpretation and decision making. The meaning can often be derived only if we know the context of the message. This is particularly true when we must interpret a message contained in natural language or *free text*. A clinician deals with the semantic aspect of information when making a diagnosis. Even when the message has been transmitted without any disturbance and is syntactically correct, the interpretation is not necessarily unambiguous, as we shall see in Chapter 7. In the case of natural language we can sometimes deduce several meanings, especially when we do not know the context. An example of the importance of context is the sentence "Time flies like an arrow,"[a] in which each word can have different meanings so that the whole sentence might have more than 10 interpretations. ("Time" has a meaning as a verb and a noun or even an adjective; "flies" is a verb with different meanings and also a plural noun; "like" is a verb and a conjunction; "arrow" is a substantive with a meaning associated with darts or archery, or a line in a diagram.)

4.3 Pragmatic Aspect

All interpretations ultimately lead to some activity; information also has an intention or a goal to be

---

[a] *After Naom Chomski.*

PANEL 2.1

Information

The history of the meaning of the word *information* reflects the different aspects of this term. We refer to the definitions offered by three pioneers in information science.

- Claude E. Shannon (1916):
  Information is the negative value of the logarithm of the probability of occurrence.
- Louis-Marcel Brillouin (1854-1948):
  Information is a function of the relation between possible answers before and after reception.
- Norbert Wiener (1894-1964):
  Information is a name for the content of what is exchanged with the outer world as we adjust to it and make our adjustments felt upon it.

Shannon's definition expresses information in mathematical terms and it relates information to its digital representation, which is primarily its syntactic aspect. Brillouin's definition refers to the fact that information may decrease uncertainty, its semantic aspect. Wiener, the father of *cybernetics*, stresses the pragmatic aspect of information, as visible in control theory and processes with feedback to the source of the information.

2

reached. Even a decrease in uncertainty when making a diagnosis or testing a scientific hypothesis is an effect of information. We refer to this last aspect as the pragmatic aspect. In health care, the pragmatic aspect of information is the effect on the therapy.

Many examples of the use of data illustrating all three aspects described here can be found in patient records. For instance, in a patient record one never sees the value "8.2" as such; rather, it is seen together with a further explanation, such as "Hb 8.2."

The syntactic rules prescribe that a value be preceded or followed by a unit. The meaning of that value for patient care (the semantic aspect) depends on whether the value is abnormal, given the context (e.g., the age of the patient or the patient's history in general). The pragmatic aspect deals with actions that need to be taken, for instance, giving a blood transfusion or prescribing a diet or drugs. In everyday health care, the semantic aspect may be the most difficult one to deal with.

In Panel 2.1 we have given three descriptions of information as defined in the early days of information science or communication theory. The definition of **Shannon** refers to the syntactic aspect, that of **Brillouin** is most related to the semantic aspect, and the defini-

tion of **Wiener** is related to the pragmatic aspect. Shannon can be considered the father of communication theory. He was the first to give a mathematical definition of the syntactic aspect of information, much related to the second law of thermodynamics to which the name of Boltzmann is connected.

4.4 Mathematical Definition of Information

Shannon gave a formula for the information content of a message that some event has occurred with a probability of occurrence p:

$I = -\log_2 p$, where $0 \le p \le 1$.

I is the information content in bits (binary digits, the bit being by definition the smallest unit of information; the bit also plays a prominent role in digital computers; see Chapter 3). The formula tells us that a message contains more bits of information when the probabili-

---

PANEL 2.2

Information Content of DNA

The double-helix structure of DNA (deoxyribonucleic acid) was discovered in 1954 by *James Watson* and *Francis Crick*. A DNA molecule is composed of four different bases, guanine, thymine, cytosine and adenine (G, T, C, and A, respectively) called nucleotide bases. The bases bind in pairs via a hydrogen bond, and the pairs of bases form a long string, shaped in the form of a double helix. The pairs can only appear as guanine opposite cytosine (G-C) or thymine opposite adenine (T-A), as sketched below:

```
T A C C G T A G G T C A . . .
| | | | | | | | | | | | | | |
A T G G C A T C C A G T . . .
```

The string of base pairs forms a coded message, in which the bases are the characters of the "alphabet." If one of the pairs of the string is known, then the other one is also known. This property is used during cell division, when the helices unwind themselves and each half is copied. This copying activity can be considered information transfer, but errors in the code may also occur.

If we consider a long string of, say, 100,000 bases, then the first "letter" may be either G, T, C, or A, or one of four possibilities. For all 100,000 characters we then have 4 x 4 x 4 x ... 4 $= 4^{100,000} = 2^{200,000}$ possible strings of codes. If the probability of occurrence of all strings of codes is equal, then the probability of finding a specific string is $p = 2^{200,000}$. By Shannon's formula, the information content of the code described by this molecule is therefore

$$I = -\log_2 p = -\log_2 2^{-200,000} = 200,000 \text{ (bits)}.$$

A DNA molecule of 100,000 base pairs has a length of approximately 500,000 Å and is 20 Å thick (1 Å $= 10^{-10}$ m), which is impressive compared to the amount of space required to store a code of 100,000 bits in a computer. A chromosome that contains on the order of 5×10^9 nucleotides, may code for 10×10^9 bits. For the 23 chromosome pairs in the human genome, this would mean on the order of 5×10^{11} bits (equivalent to about 60 gigabytes).

---

ty of its occurrence is lower. For instance, for an event that occurs with a probability of 1 in 1,024, the information content is 10 bits (i.e., $-\log_2 2^{-10}$). However, if we have to describe in a patient record the gender of one person in front of us, we need only 1 bit of information (e.g., by using 1 and 0 or the symbols M and F for male and female, respectively). The information content of a rarely occurring event or disease is larger than that of an event that is highly probable. Because a probability p has a positive value of between 0 and 1, the information should be a real, nonnegative number. (If we deal with a situation in which N events i may occur with probabilities p_i, where $\Sigma p_i = 1$, then the information content can be expressed as a weighted sum of all individual information contents:

$I = - \Sigma p_i \log_2 p_i$). Some examples of the use of Shannon's formula for the calculation of information content are given in Panels 2.2 and 2.3.

PANEL 2.3

Information Content of a Biological Signal

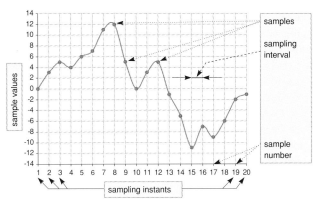

Figure 2.3
Sampling of a signal. The analog signal is converted to numbers. In the time domain, samples are taken with a rate of $1/\Delta T$, with ΔT being the sampling interval. The amplitude is converted to binary numbers, with a resolution of Δq, which is equal to (amplitude range)$/m$, with m being a power of 2 (i.e., $m = 2^n$, with n being the quantization in bits; e.g., for $n = 10$: $m = 2^{10} = 1,024$). (See also later in this Handbook Table 8.1 for examples of biosignals in which the quantization m and the bandwidth are shown.) The sampling rate must be at least twice the rate of the highest-frequency component that occurs in the signal.

We want to calculate the syntactic information content of a signal that has been *sampled* during a certain period with a total of N independent (uncorrelated) samples (see Fig. 2.3 and Chapter 8). The signal amplitude has been digitized with n different levels. For the first sample we then have n different possibilities that some amplitude may occur, and for the N samples in total $n \times n \times n ... \times n = n^N$ possible signal shapes. Apparently, the probability that a signal of some shape occurs is $p = n^{-N}$.

If we further assume that n has a value that can be written as $n = 2^m$, then the probability becomes $p = 2^{-mN}$. By Shannon's formula, the information content of a signal with N independent samples, digitized with 2^m levels, then becomes:

$$I = -\log_2 p = -\log_2 2^{-mN} = mN \text{ bits.}$$

(This can be derived much faster by realizing that the 2^m levels for one sample can be expressed by m bits, so that for N samples we need mN bits of computer storage.)

For instance, for an EEG signal that was sampled during 100 seconds with 100 samples per second and that was digitized with 128 (2^7) levels, we need a storage capacity of $100 \times 100 \times 7 = 70,000$ bits, or about 9,000 bytes.

5 Information Entropy

The formula of Shannon for the information content has an important implication for the acquisition and transmission of data in health care. We have seen that in all situations there is a transmission channel between sender and receiver. In this channel, disturbance is superimposed on the signal s. This means that it is often difficult at the receiver's site to extract the correct signal s from the mixture m. In the case of more disturbance this extraction will be more complicated or even only partly successful. This can now also be expressed in terms of information content. If the information content at the sender's site is I_s, then I_R at the receiver's site can never be larger than I_s. In the case of more disturbance, I_R becomes lower. The negative value of I is called information *entropy*, in parallel to entropy in thermodynamics. Entropy is a quantity related to the disorder of a system and cannot decrease within a closed system.

The information content I of a message transmitted from sender to receiver can also never increase. To be more correct one should add: the information content I can never increase within a closed information system. We can only increase I if we are able to use other, external information or knowledge for the extraction of the message from the mixture. The similarity between thermodynamics and Shannon's formula for information entropy concerns the statistical aspect of energetic and information-theoretical processes, respectively. Energy and information are, however, different entities. The implication of this law is that we must strive to have a maximal information content (a minimal information entropy) at the sender's site, and we should take all possible measures to keep the disturbance in the transmission channel as low as possible.

For applications of this law for situations in health care we give some practical rules that will keep the disturbance (and thus the information entropy) low:

1. Use an optimal transducer
Take care that the messages generated by the sender (the patient or the organ) are optimally recorded. Also, make sure not to add disturbance to the transmission channel. Some suggestions:

- ECGs: use noise-free electrodes (e.g., stainless steel with a silver-silverchloride paste);
- X-ray pictures: use high-resolution film material or photosensitive devices.

2. Keep the transmission channel short
Move the transducer as close as possible to the sender. Examples:

- blood chemistry: measure the PO_2 preferably directly in the blood instead of transcutaneously;
- intracardiac conduction: recording of *His*-bundle electrogram instead of a body surface ECG;
- fetal cardiac intervals: preferably put electrode directly on fetal skull instead of on maternal abdomen.

3. Reduce the transmission channel disturbance
This is to ensure that the information entropy is kept low during transmission from sender to receiver. Examples:

- EEG: screening off of external electric or magnetic fields;
- ECG: reduce disturbances caused by respiration and muscle activity.

4. Use, where possible, redundant information
If a single observation of a biological process may be distorted, then the subsequent ones may contain fewer or different distortions. Examples:

- Record a series of parallel ECG complexes. For instance, by *coherent averaging*, the disturbance can be decreased by using the repetitive character of the signals (see Chapters 8 and 25).
- Observations of the heart by independent methods, such as by echocardiography, ECG, and *catheterization*, may offer complementary information.

5. Use prior knowledge for interpretation as much as possible
The intent of this measure is for the receiver to use the knowledge and experience in helping to understand the message. Examples:

- Patient history: Use available (clinical) knowledge to obtain the necessary information for decision making; if possible, apply feedback to the sender;

- Signals and images: Use knowledge of signal and image properties, such as knowledge of the frequency domain and occurrence of events as a function of time.

6 Data in Computers

From the preceding sections it is clear that information can reach us in many different shapes and by all kinds of different media and carriers. We give a summary of the different types of carriers that transport information (Table 2.2):

1. *integers*: a *discrete number* (e.g., the number of premature ventricular contractions per time unit, or the number of leukocytes in a specimen, as seen through a microscope);
2. *reals*: a *measured variable* (e.g., a temperature or a blood pressure, but also a biosignal or a medical image);
3. *codes*: an *observation* (e.g., pain or a swelling); and
4. text: *natural language* (e.g., text in the patient history or the documentation of an event during patient monitoring).

The unambiguous computer storage of physical or chemical values offers no problems. The **coding** of drugs, diseases, or therapies can, in principle, also be agreed on, but it does not follow any natural process and is fully defined by people and is sometimes ambiguous. The coding of personal observations, let alone feelings or pain, is much more difficult and is often highly subjective, on the part of both the sender (the patient) and the receiver (e.g., the nurse). In some instances, no coding of observations is possible and only free text remains to document findings in the patient history (for that reason, all computerized patient history systems should be able to document narrative text as well; see Chapter 7).

A most important issue related to the documentation of data in a computer is the completeness and reliability of the four different types of data. For instance, is a

Variable	Example
Integer numbers	Age (in days, months or years) Heartbeats/min Number of hospital visits/month
Real numbers	pH Blood pressure (mm Hg) ECG (mV)
Codes	Diseases Drugs
Natural language	Events Patient history Some treatments

Table 2.2
Four Types of Variables Used to Document Observations in Health Care.[a]

[a] The error rates in the data tend to increase from integer numbers to natural language (see also Fig. 2.3).

manually measured blood pressure as reliable as a blood pressure measured by a transducer? Will a disease code given by one clinician be similar to the one given by another?

We will briefly discuss data completeness, accuracy, and precision, to be followed by some preliminary remarks on the coding of data and free text (more information on these topics appear in Chapters 6 and 7).

6.1 Completeness

Incomplete data may result in uncertainty. In a patient record it is not always clear whether data are missing or are absent because they were considered to be irrelevant, or were just not documented in the patient record. In the practice of patient care, generally only abnormal findings are recorded. So, when data are not found in the patient record this might mean that no abnormalities were found or that the data were not available or collected. Most of the time, the clinician who uses the data on his or her own patient knows the difference between irrelevant and missing data. However, data in computer-based patient records are also used by people other than the responsible clinician, and therefore, in such records this difference should be made explicit. In Chapter 7, much attention is given how to obtain complete patient data without overburdening the clinician.

6.2 Accuracy

Accuracy is the ability to perform a task without making mistakes or errors, or it is the degree of conformity of a measure to a certain standard or a true value (as defined in Webster's Collegiate Dictionary). The former meaning can be characterized as *correctness*; the second one can be characterized as *conformity* or *exactness*. We discuss both meanings in the following.

• Correctness
Correctness is a measure of the error rate of the data. Errors are first made during data collection, either in observations or in measurements. When measuring a

value, for example, a blood pressure, the aim is to express the blood pressure in mm Hg, but we know that the measured value is only an estimation of the "true" value and that there is an inherent inaccuracy. The observed value also has a deviation due to reading or measuring errors. We distinguish *systematic* and *statistical* errors.

When the blood pressure is measured with a cuff around the arm, we actually measure the pressure in the cuff and not in the artery. This cuff pressure is only an approximation of the arterial pressure. Furthermore, the moment that the pressure is read is determined by the moment that the sounds disappear because of the obstruction of the blood flow in the arteria brachialis. The true blood pressure is therefore usually lower than the external pressure exerted by the cuff, although we do not exactly know how much. This deviation is called a **systematic error**. If the calibration of the manometer is not correct, this will also cause a systematic, although different, error.

Variations in the blood pressure and variations in reading the mercury column mean that two successive measurements will never give exactly the same results. This is called the **statistical error**.

A special type of error are the *reading errors*, for example, reading the height of the mercury column on a blood pressure manometer. They can have both a systematic and a statistical character.

• Conformity
Conformity of data pertains to following standards or classification systems for data recording. When classification and coding systems are used to document patient data, we need to follow the rules and use the definitions of the classification system to select a proper code. For instance, when we want to classify the mental condition of a patient by using a system with only three classes, namely relaxed, normal or stressed, we can make an error by assigning the patient to the wrong category. In that case the true condition of the patient does not match the definition of the selected class. In other words, the clinician who classifies the patient does not conform to the instructions of the classification system. This source of error will be discussed more extensively in Chapter 6.

6.3 Precision

Precision deals with the degree of refinement or granularity by which a measurement is expressed, such as the number of decimal places. A body weight expressed as 89.12 kg expresses a higher precision than a weight expressed as 89.1 kg. It is misleading to specify a value with a higher precision than the accuracy with which the value is obtained. It is equally misleading that the weight of an adult should be expressed with two decimals if this precision does not bear any meaning, except for circumstances in which the body weight is continuously monitored, for example, to follow changes in the fluid balance of a patient in an intensive care unit. When the uncertainty in obtaining the body weight is ± 0.1 kg, we should specify the value as 89.1 kg. A notation of 89.12 kg suggests that the value is between 89.11 and 89.13 kg. When storing the measurements in the computer, we must ensure that the level of precision is sufficiently high.

6.4 Coding

In **coding** data, the user should first interpret the data and then assign a code. Interpretation errors are inherent to coding. Other errors caused by using codes, as well as ways of largely preventing these errors, will be discussed in Chapter 6. On the one hand, the coding of data limits the way of expressing oneself, but on the other hand, it enforces standardization of terminology, which is extremely important if the patient data are to be used by people other than only the treating clinician. Clinicians have often felt restricted by the limited degree of expression when coding medical data. However, too much detail in specifying data is also disturbing, giving false impressions of correctness. It can be misleading when the details of the code are unnecessary for the purpose for which the data are used.

6.5 Free Text

Free text (or **natural language**) gives the user the greatest liberty to express details. However, free text is essentially nonstandardized, which makes computer

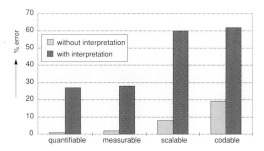

Figure 2.4

The percentage of errors in a large database of obstetric patient data as a function of the different types of data in patient records. Errors are indicated for quantifiable data (e.g., the patient's age), measurable data (e.g., a blood pressure), scaleable data (e.g., the height of the uterus above the symphysis), and codable data (e.g., a drug, a coded disease, or an event). The data were entered in a computer by a large group of physicians, after extraction from paper-based patient records. The error percentages with interpretation are far higher than those without interpretation. When interpretation was required, the physician had to perform some processing in his or her brain (e.g., calculation of the duration of the pregnancy from the date of the last menstruation and the present date) (after Van Hemel).[a]

[a] Van Hemel OJS. An Obstetric Database: HumanFactors, Design and Reliability. Amsterdam: Free University, 1977.

2

processing difficult. Free text can be seen as the personal interpretation of observed facts. If some other user needs these free text data, he or she will read the text, interpret it, and mentally reconstruct the medical object described from the interpretation. Therefore, semantically, free text has insufficient structure and is open to multiple interpretations. Such interpretation errors are unlikely to be reduced by computers.

Earlier in this chapter we discussed information entropy, which can only increase on the way from the sender to the receiver. In this respect we want to stress that the information entropy tends to increase from discrete numbers, via measurements and codes, to free text. In other words, the information in free text is probably less reliable than the information contained in integer or real numbers. The reason for this decreasing reliability is the fact that human interpretation is more difficult in coding free text expressions, and consequently, errors occur more often in coding and findings in free text than in discrete numbers or measurements. This is illustrated in Fig. 2.4, which is the result of an analysis of the reliability of data in a large-scale study of data in the records of obstetrics patients. The lesson from this study is that one should avoid human interpretation as much as possible when documenting patient data and one should always store the "raw" primary patient data, whenever possible, even if interpretations of those data are also stored. This underlines our statement earlier in this chapter that we should record data as close to the source of the data as possible.

6.6 Conclusions

In conclusion, several important rules can be phrased, partly based on the information presented above, for the documentation of patient data in computers:

1. Data should be acquired as close to the source of the data as possible.
2. Data should be recorded by obeying strict rules of standardization.
3. The original data should be stored, and if possible, human interpretations should be stored only if the raw data they are based on are also stored.

4. Coding of data should be done only if there is no other way to present the data, and it should preferably be done by the person making the observation.
5. For all data entered, there should preferably be an on-line *feedback* to the user to signal possible deviations from what should be expected.
6. Persons who enter the data should ideally benefit from this data entry, either because they will use the data later on or because it will improve the quality of their work.
7. *Authentication* (adding the coder's name and signature) and time stamping of data improves the data quality.

Key References

Komaroff AL. The variability and inaccuracy of medical data. Proceedings of the IEEE 1979;67:1196-1207.

Koran L.M. The reliability of clinical methods, data and judgments. N Engl J Med 1975;293:642-646 and 695-701.

See the Web site for further literature references.

II

Data in Computers

Authors of Part II

Chapter 3: Data Processing
    J.S. Duisterhout, E.M. van Mulligen, J.H. van Bemmel, Erasmus University Rotterdam

Chapter 4: Database Management
    J.S. Duisterhout, E.M. van Mulligen, J.H. van Bemmel, Erasmus University Rotterdam;
    with contribution of A.A.F. van der Maas, University of Nijmegen

Chapter 5: Telecommunication, Networking and Integration
    E.M. van Mulligen, P.J. Branger, Erasmus University Rotterdam

3 Data Processing

1 Introduction

The purpose of data collection from patients is to provide the clinician with information. For instance, the body temperature may give information about fever, laboratory tests may provide information on the functioning of organs such as the liver or the kidneys, and an electrocardiogram (*ECG*) may provide information on ventricular hypertrophy or an infarction. Together with knowledge about diseases and possible interventions, these data are the basis for decision making and further action (see Fig. 1.1). However, raw data acquired from the patient are not always presented in such a way that the required information can be inferred for decision making.

The derivation of *semantic* information (Chapter 2) from the data therefore requires data processing. For instance, to answer the question, "What drugs are being used by the patient?" the physician or another care provider must read all the prescriptions, calculate the period for which the drugs were prescribed, and compare this information with the current date. When data are stored in a computer, data retrieval, calculations, and decisions can be supported by computer processing. This means that, in principle, the computer can support the three stages of the diagnostic-therapeutic cycle, as discussed in Chapter 1. This cycle has the following three stages:

1. observation,
2. *diagnosis*, and
3. *therapy*.

Computer support generally becomes more complex as we climb the six levels of complexity (shown in Fig. 1.4) in Chapter 1. In this regard computers are better able to provide data acquisition, storage, and processing support than decision making and treatment support. The observation stage itself can be split into:

- data acquisition and transmission,
- data storage and retrieval, and
- data processing and presentation.

The following sections outline the hardware and software required to shape an information processing system and describe the different building blocks, tools, and peripherals of such a system.

2 The Information Processing System

Before a computer can do anything, it needs to be given *instructions* on how to handle the data. These instructions are composed in a computer *program*, which is stored in the computer *memory*. The data are also stored in the computer memory. The program "knows" what to do with the data, where to find them in its memory, and where and how to present the results; the designer of the program has defined how these are to be done. This brief description already shows that for a computer to process data, equipment and a program are needed. Therefore, we prefer to speak of a computer *system* rather than of a computer as such. The equipment (what one can touch) is called the **hardware**, and the programs are called the **software** (i.e., one cannot touch it). Hardware and software together make up the computer system.

Computer systems can be used for different types of operations. In addition to the illustrations presented in Chapter 1, take the following examples:

- Computer systems assist in the diagnostic-therapeutic cycle, especially in the observation stage, but also partly in the diagnostic and therapeutic stages. Here, computer systems are used to provide the user with the data needed to make decisions and take actions. In this situation we speak of **information-processing systems**.
- When a computer system is used to control the automatic landing of an aircraft or the therapy of a patient in an intensive care unit, we call it a **process-control system**. The computer system senses process variables and adjusts process parameters to let the process proceed safely.

The difference between process-control systems and information-processing systems is that in process-control systems the decision-making process is part of the computer system; that is, the user of the system is not part of the observation-decision-action cycle. In information-processing systems the user is the decision maker who uses the computer system to obtain the appropriate information. In an environment of an information-processing system, therefore, we discern people and computer-system activities:

1. the user,
2. data entry,
3. the user interface,
4. data-processing software, and
5. data presentation.

Each of these processes and components (some involving the user) needs hardware and software. We shall discuss the components consecutively, but we will first focus on the user.

2.1 The User

Users are essential in any information-processing system. They are responsible for entering data into the system and controlling the processing. In health care we can distinguish different types of users. Each type of user has a different behavior and requires a different support from the information-processing system. The users can be grouped into:

- occasional users,
- routine users,
- experts.

The three groups of users will be discussed in this order (see also Fig. 3.1).

- Occasional users

Occasional users are familiar with the functions that the information system provides, but they do not need to know all possibilities in great detail, such as the meaning of function keys. For these users it is important that the computer provides assistance in navigating through the system and that it protects the user against catastrophic events, such as the loss of data. If desired, the system should at any time inform the user which steps are to be taken, and it should give global or detailed "help" information on demand. Such help should always be invoked with the same command or key and it should be relevant to the user. Therefore, help needs to be context sensitive, meaning that the type of help that is displayed should depend on the phase of the program that the user has reached at the moment the user presses the help key.

- Routine users

Routine users have detailed knowledge of all functions of the **applications** that they use, and they know exactly how the system behaves in their own application. This means that offering on the computer screen too much nonessential information can be disturbing and not helpful. Superfluous information on a screen makes

3

the entire content of the screen harder to read at a glance and, moreover, occupies space that could be used for essential data. The support offered by help messages is usually not appreciated by this type of user. A smooth interaction between user and computer system is what counts, and as part of this interaction speed and ease of data entry are most essential. If such users enter data into the computer, they do not always wait for the immediate reaction of the computer system. Often, the computer cannot keep up with the user's data entry speed, and the system should allow for unprompted data entry, for instance, "*typing ahead*". Typing ahead is a feature that allows users to enter data even before the computer asks for it. Such systems often have to make a compromise between operational speed and user-friendliness.

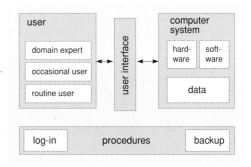

Figure 3.1
Different users of an information system. The computer system consists of hardware and software and interacts with the user through an interface. Procedures take care of logging in of the user and backing up the data.

• Experts

Domain experts are interested in getting a specific and often highly specialized job done. A researcher, for instance, will constantly change his or her requirements and will often write and modify his or her own programs. A researcher is not primarily concerned about the efficiency and the user-friendliness of the programs and the computer system; but the researcher's main interest lies in the functionality of the program and its outcome. Help information is seldom needed by such users, except when they wish to familiarize themselves with new programs.

In practice, computer users in health care are represented by all three types of users mentioned above.

2.2 Data Entry

Information is derived from data. Low-quality data result in unreliable or even erroneous information. Computers can process data and can help to extract the information from the data, but they can never generate information that was not contained in the data: the strength of a chain is determined by its weakest link. In our situation, the chain is the diagnostic-therapeutic cycle and the first link in the chain is data acquisition. Data can be entered manually or by automatic measuring devices, such as *autoanalyzers* in clinical labora-

tories, ECG recording equipment, or patient-monitoring devices that operate without human interference. In manual data entry, the user is the "transducer" who converts the data into a computer-readable format. This can, for instance, be done by filling in forms on computer screens. More advanced technologies are, among others:

– *bar code* reading devices,
– *automated character recognition* devices, or
– systems that allow data entry by *voice input*.

Systems that automatically recognize handwriting are also available, but these require user training, and they still have an error rate too high for routine clinical use. On-line *feedback* on detected or suspected errors can significantly reduce the error rate during data entry. In this respect it is important that data are entered as closely as possible to the information source, and by the person likely to know the correct information (see Chapter 2). When patient data are entered while the patient is still present in the clinician's office or surgery, any missing, ambiguous, or erroneous data can be corrected by asking the patient directly. However, when data are first written on paper and later entered into the computer by another person, errors detected in the data cannot always be corrected without referring to the information source. Moreover, a second source of errors is introduced because the message is

3

first written down, with possible errors, and is then read and entered by the data-entry typist, who might introduce new errors. Therefore, it is important to avoid situations in which there can be multiple independent points of unverified data entry.

The computer can assist in the data-entry process by detecting errors in the input data or by offering help. Examples of error detection and correction are, for instance:

- *syntactic* error checking,
- *semantic* error checking, and
- on-line help.

• Syntactic error checking

The computer can detect errors on the basis of the syntactic aspects of the entered data. All data items have a domain and a value. The domain can be, for example, calendar date or phone number. A domain defines the pattern of characters that may be expected. A calendar date, for example, 11/17/1938 (United States) or 17/11/1938 (some other countries), can be defined as "two digits, a slash, two digits, a slash, four digits"; or body weight can be expressed in kilograms, and in one, two, or three digits. The computer can easily check such data formats. When the syntactical check fails, the computer should inform the user. In a user-friendly system, the system should give information about what type of error was made and, if possible, give advice on how to correct the data and, if required, give examples.

• Semantic error checking

The semantic aspect of data is its meaning. For instance, when entering a blood pressure value, we can check for *possible* and *plausible* minimal and maximal values, but we can also check the possibility and the plausibility of the entered data in relation to already available data. For instance, entering 75 kg as the weight of a 10-month-old child is not very plausible.

• On-line help

As mentioned above, pressing the help key (or, in windows environments, a 'soft' key) should always give advice and offer examples about the question at issue.

If the user is required to choose from a limited list of options, this list should be presented in such a way that the user can select an appropriate entry. User-friendly systems will show such a list when the entered data do not match one of the possible options.

2.3 User Interface

The user interface is that part of the computer system that communicates with the user. It is used for controlling the execution and the flow of the program and for interactive data entry. The requirements for the user interface depend on the kind of user, as we have seen above. In all cases, a consistent "behavior" of the system is essential, which means that once the user has learned about the behavior of the system, it should always respond in a consistent manner. To achieve this consistency, even from one program to another, standards and style guides for building user interfaces have been developed (see also Chapter 31). We can distinguish two basic types of user interfaces:

- *character-based interfaces*, and
- *graphical* user *interfaces*.

• Character-based interfaces

In character-based interfaces, only *keyboard* symbols are used to communicate with the user. Such interfaces are normally used for a traditional programming style, in which the program determines the next step to be taken. The user then answers questions asked by the program. These questions can either be requests for data input or a choice from a limited list of options to control the program flow. Character-based interfaces require only a very low transmission rate from computer to terminal device and vice versa, that is, only character codes and character position information. Therefore, such interfaces are useful in situations in which the user is remotely connected to a system by a transmission channel with a low capacity, such as a conventional telephone line. Another reason for using a character interface is the low price of a device that handles the interaction (often called a "dumb" terminal). Character-based interfaces are efficient, but they are not very user-friendly.

- Graphical user interfaces

Graphical user interfaces (often called "windows-based interfaces") have rapidly replaced character-based user interfaces. The reason is that instead of the so-called dumb terminals, the more powerful functionality of a personal computer (*PC*) is used. Nowadays, most users are familiar with PCs and **windows**. This section will not describe the windows-oriented interfaces in great detail, but will outline their basic principles.

A window is an area on the computer screen with a border and a title bar on top that contains text fields, pictures, buttons, selection boxes, and so forth (Fig. 3.2). Buttons are graphically presented in quasi three-dimensional format (a shadow is generated by the computer to suggest a three-dimensional presentation) and appear as if they have been pressed or released, by changing the shadow. A user can "press" a button by positioning the **mouse** pointer and clicking on the button of the mouse (see Section 3.3). These elements in a window are called window controls. Window controls are used for controlling the program flow and for data entry. Behind each separate window there are one or more programs that can be invoked (i.e., activated) by the user.

Windows and their controls form a hierarchy, which means that when a window is "destroyed" (i.e., the user "closes" the window because he or she is no longer interested in using the program that is attached to it), its controls are also destroyed. A PC screen can display several windows at the same time. This is also expressed by saying that several windows can be "open" at the same time. These windows may also overlap, but only one window is active and fully visible at a particular moment. The color of the title bar generally changes automatically to indicate which one of the open windows is active. All keystrokes and mouse clicks within the window act only on the open window. In a window, only one control can be focused on at a given moment in time. All commands are then sent to the program that is attached to that control.

The programming style for software that uses windows differs greatly from the traditional programming style, as discussed under character-based interfaces. We call this type of programming *event-driven* programming.

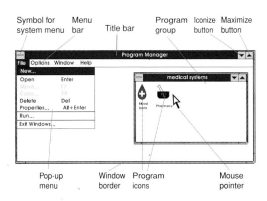

Symbol for system menu — Menu bar — Title bar — Program group — Iconize button — Maximize button — Pop-up menu — Window border — Program icons — Mouse pointer

Figure 3.2

Example of a windows-based interface, with the window itself, its border and title bar, buttons, and icons. The arrow is controlled by the mouse. Several windows may be open at the same time, but only one is active, and the open window is usually indicated by the different color of the title bar. The user selects functions by placing the arrow over a button and clicking with the mouse. A button may appear as pressed or released, by a change in appearance. (There are several standards in window interfaces, such as windows for PCs and X-windows. X-windows are mainly for graphical workstations with other operating systems, such as UNIX.)

3

An example of an event is clicking on a control with the mouse or pressing a key on the keyboard.

Window systems introduce a very important aspect of information systems: they make all systems look alike. A limited set of controls is sufficient to build a complex windows interface. This gives windows applications a standard behavior for the user interface, which makes it easier for users to learn a new system once they know what the behavior of a windows-based system is.

For information systems to be used by, for example, physicians and nurses, it is an imperative condition that all parts of an application (and, preferably, all parts of all applications) use the same type of interface.

2.4 Data Processing

During **data processing**, the data are analyzed and transformed in such a way that the required information can be presented to the user. The following paragraphs describe some examples of data processing (see Fig. 3.3 for an overview of the different terms):

- Data sorting

Computer programs can effectively order or **sort** data in different ways. For numbers this ordering may be evident (e.g., from low to high), but computers can also easily order data by alphabetic characters in a lexicographical way. Using additional sorting criteria, computers also effectively group data, for instance, ordering of patient data according to disease, gender, and age in an age-disease register.

- *Data storage and retrieval*

Data are seldom stored as independent items, but are most often grouped together, for example, as data belonging to the same event or to the same type or class (e.g., all patients who have been admitted to the department of oncology or all patients that have to be contacted by their general practitioner for screening for breast cancer). All these groups may, in turn, be related to each other. In a *database* system (Chapter 4) the data are stored in a structured way (e.g., all patients who were admitted to the cardiology department or all patients for whom a laboratory test was requested). The structure of the database and the relation between the different data are defined by the user, using the database system.

If the database lacks structure, retrieval of data would be extremely difficult and time-consuming.

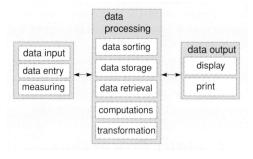

Figure 3.3
Examples of some processing actions on data, as described in the text.

Such structured databases allow us to define instructions for the computer, such as, "Give me a list of all patients younger than 12 years who were admitted to the pediatric clinic by dr. Koop during 1995 and 1996 and who were hospitalized for more than 10 days; present the data grouped according to treating clinician and sorted by name of the patient." (The organization of data in databases is described in more detail in Chapter 4.) Special query languages have been developed for retrieval of data from databases. An information system equipped with such a *query language* can produce the desired result instantaneously.

- Computations

Mathematical (algebraic, logical, statistical) and any other operations involving numbers can easily be described by algorithms, which can be translated into a computer program. In fact, all mathematical operations can be expressed by a few simple instructions, such as the addition of two numbers. Subtraction then becomes adding the negative value of a number, and multiplication of a number n by a multiplier m just becomes m additions of n. Computers can handle such operations at high speed (i.e., within a tiny fraction of a second). All of these operations are handled by the so-called *central processing unit* (see Section 3), but many computers have special built-in processors for numerical computations to further increase speed.

Computers can perform complex numerical computations, such as those used in image processing (Chapters 9, 10, and 26) or *biosignal* analysis (Chapters 8 and 25) or those used for solving differential equations in biophysical *modeling*.

- Data transformation

Humans have a limited capacity to recognize patterns. In an *X-ray* picture, for instance, we see only a two-dimensional shadow of an object. This means that two objects that are located behind each other in the X-ray beam are difficult to distinguish. The shadow of one object will overlap that of the other partly or completely. It is also impossible to determine which object is located closer to the X-ray source. Only a trained radiologist is able to build a mental model by which he or she can interpret two-dimensional pictures in three

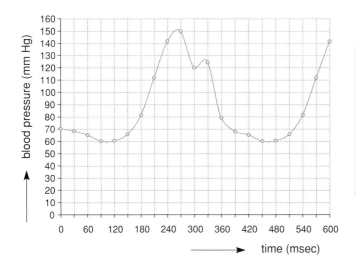

time	sample value	time	sample value
00	70	330	125
30	68	360	80
60	65	390	70
90	60	420	65
120	60	450	60
150	65	480	60
180	80	510	65
210	110	540	80
240	140	570	110
270	150	600	140
300	120		

Figure 3.4
Blood pressures in alphanumeric (a) and graphical (b) form. The information needed for decision making can be derived at a glance from the graphical presentation; it is more difficult for the user to come to the same conclusion by interpreting the alphanumeric data.

dimensions. Therefore, we prefer to have a three-dimensional picture. This can be realized by taking a series of X-ray pictures around the exposed object at different angles, as is done in *computed tomography* (see Chapter 9). The computer is then able to compute a three-dimensional picture from these two-dimensional X-ray pictures.

2.5 Data Presentation

Correct presentation of information to the user is essential for proper understanding. Information processing should enable the user to extract relevant information in the most convenient and unambiguous way. Only the information on which the user wants to base his or her decision should be presented. We can judge, for instance, whether an antihypertensive drug therapy is effective by presenting a list of blood pressure measurements that were taken four times a day during a few months, but it would be easier if we were given the average blood pressure before the therapy and after 1 month of therapy, after 2 months of therapy, and

so forth. It would be even better if the information was presented not as a list of numbers but in a graphical way (see Fig. 3.4).

It is important that users be able to specify how they want the information to be presented so that the computer can be used as a data presentation tool. The user then specifies which data he or she wants to see and how the data should be presented (e.g., as a list or in graphical form). For data presented in graphical form, users may define their own parameters, such as the time period of interest and vertical and horizontal scales.

The computer can then reorder the data in the most convenient way for the user.

Modern computer technology is not restricted to displaying data in tables and graphs, it can also present data in a multimedia format, such as through sound and movies. For instance, a computer-based patient record in cardiology not only contains alphanumeric data, as in the patient history or the physical examination, but also laboratory test results in the form of numbers, pictures such as X-ray images and cine-angio videos, together with heart sounds and ECG signals.

3

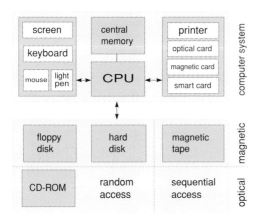

Figure 3.5
Overview of hardware components of a computer, as described in the text.

The resolution of the computer screen may present some problems here. The computer screen of a normal PC does not yet have the fine resolution required for an X-ray picture, but by zooming in on the relevant parts of high-resolution digital images, the same diagnostic detail obtained in a conventional X-ray film can be obtained. The advantage of storing X-ray pictures in a computer is that the pictures can be viewed at different locations at the same time and that they can be processed to get a better view (by zooming) or intensity (e.g., by changing the contrast) or by improving the quality of the image, by *image-processing* techniques.

3 The Hardware

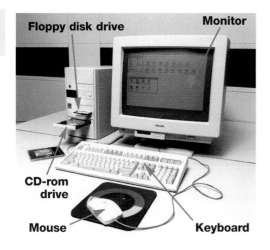

Figure 3.6
The components of a PC system. The basic parts are the CPU with its arithmetic unit and registers, the display screen, the keyboard, the central memory, and the background memory. Other special devices, such as peripherals (e.g., a printer or a modem), can be added.

The hardware of a computer system consists of a number of main components:

- the *central processing unit*,
- computer *memory*, and
- *peripherals*.

We discuss these components in the following sections. A comprehensive overview of the hardware is found in Fig. 3.5.

3.1 The Central Processing Unit

The heart of the computer consists of the central processing unit (*CPU*) and the internal or central memory (see Fig. 3.6). The computer memory contains the instructions and the data relevant to the execution of the active program.

The CPU retrieves the instructions from the internal memory and executes them. In principle, this execution occurs sequentially. The basic operations of a

---

PANEL 3.1

Multiuser, Multiprocessing, Time Sharing

* *single user, single program*
The most primitive operating system can service only one user at a time and can handle only one program at a time. This is called a single-user, single-processing system.

* *single user, multiprocessing*
The next level of operating system complexity is a single-user, multiprocessing system. In this case one user can start more than one program simultaneously and the programs will be executed concurrently. The processor divides the time between the different programs.

* *multiuser, multiprocessing*
The next higher level is the multiuser multiprocessing system. In this case a mechanism is needed to protect the data and the programs from unauthorized use by other users. Several mechanisms are used to divide the time of different users over concurrent programs:
– a program can be serviced while it is waiting for input or output and then the next program will be allowed to start its execution;
– another well-known mechanism is time sharing, in which the operating system divides the available CPU time over a number of concurrent processes.

CPU can be divided into *arithmetic* **instructions** (such as adding the contents of two memory locations) and *control* instructions (such as retrieving the next instruction). In principle, these two basic types of CPU operations are sufficient to program very complex operations. In reality, a CPU may be more complex to speed up the processing.

The CPU consists of an *arithmetic unit* and a set of *registers*. The CPU registers are used to store instructions or data once they have been retrieved or to store the intermediate results of operations. The CPU executes the instructions of a program sequentially unless a control instruction changes the order (e.g., as a result of an earlier computation). The normal sequence can also be interrupted by an external event, such as a keystroke on the keyboard. The processor may then start a program from another memory location to handle that interrupt. By switching quickly from one program to another, a single CPU can behave as if it is executing multiple programs. This is called **multiprocessing** (see also Panel 3.1).

Although the electric signals that control the computer internally operate very quickly, the time needed to send a signal from A to B, even on a computer chip, is not zero. Therefore, a CPU needs to synchronize its internal steps. For this purpose it uses a 'clock' that generates electrical synchronization pulses at extremely high speed. Each computer vendor usually advertises the speed of its CPU by this clock speed. A 100-megahertz (MHz) processor, for example, is faster than the 60-MHz version of the same CPU, but the clock speed is not the only important factor. The speed is also influenced by the complexity of the instructions that the CPU can handle and the presence of special arithmetic processors, for instance, for carrying out multiplications.

Another important factor for the speed of a computer is the number of bits that the CPU simultaneously handles during one operation, that is, during one "tick" of the clock. A CPU that can handle 16-bit numbers can also add two numbers of 32 bits each, but it has to do this in a "smart" way by splitting the operations into parts and then combining the results. Of course, this requires more steps than a 32-bit CPU needs. Modern computers have a 32-bit (e.g., modern PCs) or a 64-bit data path for internal data transfer and computations.

3.2 Computer Memory

The CPU retrieves its instructions and data from the computer memory, which is the so-called **volatile memory**. The contents of this memory are lost when the computer is not powered. This type of memory is also referred to as random access memory (**RAM**). Computer memory consists of **bytes** of 8 bits each. The bytes have a memory address, and their contents can be directly retrieved by the CPU by referring to this memory address in the address register of the CPU. To increase speed, some computers simultaneously transfer more bytes to and from the CPU within one memory cycle; for example, a 32-bit CPU transfers 4 bytes simultaneously.

3.3 Peripherals

All the devices needed for data entry, external storage, or presentation of the data are called **peripherals**. Peripherals can be divided into input and output devices (**I/O** devices) and external mass storage devices. First, we briefly describe the most frequently used Output device.

* The computer screen

The best-known output device of a computer is undoubtedly the **screen** of a PC or a workstation. It allows for character-based as well as graphical output. The format of most screens does not match the common format of paper. Early computer screens could contain at most 80 characters per line and usually 25 lines. This means that pages printed on paper and shown on a computer screen required different formats. Modern computer screens are more flexible and show partial views on a virtually unlimited document area. Moreover, a screen can display only one page at a time, which means that backward and forward scrolling is required when a document is read from a screen. Therefore, computer-stored documents are often printed before they are read; until now the com-

puter has not diminished the use of paper -- on the contrary. This is the main reason why the so-called paperless office that was predicted with the advent of PCs often generates more paper than ever before.

Modern display screens are usually much larger in size, for example, 21 inches (53 cm) on the diagonal, and can easily contain a whole page of printed text and more graphical windows. These screens, however, require more desk space and are more expensive than standard PC screens.

Input Devices

In this section we outline the devices through which data can be entered into the computer. This is done either manually or automatically (by an input device). The following describes the most important input devices.

* The keyboard

The best-known input device is the **keyboard**, which is part of PCs and all video terminals. The video terminal consists of a video **screen** plus a keyboard connected to a computer. A video terminal is in fact the combination of an output device (the screen) plus an input device (the keyboard).

The keyboard of modern video terminals or PCs is inherited from the typewriter. The layout of the character keys on a computer keyboard is identical to that on a typewriter. The old, mechanical typewriters had a handle by which the carriage that contained the sheet of paper could be returned to start a new line. The later electric typewriters and video terminals had a special key, the return key, which simulated this carriage return function. This key was used to send the characters that had been typed on a line to the computer or to signal the end of a typed line to the computer. This key is now usually marked "enter" instead of "return", although the arrow on the key sometimes reminds us of the old carriage return.

When a key on the keyboard is pressed, the code for that key is sent to the computer and is interpreted by a program in the computer. In most instances users will want to see the characters they have just typed on the screen. Therefore, the computer program will usually show those characters on the screen. The position on the screen where the typed character appears is indi-

3

cated by the *cursor*, which is a blinking rectangle or an underscore symbol on the screen that proceeds while the user is typing. Some applications change the shape of the cursor, depending on the typing mode, for example, typing over existing text or inserting new text at the position indicated by the cursor.

Apart from letter keys, number keys, and punctuation keys, a keyboard has so-called modifier keys that must be pressed simultaneously with a letter, a number, or a punctuation key. Modifier keys are SHIFT, Alt and Ctrl (Control). Depending on the keyboard type, there can also be a set of special keys for controlling the program flow, such as the so-called *function keys*, labeled F1 to F12, and some dedicated keys, such as PgUp (page up), End, and Home.

Screens can be made interactive when they are used in combination with a so-called pointing device, which can instruct the computer to react by pointing at the screen. The most important pointing device available for most screens is the mouse, described below.

- Mouse

The *mouse* is the most common *pointing device*. It consists of a small, rounded box that can be held in the palm of the hand. It has a roller ball at the bottom. The mouse is moved by hand over the table or a special mouse pad. The mouse translates the movements of the ball into movement codes and sends them to the computer. The position of the mouse is usually projected on the screen by a special drawing called the mouse cursor. When one moves the mouse, the mouse cursor moves correspondingly. The computer program that controls the position and shape of the mouse cursor is called the mouse driver program. The mouse cursor has the shape of an arrow when we are allowed to move the mouse, and it has the shape of an hourglass or a clock when the computer is busy performing a task. A mouse has one, two, or three buttons that can be used to request specific actions from the computer by clicking it. The computer can sense whether the mouse button is pressed or released.

Output Devices

Laser *printers* and *ink-jet* printers can produce hardcopy output on plain paper. The hardware is capable of producing dot matrix images with resolutions of from 150 x 150 up to 600 x 600 dots per inch (dpi). These printers contain an internal computer that converts the data input to the dot matrix. For printing plain text, the computer sends character codes to the printer, along with instructions for controlling the printing and information about the character font to be used, as well as the color, the position on the paper, the paper size, and so forth. The printer itself generates the "images" for the characters (i.e., the transformation of the desired character into a pattern of dots). In most printers the font information can be downloaded from the computer, which means that the number of fonts is virtually unlimited.

The computer can send images to the printer as bit images or in some special high-level language. The advantage of sending text and images in a high-level language is that the computer can generate output independently of the type of printing device. The internal processor of the printer translates the instructions and deals with all the instructions for the selected printer. Examples of such widespread high-level languages are *Postscript* and *PCL* (printer control language). Postscript is now the only printing language that really matters.

3

External Data Storage Devices

External storage devices allow us to store data separate from the computer memory (e.g., for security and safety reasons) or to move the data physically from one place to another. This section describes only the most common external storage devices (see also Fig. 3.6).

We can distinguish these external storage devices in the way that they can be accessed (i.e., randomly or sequentially) or by the type of technology that is used to store the data.

Random access means that the computer system can access data in any order simply by sending to the device the address where the data are stored. This is usually achieved by maintaining some *directory* structure; the actual address where the data are physically located on the external storage device is computed by using the information from the directory. A database that is continuously used for updating and retrieval will normally be stored on a randomly accessible device.

Sequential access means that data are read one after the other. Sequential storage devices should be used when it is acceptable to read the records in the sequence they are stored on the storage medium. Sequential storage devices are used, for instance, for archiving purposes or when a so-called *backup* is made of programs or data from a randomly accessible storage device. Sequentially accessible storage devices are cheaper than randomly accessible devices because the hardware involved is less complex.

The next section describes an important family of external storage devices: the magnetic storage media.

Magnetic Storage Media

Magnetic storage media use a magnetic surface to store the binary data. A bit can be represented by either a "1" or a "0," so the orientation of the magnetic field can be used for this purpose. The surface of a magnetic storage medium can be split into a multitude of magnetic cells at an extremely high density. The magnetic orientation of a cell then represents either a "1" or a "0." By moving a reading head over the surface, the magnetic orientation of

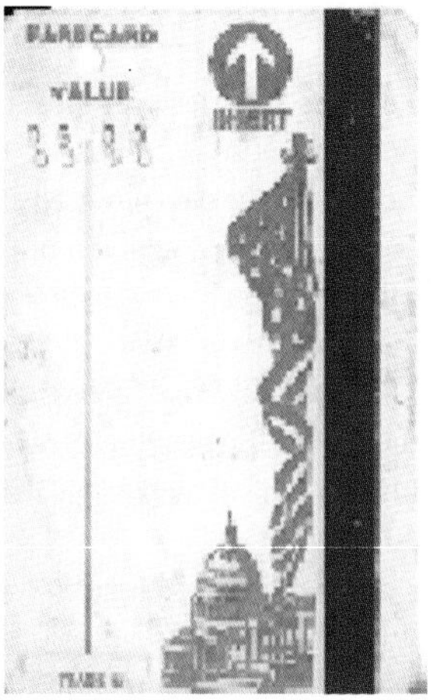

Figure 3.7
Magnetic card used by the Washington, D.C., Area Metro subway system.

the cells can be detected, and a writing head can be used to change the magnetic orientation. Various magnetic storage devices of this type are described below.

• Magnetic tape

Magnetic tape is a sequential storage device. There are several systems and standards on the market for magnetic tape storage. They all use parallel magnetic tracks to store the information. However, the number of tracks, the coding technique for the bits, and the format in which the data are stored may vary. Tapes are frequently used as a backup medium to make copies of more expensive randomly accessible devices. The storage capacity ranges from tens of Mbytes to several Gbytes. Tape media are relatively inexpensive.

• Magnetic disk

A *magnetic disk* is a randomly accessible storage device. A magnetic disk contains tracks on its surface that go in circles around the center, and it is divided into sectors. The disk spins under read/write heads that can move from the perimeter to the center of the disk. Data are addressed by the track number and the sector number on the disk. Magnetic disks are fast and are therefore ideal for active databases and for storing computer programs. The magnetic disk is also a convenient medium for temporary storage of data.

We can divide magnetic disks into nonremovable disks (e.g., the built-in, so-called hard disks) and removable disks (e.g., a *floppy* disk or a ZIP disk). Once they are installed from other media, operating systems and program libraries are typically stored on nonremovable disks.

• Magnetic cards

Data can also be stored on a card the size of a credit card (Fig. 3.7). Such a *magnetic card* can be read by a special reading device that has been connected to a computer. An advantage of these cards is that they can be carried around. The data are stored on a magnetic strip on the card. Such cards are used as banking cards, telephone cards, and so forth. The cards are cheap, but they cannot contain many data.

Although the cards can be protected by a password, they are not completely safe from fraud or misuse.

Besides the magnetic storage devices there is another family of devices: the *optical storage* devices. These devices store the data optically by using laser beams for writing and reading.

- CD-ROM

CD-ROMs (compact disk - read only memory) are disks that store bits as very tiny holes on a flat surface. These holes can be both made and detected by laser beams. CD-ROMs are used in the same way as magnetic disks and can contain both programs and data. A CD-ROM contains approximately 600 Mbytes (higher-density CD-ROMs, e.g., with a 5- to 10-fold greater storage capacity, are also becoming available). CD-ROMs can contain video images, sound tracks, and data. The latter disks are used in multimedia applications. The hardware device that is connected to the computer, the CD-ROM drive, can accept both types of disks, but requires different software. Most CD-ROM drives in PCs are used as read-only devices. The read/write version of the

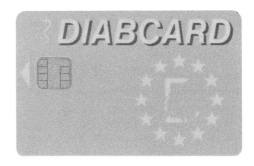

Figure 3.9
Example of a smart or chip card (DIABCARD, Siemens-Nixdorf).

CD-ROM device usually has a slow writing capability.

- Optical cards

Data storage on *optical card*s is similar to the way in which they are stored on CD-ROMs (Fig. 3.8). Optical cards can store more data than magnetic cards, but they are more expensive and are of the read-only type. Protection against improper use is almost impossible.

The next family of external storage devices are the smart cards or chip cards. Sometimes they combine the possibilities of the magnetic, optical, and chip card technology.

- Smart cards

Smart cards (Fig. 3.9) contain a chip, and therefore they can be made "intelligent" and be much better protected against improper use than magnetic or optical cards. The data can only be accessed through the chip on the card, which requires a password or a code. Different layers of protection can be built in. If the *chip card* is improperly used, the chip may even provide an instruction for the data to be destroyed. Smart cards are more expensive than magnetic and optical cards.

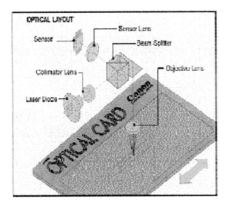

Figure 3.8
Example of an optical card (Canon).

3

4 The Software

Computers cannot operate without a **program**. Programs must be loaded from the external into the internal memory before they can be executed. When a computer is switched on, a built-in program, the so-called boot program, is automatically started. This program is permanently stored in a special small memory, called a read-only memory (**ROM**). The ROM is not *volatile*, and its contents cannot be changed by the user. For PCs this program always starts by checking the hardware. When this check has been successfully completed, it starts looking for the operating system of the computer from a floppy disk, hard disk, or CD-ROM. The following sections describe some important aspects of the software: the operating system and the user programs (purchased or written by the user). An overview of the different types of software is given in Fig. 3.10.

4.1 The Operating System

The **operating system** is the basic software of the computer and is essential for all operations. It is always present in the internal memory once the computer has

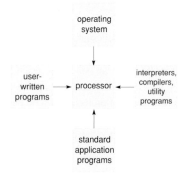

operating system

user-written programs → processor ← interpreters, compilers, utility programs

standard application programs

Figure 3.10
Different software components of an information processing system.

been started by the **boot** program. The operating system is responsible for the interaction with the peripherals, for loading and unloading user programs and data, and for all internal communication in the computer. It also controls the sharing of the computer resources between concurrent user programs. The operating system can be viewed as a layer between the computer hardware and the user programs (Fig. 3.11). Once the operating system is loaded, control of the computer is transferred to the operating system. The operating system signals its readiness by showing a so-called prompt (such as "→") on the screen in character-oriented interfaces. A **prompt** is a special character string to "prompt" the user to supply input. The user can communicate with the operating system by a special command language. Several standard operating systems are used on different hardware configurations, also called *hardware platforms*. Well-known operating systems that use character-oriented interfaces are, for example, **PC-DOS** (disk operating system for PCs) and **UNIX** for all kinds of hardware platforms, including PCs. DOS has nowadays generally been replaced by graphical platforms such as **Windows**.

After starting up, graphical or windows-oriented operating systems show their basic control window and an active mouse cursor when they are ready to accept commands. The user can give commands to the operating system either by the keyboard or by the mouse. Simple tasks are, for example, giving an overview of the data files and programs stored on disk (the directory listing) or showing the available amount of memory, expressed in bytes. These simple tasks are actually small programs that are considered part of the operating system. The operating system can also be told to load and execute a user program. However, an operating system always wants to remain in control, so it will not allow a user program to do everything it wants.

The operating system is also responsible for protecting the security of the system. Especially in a multiuser environment, users must identify themselves with a user name or identity card and type the user **pass-**

PANEL 3.2

Object-oriented Programming

The intent of object-oriented programming is to improve the development of computer programs. The first computer programs for solving mathematical problems were written as a single list of instructions. Soon, it became clear that writing complex programs in this way would reduce both the productivity of programmers and the reliability of computer programs. A first step in enhancing the development of computer programs was the introduction of the concept of a *function* or *procedure* (or subroutine). Computer languages that support this concept are referred to as *procedural languages*. A function allows a programmer to break a large list of instructions down into smaller units that can be executed repeatedly. Ideally, each function has a clearly defined purpose and interface to other functions in the program. Each unit is given a name that is comprehensible to computer programmers.

The relation between data structures and functions is not visible in procedural programming languages. Since data structures can be accessed by different functions in a program, it is important that changes to the data structure be reflected in all functions that access the data structure. Object-oriented programming alleviates the problem of maintaining consistency between data structures and functions that access those structures. With object-oriented programming, the data structure and the functions that operate on the data structure are located in one *object* (i.e., a logical software entity). The term *object-oriented programming* indicates that the software is organized as objects rather than as functions. In most object-oriented programming languages, access to individual elements of the object's data structures can be limited: private elements can only be accessed by the functions belonging to the object, and public data elements can be accessed from all functions. The changes to the object's data structures can be limited by restricting access to the data elements via the object's functions.

An important feature of object-oriented programming languages for programmers is operator overloading. This means that the meaning of an operator or function depends on the object for which it is used. For instance, an add operator applied to two *number objects* will calculate the sum of the two numbers contained in those objects. When applied to two *text objects*, the add operator will yield the concatenation of the two texts.

Object-oriented programming languages are often used to implement graphical user interfaces. Each screen element (list, button, label, etc.) is associated with an object, and the user interaction is arranged through the functions that belong to the object. An event that happens in the user interface (for instance, pressing a button or moving the mouse) will be handled by an object's function that is associated with the user interface element.

Example

A patient's physical examination (height, weight, blood pressure, etc.) can be represented as an object that contains functions to compute, for example, the *quetelet index*, to draw trends, and to support risk assessment. The following example represents an abstracted implementation:

```
start object definition "Physical Examination"
private data structures:
    ExamDate:          date
    PatientId:         number
    Height             number
    Weight             number
    BloodPressure      number
    SmokingHabit       boolean
    ChestPain          string
public functions:
    function Quetelet
    function DrawTrends
    function AssessRisk
end object definition "Physical Examination"
```

3

word or PIN (personal identification number) code to gain access to the computer system.

A special part of the operating system is the user interface, by which the user can communicate with the computer (as discussed earlier in Section 2.3).

4.2 User Programs

The development of user programs requires programming tools and tools that are used to install these programs on the computer. The first tools support users in developing programs, preferably in a high-level computer language and, if possible, programs that are computer platform independent. The latter means that the user programs can be implemented on different operating systems and on different hardware platforms. Programs that have been developed in a language that is understandable to the user, are said to be written in *source code*. There are many programming languages, and these have all been developed for special problem areas, such as computer languages for financial problems, for textual manipulation, for database operations, or for computerized public telephone switching. A *compiler* converts the source code to computer instructions that are understandable to the computer. This distinction between operating system, programming tools, and user programs is not always clear to the user. However, for most users it is not essential that they understand the distinction. Modern programming languages such as *C++*, use a programming method which is known as object-oriented programming. Panel 3.2 describes some aspects of OO programming.

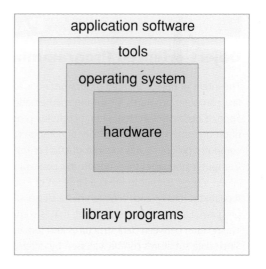

Figure 3.11
The software is organized in layers around the hardware. The operating system is responsible for controlling the hardware. The application programs make use of the supplied software tools, library programs, and utilities to build a complete application. The programs in the outer squares are more portable from one computer system to the other than the programs in the inner squares.

Key References

See Chapter 5

4 Database Management

1 Introduction

Data are at the center of all decision making in health care. Data should therefore be reliable, complete, and well structured (see also Chapters 2 and 3); computers may assist in fulfilling these requirements. This chapter deals with the structuring of data in computers.

A software *shell* around the data assists the user in all storage and retrieval operations, controls the access to the data, and keeps a *log file* of all data transactions. This software shell is called a *database management system* (*DBMS*). The application programs in an advanced information system do not themselves retrieve data from the computer but operate via the DBMS, which handles all data operations for the programs.

In this chapter, various terms are used. Therefore, we first summarize these terms (see also Fig. 4.1).

- Data are usually stored in a *database*, which structures data that belong together. A database is a collection of files.
- A *file* is a data storage entity that has a name, the file name. Files are created and deleted by the computer's file system. Files are accessed by giving the file name as one of the parameters of a command.
- A file is further subdivided into logical data *records*, which are the smallest units for data storage in the database.
- The computer's file system is responsible for the *physical storage* of the data onto a disk, which is called a *mass storage device*

Before further discussing data structuring in computers, we make a parallel with data documentation in paper-based patient records. The terminology used for paper-based records shows some similarities with the terminology used for computer-based records. After that, a further description of data structuring in computers is given.

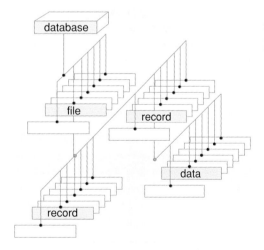

Figure 4.1
A database consists of a set of files managed by the DBMS.
A file is a named storage entity and consists of a set of records.
The file management system of the computer manipulates the files by transferring records to and from application programs.
Each record contains different data fields.

1.1 Data Structure in Paper-Based Patient Records

A paper-based patient record is an ordered set of documents that contain all medical, patient-related data collected for the care of one patient (see Chapter 7 for a more extensive description). Such a paper-based patient record is organized in a special way, in which we can distinguish administrative data such as name, birth date, patient identification, and health insurance; permanent medical data such as gender, blood group, and allergies (single occurrence); and variable and other medical data (multiple occurrences of data or time-dependent data).

The variable data can be further split into different subgroups (see also Chapter 7), such as:

- patient history,
- physical examination and follow-up examinations,
- laboratory results,
- drug prescriptions,
- images (such as *X-ray* pictures and *scintigrams*), and
- biological signals (*electrocardiograms*, *spirograms*, etc.).

In the paper-based patient record these data are grouped together in different sections, such as a section containing the patient history, collected during the first patient visit, and subsections for each follow-up visit, a section for laboratory results, a section for drug data, and so forth. In the section for patient history and follow-up visits the data are ordered chronologically. This structure of the paper-based patient record implies that users of these records must go through all sections and look for the latest available data, for example, the last laboratory results or the last medication used, if they want to know the actual status of a patient.

1.2 Data Structure in Computers

When patient data are stored in computers it is not important to keep all data for one patient physically together as long as the data can be quickly retrieved when, where, and in the format that they are needed for patient care. For reasons of efficiency and quality control it may even be better to leave the laboratory results for all patients in one laboratory database, all drug data in a pharmacy database, all diagnostic codes in a separate database, all *ECGs* and their interpretations in an ECG database, or all X-ray pictures in a radiology database. Therefore, the ordering of patient data in a computer-based record should not necessarily mimic that in the paper-based record.

Data may be organized differently in computers than in paper-based records. The reasons are as follows:

- A paper-based record is static; a computer-based record is not.
- A paper-based record can only be at one place at a time; computer-based data can be presented at multiple locations.
- Paper-based records have a fixed ordering of the data; computers can retrieve data in different sorting orders and can retrieve data selectively on the basis of user-defined criteria.
- In a paper-based record the user must browse the pages to search for the data he or she wants to see; a computer enables the user to retrieve instantly all data related to the actual health status of the patient (e.g., by retrieving the last available and still valid data).

A DBMS solves the problem as to the computer and the memory location where the data are located.

1.3 The DBMS for Data Structuring

In computer terms, the *file* is usually considered the smallest named storage unit in which data are grouped together (Fig. 4.1). A file could be, for instance, a patient history taken at some earlier date or laboratory results reported on some other date. Such files could be stored either in different databases (e.g., a database of all laboratory results) or together in one database (e.g., a database of all patients in a clinical department).

4

Information systems make use of a DBMS to store, modify, or retrieve data. By using a DBMS, users can access and modify data for different purposes. Each purpose requires a separate view of the data and specific rules for achieving consistency and maintaining the integrity of the data (see Section 2.3 of this chapter, and Chapter 33 for further discussions of these terms). The quality of the data (*correctness* and completeness; see Chapter 2) is of vital and even legal importance for the correct interpretation of the data in an information system. Therefore, it must be guaranteed that no program can delete or modify data in a way that violates the correctness, completeness, consistency, and integrity rules of the database. This is also a task of a DBMS. The next section discusses in more detail some functions of the DBMS.

2 DBMS Functions

As mentioned above, a DBMS is a software system that takes care of the storage, retrieval, and management of large data sets. All data are stored in files managed by the computer's file system, which is used by the DBMS. In order to optimize data retrieval and to provide fast access to the data, detailed knowledge of the computer's operating system and its file system organization is essential. However, the user does not need to know this, because the DBMS takes care of it. The file system organization is different for the operating systems of different computers. In fact, the DBMS shields the physical implementation of the data files from the user, and provides an operating system-independent interface that makes storage, retrieval, and data management much easier (see Fig. 4.2).

Different models can be used to look at the data in a computer, depending on the perspective or *view* one has in mind. A user may look at the data differently than a programmer, and the designer of the computer system's file system may have an even different view. In the next sections we discuss such different views or data models. The main tasks of a DBMS are summarized in Panel 4.1.

2.1 Data Modeling

In information systems we need, depending on the user requirements, specific data models to view and process the data. We can distinguish the following data models:

- **External data model**

The user of the information system is primarily interested in data associated with his or her current interest. Generally, he or she uses the computer for data entry, data presentation, and data processing. Take the following examples:

- An administrative assistant who must make an appointment for a patient wants to view in one display screen part of the administrative data for the

4

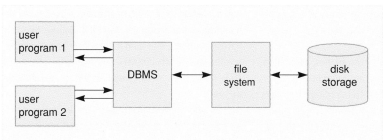

Figure 4.2
A DBMS isolates the user programs from the file system. It takes care of all data transfer to and from the database while maintaining the integrity and consistency of the database. For each database transfer request the DBMS checks whether the user has permission to perform the requested action.

PANEL 4.1

Main Tasks of a DBMS

- Taking care of all database storage, modifications, and retrieval operations:
  - mapping of the data from the user environment (the external data model) to the conceptual data model, and
  - mapping of the data from the conceptual data model to the physical file structure (the physical data model) of the computer;
- Checking the data integrity rules and the data consistency rules;
- Access control (authorization);
- Concurrency control (multi-user access); and
- Facilities for data protection (transaction logging).

---

patient, the name of the clinician and the department, and the time slots available for appointments.
- Clinicians may want to obtain an overview of the actual health status of a patient. They then ask the computer to present in one display screen the actual patient data in alphanumeric and/or graphical form.

These views of the data in which the user is interested make use of an external data model, that is, a model that offers an external view of the data.

- *Conceptual data model*

Data in a computer may have various properties. Patient identification data are different for laboratory data, or for computed tomograms. For instance:

- To identify a patient we want to store the properties name, address, patient number, etc.;
- For a laboratory test we want to store the type of test, when the sample was collected and by whom, and by whom or by what instrument the sample was analyzed.

Data groups that have similar properties are called data *entities*. For instance, patients, laboratory tests, or appointments are data entities. Data entities are often interrelated: a laboratory test is related to a blood sample derived from a patient with a certain identification. Such relations are described in *entity relation* diagrams (*ERDs*). Together, the entities and the different relations between the data entities shape the conceptual data model. Graphical tools that assist the user in defining the conceptual model are available.

Now that we have the user's view defined in the external data model and the relationships between the data have been documented in the conceptual data model, the definitions can be implemented in the DBMS. This is done by the implementation data model.

- Implementation data model

From the conceptual model the *implementation data model* can be derived. The implementation data model is the data model used by the DBMS. Many implementation models can be designed, but the user does not need to know how they operate. Some implementation models, of which the relational model is the most widely used, are described in Section 4. To realize the implementation data model in the DBMS, a *data definition language* (*DDL*), which is provided by most modern DBMSs, is used. In a relational model, for instance, the DDL defines the database as a set of tables, and it also describes constraints on the data. Some DBMSs automatically generate a DDL script from a conceptual model as specified by the user.

Above, we moved from the user-defined external model and the user-defined conceptual model to the implementation model, which is realized by the

4

DBMS's DDL. Now we have gradually approached the inner core of data storage in a computer: the internal data model and its concrete realization by *the physical data model*.

• Internal data model

The DBMS maps the implementation model onto a model consisting of computer files and logical data records. We call this the *internal data model*. This mapping is completely handled by the DBMS, and the user has no need to be concerned about this, except to know that some practical realizations of an internal data model are more efficient than other ones. This efficiency is largely determined by the computer's file system, which is described by the physical data model.

• Physical data model

The file system of the computer takes care of the physical storage of data files in disk blocks, that is, the storage of data in groups of bytes on a mass storage device. The organization of the data files on disk is called the **physical data model.**

The user should be involved in the design of the DBMS, but only with respect to the external model and the conceptual model. The designer of the DBMS is responsible for mapping the conceptual data model to the implementation data model. The internal data model and the physical data model are only of interest to computer experts and the designers of the computer system and its operating system.

2.2 Data Control

The following sections describe some important aspects of a DBMS that are essential for its proper functioning. They are, consecutively:

• *concurrency control*,
• *access control*, and
• *integrity* and consistency *control*.

Two other aspects also deserve attention:

• *transaction processing*, and
• *data security*.

• Concurrency control

Concurrency control deals with conflicts between simultaneous use of the database by different users who are, for instance, entering or updating data in identical data files. A DBMS provides automatic concurrency control to prohibit the same data from being entered or changed by different editors at the same time. An example is making an appointment for the same diagnostic test at the same time by administrative personnel. Suppose, for instance, that a clerk tries to make an appointment for a patient with the X-ray department on a certain date and time and that, at the same time, another clerk wants to make a similar appointment for another patient on the same date and time. This would lead to a conflicting situation. A DBMS will solve this conflict by limiting the concurrent entry of data: Only one user at a time may access the data for data entry or data modification; the system is then blocked for other users who want to use the same time slot. However, someone else who only wants to retrieve data, for example, to make a count of the number of planned X-rays on a certain day, should have the right to retrieve all data, regardless of the activities of other users.

This example seems simple, but there are even more complex situations, for example, when a hospital admission of a patient involves several consecutive appointments, such as with a clinician, with the laboratory, for a catheterization examination, for an ECG recording, and so forth. All such conflicting problems are, in principle, dealt with by the DBMS as part of a system for patient admission and scheduling of examinations.

• Access control

Another important issue taken care of by a DBMS is the protection of data against unauthorized use (see also Chapter 33). Not all users are entitled to see or modify the same data. A clinician is allowed to see all data on his or her own patients, but an employee of the financial department of a hospital has access only to the administrative and financial data. The latter type of employee is also allowed to see the list of medical actions that have financial implications, such as laboratory tests, but has no access to the results of the laboratory tests. DBMSs force users to register ("*log on*"), by having the

4

users make themselves known to the system and provide a secret password. The DBMS will grant the user only those access rights (i.e., for data entry and/or retrieval) that were given to the user and that are related to the user's name and the patient (see also Chapter 33).

• Integrity and consistency control

To keep the data in the database correct (by formalisms that are called *integrity* and *consistency* (see Chapter 33), the designer of the DBMS's conceptual data model can define rules or constraints that should be fulfilled. For instance, when entering the date of a hospital admission, the DBMS should check whether it is a valid date (for instance, not a holiday) and whether a time slot is free to make an appointment. The DBMS should also check, at the time that the name of a clinician is removed from the database, whether any appointments made with that clinician are still scheduled. The DBMS will, in general, check all entered data against specified constraints.

• Transaction processing

To handle a set of database operations as one indivisible operation, a DBMS supports the **transaction** *concept*. For instance, a surgery plan involves the availability of a surgeon, the reservation of an operating room, and the presence of an anesthetist. An operation cannot be planned before all three reservations have been made. In a similar way, a database transaction is only fully committed (that is, the data are actually stored in the computer) if all the necessary instructions for the DBMS that belong to that transaction have been honored. If database transactions would only partly be executed, this would leave the database in an inconsistent state. If one of the database instructions belonging to a transaction cannot be executed, the database is reset to the state just prior to the transaction or, at least, the user is notified of the inconsistent state.

• Data security

Data may be corrupted not only by users or user programs but also by external causes, such as a power failure or problems of the computer hardware (e.g., a disk crash). A solution to this type of problem is to regularly make copies of the data and keep them in a safe place. We call such a copy a **backup** of the database. When a catastrophic failure occurs, the situation prior to the failure can always be restored with the help of the last backup. A disadvantage is that all the data additions and modifications that were made between the last backup and the time of the crash, are also lost. However, with a **log file** – a mechanism that stores on a separate storage device (e.g., a magnetic tape or a separate disk) all database modifications after the last backup – all earlier transactions made after the last backup can be repeated and restored. We call this type of database **roll forward** *recovery*. For a systematic discussion of the measures to be taken, see also Chapter 33.

3 Physical Data Storage

Sections 1.2 and 1.3 described the organization of data in a computer-based record and showed that they do not necessarily reflect the data organization in a paper-based patient record. The implementation data model in a computer may be totally different from the model that underlies the paper-based patient record. In this section we first briefly discuss the data organization in a file cabinet of paper records and in a database of computer-based records to better illustrate the differences between storing paper-based records and computer-based records.

3.1 File Cabinet

The easiest way to explain a database model is to compare the database with a file cabinet that contains a set of drawers, with each drawer containing a set of cards (see Fig. 4.3). Assume, for instance, that one drawer contains cards that have the name, gender, birth date, identification (ID) number, address and telephone number of a patient, with one card for each patient (these cards then contain the patient's administrative

4

data). The cards in the drawer are usually ordered alphabetically.

Another drawer (or file) contains cards with laboratory results, with one card for each laboratory test. These cards are not ordered by patient name but by patient *ID* number. Similar drawers contain cards with given medications, X-rays, ECGs, and so forth. A special drawer contains cards that describe the relationship between ID numbers and names; these cards are also ordered by ID number but contain only the name of the patient. This drawer is, in fact, an *index* to the cards in the drawer with the administrative data, which are ordered by name. If we know only the patient's ID number, we can quickly find his or her name without browsing through the entire administrative card drawer. When organizing the patient data in this way, the file cabinet with all its drawers allows us to:

- Find the patient's ID number, given his or her name. This is done by referring to the administrative file, where we find the patient's ID number.
- Retrieve the patient's name, given his or her ID number. This is possible by using the index file.
- Retrieve all data for one patient, given the ID number. This is done by retrieving data from files that contain the different patient data, such as laboratory tests and X-rays. These data are used to support patient care.
- Retrieve data for many patients. This is done by directly referring to the file that contains, for example, the prescribed drugs, from which one may selectively retrieve data that fulfill certain criteria. This approach is followed when statistical overviews must be computed for periodic reports, the quality assessment of care, or research.

The file cabinet outlined above is the physical realization of a model for storing patient data. It differs in many respects from the common patient-based record archives in hospitals. Such archives are usually organized by patient name and birth date. The file cabinet model could, in principle, be realized in the way described above, although it looks somewhat artificial and cumbersome. We described this model, however, because it is factually a paper-based replica of the **relational database model**, which will be used in

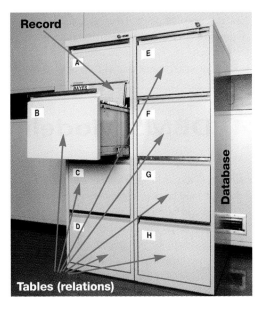

Figure 4.3
The file cabinet as a metaphor for a database model.

Section 4 to further explain some database concepts. Before doing so, we provide a brief description of physical data storage in computers.

3.2 Computer Storage

As seen in Section 2, the DBMS is responsible for mapping the conceptual data model onto the computer file system. The internal computer file organization determines where exactly the data are physically stored on disk. Data transfer to the computer file system is organized in blocks of data, also referred to as *logical data records*. The transfer of these logical data records to memory is handled by the computer file system.

Processing of data is always done for data in the main memory, the so-called primary storage. To improve its processing speed, a DBMS will try to keep frequently referenced data as much as possible in primary storage so that unnecessary data transfer to the secondary storage (the disk) can be avoided.

However, data in primary storage are **volatile** (see Chapter 3), that is, they are lost when the computer crashes or when the power is switched off. Data storage on disk provides more secure permanent storage.

The computer file system reads and writes blocks. A block may contain several data records, or a record may span several blocks. So, data records are the logical storage units, and blocks are the physical storage units. In the following section we describe some conceptual data models that may underlie a DBMS.

4 DBMS Modeling

Before a DBMS can be used to store and retrieve data, a database must be created, the data to be stored must be defined, and the relationships between the data and their constraints must be given. All this is done by the conceptual data model and its entity relation diagram. As mentioned in Section 2, a data definition language can be used to define the implementation data model. The DDL script can be translated by the DBMS into file structures. Several data-modeling techniques have been developed over the years, with the relational data model being by far the most important. We will therefore primarily refer to the relational model and only briefly address other models, such as the hierarchical model and the network model.

4.1 Relational Data Model

In Section 3 we gave an example of data storage in a file cabinet as an introduction to data modeling in general and to a *relational model* in particular. A relational data model consists of a series of tables. In each table different types of data are stored; for example, there is one table for the administrative data (name, address, gender, etc.) and one table for physical examination results. The drawers in the example described in Section 3.1 can therefore be compared with the tables of a relational data model. All *tables* together

4

Demographic Data

Pat.No.	Name	Gender	Birth date	Address	City	Phone No.
12	Johnson, M.	male	Aug 12-1934	4808 Main St	New York	(123) 456-789
66	Smith, A.F.	female	Mar 13-1950	12 Hill Lane	Baltimore	
45	Brown, M.	male	Dec 03-1960	234 New Rd.	Boston	(987)-654-321

Physical Examination

Pat No.	Date	Height (cm)	Blood Pressure		Smoking	Chest Pain
12	May 15-1996	185	80	120/80	Yes	Never
66	Feb 07-1996	180	75	117/85	No	Often
45	Apr 18-1996	175	90		Yes	Seldom

Figure 4.4
Example of a relational database with two tables, Demographic Data and Physical Examination, each with three records. Note that data fields can be numeric (Height and Weight), or textual (Name, Chest pain). Textual fields can be either free text (Address) or a list choice, for instance Gender. Some fields are left blank, indicating an unknown or missing data value. It can be important to make a distinction between unknown values (asked, but not known) and missing values (not filled out). A special marker or symbol such as a dash is often used to indicate unknown values. The more darkly shaded columns in both tables are the primary-key fields. A primary key uniquely identifies a record in a table.

PANEL 4.2

SQL

One of the best known data definition and query languages for relational databases is *SQL*. SQL contains statements for database definition (*DDL*) and data manipulation (*DML*).

DDL
The most important operation of DDL is the create table operation. With create table, a new table can be defined by specifying a name for the table and its data fields with their types. Examples of data types that can be used in SQL are:

- numerics of various sizes (INTEGER or INT and SMALLINT),
- character-string (CHAR(*n*) or CHARACTER(*n*), and varying-length, with *n* being the maximum number of characters VARCHAR(*n*), CHAR VARYING(n), or CHARACTER VARYING(*n*)), and
- real numbers of various precisions (FLOAT, REAL, DOUBLE PRECISION) and DATE and TIME.

Below is an example of a create table statement that creates the table DemoGraphics and that also specifies per data field a name and a data type. Note that PatNo is defined as an integer with the restriction that this field cannot be null (it cannot be left blank).

```
CREATE TABLE DemoGraphics (
    PatNo Integer NOT NULL default 1,
    Name char(40),
    Gender char(1),
    Bdate date,
    Address char(50),
    City char(30),
    PhoneNo char(10)
    );
```

The DDL of an SQL also contains a statement to remove a table definition from the database.

4

constitute the **domain** of the database. In a database of patient data different tables contain demographic data, patient histories, physical examinations, diagnoses, therapies, and so forth (comparable to the different drawers in the file cabinet).

A table is, in fact, a matrix of data consisting of columns (or *data fields*) and rows (Fig. 4.4). Each column corresponds to a specific data item (in database terms, an **attribute**). The item Patient Name, for instance, could be a column in a table. A table contains one row for each patient in the database. Each row (often referred to as a *record*) contains one value for each column, and all values for all columns in a row conceptually belong together. In Fig. 4.4, demographic data about patient Johnson are stored in a single row in the table labeled Demographic Data. The database consists of two tables, one for storing demographic data and one for storing data found during

---

PANEL 4.3

Conceptual Schema of a Relational Database

A conceptual schema is the grammar of a relational database. It basically represents *relations* between *entities*. According to the schema of Fig. 4.4 the following facts are grammatically correct:

- "Patient 12 has date of birth of Aug 12,1934,"
- "Patient 12 is Male," and
- "Address 234 New Rd is of Patient 45."

It appears that this conceptual schema rules out the combination of facts:

- "Patient 12 is Male" and
- "Patient 12 is Female"

because a graphical exclusion constraint is adopted. A constraint rules out specific facts or combinations of facts. Constraints, therefore, underlie integrity control (see Section 2.2). The arrow also is an example of a graphical constraint. One of the arrows is used to avoid combinations, such as:

- "Patient 12 has Name Johnson, M.," and
- "Patient 12 has Name Brown, M.,"

because this constraint states that "Patient" can occur only once in the "has Name" relation.

4

physical examinations. It also shows a representation of the conceptual data model.

The relational data model was introduced by Codd in 1970. It uses a simple and uniform data structure – the relational or database table – and it has a solid theoretical foundation. The relational model represents a database, structured by means of a collection of relations. By means of the DDL, a relational data model can be defined. Panel 4.2 gives an example of a DDL that will create the table DemoGraphics with the data fields PatNo, Name, Gender, Bdate, Address, City, and PhoneNo.

SQL (Structured *Query Language*) is one of the most well-known and standardized database languages for relational databases. It contains a DDL for the description of the implementation data model, as well as a DML (data manipulation language) for the storage and retrieval of data in the database.

In developing relational databases the formulation of tables is preceded by a conceptual analysis to identify elementary relations. In this way, concepts are separated from representations. The result, a conceptual schema, is part of the functional design (see Chapter 35). Panel 4.3 shows part of a *conceptual schema* of which the demographic table in Fig. 4.4) is an occurrence. Nowadays, DDL statements of SQL (see Panel 4.3) can be generated automatically from conceptual schemas.

4.2 Hierarchical Data Model

The hierarchical data model uses two main data structuring concepts: *records* and *parent-child relationships* (*PCR*s, see Fig. 4.5). The PCR defines the hierarchy in

---

PANEL 4.4

Object-oriented Database Management Systems

Relational DBMSs have gained popularity because of their performance and the simple underlying concepts and query languages that have made the development of applications much easier. For more sophisticated applications than the traditional record-keeping applications (e.g., computer-based patient record systems, see Chapters 7 and 29), more semantics about the data are necessary than in simple relational databases. When using relational DBMSs, these semantics can only be provided by applications programs. Separation of data storage and semantics yields a variety of problems in maintaining the DBMS. An *object-oriented DBMS* has been designed to provide richer mechanisms both for specifying data semantics and for implementing methods that perform database operations. In fact, a set of related records can be seen as one object; and associated with the object are methods for setting and updating fields contained in the object, for preserving its integrity, and for doing special computations. Two approaches to implementation exist for object-oriented DBMSs:

1. A layer that extends an existing relational DBMS with an object-oriented flavor, and
2. A new, fully object-oriented implementation.

For the example in Section 4.2, an object-oriented implementation could be represented by two objects, as depicted in Fig. 4.6, interconnected by a pointer. These objects could contain methods or procedures for setting data fields and for doing some simple computations (e.g., computing the *quetelet* index).

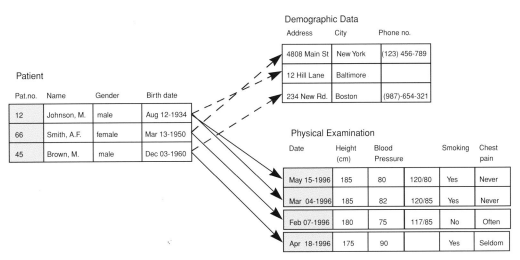

Figure 4.5
Example of a hierarchical database with three record types, Patient, Demographic Data and Physical Examination. The record Patient is the parent record; Demographic Data and Physical Examination are the child records. The Johnson patient record has two child records of the type Physical Examination.

the hierarchical data model. A record here is a collection of data that provide information on an entity, (e.g., a patient). This is similar to the rows in the relational model.

In a hierarchical data model, records of the same type are grouped into *record types*. A record type is given a name, (e.g., "patient record"), and its structure is defined by a collection of data items, such as demographic data and physical examination data.

Each field in the record has a certain *data type*, such as *integer*, *real*, or string (text). For instance, a birth date can be expressed as an integer value, but free text can be expressed only as a string. The PCR expresses the relationship between one parent record type and a number of child record types (Fig. 4.5). A parent record type can, for instance, be the record that contains the patient's name, ID number, and birth date. Child record types are, for example, records of prescribed drugs or laboratory data. A realization (or ***instantiation***) of the PCR consists of a certain parent record and some child records. In Fig. 4.5, a hierarchical data model is shown with three record types: a parent record and two PCRs.

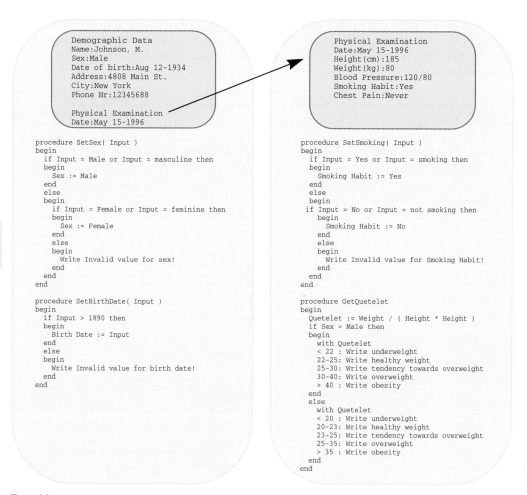

```
           Demographic Data                          Physical Examination
           Name:Johnson, M.                          Date:May 15-1996
           Sex:Male                                  Height(cm):185
           Date of birth:Aug 12-1934                 Weight(kg):80
           Address:4808 Main St.                     Blood Pressure:120/80
           City:New York                             Smoking Habit:Yes
           Phone Nr:12345688                         Chest Pain:Never

           Physical Examination
           Date:May 15-1996
```

```
procedure SetSex( Input )                    procedure SetSmoking( Input )
begin                                        begin
  if Input = Male or Input = masculine then    if Input = Yes or Input = smoking then
  begin                                        begin
    Sex := Male                                  Smoking Habit := Yes
  end                                          end
  else                                         else
  begin                                        begin
    if Input = Female or Input = feminine then   if Input = No or Input = not smoking then
    begin                                        begin
      Sex := Female                                Smoking Habit := No
    end                                          end
    else                                         else
    begin                                        begin
      Write Invalid value for sex!                 Write Invalid value for Smoking Habit!
    end                                          end
  end                                          end
end                                          end

procedure SetBirthDate( Input )              procedure GetQuetelet
begin                                        begin
  if Input > 1890 then                         Quetelet := Weight / ( Height * Height )
  begin                                        if Sex = Male then
    Birth Date := Input                        begin
  end                                            with Quetelet
  else                                           < 22 : Write underweight
  begin                                          22-25: Write healthy weight
    Write Invalid value for birth date!          25-30: Write tendency towards overweight
  end                                            30-40: Write overweight
end                                              > 40 : Write obesity
                                               end
                                               else
                                                 with Quetelet
                                                 < 20 : Write underweight
                                                 20-23: Write healthy weight
                                                 23-25: Write tendency towards overweight
                                                 25-35: Write overweight
                                                 > 35 : Write obesity
                                               end
                                             end
```

Figure 4.6

An object-oriented representation of the example in Section 4.2. The objects include methods for setting the data fields and testing the integrity of the data fields and for doing simple computations, such as computing a quetelet.

The record types are Patient, Demographic Data, and Physical Examination. Record field names can be displayed under each record type name. Although it is particularly convenient to express PCRs when using the hierarchical data model, such relationships certainly can be expressed within the relational model as well. The relational model does not give any special status to such relationships, however. Neither the relational model nor the traditional hierarchical model supports the automatic inheritance of attribute values along PCRs – unlike some modern object-oriented data models (see also Panel 4.4 and Fig.4.6).

4.3 Network Data Model

A *network data model* is a different way of representing the data structure necessary to store patient data in a computer. The network model was in the past an important model for numerous commercial DBMSs. In fact, the network data model is an extension of the hierarchical data model. It uses a structure similar to that used in the hierarchical model, but it allows for relations other than only PCR. For instance, a child record can have more than one parent, which is impossible in the hierarchical data model. The network data model may also contain circular references (i.e., the relationships form a cycle), such as a child record referring to a parent record from which it was derived. Such network connections are allowed in relational databases as well although, again, the pure relational model does not recognize predefined connections. (Nevertheless, commercial relational database products do allow database designers to designate such connections in advance to improve system efficiency.)

The following sections describe special structures used to optimize database access and future developments in database structuring.

4.4 Index Structures

An important aspect of DBMSs is to provide fast access to data, irrespective of the size of the database. Typically, the access speed to data depends on the way

that the data are physically ordered in a computer file. However, data can be ordered according to one sorting mechanism only. In the example of the file cabinet, the demographic data were sorted by patient name. To retrieve data in a different sorting order, an alternative ordering is required. This can be achieved by creating index files or tables. In the example of the file cabinet we created an index file, with the patient's ID number as the *key* and with the file containing the patient name.

The idea of an *index file* is similar to the index in a book: for each term in the index, a page number specifies the page or the paragraph where the term can be found. A database index specifies per key an indexing field where the corresponding records can be found. Similar to the keyword index in a book or the index file in our example of the file cabinet, a database index file is much smaller than the actual database file. The ordering used in the index file provides for a more efficient access for some data retrieval. Of course, more than one index file may be created, with each index file serving a different purpose.

In a relational data model each row in a table can be identified by a unique value of the combination of one or more column values, the primary key. The *sorting* of the table is done according to that specific data-field combination. The ordering is based on the first field of the combination of the column values (called the primary index), with further subordering based on the second field (the secondary index) of that key combination and so on.

An alternative sorting can now be created by using an *index file* (also a table) that contains the data field or combination of fields to be used as an alternate index, plus the data-field combination that constitutes the primary key of the table to be indexed. The index file is sorted according to the alternate index fields. Of course, the index file has the same number of rows as the table that it refers to, but the index file is much smaller than that table. Accessing rows in the sorting order of the index file requires two accesses in sequence; one is from the index file, which returns the primary key to be used, and the second is used to access the table itself. For each different ordering, a new index is required. This is similar to the example of the paper file cabinet that we gave earlier.

4

4.5 *Future Database Structures*

Database technology is still in full development. A major trend is the development of *object-oriented data models* and **object-oriented** *DBMSs* (see Panel 4.4). Distributed, heterogeneous database environments, that is, databases located on several computers, will replace the present large centralized DBMSs. This increases the flexibility and the scalability of the database needs of large institutions. Many DBMS providers are focusing on standards for **open** *databases*. With open databases it will be possible to replace the DBMS of one provider with a DBMS of another provider without having to adapt the application(s).

So-called *active databases* will also become of growing importance. Traditional DBMSs only respond to an instruction from the user, whereas an active DBMS makes assumptions about the user's information needs and tries to collect the data that he or she requires automatically.

Further applications are the development of **multimedia** *databases* that can store alphanumeric data, signals, images, movies, and sound. These will be useful because multimedia applications have great potential utility for computer-based patient records (see also Chapter 20).

Key References

Date CJ. *An Introduction to Database Systems* (6th ed.) New York, NY: Addison-Wesley Publ Comp, 1997.

Elmasri R, Navathe SB. *Fundamentals of Database Systems* (2nd ed.). New York: Addison Wesley, 1997.

Card P, Yourdon E. *Object Oriented Analysis* (2nd ed.). Englewood Cliffs: Prentice Hall, 1992.

See the Web site for further literature references.

4

5 Telecommunication, Networking and Integration

1 Introduction

The number of computers and health care institutions has grown dramatically over the past decade. The low-priced personal computer (*PC*) with its *windows-based* interface is rapidly gaining a place in many health care institutions. Initially, the PC was used to run stand-alone software, such as *word processors*, *spreadsheets*, *database* software, statistical packages, and graphical presentation packages. PCs are now increasingly used by clinicians to write patient letters, reports, and articles, for bibliographic retrieval, and to store and process research data. The stand-alone usage of PCs, however, requires cumbersome data transfer (for instance, by *floppy disks*), and seldom can such data be smoothly transferred from one system to another because of differences in *operating systems*, *file* storage methods, or *application programs*. Therefore, the demand for network communication, growing. In this respect, communication is required between PCs and *hospi-*tal *information systems*, departmental information systems, and other systems inside or outside the institution.

Once patient data have been collected in information systems in the hospital or elsewhere, the clinician wants to use such data for compiling referral or discharge letters, planning and management, and research or quality assessment of care. Through network communication, a PC can access data from the hospital systems and process them locally by user-friendly software available for PCs and workstations. Many hospitals have now installed or are installing computer networks that connect the *workstations* and PCs to the central computer facilities (see also Chapters 20 and 21).

In this chapter we describe the way that patient data can be exchanged by electronic communication, either in the hospital or throughout the health care system in general.

2 Communication in Health Care

The quality of communication between health care providers strongly influences the quality of care. Communication is essential for those patients who are under the shared care of several clinicians (see Chapter 11). Inefficient communication between these care providers may have undesired effects such as the provision of conflicting therapies or the duplication of diagnostic tests, thereby wasting financial resources and negatively influencing the quality of care.

At present, paper letters are the most common and, in most cases, the only means of communication between care providers. Studies have indicated that this way of communication is too slow for follow-up messages to be sent and often does not satisfy the information needs of the care providers involved. Problems in communication between, for instance, general practitioners (*GPs*) and specialists in hospitals include the following:

1. The outcome of a completed treatment is not reported to the GP in time.
2. Intermediate reports from the specialist to the GP are insufficient.
3. A patient's hospital discharge is not reported in time to the GP.
4. Changes in medical therapy are not reported to the specialist by the GP.
5. Questions in referral letters remain unanswered.
6. The referral letter from the GP to the specialist contains insufficient information.
7. The death of a hospitalized patient is not reported to the GP.
8. The clinician can be difficult to reach by telephone.

The content of a letter is not the only thing that determines its usefulness; most clinicians prefer structured and well-designed summaries to narrative reports. It has been demonstrated that the presentation style of the information in a message, in which headings, underlining, and capital letters are used, adds to the accessibility of the information contained in a letter.

In fact, communication does not necessarily have to occur between clinicians only. Systems that can measure, collect, and record health care data at a patient's home and then subsequently send these data to hospital-based specialists for remote monitoring of these patients (using a normal telephone connection) have been developed.

Nowadays, in addition to traditional means of communication, such as the telephone and paper mail delivery, several new possibilities for supporting communication have become available. The most well-known of these new means of communication are the facsimile (*fax*), electronic mail (*e-mail*) and electronic data interchange (*EDI*). We briefly describe these means of communication.

2.1 Fax

With the *fax* it is possible to send documents via the telephone line to a receiver, where the message is printed, thus speeding up communication considerably. Faxes are widely used in health care. Examples are the transmission of referral letters from a GP to a specialist, information about drug interactions, or literature references. Even *computed tomography* pictures are transmitted, for example, from a peripheral hospital to a university hospital, for on-line diagnostic support. In several countries, faxes are routinely used for transmission of prescriptions, referral letters and discharge summaries. In most cases, however, for this transmission to be legal, the original document (signed by the sender) needs to be delivered by regular mail to the receiver. This is especially true for prescriptions.

The fax has a number of advantages: it is an easy-to-install and easy-to-use communication tool, it is relatively inexpensive, and it fits smoothly into organizational routines. Transmission of text, drawings, and images, although with diminished quality, can easily be done via fax. It closely resembles regular mail, and existing fax communication protocols have been widely accepted. Faxes have several disadvantages, however. One is the relatively low quality of the print outs. In addition, although a fax speeds up communication, it remains merely a sheet of paper, so although a computer can be used for the composition of fax messages, the data cannot be used directly in computer applications.

2.2 E-Mail

E-mail was introduced earlier than the fax machine, although already in the late 1800s there were prototypes for the fax machine. The basic principles for e-mail have been used in telex communication for many years. E-mail is mail in electronic form; when using e-mail, the sender composes a message on his or her computer, for example, using a word processor, and sends it via a communications network (for instance, the telephone system or the *Internet*) to the

---

PANEL 5.1

Health Care Message Protocol MEDEUR

An example of a message protocol used for health care applications in The Netherlands is called MEDEUR.

When referring a patient, a clinician can send a referral letter electronically using the MEDEUR protocol. To do so, the clinician first specifies the patient and the period about which he or she wants to report. The system then automatically creates a MEDEUR message, based on the data stored in the computer-based patient record (*CPR*). Before actually transmitting the message, the clinician may want to edit the message by specifying what data to discard, or he or she can add free text to the message.

The clinician receiving such a MEDEUR messages can directly store the patient data in the CPR, without the need to retype the data. Before storing the data, the clinician may want to select or discard the data from the received message. The system keeps track of the patients who are also treated by another clinician. At the end of a patient encounter, the system prompts the clinician to let the CPR compose a message to a referring colleague, thus enabling shared care.

A typical MEDEUR message is shown in the following example, describing a patient consultation. The message can be divided into four parts:

1. E-mail numbers (UNB), the names and identification (ID) numbers of the sender (NAD, first oc-currence) and the receiver (NAD, second occurrence), and patient name and ID number (PNA);
2. The patient's medical problems, with a sequence number (SEQ), starting date (DTM), International Classification of Primary Care (*ICPC*) code, and description (CIN);
3. Data gathered during the consultation, such as laboratory test (INV), the problem that the test relates to (RFF; in this case, to diabetes mellitus), the test result (RSL), the range of normal values (RNG), prescribed medication (CLI), and the problem that the medication relates to (in this case, insulin for the diabetes and capoten for the high blood pressure); and
4. *Authentication* data and the message trailer.

If coded, this message may appear as follows (the computer takes care of all coding and decoding):

---

1. UNB+UNOA:1+500011774+500003170+940731:2127+108E'UNH+2100+
   MEDEUR:1:1:IT'BGM+UPD'DTM+ 137+1994:07:24'NAD+EMP+123456+ Dr. Sending'
   NAD+EMP+654321+Dr. Receiving'PNA+PAT+999999+ Patient name'
2. SEQ+P+1'DTM+194+1989:10:22'CIN+DI+T90.1+ICP++Insulin dependent Diabetes Mellitus'
   SEQ+P+2'DTM+194+1991:03:27'CIN+DI+K86.0+ ICP+Primary hypertension'
2. GIS+C'DTM+007+1994:08:08'INV+LM+102:LOC: Glucose'RFF+G3:1 'RSL+N+
   17.2+mmol/l'RNG+NRM+:3.5:4.5'DLI+O+0'CLI+MED+ 13617893:KMP::Ins mixt 10/90
   novolet 3M'RFF+G3:1'DLI+P+0'CLI+ MED+13180789: KMP::Capoten 25MG
   Tablet'RFF+G3:2'DLI+P+0'
2. AUT+1234+4321'UNT+2100+27'

5

computer of the receiver. This can be done directly, from computer to computer, or indirectly, via a so-called e-mail mailbox. The receiver can read, print, or edit the message because, unlike the fax, the message is still in electronic form. E-mail messages are usually in free-text format. This impedes automated processing of data by the receiving computer system, for which standardization of messages is essential.

Several e-mail protocols have been implemented in health care. E-mail operates reliably, saves secretarial time, and eliminates transcription errors. E-mail systems are increasingly used in health care for routine communication between clinicians and hospitals. However, the percentage of clinicians routinely using e-mail is still small.

2.3 EDI

EDI is a special form of e-mail. It can be defined as the replacement of paper documents by standard electronic messages conveyed from one computer to another, without manual intervention. The central, most important aspect of EDI is the use of widely supported message standards (see Chapter 34). These standards are needed to describe the syntax and semantics of the message. In commercial environments and in trade and transportation, the *EDIFACT* standard (Electronic Data Interchange for Administration, Commerce and Transport) is used. In health care, EDI is also in use, especially for financial, administrative, and logistic activities. EDIFACT is a standard that is primarily used in Europe; its counterpart in the United States (which is also widely used in Europe) is called *HL-7* (Health Level 7). Half of all hospitals in the United States are using EDI.

Message standards based on EDIFACT (see Chapter 34) have been and are being developed in the European Union (EU) and several other countries. A standardized laboratory message, for instance, can electronically transmit test results from a clinical laboratory to a GP's computer system, which can then automatically store the data in the computer-based patient record. An example of a generic message protocol, written in EDIFACT, widely used in The Netherlands and called MEDEUR, is described in Panel 5.1. Panel 5.2 gives a message protocol in HL-7 format.

When standardized messages are used to transmit data, this data exchange is system and application independent, thus reducing the costs of building interfaces between different computer systems. EDI reduces the amount of paper documents, it enables automatic handling of data, and consequently, it reduces the number of errors in data processing. Once data are entered into one system, they do not have to be reentered manually into another system. Studies have shown that the use of EDI improved the speed of communication, decreased the workload, and increased the clinician's understanding of the care delivered by other health care workers. It was also demonstrated that substantial financial benefits can be achieved. In Denmark, for instance, savings of up to 20% on message handling costs are estimated when converting to EDI.

Similar to e-mail, EDI offers a fast exchange of data, but in addition, it facilitates fully integrated data exchange between computer systems. Sophisticated computer hardware and software and a well-organized, national message standardization body are necessary. Initial investments for EDI are therefore higher than those for fax or e-mail. Another difficulty is the shift in costs that occurs with e-mail and EDI. When using paper mail, the sender pays all the costs, whereas when using EDI, the receiver is also charged. Organizations that have a considerable amount of outgoing mail (for instance, hospitals) might especially benefit from the use of EDI. GPs, on the other hand, receive more mail than they send out. This unbalanced situation will not stimulate the use of EDI unless ways are found to even the score financially.

5

PANEL 5.2

Message Protocol in HL-7

An HL-7 (Health Level 7) message can be used, among other things, to exchange data with a laboratory system. A message is separated into a number of segments:

- a message header segment (MSH),
- a patient identification segment (PID),
- an observation request segment (OBR),
- an observation result segment (OBX), etc.

Each segment contains a number of data fields. HL-7 defines the data type, the composition for fields with multiple values, and when applicable, the possible values for a data field. The example message shown below is used to retrieve information about electrolytes and complete blood count (CBC) from a given laboratory information system. After the headers MSH and PID, the OBR for electrolytic information is depicted together with the corresponding OBX lines. Subsequently, the OBR for CBC and the results are shown.

```
MSH|...
PID|...

Electrolytes:
OBR|1|870930010^OE|CM3562^LAB|80004^ELECTROLYTES|R|198703281530|198703290800|||
401-0^INTERN^JOE^^^^MD^L|N|||||SERI^SMITH^RICHARD^W.^^^DR.|(319)377-4400|
This is requestor field #1. Requestor field #2|Diag.serv.field #1.|
Diag.serv.field #2.|198703311400|||F<CR>
OBX|1|ST|84295^NA||150|mmol/l|136-148|H||A|F|19850301<CR>
OBX|2|ST|84132^K+||4.5|mmol/l|3.5-5|N||N|F|19850301<CR>
OBX|3|ST|82435^CL||102|mmol/l|94-105|N||N|F|19850301<CR>
OBX|4|ST|82374^CO2||27|mmol/l|24-31|N||N|F|19850301<CR>

CBC:
OBR|2|870930011^OE|HEM3268^LAB|85022^CBC|R|198703281530|198703290800|||401-0 ^
INTERN^JOE^^^^MD^L|N|||||BLD|^SMITH^RICHARD^W.^^^DR.|(319)377-4400|This is
requestor field #1.|This is Requestor field #2.|This is lab field #1.|Lab
field #2.|198703311400|||F<CR>
OBX|1|ST|718-7^HEMOGLOBIN:^LN||13.4|GM/DL|14-18|N||S|F|19860522<CR>
OBX|2|ST|4544-3^HEMATOCRIT:^LN||40.3|%|42-52|L||S|F|19860522<CR>
OBX|3|ST|789-8^ERYTHROCYTES:^LN||4.56|10*6/ml|4.7-6.1|L||S|F|19860522<CR>
OBX|4|ST|787-2^ERYTHROCYTE MEAN CORPUSCULAR VOLUME:^LN
   ||88|fl|80-94|N||S|F|19860522<CR>
OBX|5|ST|785-6^ERYTHROCYTE MEAN CORPUSCULAR HEMOGLOBIN:^LN
   ||29.5|pg|27-31|N||N|F|19860522<CR>
OBX|6|ST|786-4^ERYTHROCYTE MEAN CORPUSCULAR HEMOGLOBIN CONCENTRATION:^LN
   ||33|%|33-37|N||N|F|19860522<CR>
OBX|7|ST|6690-2^LEUKOCYTES:^LN||10.7|10*3/ml|4.8-10.8|N||N|F|19860522<CR>
OBX|8|ST|764-1^NEUTROPHILS BAND FORM/100 LEUKOCYTES:^LN||2|%||||F<CR>
OBX|9|ST|769-0^NEUTROPHILS SEGMENTED/100 LEUKOCYTES:^LN||67|%||||F<CR>
OBX|10|ST|736-9^LYMPHOCYTES/100 LEUKOCYTES:^LN||29|%||||F<CR>
OBX|11|ST|5905-5^MONOCYTES/100 LEUKOCYTES:^LN||1|%||||F<CR>
OBX|12|ST|713-8^EOSINOPHILS/100 LEUKOCYTES:^LN||2|%||||F<CR>
```

(This example is taken from the Duke University web-server (http://www.mcis.duke.edu/standards/HL7/pubs/version2.3) with information about the current version 2.3 of the HL-7 standard)

5

3 Shared Care Protocols

When health care providers use systems with **compu-ter-based patient records** (see Chapter 7), communica-tion between these systems can be highly automated, which offers several advantages. For a number of health care problems, **shared care** protocols have been devel-oped. Such protocols involve the division of tasks between health care providers from different disciplines. Optimal communication is considered to be vital for shared care from both medical and cost-effectiveness points of view. **Standardization** of messages is necessa-ry not only with respect to the syntax of the messages but also to the semantics and to medical procedures.

The use of computer-based patient records and EDI can facilitate shared care, because they can assist cli-nicians in maintaining high-quality communication by automatically generating messages for the other clinicians providing care. The contents and frequency of these messages are defined in a shared care proto-col, and the information systems take care of timely exchange of the relevant data. However, clinicians often lack the time to comply with the protocols for shared care support.

Communication links in health care can roughly be divided into intramural (*within* the walls of a hospital) and extramural communication. In extramural com-munication there is a trend for the fax to be replaced by EDI, allowing for a higher degree of automation of communication and guaranteeing better protection of privacy. **Smart cards** (also called: **chip cards**, see Chapter 3) can also play a role in this situation, but they have a severe drawback in that transportation of the information is still manual.

4 Communication Hardware

An information network within a health care institu-tion consists of hardware and software and a network that physically interconnects computers. It is not necessary to install wires for each required connec-tion between PCs, workstations, or computers (point-to-point connection, see Fig. 5.1 and 5.2). This type of **point-to-point communication** is secure but very expensive. Instead of many point-to-point connec-tions, a network is set up and the various computers are connected to the **network** (Fig. 5.3). The network takes care of the required connections.

The network makes it possible for a message to be de-livered from one computer to the requested addressee computer and that the messages can be read and under-stood by all parties. The first step in building a compu-ter network is the actual wiring between two or more computers and the installation of a network device (e.g., a card in the PC) that provides a plug to the network. There are a number of standards for the cables and the connectors in a network, for example, **Ethernet** **twisted pair**, **ISDN** (Integrated Services Digital Network), or **ATM** (Asynchronous Transfer Mode). Each of these communication networks has its own frequency **bandwidth** limitations (which determines the capacity for information transmission). For Ethernet, for instance, a typical communication speed is 10 megabits per second (Mbits/s; 10,000,000 bits/s)

4.1 Public Telephone Network

A simple example of a network is the switched telephone network, which is frequently used for low-speed data transmission as well as for speech transmission. A special device, a **modem** (modulator-demodulator), is needed to transform the computer's digital signal into a modulated analog signal that is used over telephone lines. The tele-phone exchange provides the switch to the addressee. The hardware setup is depicted in Fig. 5.1.

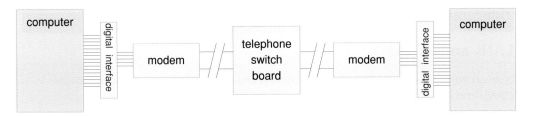

Figure 5.1
Hardware setup for data interchange by a public telephone network. A special device, a modem (modulator-demodulator), transforms the computer's digital data into a modulated analog signal that is transmitted over telephone lines. At the sender's side the digital signal is modulated into an analog, frequency-modulated signal, and at the receiver's side the reverse is done. The telephone company provides the switch to the addressee.

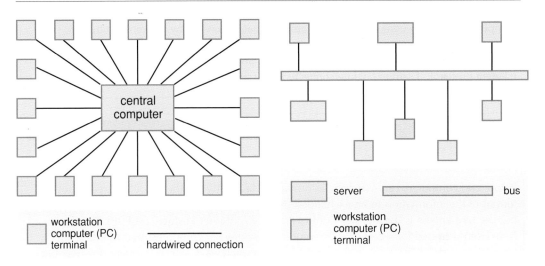

Figure 5.2
Star-like network. Each unit has its own connection with the central computer.

Figure 5.3
Network in which a bus structure is used.

5

4.2 Digital Networks

Because public telephone networks have only a limited bandwidth, special digital networks dedicated to data transmission have been designed (Fig. 5.2). Used locally, they are called local-area networks (*LAN*s); used over long distances they are called wide-area networks (*WAN*s). (Panel 5.3 provides more details on LANs and WANs.) Computers belonging to the network take care of addressing, error detection and correction, and so forth. Ideally,

network provisions should be transparent to the user, which means that, except for communication speed, the user should be unaware of the network in use, the geographical distance of connected computers, and so on.

With respect to the hard wiring used, it does not matter whether this is a simple twisted pair, a coaxial cable, or a glass fiber cable. If standard communication protocols are used, such as Transfer Control Protocol/Internet Protocol (*TCP/IP*) (see Panel 5.4), users will not have to write their own software for data communication. Even wireless connections are,

---

> ## PANEL 5.3
>
> ### LANs and WANs
>
> Network communication within an organization is often referred to as a local area network (*LAN*). Its characteristics are as follows:
>
> - the physical distance between the computers is restricted (<2 km),
> - it generally implements one network protocol, and
> - the communication bandwidth is high.
>
> Wide area networks (*WANs*) span much larger areas, even world wide, and they provide less bandwidth than a LAN. Several LANs can be interconnected to allow for communication between computers that are geographically farther apart or that are owned by different institutions. These LANs can be interconnected by means of gateways. Gateways are special computers that reside on both networks and that are equipped to forward and translate data if the two networks run different protocols. Examples of interconnected LANs are BITNET, ARPANET, and Internet.

> ## PANEL 5.4
>
> ### TCP/IP
>
> Before two computers can exchange information via a network, they should agree about the format of the information to be exchanged. Nowadays, there are several standard protocols, but the best known is the Transfer Control Protocol / Internet Protocol (TCP/IP). Solutions have been provided for worldwide communication between computers that use different network protocols. These are in the form of network gateways, which translate one network protocol into another.

5

in principle, fully transparent to all electronic communication. Of course, the speed of one way of communication will be higher or more expensive than the speed of another one. For images, a high communication bandwidth (high speed) is required; for reporting of laboratory results, a low speed may be sufficient.

---

5 Communication Software

When the computer is connected to a network, it is essential that the required communication software be installed before EDI can take place. This communication software deals with:

1. addressing and routing software,
2. creating and maintaining reliable data communication,
3. correct termination of connections,
4. authentication and security, etc.

The International Standards Organization (*ISO*) has developed a reference model for open systems interconnection (*OSI*) that describes all the functionality included in communication software and also how all tasks interrelate (see also Chapter 34).

5.1 Addressing and Routing

In general, computer networks interconnect more than two computers, so that the sending computer needs to know the exact address of the computer that should receive the message. The address of each computer must be unique in the computer network. If the computer network is large, it is virtually impossible to maintain a correct list of all addresses at all host computers. In that case, the network can be subdivided into subnetworks. If the receiving computer is in the same subnetwork, the address is locally known at the sending computer and the message can be sent directly. If not, the message is forwarded to the subnetwork's *gateway*. This computer interconnects several subnetworks and will decide to which gateway of which subnetwork the message should be forwarded. This gateway will check if the requested computer is in its sub-network. If so, it will forward the message to the requested computer; otherwise, it will select a gateway of another subnetwork. Usually, the gateway role is fulfilled by an ordinary computer. In large organizations, such as a hospital, it is common to use computers that are dedicated to this network routing task, the so-called network routers.

In the network configuration described in Fig. 5.3 (a bus network system), the connections between computers are shared by all computers in the network. The messages on the network bus to be exchanged between computers can have different senders and receivers. Between two computers there can even be several open connections at the same time for different applications that are simultaneously operational. In this situation messages from different applications to and from the same computer are using the same physical connection.

5.2 Reliability of Communication

The communication software is responsible for delivering the right messages to the right connection (i.e., to a specific computer). Another task of the communication software is to break messages apart into equally sized packets and to reconstruct the original message from the packets at the receiving side. The size of the packets is imposed by the network protocol that has been implemented. If a packet is corrupted, for instance, by electrical interference, the communication software will automatically detect the error and request a retransmission of the packet. All other packets that arrive on that connection in the meantime are queued by the communication software so that the original message can still be reconstructed.

5.3 Authentication and Security

Important aspects in the communication software are *authentication* and *security*. By authentication we mean verification that the address of the sender, as contained in the messages, is really the address of the computer that composed the message. With the increasing use of network technology and specifically of the public network referred to as the *Internet*, this is becoming more and more important. A related issue is security, that is, the information contained in a message should only be understood by the sender and the intended receiver of the message. There are several approaches to *encrypt* the data of a message with an encryption key that is known only to the sender and the receiver.

5.4 Clients and Servers

In network technology, the application that initiates network communication is called the *client* (usually the one who requests information), whereas the

5

PANEL 5.5

World Wide Web

The *World Wide Web* (WWW) is an on-line document system that supports links between documents. There are several client applications, called *browsers* (e.g., Mosaic, Netscape, Explorer), which facilitate the network connection to WWW services and display the documents provided by a WWW server. When a WWW document is displayed to a client, all words in the document that provide links to other documents are highlighted. Selecting such a highlighted word results in a message to a WWW server indicating that the linked document should be retrieved and sent to the client. WWW documents may consist of text, images, video, or sound. For all these types of information, the browser must provide means of viewing or playing the information. An attractive feature of WWW documents is that a phrase can be linked to a document on another server. For example, a WWW document on a server in New York can have a link to a document on a server in Amsterdam. The user of WWW is, however, not aware of the physical location of WWW servers in the Internet. An example of a WWW server is the Virtual Hospital. This WWW server provides a large number of documents and a large number of hypertext links relevant for health care.

Because the WWW has proven to be very successful and because it is accessible to a large public, many providers of on-line information are now making their information available on a WWW service. An example is *MEDLINE*, a large database with abstracts of all medical articles that appear in the international refereed medical journals. It is also available as a WWW server called Internet Grateful Med. Via ordinary WWW browsers, the MEDLINE database can be searched by entering *keywords*. The retrieved abstracts are then formatted as WWW documents and sent to the browser.

• E-mail

Apart from the WWW explosion, there are other typical network applications on the Internet, such as e-mail, transfer of files, and network terminal emulation (*telnet*). With e-mail, one can compose a message and send it to an addressee. All users of Internet have a unique name consisting of their name and computer name, for example, handbook@mi.fgg.eur.nl. By using that address in an e-mail message, Internet's mail servers are capable of delivering the message to the addressee.

• Java

With *Java* it is possible not only to retrieve a document or data from the WWW server but also to retrieve a small application (that is, software) with which the document or data can be made visible. This allows for a more dynamic presentation of data than as a plain document only. Early examples of Java applications, called applets, are the visualization of Pythagorean theorem, browsing of three-dimensional molecular structures, and visual comparison of different sorting algorithms. The technology is still in rapid development. Some examples on the Web site of this Handbook have been written with Java.

• FTP

A file transfer protocol (*FTP*) is used to copy a file to or from another computer on the network. The network terminal emulator is used to log in remotely on a computer and start applications. For FTP, as well as for telnet, access to a remote computer is granted on the basis of a user name and password to that computer. For some servers there is an *anonymous log-in* account that has been created for FTP, which allows anyone to copy files. Software that is in the *public domain* is distributed in this way by using computers that have an anonymous log-in account for FTP.

receiving party is called the *server* (usually the one who provides information). The application that runs on the server and handles incoming requests is called a *service*. Applications can implement different *client-server* modes of using the network.

If an application uses the network *asynchronously*, it will not wait for confirmation of the server. This type of communication is generally used for e-mail. The composer of an e-mail message is usually not willing to wait for a confirmation of a computer, possibly somewhere at the other end of the world, because it might take an hour or more to get a message there and back.

Synchronous applications require the server to confirm the receipt of a message, either by sending an explicit confirmation message or by sending a preliminary reply that the message has arrived. This connection mode is used by database applications, in which the client sends out a request for data to the database server and subsequently waits for an answer. Real-time connections require the server to respond within a certain time frame so that the information displayed to the client is almost instantaneously. A specific example of the use of this mode are client computers that register *vital signs,* provided by monitors on an intensive care unit. The continuous registration of the arterial blood pressure by a monitor device, for instance, requires a real-time communication with a ward station computer that displays the blood pressure.

6 Internet

Network technology is one of the fastest-growing areas in technology. The growth of network communication can best be demonstrated by the exponential growth of the *Internet*. This *WAN* connects a large number of computers worldwide and offers a large number of public services that can be freely accessed. Each institute or company that is connected to the Internet maintains a part of the network. As a consequence, the use of the Internet network is free, although sometimes one must pay for the connection to the Internet. The worldwide Internet consists of a large number of networks that have been interconnected by gateways, and each subnetwork can use a different communication medium. Internet is based on the *TCP/IP* (see Panel 5.4) and supports synchronous and asynchronous applications. The most prominent application on the Internet is the *World-Wide Web* (see Panel 5.5).

Key References

Tanenbaum AS. Computer Networks (3rd edition). Englewood Cliffs, NJ: Prentice Hall, 1996.

Branger PJ, Duisterhout JS. Communication in health care. Meth Inform Med 1995;34:244-252.

See the Web site for further literature references.

5

III

Data from Patients

Authors of Part III

Chapter 6: Coding and Classification
    J.S. Duisterhout, Erasmus University Rotterdam; P.F. de Vries Robbé, F.J. Flier,
    A.A.F. van der Maas, University of Nijmegen; with contribution of A.T. McCray, National Library
    of Medicine, Bethesda

Chapter 7: The Patient Record
    A.M. van Ginneken, P.W. Moorman, Erasmus University Rotterdam; with contribution of A.A.
    Becht, Technical University, Delft

Chapter 8: Biosignal Analysis
    J.H. van Bemmel, Erasmus University Rotterdam

Chapter 9: Medical Imaging
    A. Hasman, Maastricht University

Chapter 10: Image Processing and Analysis
    E.S. Gelsema, Erasmus University Rotterdam

6 Coding and Classification

1 Introduction

In the traditional patient record, data are available in written format only, mainly as free text, but sometimes also as numeric data, such as laboratory test results. The patient record is primarily used for patient care itself, that is, for diagnosis, therapy, and prognosis. Reconstructing the patient history from such a handwritten patient record by a clinician other than the original author is hindered by the fact that many medical terms are ill-defined and are perhaps even ambiguous.

Since many patient data are becoming available in computer-based patient records (*CPRs*) (see Chapter 7), use of these data for purposes other than traditional archiving and reporting is becoming feasible. Reasons for storing medical data in a computer are given in Panel 6.1. *Decision-support* systems may support care providers in making decisions based on CPR data (see Chapters 15 and 16). For instance, prescription of a drug may trigger a decision-support system that checks for *contraindications* or *drug interactions*. Such a system will be able to operate properly only if all the diseases and symptoms of a patient are recorded in a standardized and consistent way. Many data in health care, such as diagnoses, patient history data, physical examination data, or the reporting of X-ray pictures, are expressed as *free text* (see also Chapters 2 and 3). This leads to an infinite list of possible expressions. However, statistical overviews and decision-support systems can cope with only a finite number of classes. Rules for assigning expressions from the patient record to classes must be well defined by objective criteria. Assigning such an expression to a class always implies data reduction (i.e., loss of information), but this is not necessarily a disadvantage.

The appropriate level of detail and the structure of the *classification* system depend on the purpose for which the classification system has been designed. A classification of diagnoses for health statistics, for example, may require categories other than classifications for planning patient care in a hospital ward. On the other hand, it must be possible to present all medically relevant expressions in CPRs without any data reduction. Therefore, standardized terminologies are used in these type of applications.

In this chapter, we will follow as much as possible the standard terminology used in the International Standards Organization (*ISO*) International Electrotechnical Commission (IEC) Technical Report TR 9789 (*Information Technology; Guidelines for the Organization and Representation of Data Elements for Data Interchange. Coding Methods and Principles*) (see also Chapter 34). This means that three basic elements are used in the so-called semantic triangle: (1) *object*, (2) *concept*, and (3) *term*.

- Objects, also called referents, are particular things in reality, and they are concrete (e.g., the stomach), as well as abstract (e.g., the mind).
- A concept is a unit of thought formed by using the common properties of a set of objects (e.g., an organ).
- A term is a designation by a linguistic expression of a concept or an object in a specific language.

Reasons for Storing Medical Data in a Computer

Application areas

- Patient care
- Quality control by:
  - uniform reporting of results
  - comparing data with those from other units or centers
  - protocol management
  - increased insight
- Medical research, including epidemiology
- Planning and management

Advantages of coding medical data

- Data reduction
- Standardized terminology
- Enabling statistical overviews and research
- Support of management and planning
- Coupling with decision-support systems

2 Classifications

The term *classifying* has two different meanings:

1. the process of designing a classification, and
2. the coding or description of an object by using codes or terms that are designators of the concepts in a classification.

Here, we use only the first meaning of classifying. A classification is an ordered system of concepts within a domain, with implicit or explicit ordering principles. The way in which classes are defined depends on their intended use. A classification is based on prior knowledge and forms a key to the extension of knowledge (see also Fig. 1.1).

The purpose of a classification is, for example, to support the generation of health care statistics or to facilitate research. Examples are the classification of abnormalities of *electrocardiograms* or diagnoses of patients into disease classes.

In a classification, concepts are ordered according to generic relations. *Generic relations* are relations of the type "A is a kind of B," for example, pneumonia is a kind of lung disease, where pneumonia represents the *narro-* wer concept and lung disease represents the *broader* concept. Classifications contain concepts within a certain *domain*. Examples of domains are reason for encounter, diagnosis, and medical procedure. In this respect the International Classification of Diseases, 9th edition (*ICD*-9), which will be discussed in Section 5.1, is a classification of diagnoses. A classification allows one to compare findings collected in different environments. For instance, if we want to compute the number of beds required per age category in a hospital, we could use the following age classes:

babies	age	0-3
children	age	4-12
teenagers	age	13-18
adults	age	19-64
elderly	age	65+

In this hypothetical example, defining the classes is a relatively simple task and the requirements for a classification are easily met (see Panel 6.2). Classifying is done according to a single criterion: age; that is, age is used as a *differentiating criterion*.

6

PANEL 6.2

Requirements for a classification

1. Domain completeness
2. Nonoverlapping classes (mutual exclusiveness)
3. Suitable for its purpose
4. Homogeneous ordering (one principle per level)
5. Clear criteria for class boundaries
6. Unambiguous and complete guidelines for application
7. Appropriate level of detail

Additional requirements for computer-assisted coding systems

1. Allow for the use of synonyms
2. Allow for the use of lexical variations
3. Insensitive to spelling errors
4. Reliability
   – consistent operation (insensitive to ordering of terms)
   – correct

2.1 Ordering Principles

In classifications that use more than one ordering principle, the situation is more complicated. In classifying diseases we deal with the following aspects, among others:

- anatomic location,
- *etiology*,
- *morphology*, and
- dysfunction.

Each of these aspects can be used for a different ordering. Such an ordering throughout a classification is called an *axis*. Multiaxial classifications use several orderings simultaneously. In the International Classification of Primary Care (*ICPC*), for instance, the diagnoses are classified along two axes, one for the *organ system* (an alphabetic character) and one for the *components* (a number; see Table 6.1). ICPC has primarily been designed for epidemiological purposes. Therefore, the classes were chosen in such a way that for health care studies in primary care, each class will contain a sufficient number of cases. This is why all tropical diseases are grouped together. This classification may be of use in areas such as Europe or North America, but it is definitely impractical for general practitioners operating in

Table 6.1 The Two-Axial ICPC.

First axis: organ systems

Code	Organ System
A	General and unspecified
B	Blood
D	Digestive
F	Eye
H	Ear
K	Circulatory
L	Musculoskeletal
N	Neurological
P	Psychological
R	Respiratory
S	Skin
T	Endocrine and metabolic
U	Urology
W	Pregnancy and family planning
X	Female genital system
Y	Male genital system
Z	Social problems

Second axis: components

Code	Component
1 - 29	Symptoms and complaints
30 - 49	Diagnostic screening and prevention
50 - 59	Treatment and medication
61 - 61	Test results
62	Administrative
63 - 69	Other
70 - 99	Diagnoses

6

tropical areas, such as Africa, Central and South America, India, or Indonesia.

2.2 Nomenclatures and Thesauri

One of the problems of uniform registration in health care is the lack of a common terminology. A **thesaurus** is a list of terms used for a certain application area or domain. Examples are a list of diagnostic terms or a list of terms for laboratory tests. A thesaurus is always intended to be complete for its domain. For practical usage, thesauri that also contain a list of *synonyms* for each preferred term have also been developed. In this way, a thesaurus stimulates the usage of standardized terminology. A restricted set of preferred terms used within an organization for a given purpose is called a *controlled vocabulary*.

In a **nomenclature**, codes are assigned to medical concepts, and medical concepts can be combined according to specific rules to form more complex concepts. This leads to a large number of possible code combinations.

The difference between a classification system and a nomenclature is that in the former possible codes are predefined, whereas in the latter a user is free to combine codes for all aspects involved. The retrieval of records for patients whose data fulfill certain classification codes from a large database is relatively easy; retrieving records for patients stored by using a nomenclature is more difficult because of the high degree of freedom, leading to very complex codes. A nomenclature, however, is useful in producing standardized reports, such as discharge letters.

In 1933, the New York Academy of Medicine started work on a database of medical terms, the Standard Classified Nomenclature of Diseases. The American Medical Association continued this work in 1961, and in 1965 the Systematic Nomenclature of Pathology (**SNOP**) coding system was published by the American College of Pathologists. SNOP formed the basis for the development of the Systematized Nomenclature of Human and Veterinary Medicine (**SNOMED**), which is an example of such a nomenclature (see Section 5.4).

2.3 Codes

Coding is the process of assigning an individual object or case to a class, or to a set of classes in the case of a multiaxial classification. In most classifications, classes are designated by codes. Coding is, in fact, interpretation of the aspects of an object. Codes may be formed by numbers, alphabetic characters, or both. The following list describes different types of codes.

- Number codes
- Number codes may be issued sequentially. This means that each new class will be given the next unused number. The advantage is that new classes can easily be added.
- Numbers could be issued at random to avoid any patient-specific information is hidden in the code.
- Series of numbers can be reserved for sets of classes. Issuing this type of number is only of use with a fixed set of classes, that is, when no expansion of the set of classes is expected.

- Mnemonic codes
A mnemonic code is formed from one or more characters of its related class rubric. This helps users to memorize codes. However, for classifications with many classes this may lead either to long codes or codes with no resemblance to the class rubrics. Therefore, mnemonic codes are generally used for limited lists of classes. For example, hospital departments are often indicated by a mnemonic code, such as ENT for the Department of Ear, Nose, Throat, CAR for Cardiology, or OB-GYN for the Department of Obstetrics and Gynecology.

- Hierarchical codes
Hierarchical codes are formed by extending an existing code with one or more additional characters for each additional level of detail. A hierarchical code thus bears information on the level of detail of the related class and on the hierarchical relation with its parent class. This way of coding bears resemblance to the structure of **hierarchical databases** (Chapter 4), with "parents" at the higher level, and "children" at the lower levels. This implies

6

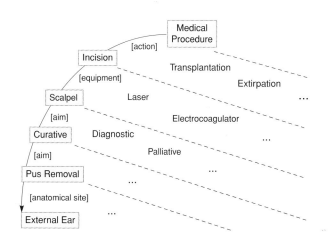

Figure 6.1
Example of a multilevel classification of medical procedures. The differentiating criteria are indicated between rectangles. The criteria for membership in each subclass are not adopted here.

that patient data can be retrieved by using hierarchical codes at a certain level, even when significant extensions or modifications are made at lower levels. An example of hierarchical codes are the codes used in *ICD*-9.

• Juxtaposition codes

Juxtaposition codes are composite codes consisting of segments. Each segment provides a characteristic of the associated class. In ICPC, for instance, a diagnostic code is formed by using a code consisting of one letter of the alphabet (a mnemonic code for the tract), followed by a two-digit number. For instance, all codes with the character "D" are related to the tractus digestivus and all codes starting with an "N" describe disorders of the nervous system. In the example of ICPC, two independent characteristics are coded simultaneously, and each characteristic has its own position in the code.

• Combination codes

Another example is a classification of medical procedures using ordering principles: action, equipment, aim, and anatomical site (see Fig. 6.1). The combination of 100 anatomical sites with 20 different actions, 10 different instruments, and 5 different purposes results in a classification system with a potential of a 100,000 classes and codes. A way to cope with this explosion is the use of a combination code. By using a six-digit combination code consisting of four segments, with segments dedicated to action (two digits), equipment (two digits), aim (one digit), and anatomical site (one digit), respectively, a coding clerk has to distinguish only 135 codes, with which 100,000 combinations can be generated.

• Value addition codes

In value addition codes only powers of 2 are used as a representation of a data item or class. Just as in a combination code, several characteristics can be coded. In this case, however, only one number instead of a segment for each characteristic is used as a code. This is easily illustrated if we code the presence or absence of risk factors, such as:

$$2^0 = 1 \text{ for smoker/0 for nonsmoker,}$$
$$2^1 = 2 \text{ for overweight/0 for no overweight,}$$
$$2^2 = 4 \text{ for increased cholesterol/0 for not increased cholesterol.}$$

By using the codes 1 to 7 we can sum all the three risk factors mentioned above. A smoker who is overweight but with no increased cholesterol level is coded as 3, and a nonsmoker who is overweight and who has an increased cholesterol level is coded as 6.

6

2.4 Taxonomy

Taxonomy is the theoretical study of classification, including its basic principles, procedures, and rules. The term *taxonomy* is known from Linnaeus's work in classifying biological organisms. The term taxonomy is also used to designate the end product of a taxonomic design process and is then frequently synonymous with classification. In this book we will use the term taxonomy for the first definition: *the science of classification.* The term *classification* is used for the end product of the design process. Taxonomy is concerned with classifications in general. All objects in a group have some features in common, that is, they fall within the boundaries of a group. All mammals form one group, to which people, cats, and whales belong. A group may be further subdivided on the basis of another feature or character. The lion, the tiger, and Felix domestica (the cat in our home) all belong to the group (or set) of cats. In a disease classification system such as ICD-9, the classification and subdivision are performed by the grouping of diseases in organ systems or by etiology. The different "chapters" (main disease categories or etiological categories) of ICD-9 are subdivided into groups, the groups are divided into three-digit classes, and so on (see Section 5.1 for a description of ICD-9).

2.5 Nosology

Nosology is usually defined as the science of the classification of *diseases.* Since nosological discussions usually involve symptoms, syndromes, disorders, and injuries, as well as diseases, it would be more appropriate to define nosology as the science of the classification of diagnostic terms, that is, the taxonomy of diagnostic terms. Increasing information needs in health care have highlighted many nosological problems. It seems that the impressive expansion of the diagnostic vocabulary during the last century has not been matched by the development of a precise meta-language for describing relations between diagnostic terms. Although meta-terms such as *disease, disorder* and *syndrome* are widely used, there is much confusion as to their proper meaning. A

Table 6.2
ARA Criteria for the Classification of Rheumatoid Arthritis, 1987.[a]

1.	Morning stiffness
2.	Arthritis of three or more joint areas
3.	Arthritis of hand joints
4.	Symmetric arthritis
5.	Rheumatoid nodules
6.	Serum rheumatoid factor
7.	Typical radiographic changes

[a] At least four of the seven criteria must be fulfilled.

meta-language for describing nosological relations is either lacking or unused.

Nosology is usually distinguished from *nosography*, which is the science of the description of diseases. The difference between the definition and the description of disease is usually explained as follows: A disease *definition* gives only essential characteristics of the disease, whereas a *description* includes accidental characteristics, that is, characteristics that are empirically correlated with the essence of the disease, such as the so-called classification criteria of rheumatoid arthritis by the American Rheumatism Association (*ARA*) (see Table 6.2). There are no essential characteristics in this definition; all characteristics are accidental. This kind of definition, in which a set of accidental characteristics is used, is called *polythetic*. Apparently, the essential characteristic of rheumatoid arthritis is something that medical science has not yet discovered.

There is a growing feeling that classifications such as ICD, SNOMED and the Diagnostic and Statistical Manual for Mental Disorders (*DSM*-IV) do no justice to the way in which diagnostic terms are actually used in health care and that a new *paradigm* is needed.

6

3 History of Classification

In health care, the most widely used classification system is ICD and the classifications derived from it. The first attempt at registration was the London Bills of Mortality in 1629. The first edition of the International List of Causes of Death, as it was then called, was presented by Jacques Bertillon at a meeting of the International Statistical Institute (ISI) in 1893 in Chicago, and it was officially accepted in 1900. This list was regularly revised under the supervision of ISI until its fifth edition in 1938. Until then, the code list was primarily used for mortality statistics. Health insurance companies, hospitals, medical services, the military, and other agencies felt a growing need to extend the list with codes for morbidity. The International Health Conference, held in New York City in 1946, entrusted the Interim Commission of the World Health Organization (**WHO**) with the responsibility of undertaking the necessary preparatory work to extend the International List of Causes of Death with an International List for the Causes of Morbidity.

A congress to discuss the Sixth Revision of the International List of Diseases and Causes of Death was convened by the government of France in Paris in 1948. Delegates from 29 countries participated in the conference and approved this classification proposal, prepared by an expert committee of WHO. This conference also recommended establishment of a comprehensive program of international cooperation, including the establishment of national committees for vital and health statistical programs. Following Revision Conferences were held under the auspices of WHO (the Seventh Revision in Paris in 1955, the Eighth Revision in Geneva in 1965, the Ninth Revision in Geneva in 1975, the latter was abbreviated to ICD-9, and the Tenth Revision in Geneva in 1989 (ICD-10). The general philosophy behind these classification systems was the classification of diseases by their etiology rather than by a particular manifestation of the disease. There was, however, a growing need for more detail and more relevance to the evaluation of patient care.

In the Ninth Revision, a special four-digit code category was added for the classification of neoplasms, with an optional fifth digit indicating its behavior. Optional classifications were introduced to allow for the use of additional codes besides the traditional etiological codes in order to code other manifestations of diseases. The mental disorders chapter was extended with codes for glossary descriptions. From the Ninth Revision, a modified version (ICD-9-CM, where CM stands for clinical modifications) was made for clinical use.

In 1990, WHO's World Health Assembly adopted the Tenth Revision. The "core" classification of ICD-10 is a three-character code, which is a mandatory level of coding for international reporting. The four- and five-digit sublevels are recommended for many purposes, such as a further subdivision or classification of other aspects, and they form an integral part of ICD.

The International Classification of Procedures in Medicine (ICPM) contains, among other things, classifications for diagnostic, therapeutic, and surgical procedures. ICPM was published in 1976. In the United States, the Current Procedural Terminology (CPT) was published, in Canada the Canadian Classification of Diagnostic, Therapeutic and Surgical Procedures (CCP) was published, and in France, the Catalogue des Actes Médicaux (CDAM) was published.

In 1933, the first official edition of the Standard Classified Nomenclature of Disease (SNDO) was published in the United States. SNDO is a system for diagnostic terminology ordered by localization and etiology. The 5th and last edition was published in 1961 by the American Medical Association and contains a third axis for surgical procedures. American hospitals used this system until it was replaced by ICD-A, the American adaptation of ICD.

In 1965, the College of American Pathologists published the Systematic Nomenclature of Pathology (SNOP) which contained four axes: topography, morphology, etiology, and function. SNOP was the basis for SNOMED, which includes even more axes. SNOMED aims at covering the complete medical terminology (see also Section 5.4).

6

4 Classification and Coding Problems

Classification problems should be distinguished from coding problems:

- Classification problems concern the ordering of concepts in a way that is logically sound, elegant, and well-suited for the potential users of the classification.
- Coding problems concern the technical support that must be provided to enable coding clerks to assign an individual case to the right class and produce the right code in an efficient and reliable way.

4.1 Classification Problems

A problem of juxtaposition, combination codes, and value addition codes is that not all combinations that can be generated are sensible. In the example of the medical procedures, a "transplantation to remove an abscess" is not sensible. Combination codes also give ambiguous results. The combination of a code for larynx, a code for removal, and a code for tube is ambiguous. It is unclear whether the tube or the larynx is removed, because the code lacks semantic information about how the items are related. In a prestandard for the classification of surgical procedures of the *Comité Européen de Normalisation* (*CEN*) (see Chapter 34), this ambiguity problem is tackled by the use of both semantic categories and syntactic categories.

When developing a classification of diseases, etiology, location, and pathophysiological mechanism can be useful ordering principles. However, we cannot always apply each ordering principle to all diseases. Using etiology as the ordering principle, we can classify "viral pneumonia" as a viral disease, but we cannot classify "pneumonia" with the same degree of certainty to any etiological class. Therefore, pneumonia will be classified, using an anatomical ordering principle, as a pulmonary disease. Most classifications combine several ordering principles on one level. The overlap of disease classes that then results violates the rule of mutual exclusiveness (see Panel 6.2). The class "pul-

monary disease" intersects with the class "viral disease." When a disease is already classified elsewhere, an exclusion statement is used to indicate that the disease is considered a member of one class only. However, this will cause problems in statistical analysis. If we want to compute the number of cases resulting from a viral disease, we cannot simply count the members in the class "viral diseases", since "viral pneumonia" is also a viral disease but those cases are classified in the class "pulmonary diseases". Adding the two classes will include cases of nonviral pulmonary diseases as well.

The dynamic nature of classification explains the continuous need for maintenance of classifications such as ICD and SNOMED. The classification of acquired immune deficiency syndrome (AIDS) as a viral disease was preceded by the classification of AIDS as an immune deficiency disease. The question whether AIDS was a viral disease was accompanied by much discussion. Nowadays, the hypothesis that AIDS is caused by infection with human immunodeficiency virus (HIV) is widely accepted. Creutzfeldt-Jakob's disease is currently regarded to be a prion disease, but it used to be regarded as a slow virus disease. Because diagnostic terms can disappear or serve different diagnostic goals over periods of time, one should be aware that statistical analysis of existing data may require a different algorithm each time a change is made to the classification scheme.

4.2 Coding Problems

Browsing large medical classifications of diagnoses and procedures is required to encode a patient's condition for medicoeconomic purposes. The basic problem with this kind of browsing is the fact that the language used in the classification is rather different from the clinical language found in the patient record. Regardless of who encodes the patient's condition, there are difficulties in terms of mismatches between the terms in the classification and the overall representation of the patient. This gap can be bridged by using

6

adequate computer programs.

Two different techniques are used to provide clinicians and encoders with intelligent help. The first type is *morpho-semantic analysis* of the input languages to extract all underlying concepts. This analysis decomposes all compound words into their parts: prefixes, stems, and suffixes. It then groups similar stems into more general categories. On this basis, an analysis of all available sentences around the classification in use is performed and a corresponding indexing is precomputed. Any future query of the browsing process will be handled in this context. The net result is a somewhat conceptual indexing of the classification, which has been shown to be much more valuable than usual lexical indexing.

The other type of assistance is the *incorporation of a*

thesaurus with synonym expressions that all point to an existing entry in the classification. Such a thesaurus, which may be hidden to the user, is part of the corpus on which the indexing is done. By using a large thesaurus, the overall performance of the browser may be dramatically increased. Local thesauri that use expressions and other medical terms specific to a language or country are also possible. In general, synonyms may include equivalent expressions (e.g., proper names) or subexpressions that represent a specialization of the initial expression. At the implementation level, browsers for medical classifications are readily available for use on personal computers, and they usually have adequate response times.

5 Classification Systems

5.1 ICD-International Classification of Diseases

As discussed in Section 3, **ICD** is the archetypal coding system for patient record abstraction. The first edition was published in 1900, and it is being revised at approximately 10-year intervals. The most recent version is ICD-10, which was published in 1992. WHO is responsible for its maintenance. Most present registration systems, however, are still based on ICD-9 or its modification, ICD-9-CM, which contains more detailed codes. ICD consists of a core classification of three-digit codes, which are the minimum requirement for reporting mortality statistics to WHO. An optional fourth digit provides an additional level of detail. At all levels, the numbers 0 to 7 are used for further detail, whereas the number 8 is reserved for all other cases and the number 9 is reserved for unspecified coding.

The basic ICD is meant to be used for coding diagnostic terms, but ICD-9 as well as ICD-10 also contain a set of expansions for other families of medical

terms. For instance, ICD-9 also contains a list of codes starting with the letter "V" for reasons for encounter or other factors that are related to someone's health status. A list of codes starting with the letter "E" is used to code external causes of death. The nomenclature of the morphology of neoplasms is coded by the "M" list.

The disease codes of both ICD-9 and ICD-10 are grouped into *chapters*. For example, in ICD-9, infectious and parasitic diseases are coded with the three-digit codes 001 to 139, and in ICD-10 the codes are renumbered and extended as codes starting with the letters A or B; for tuberculosis the three-digit codes 010 to 018 are used in ICD-9, and the codes A16 to A19 are used in ICD-10. The four-digit levels and optional five-digit levels enable the encoder to provide more detail. Table 6.3 gives examples of some codes in the ICD-9 system.

The U.S. National Center for Health Statistics published a set of clinical modifications to ICD-9, known as ICD-9-CM. It is fully compatible with ICD-9, but it contains an extra level of detail where needed (see Table 6.3). In addition, ICD-9-CM contains a volume III on medical procedures.

6

Code		Disease
001	- 139	Infectious and parasitic diseases
001	- 009	Infectious diseases of the digestive tract
003		Other Salmonella Infections
	- 003.0	Salmonella gastroenteritis
	- 003.1	Salmonella Septicemia
	- 003.2	Localized Salmonella Infections
	-	003.20 Localized Salmonella Infection, Unspecified
	-	003.21 Salmonella Meningitis
	-	003.22 Salmonella Pneumonia
	-	003.23 Salmonella Arthritis
	-	003.24 Salmonella Osteomyelitis
	-	003.29 Other Localized Salmonella Infections
	- 003.8	Other Specified Salmonella Infections
	- 003.9	Salmonella Infections, Unspecified

Table 6.3
Example of a Four-Digit Code Level in ICD-9 and the Five-Digit Code Level as Extended by the ICD-9-CM.

5.2 ICPC–International Classification of Primary Care

The World Organization of National Colleges, Academies and Academic Associations of General Practitioners/Family Physicians (WONCA) did not accept ICD-9, but came up with its own classification. The granularity of this system is less than that of ICD-9. It is not only used for coding diagnoses but it also contains codes for reasons for encounter (RfE) and for therapies and laboratory tests. In most primary care information systems, the laboratory test results are directly entered as coded numerical values, so there is no need for manual coding, and a drug prescription module automatically stores the generic code for the drug and other prescription data.

ICPC is compatible with earlier WONCA classifications, such as the ICHPPC-2-Defined (International Classification of Health Care Problems in Primary Care) and the IC-Process-PC. For codes derived from ICHPPC-2-Defined, inclusion criteria (for further spe-

cification of the code) are used.

ICPC is a two-axis system (see Table 6.1). The first axis, primarily oriented toward body systems (the tracts), is coded by a letter, and the second axis, the component, is coded by two digits. The component axis contains seven code groups. In this system the diagnosis pneumonia is coded R81 (R for respiratory tract and 81 for the diagnostic component). Codes that can be applied to more than one tract are described only as a two-digit component. For instance, the procedure code 42 (electrical tracing) can be used for electrocardiograph registration by using the code K42. These codes require the combination with a tract letter.

ICPC is used to encode encounters structured according to the *SOAP* principle (S for subjective information, e.g., complaints; O is for objective information, e.g., test and lab results; A is for assessment, e.g., diagnosis; and P is for plan, e.g., diagnostic tests, treatment, medication, etc.; see also Chapter 7) Optionally, a fourth digit is used for some cases when an extra level of detail is required or to specify synonyms, which is a mixture of coding principles. ICPC

6

can be used in the RfE mode (i.e., for coding the reason for encounter or the complaints), the diagnostic mode, or the process mode, where further actions, such as laboratory tests and therapies are coded. The process mode is not coded directly, since most of its components are already incorporated as alphanumeric values.

An attractive way to organize patient-oriented information is by *disease episodes*. ICPC can be used to organize the registration of a disease episode over time, from its onset to its resolution. A disease episode may include several encounters. Each problem in an encounter should be coded separately. The same holds for complications of primary diseases. The committee that developed ICPC also produced conversions to and from ICD-9 and ICD-10. For several diagnoses of ICPC, criteria derived from ICHPPC-2-Defined have been defined.

5.3 DSM-Diagnostic and Statistical Manual for Mental Disorders

A specialist code designed by the American Psychiatric Association is the Diagnostic and Statistical Manual for Mental Disorders (*DSM*) coding system. The first edition (DSM-I) was published in 1952. In developing DSM-II the decision was made to base it on the then newly developed ICD-8. Both systems became effective in 1968. DSM-IV has been coordinated with the development of ICD-10.

The chapter on mental disorders of ICD-9-CM was compatible with DSM-III-R, its revised third edition. The fourth edition, DSM-IV, is compatible with the chapter on mental disorders in ICD-10. The classification is intended to be used by psychiatrists. However, the etiology or the pathophysiological processes are only known for some mental disorders. The approach taken in DSM-III, DSM-III-R, and DSM-IV is nontheoretical with regard to etiology or the pathophysiological process except for disorders for which the etiology or the pathology is established. In these cases etiology and pathology are included in the definition of the disorder. For instance, it is believed that phobic disorders

represent some displacement of anxiety, resulting from the breakdown of defense mechanisms that keep internal conflicts out of one's consciousness. Others explain phobic disorders on the basis of acquired or learned avoidance responses to conditional anxiety. Still others believe that certain phobias result from a dysregulation of basic biological systems that mediate separation anxiety. Clinicians, however, agree on the clinical manifestations. Since it is not possible to define a theory for each disorder, let alone know the etiology, DSM is designed to describe the clinical manifestations of the disease along several axes. Therefore, DSM is a multiaxial classification system. Like ICPC, DSM also uses definitions for the disorders, including criteria for assigning a diagnosis.

Disorders in the DSM systems are classified along five axes:

- clinical syndromes,
- personality disorders and special developmental disorders,
- relevant physical conditions,
- severity of psychological stressors, and
- overall psychological functioning.

5.4 SNOMED-Systematized Nomenclature of Human and Veterinary Medicine

SNOMED allows for the coding of several aspects of a disease. SNOMED was first published in 1975 and was revised in 1979. Its current version is called *SNOMED International* (Systematized Nomenclature of Human and Veterinary Medicine). SNOMED is also a multiaxial system. SNOMED II was a code with 7 axes, and SNOMED International has 11 axes or modules. Each of these axes forms a complete hierarchical classification system (see Table 6.4). A diagnosis in SNOMED may consist of a topographic code, a morphology code, a living organism code, and a function code. When a well-defined diagnosis for a combination of these four codes exists, a dedicated diagnostic code is defined. For example, the disease

6

Axis	Definition	Description
T	Topography	Anatomic terms
M	Morphology	Changes found in cells, tissues and organs
L	Living organisms	Bacteria and viruses
C	Chemical	Drugs
F	Function	Signs and symptoms
J	Occupation	Terms that describe the occupation
D	Diagnosis	Diagnostic terms
P	Procedure	Administrative, diagnostic and therapeutic procedures
A	Physical agents, forces, activities	Devices and activities associated with the disease
S	Social context	Social conditions and important relationships in medicine
G	General	Syntactic linkages and qualifiers

Table 6.4
The 11 Axes of SNOMED International.

code D-13510 (Pneumococcal pneumonia) is equivalent to the combination of:

- T-28000 (topology code for *Lung, not otherwise specified*),
- M-40000 (morphology code for *Inflammation, not otherwise specified*), and
- L-25116 (for *Streptococcus pneumoniae*) along the living organism axis.

Tuberculosis (D-14800), for instance, could also be coded as Lung (T-28000) + Granuloma (M-44000) + Mycobacterium tuberculosis (L-21801) + Fever (F-03003). However, this can be confusing since tuberculosis is not only restricted to the lung. SNOMED is also able to combine medical concepts, using so-called combination or juxtaposition codes, to form more complex concepts. Linkage between concepts, for instance, can be expressed by "is caused by." In SNOMED International, almost all diagnostic terms of ICD-9-CM are incorporated in the disease/diagnostic module (D-codes). Rules for combining SNOMED terms to form complex entities or complex concepts have not yet been developed.

Any SNOMED term may be combined with any other SNOMED term. This means that there are often multiple ways to express a code for the same valid concept; however, these are not always meaningful. This freedom of combining codes for all axes allows for meaningless codes; checking such codes for correctness by a computer is almost impossible.

5.5 ICD-O-International Classification of Diseases for Oncology

In 1976, WHO published the first edition of the International Classification of Diseases for Oncology (*ICD-O*) after extensive field testing. It was based on ICD-9. The second edition, published in 1990, is an extension of the draft neoplasm chapter of ICD-10. ICD-O combines a four-digit topography code based on ICD with a morphology code that includes a neoplasm behavior code and a code for histological grading and differentiation. These neoplasm morphology

6

codes have been adopted in the morphology axes of SNOMED and SNOMED International. ICD-O is widely used for cancer registrations.

5.6 CPT-Current Procedural Terminology

Another coding system used in the United States for billing and reimbursement is the Current Procedural Terminology (**CPT**) code. It provides a coding scheme for diagnostic and therapeutic procedures that define procedures with codes based on the cost.

5.7 ICPM-International Classification of Procedures in Medicine

ICPM was published in 1976 by WHO for trial purposes. It contained chapters on diagnostic, laboratory, preventive, surgical, other therapeutic, and ancillary procedures. Originally, WHO planned to add chapters on radiology and drugs and to revise the classification after some years on the basis of comments received from users. Unfortunately, this never happened. Nevertheless, ICPM has been a source of inspiration for a number of other procedural classifications. The procedural part of **ICD-9-CM** and **CCP** were both based on ICPM. In Germany and The Netherlands, extensions of ICPM are mandatory in hospitals for reimbursement and administration purposes.

5.8 RCC-Read Clinical Classification

The Read Clinical Classification (**RCC**), or Read code, was developed privately in the early 1980s by a British GP (James Read), and was adopted by the British National Health Service (NHS) in 1990. RCC has been further expanded by the Clinical Terms Project. The Clinical Terms Project is a working group chaired by

the chief executive of NHS, which consists of representatives from the Royal College of Medicine, the Joint Consultants Committee, the General Medical Services Committee of the British Medical Association, and the NHS executive. RCC tries to cover the entire field of health care (see Table 6.5).

RCC has especially been developed for use by CPR systems. It aims to cover all terms that may be written in a patient record. They are arranged in chapters that cover all aspects of care. Each code represents a clinical concept and an associated "preferred term." Each code can also be linked to a number of synonyms, acronyms, eponyms, and abbreviations, which allows for the use of natural language. The concepts are arranged in a hierarchical structure, with each successive level representing greater detail. RCC uses a five-digit alphanumeric code which, in principle, allows for more than 650 million possible codes. RCC is compatible with and is cross-referenced to all widely used standard classifications, such as ICD-9 (see Table 6.6), **ICD-9-CM**, OPCS-4, **CPT**-4, and Diagnosis-Related

Table 6.5
Domains Covered by the British RCC.

Diseases

Occupations

History/symptoms

Examinations/signs

Diagnostic procedures

Radiology/diagnostic imaging

Preventive procedures

Operative procedures

Other therapeutic procedures

Administration

Drugs/appliances

Health status measurements

Diagnosis Related Groups (DRGs)

6

Level	Term	RCC	ICD-9-CM
1	Infectious/parasitic diseases	A	001-139
2	Viral disease with exanthem	A5	050-057
3	Rubella	A56	056
4	Rubella + neurological complications	A560	0560
5	Rubella + encephalomyelitis	A5601	056.01

Table 6.6
Example of RCC mapping to ICD-9-CM.

Groups (*DRGs*). RCC has a one-to-one cross-reference, or mapping, to all the terms in the classifications mentioned (Table 6.6). This hierarchy in coding detail is found in all code categories. In RCC version 3, terms may have multiple parents in the hierarchy. Version 3.1 adds the ability to combine terms in a specific, controlled way.

5.9 ATC-Anatomic Therapeutic Chemical Code

The Anatomic Therapeutic Chemical Code (*ATC*) has been developed for the systematic and hierarchical classification of drugs. In the early 1970s, the Norwegian Medicinal Depot expanded the existing three-level anatomic and therapeutic classification system of the European Pharmaceutical Market Research Association and added two chemical levels.

Later, the WHO Drug Utilization Research Group accepted the ATC classification as a standard. Presently, the WHO Collaborating Center for Drug Statistics Methodology in Oslo is responsible for maintaining the ATC codes. ATC is an acronym for anatomical (A), the organ system in the body for which the drug is given; therapeutic (T), the therapeutic purpose for which the drug is used; and chemical (C), the chemical class to which the drug belongs. Table 6.7 provides an example of an ATC code and its composition, while Table 6.8 provides a listing of the definitions used in the ATC code.

All classifications have disadvantages. No coding system fulfills all needs of all users. The advantages of the ATC are as follows:

- It identifies a drug product, including the active substance, the route of administration, and if rele-

6

Code	Description
C	Cardiovascular system (1st level, anatomical main group)
C03	Diuretics (2nd level, therapeutic main group)
C03C	High-level diuretics (3rd level, therapeutic subgroup)
C03CA	Sulfanomides (4th level, chemical/therapeutic subgroup)
C03CA01	Furosemide (5th level, subgroup for chemical substance)

Table 6.7
Five Levels of the ATC Code Illustrated by the Code for Furosemide.[a]

[a] At the lowest (5th) level the code also contains information on the defined daily dosage (DDD), the unit of measurement, and the route of administration.

Unit	Unit Abbreviation	Route of Administration	Abbreviation for Route of Administration
gram	g	Inhalation	Inhal
milligram	mg	Nasal	N
microgram	mcg	Oral	O
unit	E	Parenteral	P
thousand units	TE	Rectal	R
million units	ME	Sublingual/buccal	SL
millimole	mmol	Transdermal	Td
milliliter	ml	Vaginal	V

Table 6.8
Units and Administration Routes Defined in the ATC code.

vant, the dose;
- It is therapeutically as well as chemically oriented, a feature that most other systems lack;
- Its hierarchical structure allows for a logical grouping;
- It is accepted as the international WHO standard for drug utilization research.

A disadvantage is that it does not cover combination products, dermatological preparations, and locally compounded preparations.

In some countries national drug databases often contain the ATC code for each drug product. This allows pharmaceutical information systems to select alternative drugs. It also provides *decision-support systems* with information to check for *drug interactions*, double medication, and dosage control.

5.10 MeSH-Medical Subject Headings

The Medical Subject Headings (*MeSH*) classification is developed and maintained by the National Library of Medicine (*NLM*) in the United States. It is generally used to index the world medical literature. Within the hierarchy of MeSH, a concept may appear as narrower concepts of more than one broader concept. For example, pneumonia is listed as a respiratory tract infection as well as a lung disease. MeSH forms the basis for the Unified Medical Language System (*UMLS*) also developed by NLM (see Panel 6.3)

5.11 DRG-Diagnosis Related Groups

The *DRG* classification is based on ICD-9-CM codes and other factors not included in ICD-9. The grouping of ICD codes is based on factors that affect the cost of treatment and the length of stay in the hospital, such as severity, complications, and type of treatment. The resulting classes are homogeneous with respect to costs and they are medically recognized. DRGs may thus be used for budgeting. Because factors related to the delivery of care are included, their usefulness for budgeting is disputable. Some disease groups are clustered further, which is called case mix.

6

PANEL 6.3

Unified Medical Language System (UMLS)

The UMLS project is a long-term research and development project at the U.S. National Library of Medicine (NLM) whose goal is to develop resources that will support intelligent information retrieval from a wide range of disparate biomedical information sources. The project is directed by a multidisciplinary team, including physicians, computer and information scientists, and linguists, and involves collaboration with many medical informatics research groups. The project work has resulted in a set of knowledge sources and accompanying programs that are updated and distributed regularly on CD-ROM. Online access to the UMLS knowledge sources is provided through the Internet-based UMLS Knowledge Source Server, which includes an application programming interface (API) and a World Wide Web interface. The Web site requires an access code and may be found at http://umlsks.nlm.nih.gov/. The UMLS Knowledge Sources are described below.

UMLS Metathesaurus

The Metathesaurus contains information about biomedical concepts and terms from a large number of controlled terminologies and thesauri. The Metathesaurus preserves the information encoded in the source vocabularies, such as the hierarchical contexts of the terms, their meanings and other attributes. The Metathesaurus is organized by concepts, which means that alternate names (synonyms, lexical variants, and translations) for the same meaning are all linked together as one concept. The Metathesaurus adds information to the concepts, including semantic types, definitions, and inter-concept relationships. The Metathesaurus contains hundreds of thousands of concepts from a broad range of vocabularies. These include, for example, all or portions of the following terminologies:

- the Systematized Nomenclature of Medicine (SNOMED International),
- the Read Thesaurus,
- the International Classification of Diseases - Clinical Modification (ICD9-CM),
- the Universal Medical Device Nomenclature System,
- the WHO Adverse Drug Reaction Terminology,
- the Classification of Nursing Diagnoses (NANDA),
- the Home Health Care Classification of Nursing Diagnoses and Interventions, ▶

6. Current Developments

The American Society for Testing and Materials (*ASTM*) is working on the standardization of an extensive nomenclature system. In Europe, standardization efforts are undertaken by the European Union (see Chapter 34). The GALEN project, for example, aims at the development of a reference model for medical concepts, which

- the Physicians' Current Procedural Terminology (CPT),
- the Medical Subject Headings (MeSH),
- the Diagnostic and Statistical Manual of Mental Disorders (DSMIV), and
- the Thesaurus of Psychological Index Terms.

In addition, translations of some of the terminologies into languages other than English are included.

UMLS Semantic Network

The Semantic Network, through its high-level semantic types, or categories, provides a consistent categorization of all concepts represented in the Metathesaurus. The links between the semantic types provide the structure for the Network and represent important relationships in the biomedical domain. There are semantic types for organisms, anatomical structures, biologic function, chemicals, events, physical objects, and concepts or ideas. The primary relationship is the "is_a" link, and there are five major categories of additional relationships: physical, spatial, temporal, functional, and conceptual relationships.

SPECIALIST Lexicon

The SPECIALIST lexicon is an English language lexicon with many biomedical terms. It has been developed in the context of the SPECIALIST natural language processing project at NLM. The lexicon entry for each word or term records syntactic, morphological, and orthographic information. Lexical entries may be single or multi-word terms and are selected for coding from a variety of sources, including lexical items from MEDLINE citation records, and a large set of terms from medical and general English dictionaries. Included with the lexicon are lexical programs, indexes, and databases which are useful for recognizing lexical variation in biomedical terminologies and texts.

UMLS Information Sources Map

The Information Sources Map contains information about the scope, location, vocabulary, syntax rules, and access conditions of biomedical databases of all kinds. Software tools are being developed whose goal it is to determine which information sources are most likely to be relevant to a particular query, to supply useful information to the user about the scope and probable utility of the information in those sources, and then to automatically connect the user to the identified information sources, retrieving and organizing the relevant information.

6

will be independent of language and existing coding systems and which will be independent of the data model used by computer-based patient record systems. NLM is developing UMLS (see Panel 6.3). UMLS contains a meta-thesaurus with medical concepts and a semantic network, which provides information on the semantic relationships between medical concepts. These concepts are taken from established vocabularies such as SNOMED, ICD-9-CM, and MeSH. NLM is developing methods to enhance the use of UMLS for encoding clinical data.

7. Conclusion

There are many overlapping classifications not only for the coding of diagnoses but also for the classification of medical events. Although most diagnostic coding systems try to be compatible with the ICD family, ICD itself represents only a limited view and is unable to fulfill the needs of all users. Another problem is that all coding systems require well-defined criteria, but a standardized medical terminology is still lacking.

Systems such as SNOMED have much more expressive power than the more rigid systems such as ICD-9-CM. In studies in which several coding schemes were compared with respect to their expressive powers, SNOMED scored much higher than ICD-9-CM. On the other hand, the use of coded data in database queries for statistical overviews and for use by expert systems is more complicated.

Wide acceptance of a coding system is essential for the development of decision-support systems. International institutions such as WHO with its recognized collaborating centers play an important role in the standardization process.

Key References

Cimino JJ. Coding Systems in Health Care. In: Van Bemmel JH, McCray AT, eds. *IMIA Yearbook of Medical Informatics 1995*. Stuttgart, New York: Schattauer, 1995.

College of American Pathologists. *SNOMED, Systematized Nomenclature of Medicine*. Chicago: Coll of Amer Pathol, 1994.

Fetter RB, Thompson JD. *The New ICD-9-CM Diagnosis Related Groups Classification Scheme*. New Haven: Yale University School of Organization and Management Publ, 1981: vol.I-V.

Gersenovic M. The ICD family of classifications. Meth Inform Med 1995;34:172-5.

Lindberg DAB, Humphreys BL, McCray AT. 1993. The Unified Medical Language System. Meth Inform Med 32:281-91.

See the Web site for further literature references.

6

7 The Patient Record

1 Introduction

The traditional paper-based patient record used in a clinical setting generally contains the notes of clinicians and other care providers. These notes are often supplemented with data from other sources: laboratory test results and reports describing the results of other tests that have been performed, such as X-rays, pathology, *ultrasound*, lung function, and *endoscopy* (see Chapters 12 and 13). With the exception of electrocardiograms, some *images*, or drawings, the majority of information in the paper-based record involves data that can be expressed in characters and digits (*alphanumeric data*). In most European countries, the nursing record is usually kept as a separate document (see Chapter 14). Most nontextual information, especially images, can be viewed only upon request, and it may even be necessary for the clinician to go to a special location to view the materials. Hence, the set of patient data is generally not yet available as a whole at the place and time it is needed.

This chapter first provides a brief overview of the history of the patient record, starting with Hippocrates, to be followed by modern views on the structure of the patient record, the development and use of computer-based patient records (*CPR*s), the entry of data into the CPR, coding and standardization, the representation of time in CPRs, and the clinical use of the CPR. Chapter 29 provides more details on structuring patient records in computers.

2 History of the Patient Record

The patient record is an account of a patient's health and disease after he or she has sought medical help. Usually, the notes in the record are made by the nurse[1] or the physician. The record contains findings, considerations, test results and treatment information related to the disease process.

In the fifth century B.C., medical reporting was highly influenced by Hippocrates. He advocated that the medical record serve two goals:

1. it should accurately reflect the course of disease, and
2. it should indicate the possible causes of disease.

With the medical insight of those times, the records contained descriptions of events that preceded disease rather than real causal clarifications. Panel 7.1 shows how Hippocrates described the course of a disease (see Fig. 7.1 for the text in Greek). The example shows

---

[1] *In some countries, both physicians and nurses have equal access to medical records, which are then most often called patient records. In other countries, there are separate medical records and nursing records.*

PANEL 7.1

Hippocrates Describes a Disease

The description starts with the patient's history prior to his request for medical help:

"Apollonius was ailing for a long time without being confined to bed. He had a swollen abdomen, and a continual pain in the region of the liver had been present for a long time; moreover, he became during this period jaundiced and flatulent: his complexion was whitish."

Hippocrates proceeds with the reason for seeking medical help:

After dining one day and drinking to excess, Apollonius "at first grew rather hot and took to his bed. Having drunk copiously of milk, boiled and raw, both goat's and sheep's, and adopting a thoroughly bad regimen, he suffered much therefrom."

Reports on the progress of the illness follow from that time onward. They are not provided daily, but are provided only at times when important changes in the symptoms occur.

*There were exacerbations of the fever; the bowels passed practically nothing of the food taken, the urine was thin and scanty. No sleep. Grievous distention, much thirst, delirious mutterings. .....
About the fourteenth day from his taking to bed, after a rigor, he grew hot; wildly delirious, shouting, distress, much rambling, followed by calm; the coma came on at this time.... About the twenty-fourth day comfortable; in other respects the same, but he had lucid intervals. .....
About the thirtieth day acute fever; copious thin stools; wandering, cold extremities, speechlessness. Thirty-fourth day: Death.*

Ἀπολλώνιος ὀρθοστάδην ὑπεφέρετο χρόνον πολύν. ἦν δὲ μεγαλό–σπλαγχνος, καὶ περὶ ἧπαρ συνήθης ὀδύνη χρόνον πολὺν παρείπετο, καὶ δὴ τότε καὶ ἰκτερώδης ἐγένετο, φυσώδης, χροιῆς τῆς ὑπολεύκου. φαγὼν δὲ καὶ πιὼν ἀκαιρότερον βόειον ἐθερμάνθη σμικρὰ τὸ πρῶτον, κατεκλίθη. γάλαξι δὲ χρησάμενος ἐφθοῖσι καὶ ὠμοῖσι πολλοῖσιν, αἰγείοισι καὶ μηλείοισι, καὶ διαίτῃ κακῇ πάντων, βλάβαι μεγάλαι. οἵ τε γὰρ πυρετοὶ παρωξύνθησαν, κοιλίη τε τῶν προσενεχθέντων οὐδὲν διέδωκεν ἄξιον λόγου, οὐρά τε λεπτὰ καὶ ὀλίγα διῄει. ὕπνοι οὐκ ἐνῆσαν. ἐμφύσημα κακόν, πολὺ δίψος, κωμα–τώδησ, ὑποχονδρίου δεξιοῦ ἔπαρμα σὺν ὀδύνῃ, ἄκρεα πάντοθεν ὑπό–ψυχρα, σμικρὰ παρέλεγε, λήθη πάντων ὅ τι λέγοι, παρεφέρετο. περὶ δὲ τεσσαρεσκαιδεκάτην, ἀφ᾽ ἧς κατεκλίθη, ῥιγώσας ἐπεθερμάνθη. ἐξεμάνη. βοή, ταραχή, λόγοι πολλοί, καὶ πάλιν ἵδρυσις, καὶ τὸ κῶμα τηνικαῦτα προσῆλθε. μετὰ δὲ ταῦτα κοιλίη ταραχώδης πολλοῖσι χολώδεσιν, ἀκρή–τοισιν, ὠμοῖσιν. οὔρα μέλανα, σμικρά, λεπτά. πολλὴ δυσφορίη. τὰ τῶν διαχωρημάτων ποικίλως. ἢ γὰρ μέλανα καὶ σμικρὰ καὶ ἰώδεα ἢ λιπαρὰ καὶ ὠμὰ καὶ δακνώδεα. κατὰ δὲ χρόνουσ ἐδόκει καί γαλακτώδεα διδόναι. περὶ δὲ εἰκοστὴν τετάρτην διὰ παρηγορίης. τὰ μὲν ἄλλα ἐπὶ τῶν αὐτῶν, σμικρὰ δὲ κατενόησεν. ἐξ οὗ δὲ κατεκλίθη, οὐδενὸς ἐμνήσθη. πάλιν δὲ ταχὺ παρ–ενόει, ὥρμητο πάντα ἐπὶ τὸ χεῖρον. περὶ δὲ τριηκοστὴν πυρετὸς ὀξύς, διαχωρήματα πολλὰ λεπτά, παράληρος, ἄκρεα ψυχρά, ἄφωνος. τριηκοστῇ τετάρτῃ ἔθανε.

Figure 7.1
Description of a disease by Hippocrates 2,600 years ago. The patient history is that of Apollonius.

PANEL 7.2

Time-Oriented Medical Record

Feb 21, 1996: Shortness of breath, cough, and fever. Very dark feces.
Exam: RR 150/90, pulse 95/min, Temp: 39.3 °C. Rhonchi, abdomen not tender.
Present medication 64 mg Aspirin per day. Probably acute bronchitis, possibly
complicated with cardiac decompensation. Bleeding possibly due to Aspirin.
ESR 25 mm, Hb 7.8, occult blood feces +.
Chest X-ray: no atelectasis, slight sign of cardiac decompensation.
Medication: Amoxicillin caps 500 mg twice daily, Aspirin reduce to 32 mg per
day.
Mar 4, 1996: No more cough, slight shortness of breath, normal feces.
Exam: slight rhonchi, RR 160/95, pulse 82/min. Keep Aspirin at 32 mg per day.
Hb 8.2, occult blood feces.

---

that he recorded his observations in a purely chronological order. We call such a record a *time-oriented medical record*. The descriptions mainly reflect the story as it is phrased by the patient and the patient's relatives. In Hippocratic medicine, it was very important to estimate the prognostic value of findings. Well-documented disease histories play an important part in achieving that goal. It is the physician's and nurse's most important task to relieve suffering, but these providers must know their limits and refrain from pointless interference. Hippocrates' vision is still the basis for the oath or promise that all physicians must take before they can start to practice their profession.

Until the early 19th century, physicians based their observations on what they could hear, feel, and see. In 1816, Laennec invented the stethoscope. This instrument contributed considerably to available diagnostic techniques. When more diagnostic instruments became available, such as the ophthalmoscope and the laryngoscope, a terminology was developed to express the new findings with these instruments. The advent of this new technology caused the emphasis of the patient record to expand the scope from the story told by the patient or the patient's family to the findings of the physician and the nurse.

Shortly after 1880, the American surgeon William Mayo formed the first group practice, which became the now well-known Mayo Clinic in Rochester, Minnesota. In the early Mayo Clinic, every physician kept medical notes in a personal leather-bound ledger. The ledger contained a chronological account of all patient encounters. As a result, the notes pertaining to a single patient could be pages apart, depending on the time intervals between visits. The scattered notes made it complicated to obtain a good overview of the complete disease history of a patient. In addition, part of the patient information could be present in the ledgers of other physicians. In 1907, the Mayo Clinic adopted one separate file for each patient. This innovation was the origin of the patient-centered medical record. The fact that all notes were kept in a single file did, however, not mean that there were criteria which the content of those records had to meet. In 1920, the Mayo Clinic management agreed upon a minimal set of data that all physicians were compelled to record. This set of data became more or less the framework for the present-day medical record.

Despite this initiative toward standardization of patient records, their written contents were often a mixture of complaints, test results, considerations, therapy plans, and findings. Such unordered notes did not provide clear insight, especially in the case of patients who were treated for more than one complaint or disease. Weed tackled the challenge to improve the organization of the patient record, and in the 1960s he intro-

7

PANEL 7.3

Source-Oriented Medical Record

Visits

Feb 21, 1996:   Shortness of breath, cough, and fever. Very dark feces.
Exam: RR 150/90, pulse 95/min, Temp: 39.3 °C.
Rhonchi, abdomen not tender.
Present medication 64 mg Aspirin per day. Probably acute bronchitis, possibly complicated with cardiac decompensation.
Bleeding possibly due to Aspirin.
Medication: Amoxicillin caps. 500 mg twice daily, Aspirin reduce to 32 mg per day.

Mar 4, 1996:   No more cough, slight shortness of breath, normal feces.
Exam: slight rhonchi, RR 160/95, pulse 82/min.
Medication: keep Aspirin at 32 mg per day.

Laboratory tests

Feb 21, 1996:   ESR 25 mm, Hb 7.8, occult blood feces +.
Mar 4, 1996:   Hb 8.2, occult blood feces.

X-rays

Feb 21, 1996:Chest X-ray: no atelectasis, slight sign of cardiac decompensation.

---

duced the **problem-oriented medical record**. In this problem-oriented medical record, each patient was assigned one or more problems. Notes were recorded per problem according to the **SOAP** structure, which stands for subjective (S; the complaints as phrased by the patient), objective (O; the findings of physicians and nurses), assessment (A; the test results and conclusions, such as a diagnosis), and plan (P: the medical plan, e.g., treatment or policy).

Besides further improvement in the standardization and ordering of the patient record, the main purpose of the problem-oriented SOAP structure is to give a better reflection of the care provider's line of reasoning. It is immediately clear to which problem the findings and the treatment plan pertain. Although Weed's problem-oriented record was readily accepted on a rational basis, it proved to require much discipline to adhere to the method in practice. Data associated with more than one problem need to be recorded several times. Panels 7.2, 7.3, and 7.4 provide three versions of the same notes in time-oriented, source-oriented, and problem-oriented formats, respectively.

3 The Present-Day Medical Record

Most modern patient records are not purely time oriented, because strict chronological ordering makes **trend analysis** difficult. Laboratory test results may be separated by visit notes, X-ray reports, and other kinds of information. In such a record, one cannot quickly obtain insight into the course of, for example, the

---

PANEL 7.4

Problem-Oriented Medical Record

Problem 1: Acute bronchitis

Feb 21, 1996   S: Shortness of breath, cough, and fever.
                O: Pulse 95/min, Temp: 39.3 °C.
                    Rhonchi. ESR 25 mm.
                    Chest X-ray: no atelectasis, slight sign of cardiac decompensation.
                A: Acute bronchitis.
                P: Amoxicillin caps. 500 mg twice daily.

Mar 4, 1996   S: No more cough, slight shortness of breath.
                O: Pulse 82/min. Slight rhonchi.
                A: Sign of bronchitis minimal.

Problem 2: Shortness of breath

Feb 21, 1996   S: Shortness of breath.
                O: Rhonchi, RR 150/90.
                    Chest X-ray: no atelectasis, slight sign of cardiac decompensation.
                A: Minor sign of decompensation.

Mar 4, 1996   S: Slight shortness of breath.
                O: RR: 160/95, pulse 82/min.
                A: No decompensation.

Problem 3: Dark feces

Feb 21, 1996   S: Dark feces.
                    Present medication Aspirin 64 mg per day.
                O: Abdomen not tender, no blood on the glove at rectal examination Hb 7.8.
                A: Intestinal bleeding possibly due to Aspirin.
                P: Reduce Aspirin to 32 mg per day.

Mar 4, 1996   S: Normal feces.
                O: Occult blood feces.
                A: No more sign of intestinal bleeding.
                P: Keep Aspirin at 32 mg per day.

---

hemoglobin level. To facilitate trend analysis, current records are generally *source oriented*. The contents of the record are ordered according to the method by which they were obtained; notes of visits, X-ray reports, blood tests, and other data become separate sections in the patient record. Within each section, those data have a chronological order. Problem-oriented recording following Weed's SOAP code affects only the clinical notes.

An important question is how well the current paper-based record is suited for its purpose. As one may rightfully expect, the patient record is used first and foremost to support patient care. However, developments in health care have made this task more complex, and there is also a greater demand for patient data for purposes other than patient care. Well-recognized ways of using the patient record today include the following:

- Supporting patient care:
  - a source for evaluation and decision making, and
  - a source of information that is shared among care providers.
- A legal report of medical actions.
- Supporting research:
  - clinical research,
  - epidemiological studies,
  - assessing quality of care, and
  - postmarketing surveillance of drugs.
- Educating clinicians.
- Healthcare management and services:
  - providing support for billing and reimbursement,
  - a basis for pre-authorization by payers,
  - providing support for organizational issues, and
  - providing support for cost management.

Although medical notes are usually recorded on paper, paper-based notes have disadvantages that mainly stem from medical progress. The enormous growth of medical knowledge has led to an increasing number of clinical specialties. Specialization leads to multidisciplinary care, so that more than one care provider is involved in a patient's treatment. In such a setting, one physical record per patient causes too many logistical problems. Therefore, there are often as many records for a patient as there are specialties involved in his or her treatment. Patient data then become scattered among a variety of sources. When clinicians want to form a complete picture about a patient's health, they may need to consult records that are kept by their colleagues. Paper files can only be in one location at a time, and sometimes they cannot be found at all. Handwriting may be poor and illegible, data may be missing, or notes may be too ambiguous to allow proper interpretation.

The rapid advances in medical technology and information make it difficult even for specialists to have state-of-the-art knowledge at their fingertips. Yet, patients may expect treatment according to the best available insight. A fundamental limitation of paper-based records is that they can only contribute passively to the decision making of the clinician (see Chapters 15-17). The record cannot actively draw the care provider's attention to abnormal laboratory values, contraindications for drugs, or allergies of the patient, for example, to iodine and penicillin.

Beside limitations that directly involve patient care, the paper-based record also has disadvantages that are related to research purposes and healthcare planning. To support these goals, patient data need to be unambiguous, well structured, and easily, but not unlawfully, accessible. Respecting the privacy of the patient is a topic of continuous concern (see Chapter 33).

It is obvious that retrospective research on the basis of large numbers of paper-based records is extremely laborious and that many data would prove to be missing or useless. This is one important reason why most studies are conducted prospectively.

In summary, paper as a storage medium for patient data has the following disadvantages:

- The record can be only at one place at a time. It may not be available or it may even be missing.
- The contents are in free text; hence they are:
  - variable in order,
  - possibly illegible,
  - possibly incomplete, and
  - possibly ambiguous.
- For scientific analysis, the contents need to be transcribed, with potential errors.
- Paper-based notes cannot give rise to active reminders, warnings, or advice.

4 The Computer-based Patient Record

The increasing demand for well-structured and accessible patient data, in combination with developments in computer science, sparked a great interest in the development of an electronic patient record. Computers have the potential to improve legibility, accessibility, and structure, but these pose

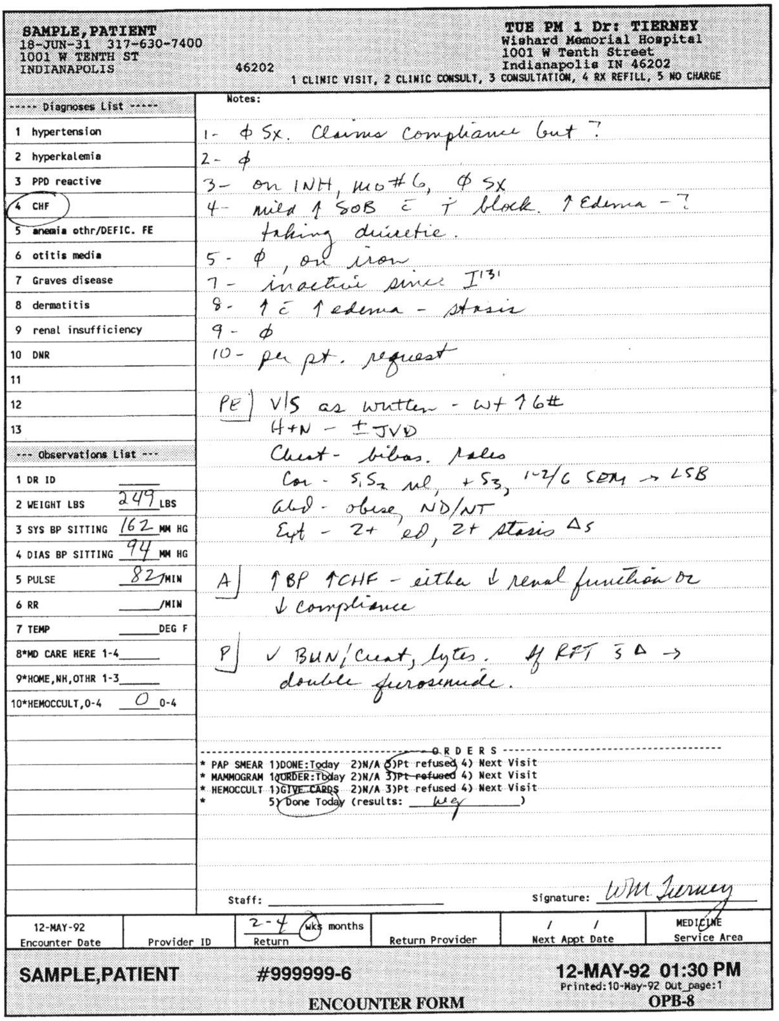

SAMPLE, PATIENT
18-JUN-31 317-630-7400
1001 W TENTH ST
INDIANAPOLIS   46202

TUE PM 1 Dr: TIERNEY
Wishard Memorial Hospital
1001 W Tenth Street
Indianapolis IN 46202

1 CLINIC VISIT, 2 CLINIC CONSULT, 3 CONSULTATION, 4 RX REFILL, 5 NO CHARGE

----- Diagnoses List -----

1	hypertension
2	hyperkalemia
3	PPD reactive
4	CHF
5	anemia othr/DEFIC. FE
6	otitis media
7	Graves disease
8	dermatitis
9	renal insufficiency
10	DNR
11	
12	
13	

--- Observations List ---

1 DR ID	
2 WEIGHT LBS	249 LBS
3 SYS BP SITTING	162 MM HG
4 DIAS BP SITTING	94 MM HG
5 PULSE	82 /MIN
6 RR	/MIN
7 TEMP	DEG F
8*MD CARE HERE 1-4	
9*HOME,NH,OTHR 1-3	
10*HEMOCCULT,0-4	0 0-4

Notes:

1- ∅ Sx. Claims compliance but ?
2- ∅
3- on INH, mo # 6, ∅ Sx
4- mild ↑ SOB c̄ ↑ block. ↑ edema - ?
   taking diuretic.
5- ∅, on iron
7- inactive since I¹³¹
8- ↑ c̄ ↑ edema - stasis
9- ∅
10- per pt. request

PE) V/S as written - Wt ↑ 16#
    H+N - ± JVD
    Chest - bibas. rales
    Cor - S₁ S₂ nl, + S₃, 1-2/6 SEM → LSB
    Abd - obese, ND/NT
    Ext - 2+ ed, 2+ stasis Δs

A) ↑ BP ↑ CHF - either ↓ renal function or
   ↓ compliance

P) ✓ BUN/Creat, lytes. If RFT 3 Δ →
   double furosemide.

--------------------------- O R D E R S -----------------------------------
* PAP SMEAR 1)DONE:Today 2)N/A 3)Pt refused 4) Next Visit
* MAMMOGRAM 1)ORDER:Today 2)N/A 3)Pt refused 4) Next Visit
* HEMOCCULT 1)GIVE CARDS 2)N/A 3)Pt refused 4) Next Visit
*   5)Done Today (results: __neg__   )

Staff: _____   Signature: WM Tierney

| 12-MAY-92 | | 2-4 wks months | | / / | MEDICINE |
| Encounter Date | Provider ID | Return | Return Provider | Next Appt Date | Service Area |

SAMPLE,PATIENT   #999999-6   12-MAY-92 01:30 PM
                                                     Printed:10-May-92 Out_page:1
              ENCOUNTER FORM   OPB-8

Figure 7.2

Encounter form of the Regenstrief Medical Record System. At the upper left is a list of diagnoses. Below this list, some structured data, such as vital signs, can be entered. The progress notes are handwritten and will be entered into the system by trained personnel. Each specialty has its own dedicated forms.

heavy demands on data collection. The following sections offer an introductory overview of the CPR. Chapter 29 provides a more elaborate description of the reasons for structuring the CPR.

For more than 25 years people have tried to develop the CPR. The first developments were in a hospital setting and focused on those parts of the patient record that were relatively easy to structure, such as those containing diagnoses, laboratory test results, and medication data. Narratives proved to be far more difficult to collect in a structured format. Typical examples of narratives are notes on the history of the patient and the physical examination. Not only do clinicians vary widely in the phrasing of their findings but they also appear to be reluctant to enter data directly into a computer, because they felt that data entry on a terminal would be time-consuming and unfriendly to the waiting patient.

Several elaborate systems developed in the 1970s continue to remain in use. Examples are *COSTAR*, *TMR*, *RMIS*, *STOR*, and *ELIAS*. For the collection of notes from physicians or nurses, these systems use so-called encounter forms. An example of a form is the one used in the Regenstrief System (*RMIS*),

7

shown in Fig. 7.2. On these forms, the system has printed part of the patient data, such as diagnoses and problems that the patient is known to have, medication prescribed at the previous visit, and test results that have become available. In the case of a new patient, only basic administrative information appears on the form. Most of the encounter forms have a number of fixed items, which the care provider is expected to fill in. Examples of such fixed items are weight, blood pressure, pulse rate, possible new diagnoses, medication, and medical decisions. The physician or the nurse can add notes pertaining to history and physical examination in writing, if they are considered to be relevant. A variety of different forms are usually available to accommodate preferences at the level of a clinical specialty or department. After office hours, the contents of the forms are entered into the computer by clerical personnel. Clinicians can consult the patient record on the computer at any time and generally do so mainly outside office hours.

Transcription of freehand dictations by clerical staff has the disadvantage that the data are not immediately available and may contain errors as a result of misinterpretations. The next sections address the use of CPRs in primary and specialty care.

4.1 Primary Care

Over the past decade, general practitioners (**GP**s) in The Netherlands and the United Kingdom have made considerable progress with respect to the use of the CPR. In 1997, more than 90% of the Dutch GPs were using an information system and more than 50% of them had replaced their paper-based charts by CPRs. GPs are far ahead of the specialists, who rarely use a computer for record keeping, and if they do, it usually involves the recording of data in the context of research. Besides electronic record keeping, primary care information systems also support the administrative and financial aspects of running a practice. Usually, the CPR is an electronic version of the paper-based patient record with options for problem-oriented record keeping. The information system is usually able to print referral letters and prescriptions, and it often provides the option to code diagnoses and findings according to the International Classification of Primary Care (**ICPC**) or the **ICD9-CM** (see Chapter 6). Although the latter requires initiative from the care provider, there is a strong incentive on the part of the clinicians to do this themselves when coding is required for reimbursement.

4.2 Specialty Care

One would expect specialists to have a far greater need for computerization of the patient record than GPs. GPs treat patients on a long-term basis and they receive reports from all other patient care providers, whereas the specialist is often confronted with fragmented patient data. Yet, there are several explanations for the fact that specialists are not as eager to adopt the CPR as GPs. In some countries, GPs either run a practice by themselves or participate in a small group practice. In such a setting, few other people are involved in decisions concerning practice management. Specialists, however, work in a complex environment, where management staff must consider the influence of information technology on a variety of future users and on available resources and logistics. This interdependence between decisions by specialists and organizational aspects is very strong in a **managed-care** environment, such as in the USA. Although GPs may be confronted with a broad spectrum of pathologies, their notes are usually less extensive and less detailed than those of a specialist. Hence, the interactive use of a CPR may be more time-consuming for a specialist than for a GP. Finally, there may be different specialties in a given clinic, each with its own requirements for the contents of the patient record. It is unlikely that one CPR could satisfy the majority of specialists. System developers must tailor the CPR for a specialist in such a way that the record can accommodate a variety of domains, while the record's contents can be merged with those of other providers to form a complete record of the patient's medical history.

5 Data Entry

Present CPRs usually support *time-oriented*, *source-oriented*, and *problem-oriented* views of the patient data, although the latter requires that clinicians explicitly specify the patient's problems and the relationships between problems and findings.

It is widely recognized that patient descriptions created via structured data entry are essential to obtain reliable patient data that are suitable not only for patient care but also for example for decision-support and research. Therefore, the entry and presentation of data in the CPR are primary topics in CPR research. Although a variety of combinations may occur, there are two main strategies for the collection of structured data:

- natural language processing, and
- direct entry of data in a structured fashion.

5.1 Natural Language Processing

Natural language processing (*NLP*) has the advantage that it can be applied to existing free text. The text must be obtained by dictaphone or a speech recognition system, but the most current CPRs allow physicians and nurses to remain fully free in the amount of detail that they provide and their choice of words. Thesauri of medical terms (see Chapter 6) and knowledge of language structure (syntax, synonyms, etc.) can assist in *parsing* sentences in free text (or natural language). The most elementary form of NLP produces an index of the terms used. Such indices are used to retrieve texts in which one or more specified terms are present. However, when the search criterion is, for instance, cough, the result will contain cases in which cough has been confirmed as well as denied.

Therefore, medically correct coding requires semantic knowledge about medical terms, their synonyms, and how the terms may be combined into meaningful expressions.

Examples of such knowledge are:

- stomach: is an organ,
- cough: is a complaint,
- AIDS: is a disease,
- dyspnea: is synonymous with shortness of breath, and
- pain: can be described by location, severity, progression, radiation, precipitating factors, etc.

These descriptors, in turn, can be defined by other terms. This knowledge, which has a semantic basis, in combination with syntactic knowledge, can be applied to the interpretation of sentences in a medically meaningful fashion. Even if terms such as "cough" and "sputum" are separated by several other words, there will be no question that they belong together since sputum is one of the descriptors of cough. Take the following sentence in a patient history: "Maximum walking distance without pain is 200 m." NLP methods can deduce that "leg claudication" is involved, provided that "maximum walking distance" is only known as a descriptor for "leg claudication." Note that the knowledge would be incomplete if "walking distance" would be the only descriptor for "leg claudication," because pain elsewhere may also limit walking distance.

Yet, numerous problems remain. Take, for example, the following phrase: "Walking distance was 200 m due to chest pain, but not to pain in the leg." The concept "maximum walking distance" may occur in several contexts, among which are angina pectoris and leg claudication. Important in the context of this sentence is the recognition of the negation regarding maximum walking distance due to leg claudication. Furthermore, a good synonym thesaurus is needed to associate "chest pain" with "anigina pectoris", and "pain in the leg" with "leg claudication." Because of the possible danger of incorrect interpretation by NLP, the results preferably need to be checked, but this additional step again requires human effort. Unfortunately, narratives often contain ambiguities that can easily be resolved by a human but not by a computer algorithm.

Important advances in our ability to obtain useful data from narrative reports have been achieved in the

7

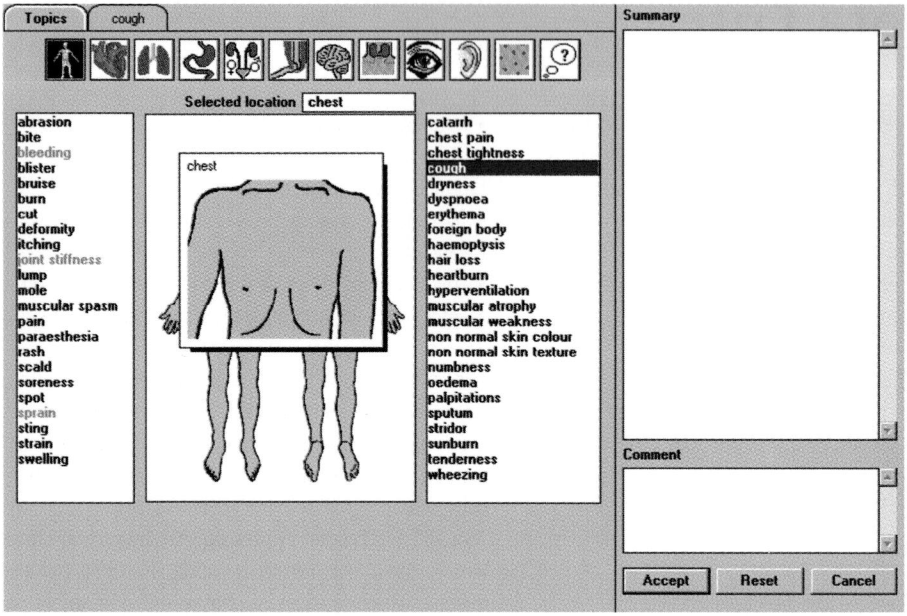

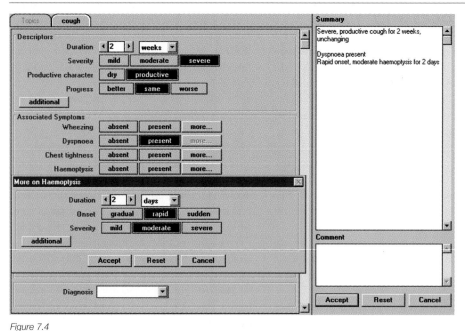

Figure 7.3
Example of a screen of the Pen&Pad system that helps the user to select the symptom or complaint to be described. The list on the left presents complaints of a general nature. The symptom list on the right has a specific focus, depending on a location selected by the user, in this case the chest.

Figure 7.4
The screen of the Pen&Pad system offers predefined options for description after a symptom has been selected. Here, "cough" can be further specified by direct descriptors and associated symptoms. More detail can be added via the buttons "more" and "additional." The user can see the result of his data entry on the right side of the screen in textual format.

domain of Radiology by the Columbia-Presbyterian Medical Center in New York. Their NLP software performs as well as coding by radiologists and internists under certain circumstances. The conclusion is that NLP, at best, will be able to extract as many data as a human colleague can but we have reached that point in only a few very limited domains. The advantage that, in principle, NLP does not restrict the clinician in phrasing his or her findings coexists with a disadvantage: NLP cannot stimulate care providers to be more complete and more explicit in their descriptions.

5.2 Structured Data Entry

The other main strategy for obtaining data in a more complete and less ambiguous format is to enter the data directly in a structured way. Therefore, this section focuses on structured data entry (**SDE**) directly by the care provider. SDE differs significantly from the present routine of patient data entry, but it has proven to result in more reliable and more complete data. It is important that care providers receive as much support as possible when they use SDE. One cannot expect them to use a bulky manual that specifies which terms may be used in which context and in which combinations. This type of information must be incorporated into the user interface in such a way that the user needs only to choose from available options. An example is the Pen&Pad interface for SDE, as shown in Figs. 7.3 and 7.4. The particular strategy that best supports SDE strongly depends on the variety of findings with which the care provider may be confronted; it depends on the size of the clinical domain.

5.3 Forms for Data Entry

In the context of a given medical specialty or of a specific study, only a limited number of items needs to be specified. It may be efficient to combine these items in one or two forms. The data entry task is then reduced to filling out these forms. The advantage of such forms is that users quickly familiarize themselves with the position of the various items and barely need to navigate through the system.

Even when a CPR user is highly specialized or is collecting data in the context of a specific study, users may still need to record patient findings beyond their primary domain of knowledge and interest. These incidental findings must also be recorded in the patient record. The wider the scope of the specialty, it is less possible to predict what will be found. A domain such as internal medicine is so vast that nearly all imaginable findings must be available to the physician. Hence, the CPR must also support SDE for large medical domains. A form-based approach is not suitable for that purpose. The number of potential findings is enormous, whereas a small, unpredictable number of findings may occur in a particular patient. A form that accommodates all potential findings would resemble a soccer field of boxes but with checkmarks in only a few of those. An all-inclusive approach would amount to a large number of forms to accommodate all potential findings. When users must browse through many forms, they may lose insight of the larger picture and conclude that SDE is highly inefficient. They will then probably decide to use the free-text option to present the bulk of their findings.

5.4 Dynamic SDE

When the domain is large and when the findings to be entered are unpredictable, forms ideally should be dynamic, which means that their options should automatically be tailored to the topic of interest. There are several techniques to achieve dynamic forms: using interactive screens, menus, icons, or combinations of these.

Menu-driven user interfaces are well known. In a menu-driven interface, the user chooses an item from a list, which may produce a new list from which another item can be chosen. This procedure repeats until the user indicates that he is finished. The menu offered next depends on the choice of the user.

When the use of sequential menus is the only way that data can be entered, the CPR user may face the problem of not knowing how to navigate through the

7

PANEL 7.5

Speech Recognition for Reporting of Medical Findings

An increasing number of clinicians are using a *speech recognition* system to streamline the reporting process. For instance, radiologists, pathologists, and other clinicians use it to report diagnostic imaging findings. Currently, most clinicians use dictation, a slow and expensive method that, due to delays in typing pools, may require days to produce a typed report. Because typing errors may be introduced, the documents must be reviewed by the clinician and mistakes must be corrected.

With a speech recognition system linked to, for example, a radiology information system, the physician can dictate, edit, and instantly create electronic reports. These reports are immediately available to other clinicians and can be integrated with electronic patient records. This leads, in principle, to a considerable saving of time, offering a better service and reducing costs.

At present, several companies provide speech recognition systems for a limited number of languages and medical professions, but each system has its own features. A speech recognition system can usually be installed on a personal computer, equipped with a microphone, with typically 16 to 32 megabytes of *random access memory*, required to run the program. The system records the speech signal; digitizes and processes the signal (see Chapters 8 and 25); compares the analyzed speech patterns with a collection of possible words, deciding which of these words is most likely to have been articulated (see Chapter 27); and finally, generates the written text. Information from three sources is used to recognize a word: a phoneme inventory, a pronunciation lexicon, and a language model, which contains syntactic and semantic information.

At present, 90 to 95% of words can be recognized correctly. Errors occur when words are wrongly classified and another word is recognized instead, words are not detected (*false negative*), or words that were not spoken are inserted (*false positive*). As a result, a certain number of errors must still be corrected. In this way the output of the system becomes more reliable. However, a number of limitations on today's speech recognition systems determine user acceptance: ▶

7

menus to reach a certain item. It is time-consuming and inefficient to have to browse through a number of menus to find the desired item. This problem can be solved by offering the option of shortcuts through the use of keywords. Although the combination of menu navigation and keywords enables "to-the-point" data entry, view of the entire record is poor: one can specify some topic in detail but must ascend the menu tree to describe the next topic.

5.5 Interfaces for SDE

A variety of methods have been applied to improve the efficiency of SDE. Some improvement to observing the entire record can be achieved by displaying several levels in the menu tree at once. Other applications use a combination of images and text. Icons can be used to symbolize an option for data entry (e.g., a stethoscope

* *Speaking rate*
A distinction can be made between discrete speech recognition and continuous speech recognition. Most existing systems can only recognize words when the clinician uses discrete speech, that is, by ensuring that each word has a clearly articulated beginning and end. This requires a slight pause between the words. Continuous speech recognition does not influence the natural speaking behavior of the user. Recent developments in speech recognition enable the system to identify the start and end of a word automatically.

* *Speaker dependency*
Speaker-dependent speech recognition systems require a training period during which the user "teaches" the computer his or her specific voice profile (see also Chapter 27). A voice profile contains information on individual pronunciation of various phonetic sounds. The recognition accuracy benefits from training the system.

* *Domain dependency*
A speech recognition system uses a vocabulary containing the words that the system needs for accurate recognition. The size of the vocabulary should be limited to obtain an acceptable speed in the speech recognition process. This is why a specific system can only recognize words within a specific domain. The vocabulary for radiology contains about 24,000 words.

* *The need for a knowledge base*
The repetitive nature of certain medical reports can be expressed in a *"knowledge base"* (see Chapters 15 to 17) by using *"triggers."* These triggers are used to produce an entire line, a paragraph, or even a full page of text by speaking one or only a few trigger words. In this case, the clinician must learn how to anticipate on what the computer is expecting to realize the most rapid report generation. Knowledge bases must be customized for each user.
In the future, speech recognition is expected to achieve a high accuracy in dictating medical reports, with an error percentage close to zero and requiring little or no special training. The clinician is then able to use free-form dictation by speaking naturally and continuously, without the need for a knowledge base. This makes speech recognition usable not only for certain standardized reports but also for all medical reports that a clinician must generate. Speech recognition should become speaker independent and work under any condition (e.g., in the presence of background noise). For the time being, our ears and brain are much better than any computer in understanding masses of analog speech information.

7

for physical examination). Images provide efficient data-entry devices for the user to indicate the location of findings, such as when the user localizes an obstruction in a picture of a coronary angiogram. No matter how the dynamic interface has been realized, it is always based on knowledge about potential medical descriptions. This knowledge has much in common with the domain knowledge necessary for medically meaningful NLP. Speech recognition can be useful in combination with SDE. Current applications for speech recognition are most reliable and effective when the domain involved is restricted, such as radiology reports (see also Panel 7.5). In combination with SDE, speech recognition can be applied to the options displayed on the screen, which constitute a very limited domain. To make a CPR efficient and attractive for physicians and nurses, it is essential to make optimal use of available interface techniques.

5.6 User-Adaptive SDE

Many clinicians describe their abnormal findings at a level of detail that they consider relevant, but they often express normal findings with phrases such as: "heart/lungs WNL" (within normal limits) or "abdomen normal." Such expressions denote a set of findings, but these may vary for each care provider. Most users develop their own style for history taking and physical examination. In daily practice, clinicians follow a certain pattern of actions, and they only go deeper into something when they encounter abnormalities during this first screening. One physician may use the expression "heart normal" to indicate a regular heartbeat and the absence of murmurs, whereas another physician may use the same expression to indicate the absence of ventricle enlargement as well.

For the collection of unambiguous data, users should be discouraged to use summarizing terms, but the presentation of an explicit description of all normal findings is extremely time-consuming and will quickly cause annoyance. The fairly constant nature of routine history taking and physical examination can be used to make an SDE application more efficient by expanding it with a feature that allows it to "learn" the meaning of "normal findings" for each physician or nurse, that is, to be user adapted. The application will ask the user to specify the meaning of a "normal statement" upon first use, and it will feed this specification back upon subsequent use of that same statement. In this way, efficiency and completeness of data input can be reconciled.

If the SDE in an application is supported in a more intelligent way, care providers will be more willing to accept it. For such intelligent support it is crucial that the program be based on semantic knowledge about potential descriptions of findings. The interface should be transparent and intuitive, and it should clearly distinguish between descriptive options and actually entered patient data.

6 Coding and Standardization

6.1 Exchangeability of Patient Data and Coded Data

Large-scale projects that involve multiple institutions, even at an international level, not only need structured and unambiguous data but also need semantic exchangeability of data. Coding systems, such as the International Classification of Diseases (*ICD*), the Systematized Nomenclature of Diseases (*SNOMED*), the **Read** code, and the **ICPC** are under continuous development in order to supply an internationally accepted vocabulary for the medical domain. The challenge is to obtain not only structured data but also a mapping of entered data onto these coding systems.

6.2 Nontextual Data

Many diagnostic techniques produce images and signals, such as X-ray equipment, CT scanning, or *magnetic resonance imaging*, *endoscopy*, anatomy, or pathology; Doppler *ultrasound* and *echocardiography*, *electrocardiograpy*, *electroencephalography*, *electromyography*, etc. So far, we have discussed the electronic equivalent of the paper-based record, which mostly contains reports of tests that also produce images and signals. All data collected for a certain patient are part of the patient's record. At present it is time-consuming for a clinician to obtain nontextual data. As a result, some clinicians only use the final reports for their decision making without referring to the source data. The availability of large electronic storage capacity at decreasing cost, as well as improvements in data transfer and exchange, brings a *multimedia patient record* within reach. Once different data formats and physical distances can be overcome, care providers will have the complete patient record at their disposal, including signals and images.

7 Representation of Time

Time plays a very important part in health care. The patient's course of disease unfolds over time, the physician's insight may evolve over time, and protocol-based care involves actions with specific intervals in between. Therefore, time stamping is essential. The patient record is a *chronological* account of observations, interpretations and interventions (see Chapter 1). The physician relies on time-related data for decision making, such as repeating a test or renewing a prescription. Time stamps are also essential for detecting trends, for example, in an intensive care unit or when following the condition of chronically ill patients. For instance, when the number of white blood cells seems to decrease, knowledge of the amount of time between two consecutive measurements is essential.

Time can be expressed in relative terms ("2 days after") or in absolute terms ("June 5th, 10:30 a.m."). Relative time is used in medical knowledge that must be applied to a particular situation and in, for example, descriptions of the course of disease. Absolute time is often associated with facts, such as the date of a visit or the date of a bone fracture.

Relative temporal expressions become practical only when they are applied to a concrete situation. Relative time can be expressed as *absolute time* as soon as the relationship with real time has been established. If a patient with measles shows the first signs of eruption on May 3, then it is expected that they will disappear between May 8 and 10. A clinical protocol often prescribes intervals for monitoring laboratory test results and the duration of certain medications. All these rules are expressed in relative time. Once the starting date of the protocol is known, it is possible to derive which steps need to be taken at what time.

Absolute time is not always preferable to relative time. On the contrary, it is often more difficult for a physician to interpret a series of calendar-oriented events than it is to apprehend the duration of various phases in a disease process. The key issue is that the relationship between relative and absolute time must

be known to offer the representation that is most suitable for the situation at hand.

For the purpose of decision making, data are interpreted within the context of medical knowledge. Interpretation of data and decision making can be difficult when time indications are inaccurate. This problem often occurs when one must rely on one's own memory. The order of a series of events can be very important, but it cannot always be derived from the available data in a reliable way. Computers can be used to perform temporal inferencing, provided that temporal data are recorded in an unambiguous fashion. Computer applications can monitor critical medical parameters and support adherence to a protocol. To take advantage of such applications, *time stamps* in the CPR must be recorded in a standardized format.

Temporal indications are also essential for the following two reasons:

1. The patient record must be a reliable reflection of reality, and because it is not legal to edit the data in a patient's record at a later date, there must be an option to record evolving insight.
2. Medical actions must always be interpreted in the proper context: a physician may not be held responsible for improper medical actions taken on the basis of insight that was available at a later time but that was not available at the time that those actions were taken.

A classic example of data where several time stamps are required are the laboratory tests:

1. the moment that the sample is taken,
2. the moment that the sample is tested, and
3. the moment that the test results are available to the physician.

A test result provides information about the sample at the time that it was taken. When too much time elapses between sampling and testing, the result may become invalid. It is also important that abnormal test results come to the physician's attention as soon

7

as possible. In short, there must be a standardized way to record the following for each piece of information in the patient record:

- when it was observed and by whom,
- when it was entered and by whom,
- the time that it begins to apply.

8 Clinical Use of the CPR

Despite all of the developments regarding the CPR during the last few decades, it is still only used on a small scale in most settings. The strong focus on the shortcomings of the paper-based record have pushed its strong aspects to the background. The paper-based record has five strong advantages and the CPR has seven principal strengths (Table 7.1). Apparently, most present CPR applications do not yet outweigh the advantages of the paper-based record. Familiarity with the current routine of using paper-based patient records plays an important part. Developers have understood that it is not sufficient to eliminate the limitations of the paper record; its

strengths must also come to expression in its electronic equivalent.

Introduction of the CPR in specialized care requires applications for use in inpatient as well as outpatient settings. Inpatient use of the CPR requires that the nursing record also become available in electronic format (see Chapter 14). An important problem of a logistic and financial nature involves data entry and display at the patient's bedside. Bedside computerized equipment is usually available only in intensive care units. Another option would be the use of portable equipment, preferably with a wireless connection to the host system.

Advantages of paper records	
1.	They can easily be carried around,
2.	Much freedom in reporting style,
3.	Easy data browsing,
4.	Requires no special training, and
5.	Never 'down' as computers sometimes are.

Advantages of CPRs	
1.	Simultaneous access from multiple locations,
2.	Legibility,
3.	Variety of views on data,
4.	Support of structured data entry (SDE)
5.	Decision support,
6.	Support of other data analysis,
7.	Electronic data exchange and sharing care support

Table 7.1
Advantages of Paper-Based and Computer-Based Patient Records.

7

8.1 Other Uses of the CPR

Nonacademic medical centers will not usually be attracted to the CPR for its potential for use in research. However, it is to be expected that hospital management, insurance companies, and government institutions will pose a greater demand on patient data (e.g., for the assessment of quality of care). A CPR is almost indispensable for the efficient delivery of data to other parties. Eventually, data for direct patient care and other purposes will have to be collected in one patient record. User acceptance requires a gradual migration from the present situation to a new one. Therefore, the collection of structured data must be encouraged, but not enforced. Users will have to be strongly involved in CPR development. They must recognize their desires and preferences in the final product. Consequently, the development of a CPR must be a concerted action of designers, implementers, and end users. Many user requests involve routine tasks such as billing, correspondence, and printouts of prescriptions. The CPR can only be used to its full potential when it has been used long enough to contain important data about the majority of a practice's patients.

Clinicians will have to make an investment before they can take advantage of powerful and flexible overviews, decision support, electronic communication, and shared records.

The greatest challenge is the tension between effort and benefit. It should be kept in mind that users will invest in the quality of their patient records only if it is rewarding.

8.2 Multimedia Patient Records

In recent years increasing interest has been shown in making the CPR more complete by adding images and signals: the so-called multimedia patient record (*MPR*; see also Chapter 20). In practice, the development and installation of one integrated solution did not appear feasible. The reason is not only the size and complexity of such a project and the required scope of expertise, but also the fact that healthcare institutions are reluctant to do away with their current equipment and invest in new systems. An MPR should be achieved as much as possible by using existing systems and software and by the gradual introduction of this new technology. This requires the integration of existing systems with new applications to supply the functionality of the MPR. Expertise in networking, communication, and integration is needed. Yet, it is apparent that currently used software varies greatly in type and age and that the task is complicated by the large number of old applications that do not meet present standards for data transfer and communication. (Integration and communication are discussed in Chapter 5.) At this stage, however, the aspects of user acceptance and financial and logistic problems outweigh the technical problems, and *NLP* and *SDE* also face many obstacles.

Key References

Dick R.S. and E.B. Steen, eds. 1991. The Computer-based Patient Record. An Essential Technology for Health Care. Washington DC: National Academy Press.

Rector AL, Nowlan WA, Kay S et al. Foundations for an electronic medical record. Meth Inform Med 1991;30:179-86.

Weed L. *Medical Records, Medical Education and Patient Care.* Cleveland OH: Case Western Univ Press, 1969.

See the Web site for further literature references.

7

8 Biosignal Analysis

1. Introduction

All living things, from cells to organisms, deliver signals of biological origin. Such signals can be electric (e.g., the **depolarization** of a nerve cell or the heart muscle), mechanical (e.g., the sound generated by heart valves), or chemical (e.g., the PCO_2 in the blood). Such biological signals – in short, **biosignals** – can be of interest for diagnosis, for patient monitoring, and biomedical research.

Throughout their lifetimes, living organisms generate an abundant stream of signals, often hidden in a background of other signals and noise components. The main goal of processing biosignals is to filter the signal of interest out from the noisy background and to reduce the redundant data stream to only a few, but relevant, parameters. Such parameters must be significant for medical decision making, for example, to solve a medical problem or to increase insight into the underlying biological process. In this respect we refer to what was said in Chapter 1 about the use of data to obtain information and to acquire knowledge (see also Fig. 1.1). The purpose of biosignal processing is the derivation of **information** from the data (the signals), as was also explained in Chapter 2.

In parallel to the stages depicted in Fig. 1.2, the processing of biosignals usually consists of at least four stages (see Fig. 8.1):

1. *measurement or observation, that is, signal acquisition,*
2. *transformation and reduction of the signals,*
3. *computation of signal parameters that are diagnostically significant, and*
4. *interpretation or **classification** of the signals.*

In the first stage, signal acquisition, we use **transducers** to obtain electric signals that can be processed by computers. At the signal acquisition stage, chemical or mechanical signals are *transduced* into electrical form, and signals that are already electric are picked up by electrodes. At that first stage it is of great importance to maintain a signal **entropy** that is as low as possible, that is, to obtain signals with low disturbance, namely, a high **signal-to-noise ratio** (see Chapter 25). Once the signals have been transduced to electrical form, they are made digital (**digitized**) so that they can be processed by computers (see Section 4 below).

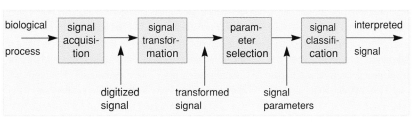

Figure 8.1
The four stages of biosignal processing. The first two stages deal with the *syntax* of the signal; the last two stages deal with the *semantic* signal properties.

8

In the second stage, we want to reshape (*transform*) the signals in such a way that we can derive semantic parameters in the third stage. The second step is also called *preprocessing*. The signals contain many more data than are actually needed to derive parameters that offer semantic information. This is called **redundancy**. For instance, to diagnose **left bundle-branch block** from an electrocardiogram (**ECG**), a physician requires only one to three ECG complexes, instead of the many complexes that are usually recorded. However, to diagnose certain types of cardiac arrhythmias, several hours of ECG recordings are sometimes needed, (e.g., those acquired during so-called **Holter** monitoring). Sometimes the data redundancy is used to eliminate the noise components, for instance, by **filtering** (see also Chapter 25). In short: during the preprocessing or transformation stage we want:

1. to decrease the disturbance, and
2. to reduce the amount of data so that we can compute the diagnostically most significant parameters.

The third stage delivers semantically relevant parameters (also called **features**) that can be used as inputs for further decision making. In a way, such parameters bear resemblance to the signs and symptoms that are used to make a diagnosis (see Chapter 15). Such signal features should therefore have discriminatory power, for example, to find out whether the patient has disease A or disease B, or whether there is a trend in the disease process. The features are extracted by sometimes rather complex signal processing methods. These methods show many parallels with the methods that are used in i**mage processing** (see Chapter 10). Once the signal parameters have been obtained, they are used for human or computer-assisted decision making in the interpretation stage.

The interpretation or classification stage of biosignal processing does not differ essentially from the methods that are used in **pattern recognition** (Chapter 27) or in other diagnostic support methods: they can have a logical basis, follow heuristic reasoning, be of statistical origin, or be a combination of different methods (see Chapter 15).

This chapter next discusses the characteristics and the different types of biosignals, sampling methods and **analog-to-digital** conversion, and application areas of biosignal analysis. The aim is to offer some insight into signal processing methods while trying to avoid the use of too complex mathematical formalisms. A more elaborate discussion of signal processing methods is presented in Chapter 25.

2. Characteristics of Biosignals

Biosignals are derived from biological processes observed in medicine. Such processes are highly complex and dynamic. Biosignals are usually (not always) a function of time. For example, they can be expressed as *s(t)*, with *s* being the signal and *t* the time. Some signals can be described by a few parameters only. A sine wave *s(t)*, for instance, could be defined as $s(t) = A \sin(\omega t + \phi)$. Only three parameters (the amplitude *A*, the frequency ω, and the phase ϕ) suffice to fully describe *s(t)*. Once we know the parameters, the signal waveshape is fully determined. However, when the signal *s(t)* is corrupted by noise *n(t)* (as seen in Chapter 2, $m(t) = s(t) + n(t)$) the behavior of the signal can then, at best, be statistically predicted.

In contrast to mathematically determined signals, such as sine waves, biosignals can seldom be described by a few parameters only, and the latter are generally characterized by a large variability. If the biological processes that generate the signals are in a dynamic state, that is, are continuously changing, their behavior can seldom be accurately predicted; the parameters describing the signals change continuously. For instance, for a patient in an intensive care unit, parameters that describe the function of the heart and circulation, the lungs and respiration, blood chemistry and the hormonal system may vary continuously. Therefore, the signals derived from such processes reflect the dynamic and **nonstationary** character of such processes.

8

A classification of biosignals according to waveshape and stationarity is related to the type of process from which they are derived, whether it is dynamic or not and whether it shows a repetitive behavior or not. The next section describes the different types of signals encountered in biological processes.

3. Types of Signals

As remarked above, this chapter primarily deals with signals that are variables as a function of time. These signals can be classified as **stationary** or **nonstationary**, and the signal waveshapes can de **deterministic** or **statistical** (or stochastic) (see Fig. 8.2).

3.1 Deterministic Waveforms

Biological processes that show some repetitive character, such as a beating heart or respiration, generate signals that are also repetitive. Such signals often show a more or less deterministic waveform. Deterministic signals can be periodic, quasiperiodic, aperiodic, or simply transient. In living organisms, purely periodic signals (such signals are essentially only mathematically defined, such as a sine wave) are not seen. Therefore, the term *quasiperiodic* or even *aperiodic* is better used to describe a repetitive biological signal. An example of an aperiodic signal is, for instance, the signal that can be picked up from the blinking eyes, the electro-oculogram. A depolarizing cell, triggered by some stimulus, also generates an electric signal (a **depolarization** and **repolarization** wave), which is called a **transient** signal.

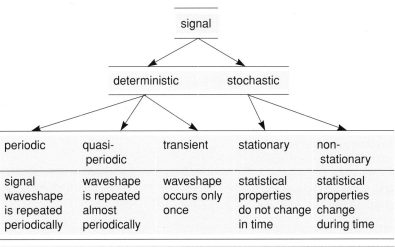

signal				
deterministic			stochastic	
periodic	quasi-periodic	transient	stationary	non-stationary
signal waveshape is repeated periodically	waveshape is repeated almost periodically	waveshape occurs only once	statistical properties do not change in time	statistical properties change during time

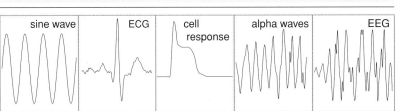

sine wave	ECG	cell response	alpha waves	EEG

Figure 8.2
Types of biological signals classified into two main groups: the deterministic and the stochastic (or statistical) signals. The deterministic group is subdivided into periodic, quasiperiodic, and transient signals; the stochastic signals are subdivided into stationary and nonstationary signals.

8

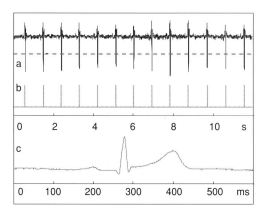

Figure 8.3
Point process (b) derived from a band-pass-filtered ECG (a). The noise-free ECG can, in principle, be restored from the point process and the waveshape of one P-QRS-T complex only (c).

A separate group of deterministic signals are the **point processes** that can be described as an impulse series $\delta(t)$. A point process can be considered a binary signal, which is most of the time "0", and, when some event occurs it very briefly becomes "1" (see Fig. 8.3b). Point processes are not generated by a biological process, although the pacemaker impulses in the **SA** and the **AV** nodes of the heart could be considered point processes. In point processes, the shape of the signal is not of interest; what is of interest is the instant that some event occurred, such as the start of the depolarization in the ventricles, indicated by the onset of a **QRS** complex in an ECG (Fig. 8.3a), or the moment that the eye blinks.

If a signal waveshape $w(t)$ reoccurs quasiperiodically, such as the **P-QRS-T** complex in an ECG, it is in principle possible to reconstruct the entire ECG from the point process $\delta(t)$ representing the times of occurrence of the ECG complexes and the waveshape $w(t)$ of one

ECG complex only (Fig. 8.3c). All other complexes can then be considered redundant since they give no extra information. This is different in case of multiple waveshapes, for example, when the ECG shows multifocal extrasystoles.

3.2 Stochastic Waveforms

Another group of signals are the stochastic, or statistical, signals. They are generated, for instance, by groups of cells that depolarize in a more or less random fashion, such as muscle cells (generating the electromyogram (**EMG**)) or nerve cells in the **cortex** (generating the electroencephalogram (**EEG**)). The waveshape of such signals bears a nondeterministic character and can be described only in statistical terms. Dependent on the type of biological process, these stochastic signals are stationary or nonstationary. In the case of stationarity, the signal *properties* do not change over time[1], for instance, when a patient is in a stable condition.

The discrimination between stationary and nonstationary signals is of interest. If the biological process is in a dynamic state, we may expect that the signals that are generated are also nonstationary. An example is the EEG derived from a patient during an epileptic seizure. The parameters that can be derived from nonstationary signals (e.g., from patients in an intensive care unit) can be plotted as a function of time, which is called **trend analysis**.

---

[1] *There are different types of stationarity, depending on the statistical parameters that do not change over time. For a* **widely stationary** *signal, for instance, the mean and the dispersion do not change as a function of time*

8

4. Analog-to-Digital Conversion

All biosignals are analog variables. Therefore, before they can be processed by computers, they must be **digitized** (quantitated or discretized). This is done by

analog-to-digital conversion. When done correctly, no information is lost, and the original analog signal can even be restored from the digital one by **digital-to-**

PANEL 8.1

Sampling of Signals: How Often?

Without exception, all biosignals are analog signals. Processing of biosignals by computers therefore requires discretization (i.e., sampling and quantification). This panel explains the *sampling process* without referring to formulas.

The *sampling theorem* mathematically phrased by Shannon and Nyquist states that a signal must be sampled at a rate at least twice the rate of the highest-frequency component present in the signal. If we use a sampling rate that is too low, the signal is distorted. If we obey the sampling theorem, the complete *syntactic information content* of the signal is retained. This is illustrated by the following example.

An EEG usually contains statistical, more or less sine wave-shaped fluctuations that may occur at a rate of up to 30 times/second. This can also be expressed by saying that the EEG contains frequencies up to 30 Hz. Higher frequencies may also be present (e.g., from other signal sources) but these are generally not of semantic interest.

The sampling theorem then prescribes that we should sample the EEG at least at 2 x 30 = 60 Hz to keep all signal properties. Table 8.1 gives the frequency bandwidths of interest and the most commonly used sampling rates for some biosignals. For instance, for ECGs (bandwidth, 0.15-150 Hz) a sampling rate above the Shannon frequency (500 Hz) is most often used. If we obey the rule of the sampling theorem it is, in principle, possible to restore the original analog signal by digital-to-analog conversion.

---

analog conversion. Based on this principle, the compact disk can store digital images or sound that can be restored to visible pictures and audible sound. Computers operate with discrete signals only. Discrete signals are derived from analog signals by **sampling** (see Panel 2.3). In sampling, the amplitudes of the analog signal are measured (in principle) at equidistant intervals and are converted to discrete values, that are

Signal	Bandwidth (Hz)	Amplitude range	Quantization (bits)
Electroencephalogram	0.2-50	600 μV	4-6
Electrooculogram	0.2-15	10 mV	4-6
Electrocardiogram	0.15-150	10 mV	10-12
Electromyogram	20-8000	10 mV	4-8
Blood pressure	0-60	400 mm Hg	8-10
Spirogram	0-40	10 L	8-10
Phonocardiogram	5-2000	80 dB	8-10

Table 8.1
Bandwidths, Amplitude Ranges, and Quantization of Some Frequently Used Biosignals.

8

PANEL 8.2

Sampling of Signals: How Accurate?

When sampling a signal, we use an *analog-to-digital converter* (A-D converter or ADC). Samples are taken at a rate at least twice the rate of the highest-frequency component contained in the signal (i.e., the mixture of signal plus noise, unless the noise has been filtered out beforehand), and the samples are quantitated and expressed as numbers. The latter is always done with a limited accuracy and may, in principle, add so-called quantization noise to the sampled signal. This quantization noise should generally not exceed the noise that is already present in the signal, or, as expressed in more general terms, discretization by the ADC should not increase the information entropy (see Chapter 2); syntactic and semantic signal properties should be left intact.

The degree of quantization can be expressed as the number of quantization steps for the range of possible amplitude values. If the signal amplitude spans a range of A volts (e.g., from $-A/2$ to $+A/2$) and the quantization step is Δq, then the number of quantization steps is $m = A/\Delta q$. In practice, let m be a power of 2: $m = 2^n$, so that the quantization of the ADC can be expressed in n bits. For instance, an ADC with an accuracy of 10 bits can discern $2^{10} = 1024$ different amplitude levels, resulting in a resolution of about 0.1%, expressed as a percentage of the signal range A. An ADC that delivers samples with 8-bit accuracy ($2^8 = 256$ steps) is called an 8-bit ADC. A 1-bit ADC only determines the sign of the signal (or whether it is larger or lower than some threshold).

For most biosignals a 6- to 12-bit ADC is sufficient; a 12-bit ADC implies a resolution of 1/4096 (less than 0.025%), related to a signal-to-noise ratio which is far superior to that attainable with most signal *transducers*.

---

expressed as binary numbers. The latter is also called *quantization* or *quantification*. This sampling and quantization is done in an *analog-to-digital converter* (ADC or A-D converter). When f_s is the **sampling frequency**, then the **sampling interval** $\Delta T = 1/f_s$. The more changes per second there are in the signal (i.e., the higher the frequency content of the signal; see Chapter 25), the higher the sampling frequency must be.

Chapter 2 gave an example of the information content of a sampled signal but did not discuss the sampling process itself. Two main questions must be answered when sampling biosignals:

1. *How often* must sampling be done?
2. *How accurately* do the amplitudes have to be quantified?

The former is expressed in samples per second, and the latter is expressed in numbers of bits. This is explained in Panels 8.1 and 8.2, which elaborate on discretization, sampling, and quantification. Table 8.1 gives the amplitude ranges and the required accuracies of some known biosignals.

4.1 How Often?

For proper sampling it is important that no information be lost (i.e., the signal entropy should not increase) so that the signal interpretation will not be hampered. A sampling rate that is too low may cause information loss (see Fig. 8.4); a sampling rate that is too high is redundant and does not offer extra information but requires more computer memory. Take the following examples:

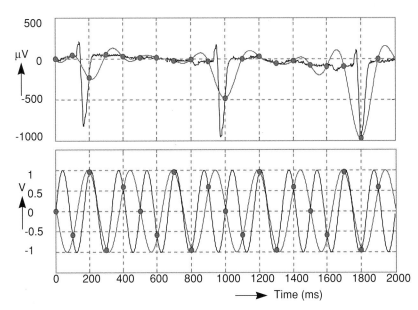

Figure 8.4
Effect of sampling frequencies that are too low to see the correct waveshapes of two signals, showing that information is lost for (a) an ECG and (b) a sine wave. The original signal is indicated with a black line, the signal that is sampled at a frequency that is too low is indicated with a red line. The sampling points that are taken with a frequency that is too low are indicated in red. As can be seen, in both signals certain amplitude values are lost.

- It is inappropriate to measure a patient's blood pressure every millisecond at a resolution of tenths of mm Hg. In healthy people, when the circulation is in a relatively stable state, it is sufficient to sample the blood pressure, at most, once a year, or even less frequently.
- When the physical condition of a patient is examined on a bicycle ergometer, the blood pressure will be measured, for example, every 3 minutes, because a higher workload causes a higher heart rate and a higher cardiac output, and consequently, the blood pressure changes faster.
- For a patient on a post-cardiac surgery unit, the blood pressure is measured arterially at every cardiac beat because of the possible unstable condition of the patient.

Apparently, the question *How often?* depends on the dynamic properties of the underlying biological process, our interest in the meaning of the signal parameters (their semantic information content; Chapter 2), and their use for therapy (the pragmatic aspect; for instance, to control the blood pressure during patient monitoring).

In determining the correct sampling frequency, we follow the **Shannon-Nyquist** theorem, which states that:

A signal should be sampled at a rate that is at least twice the rate of the highest frequency component present in the signal.

A higher sampling frequency causes **redundancy** (i.e., higher cost but no information loss), and a lower frequency causes signal distortion and a possible loss of semantic information content. Panel 8.1 further explains the relationship between sampling rate and frequency content of some biosignals.

Sometimes, the true frequency content of biosignals cannot be estimated because small waveforms cannot be discriminated from the noise. Furthermore, small waveforms (such as **Q-waves** in ECGs) contribute almost nothing to the power of the signal. To keep the error of the peak amplitude of a small waveform component in a signal less than 10%, as a rule of fist, the sampling interval should be shorter than about 10% of the duration of this small waveform component.

4.2 How Accurate?

For some biosignals, the amplitude must be measured with a resolution of about 1% of the amplitude range

8

of the signal; for others a resolution of even 10% is sufficient. We give some examples:

- For ECGs, Q-wave amplitudes should be measured with a resolution of 20 mV or less, because the presence of a Q-wave (e.g., in lead I or aVF) can indicate the presence of an infarction.
- For EEGs, the amplitude itself is generally not of interest, but changes in average amplitudes over time might reveal changes in the underlying process.

If signals are not sampled at a sufficiently high sampling rate and if the amplitudes are not measured accurately enough, the signals will be distorted and it may then be impossible to derive the necessary parameters. Figure 8.4 shows the effects of a sampling frequency that is too low.

This short description of analog-to-digital conversion can be concluded as follows:

Discretization of analog variables, such as biosignals, is possible without a loss of information. The sampling rate is determined by the frequency content of the signal and should be at least twice the rate of the highest frequency component present in the signal. The degree of quantization is determined by the required accuracy of the parameters that are to be computed from the signal. Panel 8.2 further explains the quantification of biosignals.

5 Application Areas of Biosignal Analysis

Methods for the processing and interpretation of biosignals are in continuous evolution, mainly due to the constantly changing information technology. Biosignal processing and interpretation comprise a wide variety of different applications. Here are a few examples:

- *Function analysis*, which is done in diagnostic units for *EMG* or *EEG* analysis, or for the *ECG*, the *phonocardiogram*, the *spirogram*, and so on.
- *Population screening*. The same type of signal processing used for function analysis is also encountered in biosignal applications for population screening.
- *On-line analysis*, which takes place in situations in which the patient is closely monitored such as in units for intensive or coronary care, peri- or postsurgical care, and perinatal care. Another example of on-line analysis is the control of prostheses by still intact nerves or muscle ends.
- *Basic research*. For more fundamental research, such as in physiology, signal processing can be used to analyze neuronal or cell depolarizations or the computation of the cardiac depolarization wavefront.

In dealing with biological processes, there are roughly four different situations in which we are confronted with categories of signal analysis (as depicted in Fig. 8.5). Figure 8.5 shows, from top to bottom, how insight into the process increases. These four categories of signal analysis are discussed below.

1. Output signals only
   The most common situation is one in which we deal with a biological process that only delivers output signals (Fig. 8.5a). We have no or only marginal knowledge of the process delivering the signals. The approach to be followed in analyzing the signals is mainly empirical. A representative example of this situation is EEG analysis.

2. Evoked signals
   Some of the inputs to the process under investigation may already be known, or we can even offer an input signal or stimulus (Fig. 8.5b). Ideally, we are then able to gain insight into the state of the biolo-

gical process. Examples of this situation are **evoked responses** in EEG examinations or mechanical or electrical stimulation of cells, nerves, and muscles.

3. Provocative tests

   A further category involves situations in which we want to test the biological process under some forced or at least known condition (Fig. 8.5c), sometimes combined with a known input stimulus. Many provocative tests fall in this group, such as physical exercise tests in which we measure ECG **ST-T** parameters or spirographic signal parameters, EEG analysis during anesthesia, or atrial pacing during catheterization.

4. Modeling

   In those cases in which sufficient knowledge about the process is available, we may be able to develop a model of the biological process (Fig. 8.5d), for example, modeling of parts of the circulation or cardiac **depolarization**. Such models are used either for research and education or for the estimation of signal parameters. The arrow indicates feedback control to the model or the process.

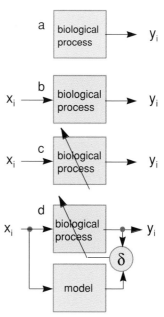

Figure 8.5
Four different situations in biosignal processing: output signal only (a), evoked signals (b), provocative test (c), and process modeling (d).

Many data flow from the patient via transducers to the nurse or the physician both for function analysis and for on-line monitoring. This flow should be reduced, channeled, and documented, for which the computer is the ideal vehicle. The sophistication level of the data acquisition equipment is steadily increasing, since most signal processing equipment is integrated with microcomputers.

Signals offer parameters that support medical decision making and trend analysis. This decision making is increasingly based on objective and numerical measurements instead of subjective observations. Biosignals are examples of objective measurements that may be used as inputs for intervention rules during monitoring. This increased objectivity may lead to the reduction of human errors.

Key References

See Chapter 25

8

9 Medical Imaging

1 Introduction

Medical imaging is to a large extent impossible without the use of computers. It is based on physical principles that immediately render an image or is based on sometimes intensive computer processing of measurements. Computers are applied in medical imaging to:

- construct an image from measurements,
- obtain an image reconstructed for optimal extraction of a particular feature from an image,
- present images,
- improve image quality by image processing (discussed in Chapters 10 and 26), and
- store and retrieve images (Chapter 13).

In medical imaging, images of organisms, organs, or of parts of organs, are generated by means of radiation. This radiation is often of an electromagnetic (*EM*) nature. After image formation, the images must be displayed for interpretation. The display medium can be the original image carrier, for example, a processed film on which the image was formed, or another carrier, such as a photograph or a computer display monitor. Figure 9.1 presents the spectrum of EM radiation and the part of the spectrum used for each type of application. Other types of radiation are also referred to in Fig. 9.1, such as ultrasound and electrons. The Figure also indicates, for instance, that electrical

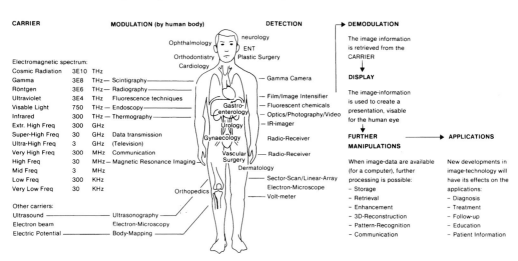

Figure 9.1
Overview of the use of electromagnetic radiation for medical applications (E4 stands for 10^4) (after Philips).

potentials can be visualized in the form of body surface maps.

It is possible to use visualization techniques to produce images of phenomena that in themselves are not directly visible. The following sections explain the principles of image formation. First, we describe ultrasound, an important example of non-EM radiation; then we discuss radiology applications using various types of EM radiation. We do not discuss imaging procedures that use visible light, such as endoscopy.

2. Ultrasound

Ultrasound is produced by *piezoelectric* crystals that transform electrical energy into acoustic energy and vice versa. These crystals can vibrate with frequencies of about 2 to 10 MHz, frequencies much higher than those present in audible sound (maximum of 20 kHz). The principles of ultrasound are similar to those of radar and sonar. Pulsed sound waves are emitted, and the energies and arrival times of the received echoes caused by the reflections are measured. The main interest lies in determining the distance between the ultrasound source and possible reflectors. When suitably displayed, anatomical images of the investigated area can be obtained.

The distance between the source and the reflector can be computed by multiplying the time interval between emission of the sound-wave pulse and the detection of the echo coming from a reflector by the sound velocity and then dividing the result by two. The accuracy of the distance measurement depends on the duration of the emitted pulse: the shorter this pulse, the higher the accuracy. A pulse contains one or two wavelengths. Reflectors that are at least this distance apart can therefore be discerned. The ability to discern two reflectors that are positioned behind each other is called the axial resolution.

The cross section of the emitted beam must be small so that the location of the reflections can be determined accurately: with a broader beam more locations at the measured distance from the source may cause a diffuse echo. However, the diameter of the crystal must be minimally 10 to 20 times the wavelength to obtain a directed beam. Further details on *echo scanners* are given in Panel 9.1.

2.1 A-Mode

Visualization of reflections can be performed in several ways. A distinction can be made between one- and two-dimensional ways of visualization. In the *amplitude mode* (*A-mode*) the energy of each echo is displayed as a function of the time interval between the pulse and the echo. The amplitude of the echo is displayed along the vertical axis, whereas the horizontal axis represents time. The time interval between the pulse and the echo corresponds to the distance between the transducer and the reflecting tissue boundary. Moving boundaries are visible as echo amplitudes that move horizontally along the time axis. The A-mode provides one-dimensional information about the location of the reflecting boundaries. The beam has a certain direction, and only the echoes of those boundaries that intersect the beam are detected.

2.2 M-Mode and B-Mode

The *motion mode* (*M-mode*) is similar to the A-mode; it also provides one-dimensional information. In this case, however, the amplitude of each echo, belonging to an individual pulse, is represented as the brightness of the point located along the time axis, corresponding to the arrival time of the echo. This is also called brightness mode (*B-mode*) which in this case provides one-dimensional location information. The other axis is now used to display the echoes of subsequent pulses. In this presentation, one coordinate therefore indicates the depth in the patient and

9

PANEL 9.1

Principle of Echo Scanners

In echo scanners, sound pulses are generated with frequencies of about a few MHz. These pulses are absorbed, scattered, or reflected in the patient. The reflections give rise to relatively strong echoes.

Reflections occur at interfaces between media that are different with respect to density and/or the velocity of sound (sound is reflected at interfaces with different acoustic impedances; the so-called acoustic impedance is equal to the product of sound velocity and density). Soft tissue and water have about equal densities and sound has about equal velocities in the two media. Therefore, most of the sound waves are not reflected at their interface. At an interface between soft tissue on one side and bone or air on the other side, a strong reflection is observed.

Scattering takes place if the dimension of the object is small (i.e, about the wavelength of the incident radiation). The beam is then scattered in all directions, and therefore, the amplitude of the signal detected by the transducer is relatively small.

The resolution of an echo scan, that is, the degree with which details located close together can still be distinguished, is determined by both the wavelength of the sound waves and the duration of the emitted pulse. The pulse is usually several wavelengths long. In practice, therefore, reflections from two points separated by a few wavelengths can be discriminated. The smaller the wavelength the better the resolution. Since the wavelength is inversely proportional to the frequency, the resolution is proportional to the frequency.

The *attenuation coefficient* (which expresses how much the beam is attenuated per centimeter of tissue because of scatter and absorption) is also proportional to the sound frequency for soft tissue and is even proportional to the square of the frequency for other types of tissues. Therefore, the depth of penetration of the sound waves is inversely proportional to the frequency. The more the beam is attenuated, the more difficult it is to measure the reflections of deeper structures, since the signal-to-noise ratio (see Chapter 25) gradually becomes smaller. Since resolution and penetration depth pose contradictory requirements, a compromise must be made: deeper structures can only be visualized with relatively low frequencies, with a concomitant lower resolution. Also, the type of tissue influences the amount of absorption of the beam. Air and bone, for example, are strong absorbers, whereas muscle tissue and water hardly attenuate the beam.

At a frequency of 3 MHz (wavelength of 0.5 mm) depths of up to 10 cm are well visualized, with an axial resolution on the order of 1 mm. For eye examinations a higher resolution is needed. In this case frequencies of between 5 and 13 MHz (wavelengths of between 0.25 and 0.075 mm, respectively) are used. For brain examinations the sound beam must first pass bone structures (e.g., the tempora). Because of the high absorption of bone, especially for high frequencies, only low frequencies can be used, implying a lower resolution.

the other coordinate indicates time, so that it is possible to visualize the movement of objects that are crossed by the ultrasonic beam. In this way, for instance, the movements of heart valves can be observed by following the corresponding points as they move along the time axis.

9

2.3 C-Scan

Boundaries that are not perpendicular to the beam axis produce weak echoes. Therefore, A-, B-, and M-mode applications that have fixed beam directions do not display all boundaries equally well. In a *compound scan* (*C-scan*) the crystal can be moved so that the direction of the beam is changed. The crystal is connected to a flexible arm that is linked to a fixed point of reference. Rotation transducers are present in the arm so that it is always possible to establish the position of the crystal and the direction of the beam. Because of the movements of the crystal, part of the boundary will probably be crossed by the beam from several directions, including a direction perpendicular to it, thus producing a large echo. Although the quality of the C-scan is high, it has the disadvantage of taking a few seconds to build up the image, making it impossible to follow moving structures.

2.4 Sector Scan

The movement of the transducer can be sped up by mechanical means. In parallel scanning the crystal is moved in such a way that the beam is continuously shifted in a certain direction until a complete area of interest has been scanned. This procedure results in a parallel scan. By another way of scanning, a *sector scan* is obtained: each successive beam makes a small angle with the previous one (Fig. 9.2). In both cases two-dimensional images are obtained, in which the intensity of the image represents the amplitude of the echo (two-dimensional B-mode).

Instead of working with a moving, single crystal, it is also possible to use a stationary probe containing a linear array of about 100 crystals. When these crystals are electrically activated one after the other, a parallel scan can be produced in any direction. The data are usually stored in a memory, and therefore, they can first be corrected and processed before being displayed. In this way, distances between certain boundaries can be obtained or displacements of vessels can be measured.

2.5 Doppler Effect

For the measurement of flow velocities the **Doppler effect** is used. When a sound wave is reflected by a target that has a velocity component in the direction of the sound beam, the frequency of the reflected sound wave is higher when the target approaches the sound source or lower when the target recedes from the sound source. The shift in frequency is proportional to the frequency of the incident beam and to the velocity of the target. In normal Doppler applications a continuous stream of sound is generated by a transmitter, and another transducer is necessary to detect the reflected sound waves. Because of the continuous transmission of sound waves the distance from the target to the transmitter cannot be determined: everything that moves inside the beam contributes to the Doppler signal. In modern equipment the Doppler shift can also be determined by pulsed sound. In that case only one transducer is necessary. By using sound pulses it is possible to take into account the reflections from a certain sample volume only. By repositioning the sample volume of the transducer in a systematic way, a two-dimensional velocity distribution can be determined (a flow map). The *flow map* can be superimposed on the echo image (color-coded flow mapping). In this way, flow information and anatomical information are presented simultaneously.

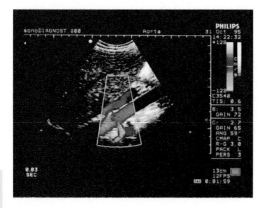

Figure 9.2
Sector scan by ultrasound of part of the aorta.

2.6 Advantages of Ultrasound

The use of ultrasound has the advantage that it has no harmful side effects. Therefore, the echo scan is an important technique for examining pregnant women and young children.

Ultrasound applications include, among others:

- determination of heart function,
- examination of the brain
- obstetric examinations,
- eye examinations,
- determination of the perfusion of tissues, and
- detection of tumors and cysts.

3. Radiology

Since their discovery in 1895 by Roentgen, *X rays* have increasingly been used for diagnostic purposes. In this section we discuss the way in which computers have enhanced the capabilities of X-ray systems. The presentation will not be in a chronological order, but will emphasize the extensions that have resulted from using computers, ranging from relatively simple applications in which an existing function is now supported by a computer to complex ones in which computers enable new applications of X rays that are unlikely to be achieved in a conventional way. The relatively simple applications include computed radiology and digital subtraction angiography (DSA). The more com-

plex applications include computed tomography (CT). Although not based on X rays, magnetic resonance imaging (MRI) will be discussed in this section as well (see Section 3.4 and Panel 9.3).

3.1 Imaging by Means of X rays

A beam of X rays is generated by an X-ray tube. The cross section of the beam is shaped by a diaphragm. The beam is directed toward the part of a patient that has to be examined. Behind the patient, the transmit-

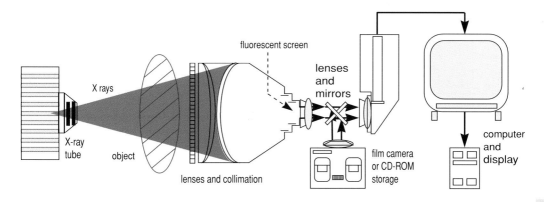

Figure 9.3

Principle of an X-ray system with image intensifier. X rays impinging on the image intensifier are transformed into a distribution of electrons, which produces an amplified light image on a smaller fluorescent screen after acceleration. The image is observed by a television camera and a film camera and can be viewed on a computer screen and stored on a CD-ROM or a PACS.

9

ted X rays are detected with the help of a fluoroscopic screen that produces visible light that in turn exposes a film (film-screen combination) or by a fluoroscopic screen that can be viewed directly or with an image intensifier.

The attenuation of the X-ray beam depends on the type of tissue (its density and its chemical composition) and on the amount of tissue traversed. Lung tissue attenuates the X rays much less than bone. The X-ray beam will have a much lower intensity behind a rib than behind an intercostal space. A silver halide film is too insensitive for X rays to record this large contrast. This low sensitivity was overcome by employing film-

screen combinations. These are sandwich-like structures with layers comprising one or two luminescent screens and a silverhalide film.

The intensity distribution of the transmitted beam can be transformed into an electric signal with the help of an image intensifier. A fluorescent screen in the image intensifier transforms the X-ray distribution into a charge distribution of electrons. These electrons are accelerated and then directed to a second, smaller fluorescent screen, on which an amplified light image appears. This image is then recorded by a television camera or by a film camera. The television signal can also be used to *digitize* the image (Fig. 9.3).

Images can also be generated on a storage phosphor plate instead of on a screen-film combination. The latent image stored on the phosphor plate can be read out by a laser scanner. In this way, digital X-ray images (in short: X-rays) are directly obtained. This is called *computed radiology* or digital radiology. The images on film can also be digitized with a laser film digitizer. The techniques mentioned above all yield so-called *shadow images*. On the film or television monitor we cannot discriminate the various structures that are successively passed by the beam. Also, the **contrast** is not always good enough to visualize, for example, blood vessels. In the next section we discuss DSA. This procedure also makes use of shadow images, but it enhances contrast by subtracting bone structures from the image.

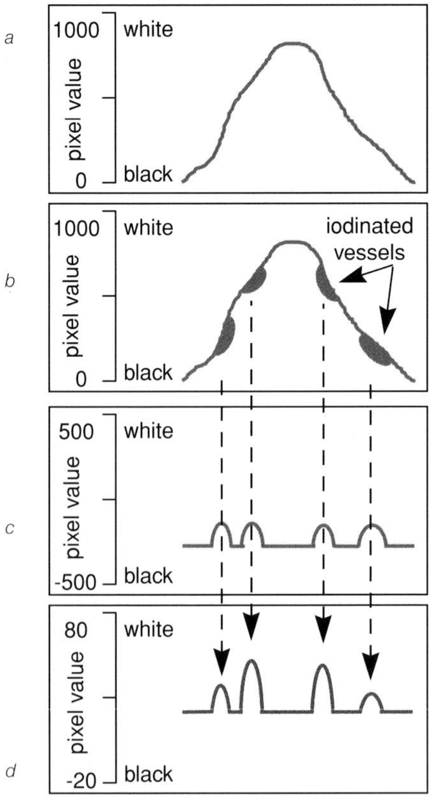

3.2 Principles of DSA

Blood vessels often absorb as much radiation as the surrounding tissues and therefore cannot be discerned on X-ray images. By injecting **contrast agents** into blood vessels, these vessels can be visualized: the contrast medium contains iodine, which absorbs X rays. Due to the presence of bone, the small contrast differences caused by the contrast medium in the blood vessels are difficult to distinguish in the presence of bone structures, since the eye is not able to detect contrast differences of less than about 3%. It is necessary to use a procedure that enhances contrast. Such a procedure is DSA.

By this procedure, an initial X-ray shadow image is

Figure 9.4
Principle of contrast enhancement (after Philips):
(a) intensity distribution along a line of an image;
(b) same distribution after injection of the contrast medium;
(c) intensity distribution after subtraction;
(d) intensity distribution after contrast enhancement.

9

obtained with the help of an image intensifier. The signal coming from the television camera is digitized and stored in the computer. Then contrast medium is injected into the veins. Again, a number of images are obtained. The precontrast image, also called the mask, is now subtracted from the subsequent images. The resulting images will only contain information that was not present in the mask, that is, information about the location of the contrast medium. Since the contrast medium fills the vessels, the resulting images will only show the vessels; bone structures that disturb the image have been removed by the subtraction procedure.

The principle of contrast enhancement is described in Fig. 9.4. Figure 9.4a presents the beam intensity along a line through the image. Figure 9.4b demonstrates how the intensity distribution is altered after the contrast medium has been injected. Note the relatively small contrast differences that result. After subtraction, the intensity distribution is only due to the vessels because of the absorption caused by the contrast medium (Fig. 9.4c). The differences in intensity can be amplified in such a way that the eye is able to perceive the blood vessels in the image (Fig. 9.4d). Figure 9.5 shows an image of the bifurcation of the aorta obtained by DSA. The spinal column is hardly visible, due to subtraction.

The quality of the image deteriorates when the patient moves. Movements can be corrected to some extent through the use of suitable software programs. These programs can shift or rotate the mask in such a way that it correlates maximally with the next image, so that movement artifacts are suppressed. Since the contrast medium is injected in the form of a bolus, the proximal part of the vessel tree is usually more visible in the first subtraction images, whereas in later subtraction images the distal part is more visible. With suitable software it is possible to construct an image that visualizes the whole vessel tree.

Apart from processing the images for visualization, it is also possible to perform measurements on the images because the image is available in digital format. Therefore, it is possible to determine the dimensions of certain details, for example, to obtain the extent of stenoses of vessels or to analyze the movement of the heart muscle.

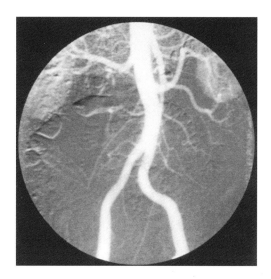

Figure 9.5
Example of digital subtraction angiography (DSA) of the bifurcation of the aorta (Philips).

3.3 Computed Tomography

Conventional X-ray images are projection (shadow) images that cannot reveal the real geometric distribution of organs. Organs that are situated behind each other are superimposed in the image so that a three-dimensional volume is projected in two dimensions. To obtain a three-dimensional impression, one must obtain a number of images from different angles. From these images the radiologist or physician can form a mental image of the three-dimensional volume in which he or she is interested.

Computed tomography is a means of obtaining images that portray the real tissue distribution in a single slice. With *CT*, therefore, a two-dimensional image of a two-dimensional slice is obtained. Hounsfield introduced CT in 1971. He was awarded the Nobel Prize for this invention in 1979.

What is the principle behind CT? Consider a cross section through the body of a patient with a thickness of about 1 mm. Now, divide the cross-section into a large

9

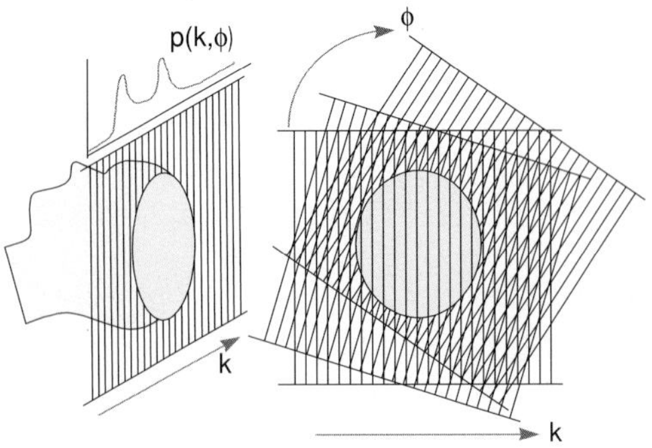

Figure 9.6
Principle of computed tomography. The combination of X-ray tube and detector is translated across the patient, producing a density profile p(k,φ). By rotating the X-ray tube-detector combination, a number of profiles will be obtained. From these profiles the attenuation coefficients of each pixel can be determined.

number of small squares, each with an area of about 1 mm^2. When a narrow X-ray beam, a so-called pencil beam, passes through the slice, each square through which the beam passes attenuates it to a certain extent. The amount of attenuation is determined by the molecular composition and the density of the tissue present in the square. The intensity of the eventually transmitted beam will be smaller than the intensity of the incident beam. The intensity reduction is caused by all the squares through which the beam passes. Each square may attenuate the beam differently because of the presence of different tissue.

To measure the attenuation of a beam, it is necessary to use a combination of an X-ray tube and a *detector*. The absorbing tissue slice is located between them. The X-ray tube produces a pencil beam of known intensity and the detector measures the intensity of the transmitted beam. For reasons that will become clear shortly, the combination of X-ray tube and detector (mounted into the so-called *gantry*) can both be shifted along a line ("translated") and rotated (see Fig. 9.6).

If the assumption is correct that by displaying the attenuation coefficients (the values indicating the amount of absorption per millimeter) we can obtain an anatomical image, we must be able to determine the atte-

nuation coefficients of each square separately. From one measurement it is not possible to deduce how much each separate square attenuated the beam. Yet, determination of the attenuation of each square in the cross-section is the purpose of the procedure.

Since one pencil beam covers only one row of squares, we must translate the beam over a distance equal to its width. In this way we can take into account the attenuation coefficients of the squares located on a neighboring row. After measuring the transmitted intensity, the procedure is repeated by translating the beam and measuring the transmitted intensity until we have covered the total cross section. It is still not possible, however, to determine the individual attenuation coefficient of each square from these data; for each position of the beam we obtain the total attenuation due to the attenuation caused by all squares that are passed by the pencil beam. What we have obtained is an intensity profile (and, therefore, a measure of the total attenuation) of the transmitted beam as a function of the position of the beam. Each point in the profile indicates how strongly the incident beam was attenuated by the row of squares that was passed by the beam in that position (Fig. 9.6). Therefore, we repeat the procedure outlined above for various angles of the beam. It is possible to compute the attenuation per square from these data. Panel 9.2 (with Figs. 9.7 to 9.10) provides a further explanation of the principle of CT and discusses the most frequently used technique: back-projection.

Since its introduction, CT equipment has gone through a number of generations. The combination of an X-ray tube generating a pencil beam with a detector that measures the transmitted beam intensity constitutes the first generation. This combination was translated and rotated to cover the whole cross section at several angles. In second-generation scanners the single detector is replaced by a frame of multiple detectors, and the X-ray tube produces a fan-shaped beam. The fan-shaped beam does not cover the whole patient cross section, and therefore, in second-generation scanners translation and rotation remain necessary. In third-generation scanners the detector array is so large that the transmission through the complete cross section of the patient can be measured simultaneously. Therefore, translation is no longer necessary. Only

9

PANEL 9.2

Principle of Computed Tomography

It is known that an X-ray beam is attenuated in an exponential way, depending on the length of the path and the attenuation coefficients of the squares, denoted here as *pixels* (picture elements) encountered along its path. If we assume that the attenuation coefficient is constant over the whole pixel and if we represent the attenuation of pixel *i* by the attenuation coefficient m_i, then the intensity of the transmitted beam *(I)* can be related to the intensity of the incident beam (I_0) in the way represented in Fig. 9.7. If we take the natural logarithm of the ratio of I and I_0, we obtain the following relation for each pixel:

$$ln\,(I\,/\,I_o) = \sum_{i=1}^{N} d_i m_i$$

Here, d_i is the length of the path that the beam traversed through each pixel *i*, and m_i is its attenuation coefficient. We have obtained an equation with, to the left, the measured intensity ratio and, to the right, N unknown quantities: the coefficients m_i. Since the geometry of the beam and the cross-section are known, the length of the path d_i traversed through each pixel is also known. Such an equation can be written for each point of the intensity profile. The number of unknown quantities therefore only increases. After the beam has covered the whole cross section, the equations contain as many unknowns as there are pixels in the cross section. By turning the gantry over a small angle and repeating the earlier procedure we obtain another intensity profile (see Fig. 9.7). The attenuation coefficients of the pixels remain the same, but the length of the paths traversed through each pixel has changed. In this way we obtain new equations with the same number of unknowns. By measuring the intensity profiles at enough angles we can, in principle, obtain as many equations as there are unknowns. With the help of a computer we can solve the equations and obtain the attenuation coefficients of each pixel in the cross section. As can be seen from Fig. 9.8, a visualization of the values of the attenuation coefficients by way of grey values indeed produces an anatomical image. The procedure of CT as explained here is not used in practice, because it would be too time-consuming, but it provides a good insight into the principles of CT. In practice, back-projection algorithms are used, since these are more efficient.

Back projection is one of the techniques that is used in practice to obtain the attenuation coefficients m_i. This technique can be used when intensity profiles that cover the total cross section under various angles are available. In an individual profile, each point represents the amount of attenuation by the pixels transmitted by the beam. Figure 9.9 shows the intensity profiles that result from a single attenuating pixel. Each profile shows ▶

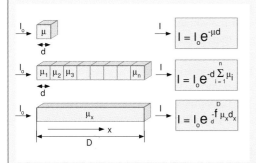

Figure 9.7
The intensity of the transmitted beam as a function of the attenuation coefficient of the pixels traversed.
Upper part, the intensity after crossing one volume element; middle part, after traversing n volume elements; lower part, the analog case.

9

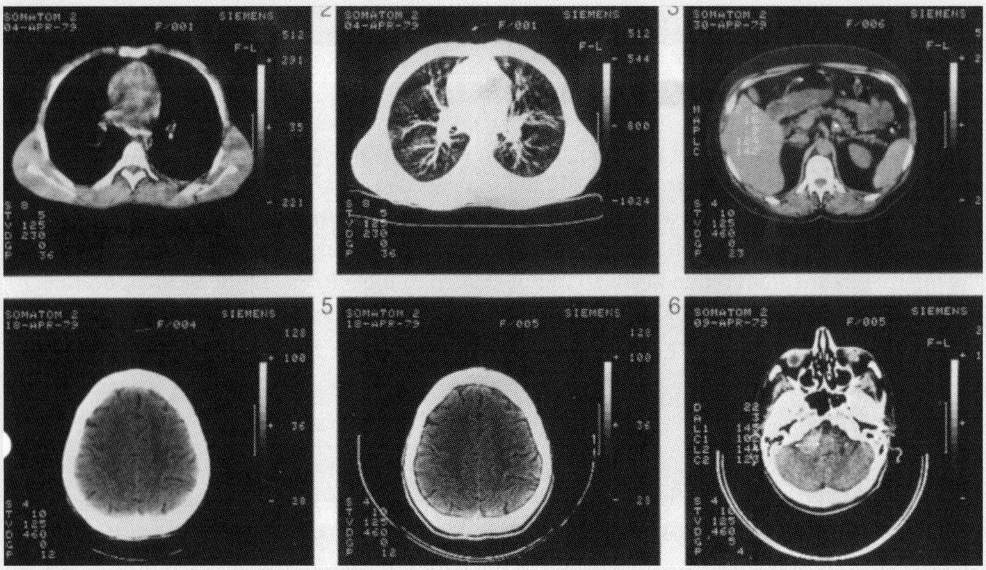

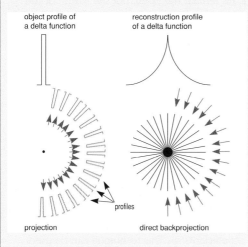

Figure 9.8
Example of cross-sections through several parts of the body: abdomen, thorax, and skull, obtained by computed tomography (Siemens).

Figure 9.9
Upper left, density distribution of a point absorber along a line through the object; lower left, the resulting intensity profiles; lower right, the back-projection; upper right, reconstructed density distribution on a line through the object (after Philips).

a dip at the location where the beam passed through this pixel.

If we have only one intensity profile we cannot determine where on the path the pixel was located. We cannot even decide whether the absorption was due to a single pixel or was due to an attenuating medium that was present over the whole path. The only inference that we can make is that the attenuating medium was present only along one line in the cross section, since the intensity profile showed a dip at only one point.

The back-projection method starts with the assumption that the absorbing medium is uniformly distributed over the line. Of course, this may be incorrect, but it will be demonstrated that the errors resulting from this assumption can be corrected. If we have several intensity profiles obtained at different angles, we get a reconstructed image, as shown in Fig. 9.9. The reconstruction has a star-like distribution. By increasing the number of angles, the intensity ▶

in the center will increase much faster than the intensity at the periphery. With the use of more angles, the back-projected image becomes more similar to the actual one, only it is less sharp; instead of an image showing one attenuating pixel, the neighboring pixels are visible in the reconstructed image as well. This blurring effect can be corrected to a certain extent by using appropriate filtering techniques, resulting in a sharper image. Since a real cross section can be considered a union of cross sections, with each one containing only one attenuating pixel, the back-projection technique can also be applied to real patient cross sections. The back-projection technique can also be used in *MRI* (magnetic resonance imaging) and *SPECT* (single photon emission computed tomography).

It appears that the attenuation coefficient is characteristic for the type of tissue (or more correctly, the chemical composition of the tissue), as is apparent from Fig. 9.10. When the values of the attenuation coefficients of the pixels are displayed on a monitor in the form of grey values, the result consists of anatomical images that can be directly interpreted (Fig. 9.8).

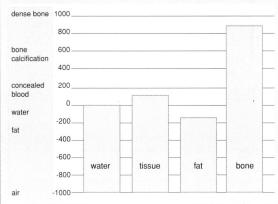

Figure 9.10
Attenuation coefficients of several tissues expressed in Hounsfield units.

rotation is necessary to obtain enough profiles. In fourth-generation CT scanners there is a stationary detector array that covers 360°. In this case only the X-ray tube rotates.

With the advent of X-ray tubes that can sustain an uninterrupted X-ray beam for a longer period of time, it became possible to scan large volumes without having to wait during the process to let the X-ray tube cool down. By rotating the X-ray tube continuously and rapidly using slip-ring power-supply technology and by slowly moving the patient table forward at the same time, it is possible to scan about 1 m of anatomical length in less than a minute. In this way, the X-ray beam traces a helical path over the patient. It is possible to reconstruct slices from the many data that can be acquired at any location.

3.4 Principles of MRI

Before explaining the imaging performed by *MRI*, a few important but difficult EM phenomena such as magnetization of the body, radio frequency excitation, and measurement of relaxations must be explained.

Certain atomic nuclei behave like a spinning top or, as stated in physics, they have spin. They behave like small magnets. One of the biologically relevant nuclei, the proton (the hydrogen nucleus), is abundantly present in all body tissues. Under normal circumstances the body is not magnetic. This is because the hydrogen nuclei (magnets) within the body point into all directions randomly, so that the net magnetic field strength, called the magnetization, of the body is zero.

When we place an ensemble of nuclei with spin in a strong magnetic field, the nuclei tend to align themselves with the magnetic field, in the same way that a compass needle aligns itself to the earth's magnetic

9

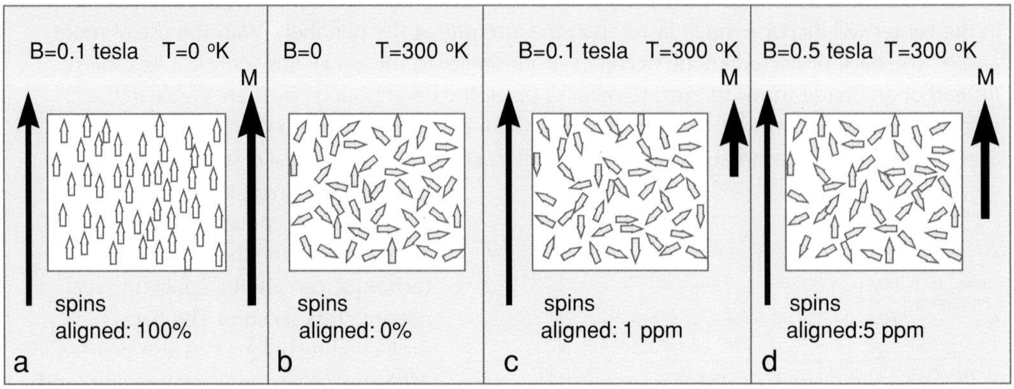

Figure 9.11
The phenomenon of spins aligning themselves to an external magnetic field. At 0 K all spins are aligned when an external magnetic field is present (a); when no external magnetic field is present the spins will point in all directions (b); at room temperature only a small part of the nuclei will align themselves: 1 per million (c) at a field strength of 0.1 tesla and 5 per million (d) at a magnetic field strength of 0.5 tesla (after Philips).

field. This alignment occurs because the nuclei prefer to be in a state with the lowest energy. Therefore, at a temperature of absolute zero (0 °K), all nuclei align themselves completely to the external magnetic field. However, at room temperature the nuclei also possess thermal energy, which is higher than the energy difference between the state in which the spin is parallel and the state in which the spin is antiparallel to the external magnetic field. Only a small excess of nuclei are pointing into the direction of the external magnetic field; the others still behave in a random way: in an external magnetic field with a strength of 0.1 tesla, the excess is only 1 in 10^6. Although this is a very small part, this can lead to a considerable number of aligned nuclei in a tissue. A milliliter of water contains 3×10^{22} molecules, so that there is an excess of about 10^{17} hydrogen atoms aligning parallel to the magnetic field. These 10^{17} atoms together cause the magnetization, because they all point into the same direction, whereas the magnetic fields of the other nuclei are canceled out. When the external magnetic field strength increases, more nuclei will align themselves, and therefore, the induced magnetization will increase (see Fig. 9.11). The magnetization is characterized by its direction and strength. The direction of the magnetization is parallel to the direction of the external magnetic field, and its strength is both proportional to the strength of the

external magnetic field and the number of nuclei present in a volume of tissue.

While the nuclei are under the influence of the external magnetic field, pulses of electromagnetic radiation are beamed into the tissue. EM radiation is characterized by an electric and a magnetic component. The magnetic component of the EM radiation exerts a force on the magnetic nuclei. When the magnetic component of the EM radiation has a direction perpendicular to the external magnetic field, it may cause the magnetization to precess around the direction of the external field in such a way that the angle between the direction of the magnetization and the external field will increase linearly with time. This only happens when the EM radiation has a certain frequency, called the Larmor frequency. This frequency is proportional to the strength of the external magnetic field and the so-called gyromagnetic ratio, which is characteristic for the element or *isotope*. The Larmor frequencies are in the range of radio frequencies (2 to 50 MHz for various isotopes at an external field of 1 tesla). The pulse of EM radiation that causes the magnetization to precess to a direction orthogonal to the external magnetic field is called the 90° RF excitation pulse (see Fig. 9.12). Since only one frequency will cause the precession of the nuclei of a certain isotope, it is a kind of resonance phenomenon, which explains the term *mag-*

netic resonance imaging.

After the termination of the RF pulse, the magnetization will gradually precess back to the original equilibrium direction. From physics we know that a changing magnetic field will induce a current in a coil, as in a dynamo. The size of the current is proportional to the strength of the magnetization component along the axis of the coil, and the frequency of the current will be equal to the precession frequency of the magnetization. When a coil is placed perpendicular to the external magnetic field the largest current will therefore be observed when the magnetization also precesses perpendicularly to the external field (see Fig. 9.13). When the magnetization returns to its equilibrium position, the component along the axis of the coil will decrease gradually, as will the amplitude of the induced current. Since the initial value of the current in the coil is proportional to the strength of the magnetization, which is the case when the magnetization precesses perpendicularly to the external field, and since the strength of the magnetization is proportional to the number of nuclei, the initial value of the current is proportional to the number of resonating nuclei. The signal observed directly after the termination of the RF pulse is called the *free induction decay* (FID) signal. This signal is the basis for imaging. The principle of MRI is further explained in Panel 9.3.

Certain factors may influence the magnetic resonance image, for example, flow phenomena in blood or cerebrospinal fluid. Flow can produce either signal enhancement (flow enhancement) or signal reduction (flow void). Magnetic resonance angiography (**MRA**) is based on signal enhancement. With MRI, arteries and veins may be selectively imaged without the need for contrast media. It is, however, also possible to use contrast agents to enhance contrast. For this purpose paramagnetic compounds such as gadolinium, manganese, or iron are used. With these contrast agents, lesions in the brain, spine, breast, and urinary tract can be visualized better.

MRI can also be used for placing so-called **fiducial markers**. This process is called tagging, and it is used in myocardial imaging. Triggered by the rising edge of the R-wave, RF pulses are produced in such a way that parallel planes perpendicular to the image plane, the tag planes, are magnetized. If slices are imaged in the

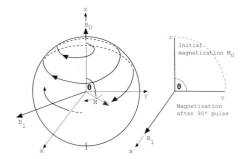

Figure 9.12
Precession of magnetization under the influence of an external magnetic field with strength B_0 and an oscillating field B_1 (due to electromagnetic radiation) during a 90° RF pulse as seen from the observer (A) and as seen from the standpoint of the rotating field (B) (Philips).

normal way directly afterward, dark lines will appear in the image where the tag planes intersect the image plane. The black lines are formed by the hydrogen nuclei that were already magnetized at the moment that the second RF pulse was generated. The second RF pulse hardly affects these nuclei, and therefore, these nuclei are invisible magnetic resonance imaging in the image. By imaging slices through the heart at different time points during the systolic interval, the deformation of the heart wall can be studied by following the positions of the dark lines .

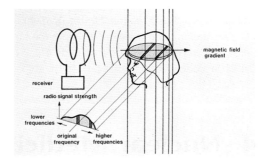

Figure 9.13
In an inhomogeneous magnetic field only protons will resonate at a certain frequency that are at locations where the magnetic field strength is in concordance with the radiated frequency. By changing the frequency, different areas will resonate (after Philips).

9

PANEL 9.3

Principle of Magnetic Resonance Imaging

The aim of MRI is to provide an image of the tissue distribution in a plane through the body, for example, by measuring the hydrogen density in that plane. The idea is, once again, to obtain a two-dimensional image of a two-dimensional slice through the body.

How can the density of hydrogen nuclei at each location of interest in the body be obtained? On the basis of the explanation in Section 3.4, it is possible to imagine the following procedure. Arrange a situation in which the strength of the external magnetic field is different at each location of interest. The hydrogen atoms at each location have their own specific Larmor resonance frequency, depending on the local strength of the external magnetic field. By irradiating the body with EM radiation at a certain frequency in a direction perpendicular to the external magnetic field, only those hydrogen nuclei that have a Larmor frequency equal to the frequency of the RF excitation pulse will resonate. The Larmor frequency depends on the strength of the magnetic field, so these nuclei are located in a small volume. The RF excitation pulse has such a duration that after the pulse the magnetization vector will precess perpendicularly to the external magnetic field (the 90° RF pulse). A current is then induced in a coil perpendicular to the external magnetic field. This current has an amplitude proportional to the number of the resonating nuclei in that volume and a frequency equal to the Larmor frequency. This frequency determines the position of the sampled volume. This procedure is repeated with other frequencies for all volumes with a specific Larmor frequency. By this procedure the density of hydrogen nuclei can be obtained at all locations of interest.

The external magnetic field is applied as follows. It consists of two parts: a strong homogeneous field and a smaller magnetic field, of which the strength changes linearly in a certain direction. The linearly changing field can be applied in three directions by three orthogonally placed gradient coils. This changing magnetic field is also called the magnetic field *gradient*. If the field gradient is directed, for instance, from head to toe, every transverse slice in the patient resonates at a different Larmor frequency. In addition, RF coils are used to produce the RF signal. These coils may also be used to detect the resultant magnetization changes. Because of the latter function, these coils are also called receiving coils.

All nuclei in a slice *orthogonal* to the gradient direction will experience the same external magnetic field strength and therefore will have the same Larmor frequency (this gradient is called the slice selection gradient). The amplitude of the current in the receiving coil after the application of a 90° RF pulse will be proportional to the total number of hydrogen nuclei in this slice. ▶

---

4 Nuclear Medicine

9

During *nuclear medicine* examination, radioactively labeled material, a *radiopharmaceutical*, is injected, for example, into the veins of a patient. The choice of the material depends on the type of examination one wants to perform. For examining thyroid disorders, an iodine compound that is taken up by the thyroid can be used, whereas in vessel examinations, erythrocytes labeled with radioactive

---

However, we are more interested in the distribution of the nuclei within this slice than in the total number of nuclei in this slice.

Therefore, we need more position selectivity, which is attained as follows. If, after the 90° RF pulse, the slice selection gradient is switched off and another magnetic field gradient is applied orthogonally to the direction of the slice selection gradient (this additional gradient is called read-out or measurement gradient, because it is applied after the 90° pulse and just before the induced current is measured in the receiving coil) the frequency of the resonating nuclei will change: nuclei in the slice located along different rows orthogonally to the readout gradient direction will experience a different external magnetic field strength (the sum of the first homogeneous field and the readout gradient field) and therefore will have different Larmor frequencies in the different rows. This means that each row of hydrogen nuclei in the slice induces a current with a different frequency in the receiving coil. The amplitude of the component with a certain frequency, again, is proportional to the number of hydrogen atoms along the corresponding row, and the frequency now determines the position of the corresponding row.

Since the sum of signals with all of these different resonance frequencies is detected simultaneously, a *Fourier transformation* (see Chapter 25) needs to be conducted to obtain amplitude and position information from the specific frequency spectrum. Each frequency corresponds to a row in the slice. The amplitude of each frequency component is proportional to the number of resonating nuclei in a certain row. The frequency spectrum therefore corresponds to a profile representing the number of hydrogen nuclei in each row as a function of the location along the direction of the readout gradient. We now have a situation similar to that for CT. By measuring the profile for different directions of the readout gradient and using a *back-projection* technique as in CT (see Section 3.3), the distribution of the hydrogen nuclei over the slice can be obtained. The procedure can be sped up by applying a second field gradient orthogonally to the readout gradient before the latter is applied and by using the resulting phase differences.

After termination of the 90° RF pulse, the magnetization gradually returns back to its equilibrium position, which is parallel to the external field. This phenomenon is called *relaxation*. Two types of relaxation can be distinguished. First, there is the relaxation caused by energy exchange with the surrounding nuclei (called the lattice). This so-called spin-lattice relaxation or longitudinal relaxation is characterized by the so-called longitudinal relaxation time, T_1, which is defined as the time that is required for 63% of the nuclei to realign themselves with the external field. The second form is the relaxation due to spin-spin interactions. Spin-spin relaxation is characterized by the transverse relaxation time, T_2, which measures the time after which the transverse component has decreased by 63%. Different tissues may have different T_1 or T_2 values, as well as different densities. This fact can be used to vary the contrast.

technetium are applied. The radiopharmaceutical (the carrier of the *isotope*) is chosen in such a way that this compound is preferably absorbed by the organ we are interested in. Its radiation is then used to create an image. The radiation emitted by the isotopes is partly absorbed inside the patient, and the remainder is detected by a so-called *gamma camera*. The gamma camera is usually connected to a computer system, with which it is then possible to construct an image.

Radioactive isotopes disintegrate into stable isotopes. For medical examinations it is better to use an isotopes with a relatively short *half-life*, which is the time in which the activity is reduced by 50%, to limit to a minimum the amount of radiation to which a patient is exposed. The radioactive isotopes with short half-lives are produced in so-called generators, that contain radioactive

9

material with a relatively long half-life that decays into the requested isotope. Over a number of days, the generator is used to produce the radioactive material needed for imaging. A technetium generator, for example, contains the radioactive isotope molybdenum-99m, which has a half-life of 67 hours. This isotope disintegrates to Technetium-99m, which has a half-life of 6 hours. The latter isotope is used for imaging purposes.

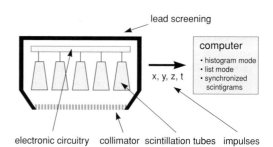

Figure 9.14
Principle of the gamma camera.

4.1 The Gamma Camera

The radiation that passes through the body is detected by a **gamma camera**. Radioactive isotopes can emit several types of radiation. In nuclear medicine, it is preferred that isotopes that emit **gamma radiation** of a suitable energy be used. Two factors determine what a "suitable" energy is. First, the emitted radioactive energy must be high enough to prevent complete absorption of the radiation within the body of the patient. The attenuation decreases with increasing energy. The second factor is that the energy of the radiation also determines the sensitivity of a detector. The higher the energy, the lower the sensitivity of a detector. Both of these contradictory requirements must be taken into account.

In early applications in which radioactive [131]Iodine was used to determine its accumulation in the thyroid, a Geiger counter was used. This detector had a low sensitivity: only 1% of the radiation was detected. By making use of scintillation detectors, the sensitivity could be increased. In these detectors the incident gamma radiation is transformed into scintillations (light pulses). A sodium-iodide (NaI) crystal activated with thallium was used as the scintillation detector. The scintillations were detected with the help of a **photomultiplier** tube and were transformed into electric pulses.

To measure the distribution of the activity inside an organ, so-called scanners were developed. To that end a **collimator** is placed between the detector and the patient. This collimator is a block of lead in which cone-shaped channels have been drilled in such a way that all channels appear to originate from one focal point. Only radiation that passes through these chan-

nels can reach the detector. This is only the case for radiation coming from a volume located in the focal point. In this way the detector is insensitive to the radiation coming from other volumes. When the detector is moved over the organ the activity distribution within the organ is measured. Scanning of the organ used to take about 30 minutes.

A new development was reported by Anger in 1957. He described a scintillation camera with a field of view of 10 inches. With this camera a whole organ could be visualized directly. The camera consisted of a NaI crystal with a thickness of 0.5 inch, and a diameter of 10 inches. The thickness of the crystal was smaller than usual by a factor of 4. Because of its thinness the sensitivity of the scintillation camera was much lower than that of earlier scanners for the radioactive isotopes that were used at that time. Regretfully, the spatial resolution of the camera was worse than that of the scanner.

The Anger gamma camera was reconsidered when Technetium-99m became available. Technetium 99m emits gamma radiation with an energy of 140 keV, and the sensitivity of the camera's crystal for this energy is much higher. A collimator is now used in front of the crystal to permit imaging. In this collimator a large number of parallel channels are present. Only gamma radiation passing through these channels reaches the crystal. Each parallel channel only passes the gamma rays that have a direction parallel to the channel walls (this means that the activity distribution of an organ can be visualized in a plane perpendicular to the channels; see Fig. 9.14).

A number of photomultiplier tubes are positioned

9

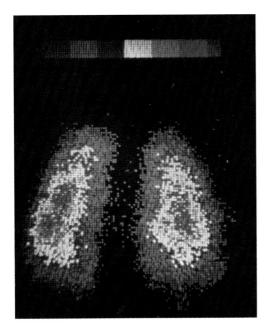

Figure 9.15
Example of a scintigram of the lungs, obtained with a gamma camera. Different intensities have been coded with different colors.

above the crystal. Each of these photomultiplier tubes delivers a pulse at the moment that a scintillation is produced within the crystal. By suitably connecting the photomultiplier tube outputs, two signals are obtained: one signal is proportional to the x-coordinate of the location where the pulse was generated and the other one is proportional to the y-coordinate. A third signal is equal to the sum of the signals produced by all photomultiplier tubes together. This signal, called the z signal, is proportional to the energy of the radiation absorbed in the NaI crystal. With the help of this signal it becomes possible to discriminate gamma radiation coming from the injected radioisotope from unwanted background radiation. When the z signal is above a certain detection threshold, the coordinates of the x and y signals are digitized and stored in computer memory. Figure 9.15 gives an example of a *scintigram*, obtained with a gamma camera, for both lungs. The coordinates can be stored in different ways. The most common ways are the so-called histogram mode and the list mode.

4.2 Histogram Mode

In the *histogram* mode the viewing area of the gamma camera is divided into a matrix of picture elements (pixels). Matrices of 256 x 256 pixels are common. As many memory locations as there are pixels have been reserved in the computer memory. Before data acquisition the contents of these memory locations are set equal to zero. After the detection of a gamma quantum at a certain location, the content of the corresponding memory location is incremented by one. This procedure is repeated until a predefined observation time has elapsed or a predefined number of counts has been detected. The contents of each memory location are now equal to the number of counts detected in the corresponding location. The count distribution represents the activity distribution over an organ, and it can be displayed on a video screen as a color or a grey scale distribution. The color or the brightness of a pixel represents a certain number of counts, for example, red for high numbers and dark blue for low numbers (see Fig. 9.15). The displayed distribution is used for diagnostic purposes in so-called static studies, which are used to examine whether the observed activity distribution is normal for the organ under consideration.
It is also possible to perform dynamic studies in the histogram mode. The computer must then store several images consecutively. After some predefined time interval, another part of the memory is used to store the next counts. This procedure is repeated for each consecutive image. In this way, it is possible to study dynamic processes. Before the start of the study it must be determined over how much time each image will be acquired. In renal studies the first images will each be acquired over 1 second. For the following images the acquisition time can be longer. This is because a radioactively labeled material usually arrives in the kidneys shortly after the injection, whereas the washout period will take more time

4.3 List Mode

If it is not known beforehand over what time interval each image should be acquired, the so-called list mode can be used. In this case, all x and y coordina-

9

tes of the counts are stored sequentially together with the times the pulses were detected. This means that much more memory is needed in the list mode than in the histogram mode. In the histogram mode, as many memory locations as there are pixels are necessary. In the list mode, as many memory locations as there are counts are needed. After acquisition, images of different formats and acquisition times can be constructed. This is possible because time information is also stored (e.g., every 10 milliseconds) between the data for the x and y coordinates. With the help of these time indications and the coordinates, many different image sequences can be constructed. Usually, the list mode is used for examinations that are not yet known, when it is not yet clear how many images with what time resolution will produce the best results.

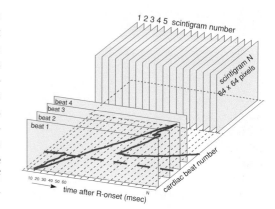

Figure 9.16
Principle of ECG-gated scintigraphy (after Robb).

4.4 Synchronized Recordings

Many physiological phenomena occur so quickly that it is impossible to produce satisfactory images with small enough acquisition time intervals. For periodic or **quasi-periodic** phenomena, a synchronized recording is possible. In cardiac studies, the **R-wave** from the electrocardiogram is used for synchronization. This technique follows a procedure that will also be discussed in Chapter 25 under coherent averaging. By dividing the RR interval into a sufficient number of intervals (Fig. 9.16), it becomes possible to obtain scintigraphic images of the beating heart. The images together show the movement of the cardiac muscle during one cardiac cycle. However, acquiring data during only one cardiac cycle does not provide enough counts to obtain interpretable images. The repetitive character of the heart beat is now used to increase the number of counts in each interval. Each time a new R-wave is detected, the acquisition sequence is repeated and all counts are added up in a memory that belongs to the appropriate interval. In this way each cardiac cycle adds counts to each image. The procedure is continued until each frame (image) contains enough counts, usually lasting several minutes. In cardiac

studies one is interested in the contraction of the cardiac muscle as a function of time and location. To that end, about 40 frames are accumulated, each covering an interval ranging from 20 to 30 milliseconds.

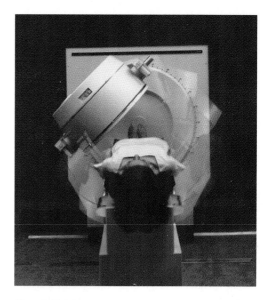

Figure 9.17
Rotating gamma camera used to determine a three-dimensional activity distribution.

4.5 Processing of Scintigrams

Computers are used not only to store images but also to further process them. With the help of computer programs, the contrast can be increased, images can be corrected for background activity and nonuniformities of the crystal, images can be filtered, and so forth.

In cardiac studies one is interested, for example, in the ejection fraction. For that purpose the contour of the left ventricle is automatically detected both in the end-systolic and in the end-diastolic phase. On the basis of the radioactivity that is left inside the heart at systole, it is possible to calculate the ejection fraction, after correction for background activity. A similar procedure can also be executed in more detail by dividing the inside of the left ventricle into a number of sectors and computing the ejection fraction for each of the sectors.

4.6 Three-Dimensional Reconstructions (SPECT and PET)

The images obtained with a gamma camera are two-dimensional projections of three-dimensional distributions of activity. By rotating the gamma camera around the patient, activity profiles can be obtained from a large number of angles. In a manner similar to that used for CT, the activity distribution in various slices of the organ of interest can be obtained from the activity profiles. In modern cameras more Anger detectors (two to four) are used to speed up the procedure. The procedure is called single photon emission computed tomography (**SPECT**). SPECT is used to make three-dimensional reconstructions of the heart, to perform brain studies, for skeletal scintigraphy, and so forth (see Fig. 9.17).

The distribution of activity in slices of the organ can be obtained in a more accurate way by another technique, called positron emission tomography (**PET**). In PET studies, radiopharmaceuticals are labeled with positron-emitting isotopes. A positron (a positively charged electron) combines rather quickly with an electron. As a result, two gamma quanta (each with an energy of 511 keV) are emitted in almost opposite directions. In PET scanners, rings of gamma-ray detectors surrounding the patient are used. Each detector interacts electronically with the other detectors in the field of view. When a photon arrives within a short time frame (in the order of a few nanoseconds), it is clear that a pair of quanta was generated and that these quanta were created somewhere along the path between the detectors. Again, reconstruction of the image takes place by using the same principles discussed for CT. In two-dimensional PET scanners, the detector rings are separated by lead septa. For three-dimensional scanning, these septa can be removed. This increases the sensitivity, but also the noise. Since the higher sensitivity permits lower radiation doses, the use of three-dimensional scanners is justified.

With the help of PET, dynamic properties of biochemical processes can be studied. A large part of biological systems consists of hydrogen, carbon, nitrogen, and oxygen. With the help of a cyclotron it is possible to produce short-lived isotopes of the last three elements that emit positrons. Examples of these isotopes are ^{15}O, ^{13}N, and ^{11}C with a half-lives of 2, 10, and 13 minutes, respectively. By using these isotopes various metabolic processes can be studied.

4.7 Functional MRI

MRI, too, is not only used to provide anatomical information; it is also increasingly used to study blood flow in the brain. This enables one to study metabolic processes in the brain indirectly, and thus MRI becomes a competitor of PET. This so-called **functional MRI** is used, for instance, to differentiate between activated and resting brain regions. In activated brain regions, the level of oxygenation of venous blood is greater than that in resting regions. Oxygen-rich hemoglobin reacts only weakly with the applied magnetic field, whereas deoxygenated hemoglobin interacts more strongly. The deoxygen-

9

ated hemoglobin therefore causes local magnetic inhomogeneities, effecting the T_2 relaxation rate.

In this way, for instance, visual stimulation causes increases in intensity in the visual cortex. A second mechanism – changes in the T_1 relaxation rate – is based on changes in the rate of inflowing arterial blood. Since the protons in the inflowing blood can still be excited, the T1 relaxation times apparently increase.

Functional MRI has introduced a new era in mapping of the human brain. Research into the function-al organization of the brain, cerebral plasticity following trauma, learning, and mental diseases will be accelerated.

Key References

Udupa JK, and Herman GT, eds. 3D Imaging in Medicine, Boca Raton FL: CRC Press, 1991.

See the Web site for further literature references.

9

10 Image Processing and Analysis

1 Introduction

Image processing and *analysis* can be defined as the application of a body of techniques to capture, correct, enhance, transform, or compress visual images. The goal of such operations is to enhance the relative quality of the information that may subsequently be extracted. Although transformations used in image *processing* are of the type *image in, image out,* operations in image *analysis* are of the type *image in, numerical information out.*

Many different image generation techniques are available, yet the image-processing techniques are to a large extent independent of the image formation process, with the notable exception of image restoration. Once images have been captured and corrected for distortions due to the acquisition process, all applicable techniques are of a very general nature. Therefore, image processing is an activity that transcends specific applications: new techniques or procedures developed to solve a specific problem will almost certainly find their way to completely different application areas.

Image processing is performed in many areas of modern society. The methods and techniques in all these areas are very similar, and the methods used in health care are therefore largely borrowed from many other applications of image processing in science and industry. To illustrate the generality of image processing, a number of applications from medicine, as well as from other areas, are given below.

• Satellite imagery

Pictures of the earth or other planetary surfaces are taken by cameras onboard spacecraft and satellites (e.g., the space shuttle photographs Earth). When images of other planets are taken, the goal is to study their surfaces to gain insight into, for instance, a planet's properties or history. Satellite imagery of the earth is used for meteorological, agricultural, environmental, and military purposes, among other things.

• Aerial imagery

Pictures of parts of the surface of the earth are taken, for instance, for crop inspection or for cartography.

• Printing and handwriting

Recognition of printed or handwritten characters is one of the earliest applications of image processing. Among the numerous applications are the automatic reading of postal codes and bank checks.

• Bar codes

The checkout counters of most supermarkets have a device that reads and interprets the **bar codes** on products. Bar coding is also used to trace documents, biochemical samples, and tissue specimens in hospitals (see also Chapter 13).

• Radiology

In medicine, radiology is one of the main users of image-processing techniques (see also Chapter 9). The application not only of conventional X-rays but also of procedures such as computed tomography (*CT*), magnetic resonance imaging (*MRI*), positron emission tomography (**PET**), and ultrasound all result in images that must be interpreted. In many of these applications, three-dimensional reconstruction is a topic of special interest.

• **Karyotyping**

Since images of chromosomes are relatively simple structures, chromosome pairing and the automatic construction of a **karyogram** were some of the earliest applications of image processing in medicine.

• Cytology and histology

The automatic or quantitative interpretation of microscopic imagery (cells and tissues) was also an early application (see Chapter 13).

2 Goals of Image Processing

10

The goals of image processing are threefold: visualization, automation, and quantification. The processing steps in image processing show many similarities to those in signal processing (see Fig. 10.1).

2.1 Visualization

When the images emerge from the acquisition device, they generally need to be improved to facilitate interpretation by the human observer. Objects of interest must be highlighted or the contrast between various parts of an image needs to be enhanced. Since the advent of three-dimensional imaging procedures, such as CT and MRI, visualization has received much attention, especially the visualization of three-dimensional structures.

2.2 Automation

Some applications are aimed at automating certain frequently occurring or tedious tasks. Examples are systems that produce a karyogram from a microscopic image of a chromosome spread or systems that automatically generate a leukocyte differential count from a blood smear. Such applications are characterized by minimal human intervention, so that the complete analysis is achieved automatically. For the leukocyte differential count application, commercially available systems were developed in the 1970s. Nowadays, this task is automated in a completely different way (by **flow cytometry**).

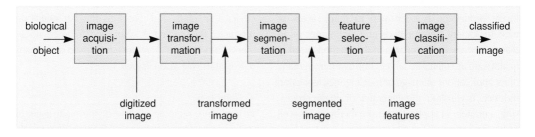

Figure 10.1
Processing steps in image processing. See Fig. 8.1 for comparison.

2.3 Quantification

Examples of image processing for quantification purposes are procedures for the measurement of stenoses in arteries or procedures for the localization and quantification of specific elements in tissue sections by electron microscopic inspection (e.g., iron in **hemochromatosis**). In such applications human intervention is allowed, since processing time is not the most important consideration.

3 Issues in Image Processing and Image Analysis

This section reviews some of the most important issues in image processing and analysis. Any real-life application is a combination of procedures, each specifically handling one of these issues (see also Fig. 10.1).

3.1 Image Acquisition and Sampling

In this section we restrict ourselves to the acquisition of images from scenes that can be observed by the human eye. Imaging procedures such as CT, MRI, and PET (see Chapter 9) are not discussed here, nor will we go into the complex processes involved in the conversion of, for example, distributions of electrons emerging from any form of electron microscopy into visible images.

• Television Camera

The most versatile image acquisition device is the television (TV) camera. It can be used to acquire images of natural scenes or photographs; light transmitted through photographic negatives (including X-ray photographic material) can be projected onto the face of a TV camera. A TV camera can also be mounted onto a microscope (Fig. 10.2). In satellite and aerial imagery, infrared cameras are often used.

For a long time, black-and-white TV cameras were the only option for high-quality scientific and quantitative purposes, but color TV technology has advanced to a stage where color cameras can be and are being used even for such demanding applications as quantitative image processing. The output of a color TV camera consists of three signals (red, green, and blue, together called the **RGB** signal), which are sampled and digitized independently (see Section 3.2) to represent the full color content of the scene in digital form.

• Charge-coupled devices

Charge-coupled devices (**CCD**s) are also used as

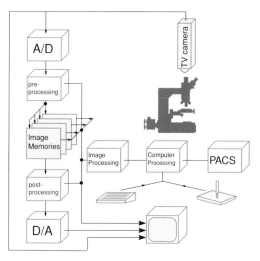

Figure 10.2

TV camera mounted onto a microscope to acquire and process microscopic pictures. A/D and D/A indicate analog-to-digital and digital-to-analog conversion, respectively. PACS indicates picture archiving and communication system.

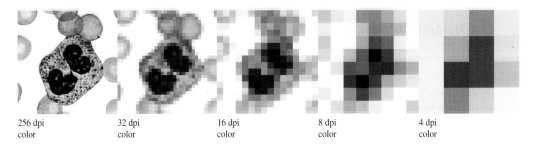

256 dpi   32 dpi   16 dpi   8 dpi   4 dpi
color   color   color   color   color

Figure 10.3
Effect of spatial resolution sampling density on the recognition of an image. In (a) a neutrophil is shown with 256 dots per inch (dpi) resolution; in (b) – (e) the resolution is decreased: 32 dpi, 16 dpi, 8 dpi, and 4 dpi, respectively. Somewhere around 16 dpi the semantic information content disappearsgets.

10

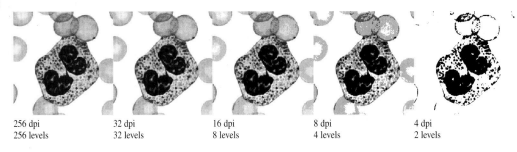

256 dpi   32 dpi   16 dpi   8 dpi   4 dpi
256 levels 32 levels   8 levels   4 levels   2 levels

Figure 10.4
Effect of using various quantization levels in the grey-scale direction. (a) Original image of Fig. 10.3 (256 quantization levels). In (b) – (e) the quantization resolution decreases: 5 bits (32 grey levels), 3 bits (8 levels), 2 bits (4 levels), and 1 bit (2 levels), respectively.

image sensors. Solid-state sensors are configured as arrays of light-sensitive silicon elements, with each element producing an electrical output of an amplitude that is related to the intensity of the incident light on that element. Solid-state arrays may be configured as line sensors or as area sensors. In the first case, the lines in the scene are scanned one at a time; in the second case, the complete image is acquired in parallel.

The sampling function in a TV camera and in CCDs is automatically accounted for by adjusting the magnification of the scene to be acquired to the line scan pattern in a TV camera or to the fixed distance between the silicon sensors in the case of CCD technology.

- Resolution

One of the most important aspects in image processing is choosing the correct **resolution** or sampling density. Since an image is just a signal in two dimensions, the same laws that apply to signal processing apply to image processing (see Chapter 8); to represent a scene faithfully, the image must be sampled at a frequency that is twice the highest relevant spatial frequency in the scene (see also Chapter 8). Figure 10.3 illustrates the effect of the sampling density on the appearance of the sampled image. A medium-resolution sensor produces images in the order of 256 x 256 picture elements (*pixels*). High resolution, which is often required in radiology, requires images of at least 2,048 x 2,048 pixels.

3.2 Grey-Level Quantization

Just as the image must be digitized along the spatial axes to arrive at a digital image, so must the image intensity be digitized. The output of a TV camera or a

CCD is an analog voltage, which is related to the intensity of the incident light. The voltage range, from zero for black to some maximum value for the highest light intensity, is divided into a number of equal intervals. The higher this number, the better the various intensity grades (*grey levels*) are preserved in the digital image. Figure 10.4 shows the effect of using various numbers of quantization levels in the grey-scale direction. Usually, 256 levels (which can be coded in one byte) are taken to cover the entire grey scale.

Taking into account the spatial resolution and the grey-scale resolution, one image of 512 x 512 pixels, with a grey-scale resolution of 8 bits, requires 0.25 megabyte (Mbyte) of storage capacity. If a representation in full color is wanted, the storage space will be three times as much (0.75 Mbyte).

3.3 Image Restoration

During image acquisition, various processes may contribute to degradation of the image. Examples are blur, introduced by a moving or out-of-focus camera, the introduction of a 50 or 60 Hz *interference* pattern, or geometric perspective distortions. Correction for such degradations is based on a model of the degradation process. The aim of image restoration is to improve the quality of the image in some way, either for visual inspection or for further digital processing. In that sense, image restoration serves the same purpose as image enhancement (see next section). The difference is that the resulting image can be expressed as the result of the inverse degradation process acting upon the original image. Therefore, image restoration is sometimes called objective image enhancement.

Restoration techniques may be global or local, and they may operate in the frequency or spatial domain. For example, removal of a disturbing pattern with a known frequency is preferably executed in the frequency domain and involves the following sequence: *Fourier transform*, *filtering*, and inverse Fourier transform (see also Chapter 25). Removal of geometrical distortions is generally executed in the spatial domain. This filtering is fully equal to similar operations in signals (see Chapter 25).

3.4 Image Enhancement

As mentioned above, the ultimate goal of image enhancement is to improve the quality of an image in some way. Depending on the application, various enhancement techniques may be applied with various goals in mind. If the image is intended for visual inspection, contrast enhancement is a sensible operation. If the image is intended for further digital processing, *segmentation* (an operation that highlights boundaries between image components and line structures in the image) may be an operation of choice, although this procedure does not necessarily produce a more effective image. Since image enhancement can be carried out with different possible objectives in mind, it is sometimes called subjective image enhancement.

Like restoration techniques, enhancement techniques may be global or local, and they may operate in the frequency or the spatial domain.

3.5 Edge or Contour Detection

Edge or contour detection techniques are used to detect line-like local structures in an image, usually as a preprocessing step to image segmentation (see next section).

Edges are the borders between two regions in an image with different average grey levels. Therefore, most edge detection techniques rely on the application of some form of gradient operator. It is possible to apply *gradient* operators that are sensitive for gradients in the horizontal, vertical, or diagonal directions, and the results may be combined to detect edges in arbitrary directions. In most practical applications, edge detection is accomplished as a local filtering operation. The detection of edges does not necessarily mean that one has also segmented the entire image: the detected edges may not be continuous and in general will not constitute a closed contour around any object of interest. On the other hand, not all image segmentation techniques depend on a previous edge detection process. Therefore, image segmentation is discussed next as an independent topic.

3.6 Image Segmentation

The goal of image **segmentation** is to decompose an image into its constituent components, possibly with the objective of performing measurements on each of them. Image segmentation is a notably difficult procedure. Yet, the quality of the results of subsequent measurements is critically dependent on the quality of the segmentation process. There are two different approaches to image segmentation. One exploits the supposed homogeneity of intensity values within components; the other is based on finding borders between components, thus exploiting inhomogeneities in the image.

- Histogram segmentation

The simplest procedure is based on an analysis of the *histogram* of intensity values. If an image is composed of light objects on a dark background, the grey-level histogram will show two maxima:

- one peak generated by object points, and
- the other generated by points in the background.

If the contrast between objects and background is sufficiently high, the two maxima in the histogram will be well separated and an intensity threshold value T may be found separating the two maxima. In the original image all grey values greater than T may then be replaced by the value 1 and all grey values less than or equal to T may then be replaced by the value 0. This produces a **binary** image in which object points are represented by the value 1. If the image is composed of more than two components, the histogram may show multiple maxima and segmentation may be achieved by multiple **thresholding**.

- Region growing

Another approach to image segmentation, also exploiting the homogeneity within regions, is **region growing**. This process starts with selecting one or more "**seed points**" in the image, the number of seed points being equal to the number of regions to be detected. Then a criterion for similarity between pixels must be formulated. In its simplest form this is a criterion based on the pixel grey value; for example, two pixels may be called similar if the absolute value of the difference between their **grey values** is smaller than a given threshold. The region-growing process is then started by inspecting all points surrounding the seed points. If a point is sufficiently similar to its seed point, it is assigned to that seed point's region. For each region the process is continued by inspecting all points surrounding the points already assigned to that region until all points in the image have been assigned.

- **Gradient** methods

A third method of image segmentation is based on discontinuities in the image. This approach is typically preceded by some sort of gradient operation (edge detection). The problem, however, is that in general the edge detection does not result in connected boundaries. It must be supplemented with procedures for edge linking to result in satisfactory continuous boundaries.

3.7 Measurements in Images

Once an image has been segmented, measurements can be made on the isolated objects. Features to be measured may be divided into several distinct groups:

1. Geometrical features, describing object properties such as area, circumference, shape, etc.
2. Intensity features, describing the distribution of grey levels in an object: mean value, standard deviation, and possibly higher-order moments.
3. Color features, objectively describing the color of objects and/or the distribution of colors within objects. It may be clear that the measurement of such features implies the availability of multispectral imagery. It is then possible to describe the color of a pixel quantitatively by a function of the pixel's grey values in the various color representations.
4. **Texture** features, describing the fine structure in the image. Such features quantify the variation in grey-level values over small distances. If objects are characterized by a repetitive pattern of grey values, texture features will be used to describe such patterns.

3.8 Image Compression

It was mentioned above that digital images take much storage space. For this reason, as well as for reasons of efficient image transmission, much attention has been paid to image *compression* techniques. The aim of such techniques is to create images that take up less space but that are sufficiently similar to the original. From these compressed images the originals may be exactly or approximately reconstructed by the application of decompression techniques.

The condition that it must be possible to reconstruct the image as exactly as possible excludes such obvious approaches as the reduction of the spatial or intensity resolution; after such operations, the original image is irrecoverable. One compression technique is called run length coding, and it exploits the fact that many images contain smaller or larger homogeneous parts. Reading the image line by line, its contents are represented by a sequence of pairs (that is, grey level and number of pixels). The factor with which the storage requirements can be reduced by this technique depends on the average run length. It is a loss-less technique (that is, it results in no loss), since it is possible to reconstruct the original image exactly by applying the inverse operation.

Another technique of loss-less compression makes use of the fact that, in general, the difference in grey levels between consecutive pixels is smaller than the grey levels themselves and that difference may therefore be stored in fewer bits.

When small degradations between a decompressed image and its original are allowed, many techniques of compression that include data loss are available. With the increase in the number of computer networks over which images are transported, for example, hospital networks or the *World Wide Web*, compression techniques have become important aspects of image processing. A standard for compressing radiological and other images is the so-called Digital Imaging and Communication in Medicine (*DICOM*) standard (see Chapters 13 and 34).

3.9 Image Registration

In some applications, two or more images are to be compared, for example, when the same scene is acquired at different times to detect possible changes. For a useful comparison, the images need to be aligned (see also the description of digital subtraction angiography in Chapter 9). This means that operations of translation, rotation, and scaling or stretching will have to be performed on one of the images, a procedure known as *image registration*. Sometimes, the parameters of such operations may be found with the help of special marker points (fiducial marks) in the images. If such points are not available, correlation techniques must be used to find the best transformation. *Fiducial marks* should be used whenever possible, since correlation techniques may be sensitive to noise.

10

3.10 Visualization

With the introduction of tomographic imaging (CT, MRI, and PET), enabling three-dimensional recon-

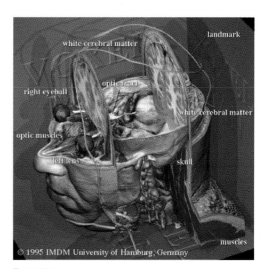

© 1995 IMDM University of Hamburg, Germany

Figure 10.5
Three-dimensional reconstruction of two-dimensional 2-D slices from a combination of CT and MRI scans (after Höhne, see Fig. 26.2).

10

struction from two-dimensional cross sections, much research has been devoted to the development of visualization techniques. Visualization is the art of rendering three-dimensional structures on the two-dimensional plane of a graphic monitor. These techniques have gone through an extremely rapid development. It is not uncommon to display three-dimensional structures (e.g., the skull or other parts of the human body) that can be peeled off layer by layer and rotated, all in real time (Fig. 10.5; see also Chapter 26). It may be clear that such sophisticated techniques require the use of very fast computing machinery.

3.11 Picture Archiving

Although strictly speaking picture archiving is not a subject of image processing, it is becoming increasingly important, especially in departments of radiology. Since modern radiological equipment yields images in digital form, the time of photographic radiology seems to be coming to an end. This, however, entails the need to store large amounts of digital images. This has been the trigger for the development of special PACS (picture archiving and communication systems). Not only must large numbers of images be stored but they should also be easily and rapidly retrievable. This implies that archiving makes heavy use of techniques of image compression, as discussed above (see Chapters 13 and 34).

4 Image Transformations

This section discusses some of the more technical details of image processing operations, with particular emphasis on operations that are used to perform image enhancement and to facilitate edge detection. As mentioned above, such image processing operations (transformations) are of the type image in, image out.

There are basically two different classes of image transformation: global and local. In both cases the intensity value in any point in the output image is a function of intensity values of a number of points in the original image. In global transformations this is a function of all points in the original image; in local transformations it is a function of only some points in a neighborhood of the corresponding pixel in the original image.

4.1 Global Transformations

The best-known global transformation is the *Fourier transform*. In signal processing, the Fourier transform results in the transformation of the signal from one domain to another: from the time domain to the frequency domain (see Chapter 25). In image processing,

the Fourier transform is a transformation of the image from the spatial domain to another domain, also a frequency domain. The Fourier transformation is often useful for frequency filtering: in the frequency domain unwanted frequencies may be removed. Back-transformation (with the inverse Fourier transformation) then results in an image in the original spatial domain from which the unwanted frequencies have been removed. Such filtering processes are sometimes used to remove, for example, an unwanted interference pattern with a known frequency (e.g., 50 or 60 Hz from an electrical power source). When low frequencies have been filtered out, back-transformation results in an image in which high frequencies are accentuated. Such an image is better suited for subsequent edge detection operations.

4.2 Local Image Transformations

In local image transformations, the intensity value of any point in the output image is a function of the intensity values of points in a neighborhood of the corre-

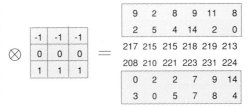

Figure 10.6
Edge detection kernel of 3 x 3 pixels, for filtering an image. The input image and the resulting output image are shown. The input image has a horizontal edge running through the middle. In the output image, this edge is clearly enhanced.

sponding point in the original image. This active neighborhood is defined by a so-called kernel.

A **kernel** usually has the shape of a square of pixels, for instance, 3 x 3 pixels, 5 x 5, or even larger, but generally $(2n + 1) \times (2n + 1)$ pixels. When using linear transformations, each element of the kernel has a coefficient associated with it. Each pixel is represented by its coordinates p_x and p_y. If the input image is written as $I0(p_x,p_y)$, the kernel coefficients as $k(i,j)$, and the output image is written as $I_1(p_x,p_y)$, the intensity of each point in the output image is expressed as a weighted sum of the intensities of the points in the active neighborhood:

$$I_1(p_x,p_y) = \sum_{i=n}^{N} \sum_{j=n}^{N} k(i,j)\, I_o\, (p_x + i, p_y + j).$$

Such transformations are often used to highlight special features (e.g., edges in an image). Consider Fig. 10.6, showing a 3 x 3 kernel, an input image, and the resulting output image. The input image has a horizontal edge running through the middle. It may be

observed that after application of the local transformation (in Fig. 10.6 denoted by the symbol $(\otimes)$ only pixels in the middle obtain relatively high values. Therefore, the kernel acts as a detector of horizontal edges. It is easy to construct similar kernels for the detection of vertical or diagonal edges. Kernels for the detection of yet other features have also been constructed, and they play an important role in the analysis chain from original image to measurements.

A special form of local transformations is the operations defined in mathematical morphology. These operations also require the definition of a kernel, called *structuring element*, but the image intensity operations are nonlinear (e.g., they involve maximum and minimum operations). Such transformations produce *erosions*, (e.g., peeling off of objects) or *dilations* (e.g., enlargements of objects) and will produce more complex transformations when they are combined. These transformations have become increasingly important in modern image processing. The details of such techniques are beyond the scope of this chapter.

5 Modern Trends in Image Processing

Procedures for digital image processing and analysis have been in development since digital computers were first used. Much has changed since the early days. First, computers have become enormously more powerful both in speed and in memory capacity. Also, the availability of disks with a capacity of gigabytes

has contributed much to the development and applicability of methods that were too complex for earlier generations of computing machinery.

Much progress has been made in the development of sensors such as TV cameras and **CCD** arrays. Modern sensors make possible spatial and intensity resolutions

10

that are much higher than those achieved by the early systems.

Whereas early applications relied on the analysis of single images, nowadays the analysis of *multimodal images* becomes increasingly important. The use of multispectral imagery has expanded to the possibility of fusion of information from different imaging modalities (e.g., in medicine the fusion of X-ray and MRI imagery). Even applications of three-dimensional analysis (e.g., series of sections or the variations of images with time) and even of four-dimensional analysis (e.g., time-dependent series of sections; see also Fig. 9.16) are now realistic goals.

As far as software is concerned, knowledge-guided methods are becoming increasingly important. When such methods are used in the top-down direction, a computerized model of the investigated object (e.g., the liver) is used to steer the image processing activity to interesting regions in the image (e.g., a liver scan). When used in the bottom-up direction, details found by image-processing procedures are checked against the model to ascertain their relevance.

Key References

See Chapter 26

See the Web site for further literature references.

IV

Patient-Centered Information Systems

Authors of Part IV

Chapter 11: Primary Care
P.J. Branger, J.S. Duisterhout, Erasmus University Rotterdam; with contribution of P. Pop, H.J. Rollema, University Hospital Maastricht

Chapter 12: Clinical Departmental Systems
A.M. van Ginneken, J.H. van Bemmel, P.W. Moorman, Erasmus University Rotterdam; A. Hasman, L.A. Plugge, Maastricht University; with contribution of N.F. de Keizer, University of Amsterdam

Chapter 13: Clinical Support Systems
J.H. van Bemmel, A.M. van Ginneken, J. Lindemans, Erasmus University Rotterdam; A. Hasman, Maastricht University; H.Y. Kwa, Cendata, Nieuwegein

Chapter 14: Nursing Information Systems
S.J. Grobe, University of Texas, Austin; P.J.M.M. Epping, Faculty of Nursing, Polytechnic Leiden; W. Goossen, Nursing Sciences, Polytechnic Leeuwarden

11 Primary Care

1 Introduction

Primary care is the area of general health care where patients are treated before they are possibly referred to a specialist or a hospital. In some countries, therefore, primary care is also called *first-line health care*, whereas primary care physicians are generally called *general practitioners* (**GPs**). In the United States, the Institute of Medicine adopted the following definition:

Primary care is the provision of integrated, accessible health care services by clinicians who are accountable for addressing a large majority of personal health care needs, developing a sustained partnership with patients, and practicing in the context of family and community.

In most countries primary care is the area where patients enter the health care system. It is often also the area of population-oriented care and the place where continuous care is given, for example, to patients with chronic diseases, elderly people, or patients who need home care and palliative care. In many countries "primary care" is done in a different setting. For instance:

- Some specialists may work in the "first-line" health care setting, for example, pediatricians in Scandinavian countries or obstetricians and gynecologists in the USA.
- In Germany, patients are allowed to turn directly to specialists who are *niedergelassene Ärtzte* ("settled physicians").
- In the United Kingdom and The Netherlands, as well as in a growing number of other countries, all patients must first contact a GP before they are allowed to go to a specialist or a hospital. In these countries the GP acts as a "**gatekeeper**" to specialized health care.

This chapter provides an introduction to the use of information systems in primary care. Section 2 describes the growing integration between primary care and shared care; Section 3 gives a historic overview of information systems in primary care. Section 4 describes the functionality of primary care systems; new developments are continuously expanding the functionality. Finally, Section 5 discusses some of the most promising developments in primary care information systems.

2 Primary Care and Shared Care

As mentioned above, primary care is not the same everywhere because it is strongly related to the structure of the health care systems in different countries. Because of the differences in the structures of

health care systems the degree of computerization in primary care may also differ from country to country. In the second half of the 1990s, the highest percentages of information systems in primary care can

PANEL 11.1

Diabetes Mellitus

Diabetes mellitus is an example of a chronic disorder that requires lifelong medical attention. There is evidence that diabetes mellitus will become an even more serious public health problem in the years to come. In The Netherlands, for instance, with a population of 15.6 million people, it has been estimated that the number of patients with diabetes will increase from 191,000 in 1980 (1.35% of the population) to 355,000 (2.2%) in 2005. This increase is partly due to the aging of the population, but it is also the result of an increasing incidence of diabetes. Furthermore, GPs are often confronted with diabetic patients with comorbidities. Researchers found that 40% of the diabetic patients over age 65 suffer from one or more other diseases, such as chronic ischemic heart disease or hypertension. These patients are likely to be involved in more than one surveillance scheme, which may lead to improperly coordinated care, and possibly to inefficient care. This was the reason to establish the so-called St. Vincent Declaration in 1989, which describes protocols how patients suffering from diabetes mellitus should be treated.

be found in the United Kingdom and The Netherlands, followed by the Scandinavian countries. Differences in the services provided by primary care, which varies from one country to another, are influenced by the following:

- the structure of the health care system, often regulated by national law, as well as by policies regarding the location and size of primary care practices and hospitals;
- the extent to which GPs act as the **gatekeepers** to the health care system and the way that patients are referred to specialists;
- the type of physician who provides primary care, for example, a GP, a family physician, an internist, pediatrician, or another specialist;
- the existence of "competitive" health care organizations, such as **managed care**;
- the financial access to care, for example, national health service, and health insurance; and
- the nearby availability and the accessibility of secondary health care facilities.

Examples of differences in health care structures between countries are described below.

- In *Finland* the entire population is covered by health insurance, which includes compensation for low income because of illness as well as high treatment costs. Most primary care is free of charge. Exceptions are dental care for adults and treatment in health center hospitals. For specialized hospital treatment, patients pay a fraction of the real costs. Patients first apply to their local health center or private practitioner for examination and treatment. If he or she cannot be treated there, the patient is referred to the outpatient department of a hospital.
- In *Belgium* a patient contacts a GP when necessary and pays immediately and directly for the provided service. There is no permanent relationship between a GP and a patient. A patient may refer to various GPs at the same time or consecutively for different health problems or even for the same health problem.
- In *Germany* a GP (*niedergelassene Arzt*) is also a person's primary contact with the health care system, but this GP is generally a specialized physician who is chosen because of his or her specialization.
- In *The Netherlands* and the *United Kingdom* each person is registered in the practice of one GP only, and that person visits only that GP or one of

his or her colleagues in the same primary care practice. The GP functions as a gatekeeper between primary and secondary care. Patients first consult the GP for any health problem. If deemed necessary, the GP refers the patient to a specialist who reports back to the same GP. The Dutch GP is increasingly considered the coordinator of **shared care**

Shared care is a situation in which clinicians (GPs and specialists) jointly treat the same patient. Patients requiring shared care are, for example, patients suffering from chronic disorders, such as diabetes mellitus, obstructive pulmonary diseases, or cardiological diseases, or patients who receive palliative care at home. To be effective, shared care requires structured coordination of medical activities, in which clinicians *know* what guidelines or **protocols** to follow and in which clinicians *trust* each other's actions and interventions. When different providers are involved in a patient's

care without proper coordination, the care process may not be meaningfully integrated; a patient receiving such care under such conditions may be subject to unjustified interventions or justified actions may not be performed.

In some countries *shared care protocols* have been developed for a number of health problems, involving the allocation of tasks between health care providers from different disciplines. Optimal communication is considered a vital aspect of shared care from both a medical and a cost-effectiveness point of view (see also Panel 11.1).

The coordination of care for chronically ill patients places large demands on the information-processing capacity of the GP and the efficiency of communication with other care providers. Many studies have demonstrated that communication between clinicians about cotreated patients is prone to be delayed, incomplete, or erroneous. Information systems may assist in improving this situation.

11

3 History of Primary Care Information Systems

In the beginning of the 1980s, at the time when the personal computer (**PC**) came on the market, the price and size of computers made it feasible to introduce computers in clinician's offices. The initial implementation of computers was driven by the need to provide administrative and medical **audit** information. In the United States, Canada and some European countries, PCs were first used in primary care in the early 1980s for administrative tasks, such as contact registration and patient scheduling, and for financial tasks, such as invoicing.

Later, basic patient-oriented data, such as **reasons for encounter,** diagnoses, and prescribed drugs, were also stored in the computer. However, these data were used for statistical reasons rather than for patient care. In several countries reporting of statistics is a task of primary care providers.

Primary care providers deliver data to several registers

of health statistics to gain insight into the health status of a population, for example, patient discharge information (diagnoses), data on newborns and abortions, and the incidence of communicable diseases and cancer. Furthermore, national registers keep identification numbers (see also Chapter 33) and classifications of laboratory procedures, surgical and rehabilitation procedures, X-ray examinations, and drugs.

However, apart from statistics, in the early primary care systems no information on the types of health problems in primary care was usually available. The introduction of the first *computer-based patient record* (CPR) systems (see also Chapters 7 and 29) in primary care in the 1980s was a major step forward in that respect. Not only did the patient data in the CPRs improve the quality of the statistics but they also made it possible for the information systems to be used for patient care itself, for the implementation of protocols, for the electronic interchange of patient data to support shared care (see Chapter 5), and for **decision-support systems** for example, drug prescription or the treatment of chronic diseases) (see Chapter 16). It is not surprising that CPRs were first introduced in primary care information systems and that they are mainly used in those countries where the GP plays a coordinating role and functions as the gatekeeper to secondary care, because in those situations, the GP coordinates the flow of all information on the patient.

Not only GPs are affected by the use of information systems in primary care. Other parties that are interested include:

- health insurance companies, which may benefit from receiving more accurate statistics on the care that has been provided as well as documentation for reimbursement in fee-for-service situations;
- the government and national health organizations, which may receive better reviews of the actual health care and health statistics;
- physicians' organizations, which may acquire data on the quality and the efficacy of care; and
- pharmaceutical industries that are interested in acquiring data on drug consumption and adverse drug reactions, for example, by **postmarketing surveillance** studies.

3.1 Gatekeepers in Primary Care

As mentioned earlier, in some countries the GP functions as the patient's entrance point to secondary care. The role of the GP, then, is to:

- authorize access to specialty, emergency, and hospital care,
- authorize diagnostic procedures, such as X rays,
- guard an individual patient from undertreatment by promptly referring the patient to the proper specialist, and
- guard an individual patient from overtreatment by trying to judge the appropriateness of treatment for referred patients.

The GP therefore needs to match a patient's needs and preferences with the correct use of medical procedures. In the United States, health maintenance organizations (HMOs), consisting of groups of hospitals and primary care providers, employ GPs as gatekeepers. In the United Kingdom, fundholding GPs hold the budget for their patients. With these budgets, the GP tries to purchase high-quality medical services for a reasonable price.

The gatekeeper's role has a number of implications for the information-processing capacity of the GP and the structuring of the GP's work. These items are discussed in the next section.

3.2 Introducing Information Systems in Primary Care: The Dutch Experience

In developed countries the reasons for introducing primary care systems are generally driven by the wish to increase the quality and the efficiency of health care. In developing countries, however, reasons are different from those that prevail in Europe, the United States, Canada, Japan, or Australia. In many developing countries maternal and child health programs have the highest priority in primary health care. For instance, the *World Health Organization* estimates that each year approximately 500,000 women die from pregnancy-related causes, and more than 98% of these women live in developing countries. There, too, primary care systems of a different kind may help to trace causes of diseases and to support epidemiological studies. Therefore, there are generally several reasons to introduce computers in primary care:

- Administration

In most countries a primary care practice operates as an independent and private enterprise, and therefore it must organize its own financial affairs. It is possible to support these financial affairs by use of information systems, which will render direct benefits to the practicing physician: reduction of the time required for administrative tasks, more accurate bookkeeping, and reduced expenses.

- Patient care

If a primary care system contains a CPR, it allows for the support of patient care by controlling drug prescriptions, incorporating care protocols and **decision-support systems**, and allowing for the electronic interchange of patient data and the performance of population-oriented tasks, such as tracing patients with certain risks and patients to be vaccinated. These functions will improve the quality of care and will possibly reduce the costs of health care on a national level.

- Research

Patient data in paper-based patient records in primary care are not accessible for health care research. In most primary care practices, patient data are still kept in handwritten paper records, with personal notes presented in a chronological order. Structured registration of patient problems, the documentation of a minimal set of patient data, and age-gender registers allow for computerized patient selection for research projects. More sophisticated research in primary care requires the introduction of a CPR with a structured registration of patient data over time.

- Shared care

In the past, most GPs in primary care operated on an individual basis. They kept their own patient documentation in their own style. Nowadays, GPs collaborate more and more, for example, in health care centers or with care providers in other institutions. Ideally, patient records are shared, which means that data must be available at different locations.

- Coded and quantified data

Handwriting does not enforce data structuring. When prescriptions or other messages must be interpreted by individuals other than the originator, an inability to read the originator's handwriting also causes errors. The use of typed data partly solves this problem. A CPR, however, invites the use of standard terminology and eases the classification and coding of data, reducing variability as a result of different interpretations.

- Quality control

Primary care systems with embedded CPRs open the possibility of comparing care profiles of clinicians within a region and between regions. Deviations are easily traced by comparing each practice with group averages and by reporting back to each clinician his or her own profile against the group average.

- Continuing medical education

The data in primary care systems can be used by teaching institutions for *case* finding and training.

3.3 Introduction of Information Systems in Primary Care

This section describes some factors that positively influenced the introduction of information systems in primary care. As an example, we give the reasons for their introduction in The Netherlands, but these reasons may equally apply to other countries such as the United Kingdom, the Scandinavian countries, Canada, and other countries with comparable health-care system structures.

- Leading role of professional physicians' organizations

In 1984, the Dutch National Association of GPs realized that information systems would have a great impact on primary care. A working group produced a reference model for a primary care information system describing its desired functionality and **data model**. Industries were invited to present their products for approval. The systems that were approved were published in the GP Association's journal.

- Training of clinicians

The Association started a training program, supported by a grant from the Ministry of Health. A course book was produced, and courses were given throughout the country. University departments of primary care together with departments of medical informatics started training courses for GPs. An annual *Symposium on The GP and the CPR* keeps GPs informed about the latest developments and trends.

11

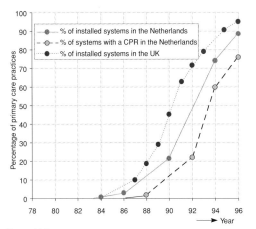

Figure 11.1
Growth of the number of installed information systems and CPRs in primary care in The Netherlands and the United Kingdom as a function of time.

11

• Reference model

The reference model was intended to be used as a guideline by both the developers and by the testers of primary care information systems. When the first developments of information systems for GPs started in The Netherlands, the Dutch association for General Practice realized that it would be important to play an active role in the development rather than to wait and see what the industry would provide. Therefore, a committee was established for the coordination of the introduction of primary care information systems in health care. This committee produced a reference model and a testing procedure for primary care information systems. The reference model describes the following functional modules:
- basic module (Section 4.1);
- medical module (Section 4.2);
- pharmacy module (Section 4.3);
- scheduling module (Section 4.4);
- financial module (Section 4.5);
- communications module (Section 4.6);
- research module (Section 4.7).

The desired functionality of each of these modules is described in the reference model; however, it does not describe the way in which it must be implemented, although it does provide guidelines for the interface and response times. A general data model describing the required data elements, including field length and data type, is provided. Data entities such as patient demographics, prescriptions or laboratory results are described by the constituting fields and the relationships between the entities. For coded data, existing standards are used as much as possible, such as the International Classification of Primary Care (**ICPC**) or the International Classification of Diseases (**ICD**) (see Chapter 6). Reference tables or thesauri are provided for all other coded data.

The reference model also contains a framework for testing systems. For systems that obtain the qualification conforming to the reference model a summary of the test report is printed in the GP Association's journal and an extensive test report can be obtained.

• Financial incentives

Not all GPs are willing to contribute financially to improve the quality of care. A reimbursement of 60% of the costs of using computers by health insurance companies in the early 1990s also stimulated the introduction of the CPR. By the end of 1996 more than 90% of all 6,500 Dutch GPs used an information system, more than 60% of which contained a CPR.

Information systems in primary care receive much attention in several other countries as well. In 1996 more than 90% of GP in the United Kingdom were using information systems, and more than 10% of these systems contained a CPR. Figure 11.1 shows the number of GPs using information systems in their practices in the United Kingdom and The Netherlands from 1980 to 1996.

4 Functionality of Primary Care Information Systems

This section discusses the functionality of a typical primary care information system that has been widely implemented in The Netherlands, where primary care physicians act as the gatekeepers in health care. The situation in the Netherlands is very similar to that in other countries, such as the United Kingdom and the Scandinavian countries. A primary care information system contains functions for the following tasks:

- practice organization and administration,
- patient care, and
- statistical overviews and research.

In the following description of a primary care information system, a modular approach will be followed. Other modular structures may also be possible, depending on the implementation in a country's health care organization. However, the modules to be described will generally be applicable to many different situations.

4.1 Basic Module

The basic module is always part of the system. It contains functions for maintaining the following data, registers, and procedures:

- Data
  - **age-gender registries** of all patients in the practice
  - **demographic data**, including health insurance data, of the patients; and
  - data on the group of people who form a household.
- Registers
  - registration of visits, examinations, and laboratory tests;
  - simple financial data, such as invoices, derived from actions and interventions (all other financial functions are supported by the financial module); and

- production of several types of standard overviews;
- Procedures
  - **data protection**: the system can only be used by authorized users;
  - use by more than one user simultaneously, for example, GPs, nurses and assistants; and
  - **log-in** control and **backup** facilities.

4.2 Medical Module

For more advanced registration of patient data the medical module is required. The core of the medical module is a CPR for primary care. To increase the possibilities for data exchange, the **reference model** describes a **data model** for all codable items. Coding tables are also specified. Data in the CPR are grouped by visit and are time stamped. A second type of ordering is made possible by using the so-called **SOAP** (subjective, objective, assessment, and plan) system (Chapter 7). Diagnoses and **reasons for encounter** are coded according to the International Classification of Primary Care (Chapter 6).

The medical module also contains facilities for **problem-oriented** registration. This means that it is possible to name and code a patient's main problems explicitly and to link the data in the CPR with one or more problems. This makes it possible to view patient data related to a particular problem or to view the complete record. Figures 11.2 and 11.3 show two examples of typical chronologically ordered patient records of systems operational in The Netherlands. The first one is an example of a system with a **character-based** interface; the second one has a graphical interface. Note the similarities between the two screens.

The CPR is the heart of the medical module. From this module most patient-oriented functions may be invoked. Drug prescriptions can be made by using a national drug database, which contains information about **contraindications**, **drug interactions**, dosages,

11

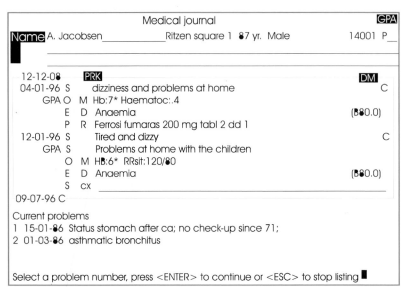

Figure 11.2
Example of a character-based primary care system. The data are ordered chronologically and are stamped with the date of data entry and the initials of the treating GP. The capital letters in the second column represent one of the SOAP (subjective, objective, assessment, and plan) codes. The contents of the line are further specified by the single capital letter in the fourth column. An optional number in the third column indicates a link to a problem number.

command CX means:
Show problem list

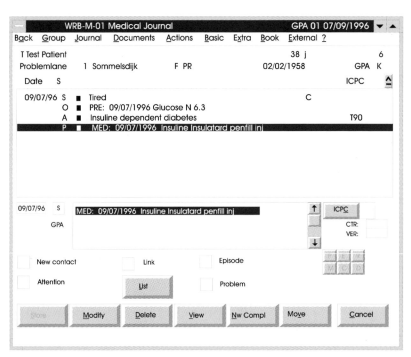

Figure 11.3
Example of a windows-based primary care information system. The screen is used to enter medical data. The top section on the screen contains display information only and cannot be changed. The middle section is the data window, and the lower section is where data are entered. Diagnostic coding in free text is done on the bottom line. From the action field on the menu bar, other windows can be invoked to enter prescriptions and laboratory data.

and prices. If diagnoses and prescriptions are properly coded, the prescription module is able to generate warnings such as the following:

- "Drug not reimbursed by insurance, select other drug."
- "This drug will interact with another drug currently prescribed, being . . .."
- "The drug . . . with a similar therapeutic effect has already been prescribed and is still being used."
- "This drug is contraindicated by diagnostic code . . .."
- "The dosage prescribed is outside the normal range for a person of age . . .."

The prescription function can be used by the GP as well as by his or her assistant; the assistant, however, is only allowed to repeat prescriptions up to a maximum number defined by the GP.

4.3 Pharmacy Module

Traditionally, in The Netherlands drug dispensing is done by GPs in villages and by a pharmacist in larger cities. The pharmacy module of a primary care information system is intended to support drug-dispensing GPs. The pharmacy module consists of two parts:

- functions for dispensing drugs, and
- functions for prescribing drugs

The prescription functionality is the same as the one in the medical module, so the essential part of the pharmacy module is the dispensing functionality, which includes financial functions. (For related functions in hospital pharmacy systems, see Section 6 of Chapter 13.)

4.4 Scheduling Module

The scheduling module supports appointment registration. It contains functions to support the practicing clerk in making appointments, producing overviews and working lists, and keeping the schedule for all GPs in a practice. It is integrated into the patient selection function (waitinglist management) of the medical module.

The modules described above are an integral part of a primary care information system. The modules for financial administration, communication, and letter-writing can be either fully integrated or linked with external modules. For the production of letters, a GP may use a standard **word processor** that is integrated into the system.

4.5 Financial Module

The financial functions for producing invoices, registering payments, and printing reminders are part of the basic module. However, these functions do not make up the complete financial administration of a health care practice. Some systems offer an integrated financial module that includes a ledger, a means for value-added tax (VAT) administration, and so forth. The software of these modules is accepted by financial auditors.

The data from the basic module can also be exported to a separate financial system.

4.6 Communication Module

GPs no longer operate in isolation, as already observed in Section 2 on shared care. When different care providers are involved in patient care, the GP remains the coordinator of the data in the network of information. Traditionally, information is exchanged by telephone, mail, or **fax**. Problems in with these forms of communication are described below:

- Lack of protocols for the exchange of messages
It is not clear for every situation when and what kind of message will be sent or will be expected. For instance, a GP is not automatically informed when a cotreating specialist changes the medication or when a hospitalized patient is discharged.

- Timely delivery
Discharge letters from specialists are often produced and delivered weeks after a patient has been discharged from the hospital.

11

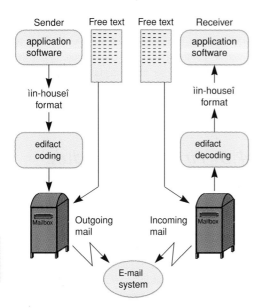

Figure 11.4
Electronic communication involves three layers of software on both the receiving and the sending sides. The top level is the application that generates the messages and stores them in proprietary format. The second layer encodes these messages by using standards for the semantics and EDIFACT for the syntax of the messages. The third layer is responsible for the technical exchange of the messages with the other side. At the receiving side decoding software transforms the EDIFACT messages to the proprietary format, which can then be further used by the application programs.

1. The first layer, the **application layer**, consists of the functions that the user can see. Messages such as referral letters or prescriptions may be sent as free or coded text. These messages are then encoded and stored in a system-dependent format, a so-called in-house format.

2. The second layer encodes these in-house-formatted messages into a standard message-type format describing the contents and the structure of the data contained in the messages. This is called the **semantic** part of the message. The **syntax** of the message is defined by a standard message format called **EDIFACT**, which is a general and international standard for electronic data interchange (Chapter 5). The EDIFACT-encoded messages are temporarily stored in an electronic mailbox for outgoing mail together with any other free-text messages.

3. The third layer is the **communication link** layer. This software layer empties the outgoing mail box and sends it to an external mail system and it receives mail in the mailbox for incoming mail.

At the receiving end there are also three layers. The first one is the decoding layer, which reads all the incoming mail from its mailbox. If a message is EDIFACT-encoded, that message is retrieved and decoded, and its contents are stored in a message in the in-house format. The user can manipulate the messages with the application layer software. For instance, laboratory results can be viewed on the display screen and can be directly inserted into the CPR with a few keystrokes. This avoids retyping and the introduction of errors.

4.7 Research Module

One of the modules, often still under development, is the research module. This module is intended to support the research of departments of primary care of universities. The module is intended to facilitate registration of extra data for patients participating in research projects and to extract data for analysis but makes the patient who is the source of the data anonymous.

At present, most departments of primary care have their own registration networks that they use to select data for research purposes. A few departments also have a proto-

- Incomplete information
Referral letters, for instance, from the GP to a specialist, generally contain unstructured information. The receiving specialist requires reliable data, which means that he or she also needs to know how the data were obtained.

- Errors in transcription of data ·
Data are read from the patient record and are typed in the referral letter or discharge letter. The receiver reads the letter and inserts the relevant data into another patient record. Errors can be made at each of these steps. **Electronic data interchange** largely overcomes these problems.

The communication module consists of three layers of software (Fig. 11.4):

PANEL 11.2

Shared Care for Patients with Benign Prostatic Hyperplasia

In all countries, primary care is emphasized to avoid patient referral to hospitals. To equip clinicians in primary care with the required diagnostic and therapeutic methods, a host of instruments and systems has been introduced in the primary-care setting. In some countries, clinicians in primary care are able to analyze urine and blood samples, record and interpret electrocardiograms, or take X-ray pictures. Many such techniques and instruments are supported by computers. If it is necessary to refer patients to specialists, the results of diagnostic tests can be electronically transmitted from the primary care setting to the outpatient clinic of the hospital.

One example of a test that is intended for use in screening patients for a possible disease, or monitoring a trend in the development of a disease is the diagnosis of prostatic obstruction due to benign prostatic hyperplasia (BPH). This test is generally carried out in a clinical setting but can now easily be done in a primary care setting.

It was proven that the degree of obstruction in BPH not only determines the choice of the type of treatment (e.g., medication or surgery), but also the clinical outcome after treatment. The presence of prostatic obstruction due to BPH is usually assessed by taking urodynamic recording of simultaneous bladder pressure and urinary flow rate, which are considered the best means of diagnosing the presence of infravesical obstruction. This test is generally done under the supervision of an urologist, since the test is invasive.

For use in the primary care setting, a diagnostic uroflow classification system was developed. This system compares uroflow parameters, obtained from patients who are generally over 50 years of age, with values derived from a database of healthy people. When a patient, being tested for BPH voids his bladder, a system computes the presence of obstruction from the measured flow rate and the voided volume, based on a decision model that uses **logistic regression**. It has been proven that this method is able to diagnose patients with severe urodynamic obstructions so that the percentage of patients referred to a urologist can be decreased by as much as one-third. Figure 11.5 shows a **ROC** of the system for the detection of prostatic obstruction in BPH, and Fig. 11.6 presents the decision tree for a typical shared care setting.

11

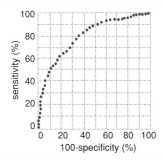

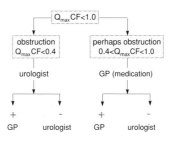

Figure 11.5
ROC for the detection of infravesical obstructions in benign prostatic hyperplasia.

Figure 11.6
Decision tree for a typical shared-care setting applying the system for the diagnosis of prostatic obstructions.

type module that allows researchers to define extra questionnaires that must be filled out at each patient encounter for patients who participate in research projects. Standardization of this functionality has not yet been achieved. To extract data from the primary care information system, a standard EDIFACT message has been developed (see Chapter 5). This message facilitates the use of data for research from different types of systems.

5 Developments

In primary care, a wide variety of patient data are collected. Together they form a very wide spectrum of complaints, findings, laboratory data, prescribed drugs, reports from specialists, and so forth, covering virtually the entire spectrum of health care. One cannot expect a GP to be able to oversee this entire spectrum of data in depth. Furthermore, medical knowledge is continuously expanding, and new diagnostic methods and therapeutic techniques become available all the time (see also Panel 11.2).

Therefore, many efforts are undertaken to develop information systems to support clinicians in primary care. These information systems should support the following tasks and functions:

- collect patient data in user-friendly and standardized ways;
- transmit patient data electronically to other clinicians for consultation;
- use data for shared care and increasingly for **evidence-based medicine**;
- receive alerts in case deviations from guidelines or protocols are detected;
- receive support in decision making, for example, by using **critiquing systems**;
- make possible communication with systems elsewhere, for example, the digital library;

- use the data for preventive purposes and **case finding**;
- be able to assess the quality and the efficacy of care;
- use the data to support practice management and planning;
- use collections of data in primary care for population-based studies; and
- use patient data for research and education.

Central to these developments is a powerful CPR (see Chapters 7 and 29).

Key References

Weed LL. *Medical Records, Medical Education and Patient Care: The Problem-Oriented Medical Record as a Basic Tool.* Cleveland OH: Case Western Reserve Press, 1971.

Van der Lei J, Duisterhout JS, Westerhof H, et al. The introduction of computer-based patient records in the Netherlands. Ann Intern Med 1993;119:1036-41.

See the Web site for further literature references.

11

12 Clinical Departmental Systems

1 Introduction

During the 1980s and 1990s continuous efforts have been made to exploit computers to enhance the collection, distribution, and interpretation of patient data. Ideally, all patient data should be integrated and should be available for consultation throughout clinics and hospitals. This has not yet been achieved completely. Considerable progress has been made in the development of computerized equivalents of the paper record, with as its main aims the support of patient care, decision support, and research. Development of the computer-based patient record (**CPR**) and obstacles in this process are discussed in Chapter 7.

Beside electronic equivalents of paper-based records, there are numerous departmental systems, that per-

form specific tasks, and these are often encountered in certain clinical departments only. These tasks are related to the collection of specific data for patient care, research, management, and planning, and to the maintenance of national data repositories. Specific tasks take place, for instance, in departments of internal medicine (oncology, nephrology, endocrinology, hematology, or endoscopy), in cardiology, neurology, obstetrics, surgery, or psychiatry. Patient monitoring and radiotherapy are special departments with specific requirements for patient care not encountered in other clinical departments.

Computers in clinical departments are generally used for the following tasks:

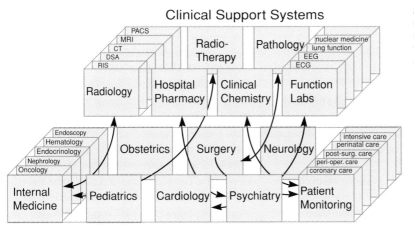

Clinical Support Systems

PACS, MRI, CT, DSA, RIS — Radiology — Radio-Therapy — Hospital Pharmacy — Clinical Chemistry — Pathology — Function Labs — nuclear medicine, lung function, EEG, ECG

Endoscopy, Hematology, Endocrinology, Nephrology, Oncology — Internal Medicine — Pediatrics — Obstetrics — Surgery — Cardiology — Neurology — Psychiatry — Patient Monitoring — intensive care, perinatal care, post-surg. care, peri-oper. care, coronary care

Clinical Departmental Systems

Figure 12.1
Overview of most patient-oriented information systems that may be found in a clinical environment.

171

- Administrative support
  This concerns the administrative and logistic planning of patient care and interventions.
- Patient data collection
  The acquisition, storage, and retrieval of patient data, examinations, biosignals, and images in CPRs; the real-time reduction and verification and the coding and processing of patient data; and the integration of all patient data into one comprehensive presentation.
- Decisions
  Simulation of interventions by using models, the support of diagnostic and therapeutic decision making, and the offering of advice and reminders to patients.
- Monitoring
  The monitoring and assessment of therapy, such as drug therapy, and the monitoring of patients in the clinic or at home.

- Reporting
  Generation of reports, for example, after the discharge of the patient from the hospital or when referring patients to other clinicians.
- Assessment
  Evaluation of the effect of the care that was provided on patient outcome.
- Research
  Studying the course of, for example, congenital or chronic diseases.

Some specific applications from this extensive and varied group of possible applications are briefly reviewed. Clinical-support systems that are found in departments such as the clinical chemistry laboratory, the hospital pharmacy, or pathology, are discussed in Chapter 13; imaging systems were discussed in Chapter 9. Figure 12.1 sketches an overview of virtually all patient-oriented information systems that can be found in a clinical environment.

2 Internal Medicine

Internal medicine may be considered the central specialty in clinical care. Within internal medicine, however, several subspecialties can be discerned, each with its own specific requirements for patient data collection and interpretation.

2.1 Oncology

In oncology, computers may offer help in the *registration* of data on the diagnosis and treatment of cancer patients and in giving *decision support* to clinicians for chemotherapy or radiotherapy (for the latter, see Section 10).
For the administration of drugs during **chemotherapy**, **protocols** that should be strictly followed have been developed. Computers may assist in both selecting and monitoring protocols.
We give some examples of both registration systems and protocol-support systems.

- Oncology registration systems
Two examples of large-scale projects in oncology are the so-called Clinical Oncology Information Network (COIN) and the National Cancer Database Project. The National Health Service (NHS) in the United Kingdom started COIN because the systems for cancer registration that were available at the time were inadequate for evaluation of the care process. In the United States, similar problems were encountered, which led to the initiation of the National Cancer Database Project in 1989.
Both projects originated from the conviction that patient data collected for patient care should also be suitable for **quality assessment,** research, and management. In the United Kingdom it proved to be impossible to reach consensus on a fully standardized oncology record. Instead, the NHS now promotes the collection of the Core Clinical Data Set, which is especially tailored to comparative research. Much emphasis is put on the alleviation of symptoms, identification

of patients with comparable prognoses, and criteria for drug dosage control.

A third example is related to the Mount Vernon Centre for Cancer Treatment, where the local cancer registry system had become obsolete. In the United Kingdom, specially trained administrative staff extracted the data from paper-based records and subsequently entered them into a computer system. This often caused delays, ranging from 3 to 6 months after the patient's first visit, because the paper-based record was almost continuously in use during treatment. For practical reasons, clinicians did not verify the extracted data. In the present system, all data are directly entered by the staff that produce the data, which has led to a large improvement in data reliability. Data entry is supported with computer forms, and personal administrative data are recorded only once. There are separate forms (screens) for the entry of data on drug prescriptions, radiation therapy, and treatment with radio-active substances. The data fulfill the requirements of the NHS and are suitable for clinical evaluation and for the creation of a variety of views. The system also allows for insight into the financial aspects of delivered care.

- Protocols for chemotherapy

Treatment of cancer patients usually proceeds strictly in accordance with a predefined **protocol**. The main reason is that the therapy of malignant disease is so aggressive that the patient's condition requires con-

stant monitoring. Criteria for interruption or changes in therapy must be explicitly available. Standardized treatment also facilitates evaluation of the treatment's effectiveness and risks. OCIS (developed at Johns Hopkins University, Baltimore, United States) and ONCOCIN (developed at Stanford University, United States), are examples of systems that offer support in adhering to the often complex protocols. Hence, the primary goal of these systems is decision support and not cancer registration as such. The systems generate reminders for the monitoring of certain parameters, draw attention to abnormal test results, and indicate the necessary adjustments to treatment.

The protocol entry system known as **OPAL,** also from Stanford University and described in Chapter 28, enabled clinicians to enter and maintain descriptions of oncology protocols that needed to be represented within the **ONCOCIN** knowledge base. Subsequent work on the **PROTÉGÉ** system (see Chapter 29) has allowed the Stanford-based investigators to generate graphical tools for the entry of knowledge related to oncology protocols as well as knowledge of protocols related to other areas of medicine (see Fig. 12.2).

2.2 Nephrology

Because of a shortage of donor kidneys, the number of patients depending on hemodialysis has risen considerably over the last decade. Many patients are, there-

12

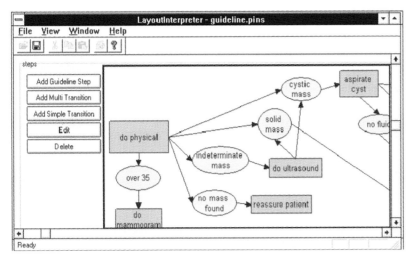

Figure 12.2
Example of a protocol entry tool generated by the PROTÉGÉ system.

fore, dependent on renal dialysis. **Dialysis** is a complex process that sometimes results in undesired effects, which must be kept to a minimum to reduce the risks of complications. During preparation of the filters, reverse flow of nonsterile fluid may lead to a variety of acute and chronic reactions. Continuous monitoring of the pressure relation between venous blood and dialysis fluid enables detection of this undesired backflow. It may also happen that ultrafiltration must be stopped because of hypotension or muscle cramps. During dialysis the following parameters are monitored: temperature, pH, pressure, flow, and filtration speed. These data can easily be stored in a computer and can be presented in graphic form.

The nephrology department in the Maria delle Croci Hospital in Ravenna, Italy, for instance, uses computers and telecommunication to monitor dialysis treatments in its own clinic as well as in clinics at other geographical locations. The system is connected to eight external hospitals and is able to monitor 16 local and 24 external dialysis machines simultaneously. Data from previous dialysis sessions are available. The available data have proven to be useful for research, and they have provided more insight into the various problems in dialysis and their possible causes.

Peritoneal dialysis offers the patient much more freedom. It is, however, difficult to evaluate the adequacy of the treatment, that is, to detect whether there is under- or overdialysis. Investigators have developed several computer programs that compute an index of adequacy, which is based on (among other things) urea, creatinine, and uric acid levels in peritoneal fluid. The index is intended to provide the clinician with information on the adjustments that need to be made on dialysis treatment. Since the various applications assign different weights to these parameters, they often produce different indices of adequacy for the same patient. Research efforts continue to determine how peritoneal dialysis can be evaluated most reliably for adequate adjustment.

2.3 Endocrinology – diabetes

The Institute for Diabetes Technology at the University of Ulm, Germany, has developed the application *Romeo* to assist diabetic patients at home by giving them therapeutic directions. The treating clinician enters the therapy plan. This includes time schedules for glucose measurements, a schema with dosages for insulin injection, dietary recommendations, and advice for physical exercise. On the basis of the complete therapy plan, *Romeo* will remind the patient at the appropriate time about certain actions that must be taken. The system is able to perform blood-glucose measurements automatically and to store the results. The patient reports data on glucose and ketone levels in the urine, insulin injections, food intake, and physical exercise. *Romeo* produces daily overviews of the patient's activities and the course of blood glucose levels, and an average profile for each 24-hour period.

The system has proven to have a stimulating effect on patients, so that their diabetes is relatively well regulated. The immediate **feedback** motivates them to achieve an optimal result. Poorly regulated patients, however, are mainly frustrated with the system. The use of systems such as *Romeo* therefore can have a strong influence on a patient's daily life. Clinicians must therefore take great care to inform their patients to avoid demotivating effects.

2.4 Hematology – hemophilia

In 1996 the Regional Hemophilia Centre at Manchester Royal Infirmary in the United Kingdom had data on more than 600 patients in its records, 450 of whom suffered from hemophilia. In addition, 100 genetic carriers of the disease had been registered. Annually, about 150 patients register for treatment. Since 1990, patient data have been kept in an information system. The data include personal details, a set of relevant test results, symptoms, and treatment, received either in the clinic or at home. Recording of site of bleeding and the type and dosage of the administered drugs, including noncoagulation medication, is emphasized. It is possible to record additional information as free text.

For each patient, the system produces cumulative reports of patient data. Within a year, cumulative printouts replace previous ones in the paper-based record. This feature provides the clinician with immediate overviews of the most recent bleeding events and the related treatments. It is immediately apparent which body sites require preventive action because of frequent bleeding. The system automatically produces reminders for patients to present themselves for regular checkups. Although data can be displayed electronically, printouts are added to the paper-based record to prevent these records from being incomplete and to avoid disruption of routine patient care. Registration of treatment helps the institution with controlling its stock of supplies. The patient database is also able to produce reports for the national hemophilia register and it supports data retrieval for scientific purposes.

2.5 Intestinal Endoscopy

Although not yet in widespread use, there are several computer applications for use in **endoscopy** departments. Most of these applications are used for reporting. The systems vary greatly in the degree to which they support structured (i.e., standardized and codable) data entry. Some applications are mainly administrative, in the sense that only patient **demographic** data adhere to a standard format, whereas the endoscopic reports are stored as free text.
Some systems permit coding of the endoscopic diagnosis or interpretation, whereas others also support standardized entry of descriptive information, (i.e., the actual findings). The largest problem is the lack of a widely accepted standard for endoscopic terminology. The matter is further complicated by the fact that subjective interpretations and objective descriptive terms are not always easy to distinguish. A term such as "acute gastritis" describes a histological finding and must be categorized as a subjective, interpretative term when based only on observations made during endoscopy. Yet, it is inappropriate to view "blood" as a purely interpretative term and to expect clinicians to use the expression "red viscous fluid" when they are describing blood that they see through the endoscope. Despite the difficulties in obtaining structured data, there are also advantages in collecting endoscopic findings in a structured fashion. A study that compared free-text reports with structured reports showed that the latter contained more information, showed more uniformity, and were less ambiguous. Not only are better-quality reports likely to improve the quality of care, but structured data are also suitable for research, **quality assessment, decision support,** and management purposes (see Chapter 7). Financial administration can easily be supported, and patients will automatically be reminded to present for follow-up examinations.

12

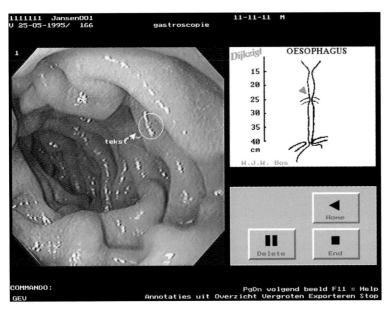

Figure 12.3
Endoscopic procedure developed in the University Hospital in Rotterdam. Physicians can select the images that they wish to store. They can also add arrows and comments to the selected images for later reference.

The introduction of the digital endoscope enables computer storage of endoscopic images. Such a means of storage allows endoscopists to retrieve images from previous examinations when a patient comes for follow-up. Since 1994, the University Hospital in Rotterdam, The Netherlands, has used a system that permits recording of endoscopic examinations (Fig. 12.3). After finishing the endoscopic procedure, physicians can select the images that they wish to store. They can add arrows and comments to these selected images for later reference. In addition, the physician may dictate text to be stored with the image. The illustrated report is stored in addition to the conventional text-based report. Network facilities permit clinicians from other departments to view and hear the illustrated reports.

Although there is no technical barrier to the digital storage of moving images, no such application is yet in use. At present, the largest bottleneck is the huge demand for storage capacity, but this problem will probably be resolved over time. Image processing techniques have not yet been applied to endoscopy.

2.6 Organ Transplants

This section provides an example of the use of computers in assisting with organ transplantation.

Eurotransplant in Leiden, The Netherlands, is a large, international organization that registers patients waiting for an organ transplantation. Eurotransplant performs donor-recipient matching and organizes the transport of organs to be transplanted. The data that Eurotransplant have collected show a large increase in the number of patients waiting for kidney transplants: the number rose from less than 500 in 1969 to more than 12,000 in 1997. The number of transplantations, however, has been about 3,000 per year over the past several years.

PIONEER is the information system of the Eurotransplant foundation. The main task of the system is to register and maintain data on patients waiting for a donor organ. The data that characterize immunological features of each patient (**HLA type**) are important. Time is crucial in organ transplants; in particular, cadaver organs need to find recipients fast, because the condition of such organs deteriorates rapidly. The HLA types of the donor and potential recipients must match in order to find the most suitable recipient. Geographical and other logistical factors are taken into account. PIONEER's central system, which carries out the matching process, is located in Leiden. At the end of 1993 it was connected to 61 different centers in Europe. In a typical year, PIONEER performs more than 5,000 matches.

3 Cardiology

Heart disease and cancer are the main causes of early disability and premature death in developed countries. Because of a continuously growing population of elderly people, the number of cardiac patients is steadily increasing. Care for these patients is provided, for instance, by general practitioners, nurses, and cardiologists. In general, four major groups of patients can be discerned: patients with ischemic heart disease (about 75%), patients with heart failure (about 20%), and patients with cardiac rhythm disturbances (about 5%); in addition, there is a growing number of children who suffer from congenital heart disease or who have undergone cardiac surgery and need continuous care.

Computers have played a prominent role in cardiology from the onset of computer use in health care. The main reason for this is the fact that it is possible to express processes in cardiac physiology in physical, biochemical, and mathematical terminologies. As a consequence, data in cardiology can often easily be quantified and coded. Early examples of this approach are **models** of the heart and the circulation, mechanical models, and electrophysiological models. Another example is the processing of signals generated by the heart, such as the electrocardiogram (**ECG**) or blood pressure signals (see Chapters 8 and 13). Furthermore, especially in cardiology, images are acquired, by

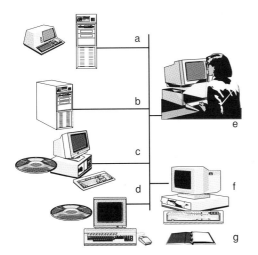

Figure 12.4
Network interconnecting systems in a department of cardiology, giving access to a hospital information system (a), an ECG management system (b), a PACS for coronary angiograms (c), a system for echocardiography (d), workstations (e), and a CPR system (f).

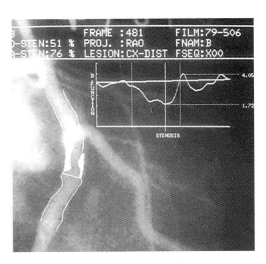

Figure 12.5
Example of image processing in a coronary arteriogram (after Reiber, Leiden University).

12

either radiology or **echocardiography** (see Chapter 25). Nowadays, departments of cardiology are often fully equipped with computers that are interconnected by networks, and they are often connected to **hospital information system**s and to the outside world (Fig. 12.4). Coronary care (see Section 9) and coronary angiography (see Chapter 9) are also areas where computers were fully integrated in cardiac care early on. We briefly summarize the main data used in cardiology.

3.1 Electrocardiography

The ECG is fully noninvasive and, therefore, is still the most frequently performed test in cardiology. ECG processing is fully supported by computers (see Chapters 8 and 13). ECG processing systems are fully integrated in **multimedia CPR**s. Systems for the processing of ECGs recorded during physical exercise are also frequently used in cardiology, as are ECGs recorded at rest. For certain patients, especially those with cardiac rhythm disturbances, so-called **Holter ECG**s (typically, 24-hour recordings) are made. The processing of Holter ECGs is fully computerized.

3.2 Coronary Angiography

The use of computers for enhancing images, such as coronary **angiogram**s or myocardial **scintigram**s, are of large interest in cardiology. The trend in coronary angiography is toward using fully digital systems. In this case, the angiographic image is stored in digital form within a computer, thereby allowing easy transfer of images from one system to another. It is possible to apply automated methods to assess the degree of stenosis in a coronary artery (see Fig. 12.5 for an example of image processing in a coronary arteriogram). Digital storage has many advantages: the radiographer does not need to develop film and the cardiologist does not need to retrieve the film for review.

3.3 Cardiac Scintigraphy

Radionuclide **scintigraphy** is a technique whereby it is possible to assess the flow of blood to the myocardium, usually following the injection of an isotope at peak exercise. The advantage of computer storage is, again, that the cardiologist is able to retrieve the scintigraphic image from the system and use it in the same way as the coronary angiogram. The myocardial scintigram may be used to assess the presence or absence of **ischemic heart disease,** and then if one is needed, a coronary angiography can be scheduled.

3.4 Echocardiography

Another imaging area in cardiology is **echocardiography.** Echocardiograms are also increasingly stored in computers and digitally processed and transmitted. Echocardiographic examinations are usually performed by medical support staff, but retrieving the digital images from a system allows the cardiologist to review the echocardiograms in the same way as the other images are reviewed.

12

3.5 CPRs in Cardiology

Applications of **CPRs** in cardiology are not radically different from those of CPRs in other clinical departments, such as internal medicine or pediatrics. However, CPRs in cardiology not only contain alphanumeric data but are also integrated with, for example, image processing systems and ECG management systems. In such so-called **multimedia CPRs,** patient data (history, physical examination, laboratory data, prescribed drugs, diagnoses, etc.) as well as cardiac images (**echocardiograms** and **coronary angiograms**) and cardiac signals (ECGs and blood pressure curves) are collected, stored, and transmitted to care providers. The data may be accessed through the workstations located in consultation rooms and integrated through networks and by electronic data interchange (**EDI,** see Chapter 5). Data can be used for patient care, as well as for quality assessment of care, research and education, or management and planning.

4 Neurology

The course of disease in patients with multiple sclerosis (MS) may be variable. Losses of function vary in severity and also in body location. Infections have an especially negative impact on the course of MS. Evaluation of treatment and clinical research require standardized data collection from multiple institutions. A special CPR called MS-COSTAR has been developed for treatment of and research with patients suffering from MS. It is based on **COSTAR,** which was developed at Massachusetts General Hospital in the United States. There are about 25 MS-COSTAR applications in the United States and a few outside the USA. On the basis of entered neurological data, the system calculates scores that characterize the functional ability of the patient. These scores are then used to determine the Expanded Disability Status Scale (EDSS). This scale plays an important part in short-term prognosis as well as in the evaluation of clinical trials.

Chronic daily headache (CDH) is the focus of an Italian system that supports standardized recording of related signs and symptoms. CDH usually has a large impact on a patient's daily life, not only because of the pain itself but also because of potential reactive depression and internal organ damage due to the extensive use of pain relievers. CDH is often preceded by intermittent headache. Headache may be related to a variety of factors such as social circumstances, menstrual cycle, familial disease, or neurological and vascular disorders. This diversity of factors requires a multidisciplinary approach to treatment and research. Potentially related factors, symptoms, and test results involve a large data set, which are collected at various locations. Standardization and combination of these data are essential for a better insight into the causes, influencing factors, and treatment of CDH.

5 Pediatrics

In pediatrics computers are used in many ways, similar to their use in other areas in clinical care, such as internal medicine, cardiology, surgery, and neurology. The differences between pediatrics and other specialties in medicine are indicated by diseases that are specific for premature infants and young children. Congenital diseases are, understandably, most seen in pediatric clinics. Therefore, large databases are often collected to study the history of children and people with such congenitally acquired diseases and the effect of interventions, either through drugs (e.g., in the treatment of growth retardation) or surgery (e.g., in the treatment of congenital cardiac diseases).

6 Obstetrics

In some countries, pregnancy and childbirth usually involve more than one clinical department. Generally, the clinics of both obstetrics and gynecology are involved. At the University Hospital in Rotterdam, The Netherlands, the clinics of obstetrics and gynecology are in separate buildings a long distance apart. The need for immediate access to patient data in the other building led to the development of an electronic obstetric record. This record supports standardized reporting regarding pregnancy and childbirth. The record contains patient data with respect to the past obstetric history, present disease, hereditary diseases, data on the current pregnancy, results of laboratory tests and ultrasound examinations, and, finally, the report of the actual delivery. To permit good insight into the course of the current pregnancy, the data from all visits preceding the delivery are displayed in a tabular format, with each row representing a summary of one visit. The application produces warnings when it is impossible or very unlikely that the entered values are correct. Most of the data are directly entered by the clinician. The system supports patient care by offering easy access to data when they are needed, but it has also led to a reduction in administrative effort. In the past, many forms had to be filled out for intake, admission, birth, report to the National Obstetric Registry, and discharge. Many of these forms contained overlapping items. The system automatically takes care of these routine, but time-consuming tasks. All gynecologists in The Netherlands have been using the system since 1993.

Recently, the system has been extended with functions for electronic requests for ultrasound examinations and patient scheduling, directly in the clinician's office, which saves considerable waiting time for the patient. It is possible to monitor cardiotocography on-line (i.e., monitoring the fetal heart rate in conjunction with contractions), enabling a quicker response by the attending clinician.

12

7 Surgery

Besides applications for the scheduling of surgery rooms, personnel, and equipment, very advanced systems for the planning and support of the actual surgical procedures are available. Other systems take care of patient monitoring during surgery (see Section 9). Most surgical planning systems are applied in the areas of cosmetic surgery and brain surgery.

An example in cosmetic surgery involves correction of

PANEL 12.1

Virtual Reality in Health Care

"Robots replacing clinicians"? Fantasy about the future impact of virtual reality on health care is rampant. However, it is hard to provide a clear definition of what virtual reality is. Virtual reality usually involves a three-dimensional representation of a computer-generated "world" that the user perceives as "real", and with which he or she can interact. Unlike watching television, in virtual reality the user is not a passive participant but rather an actor: the user can walk through a virtual house or drive a virtual car. When we deal with virtual reality applications in health care, however, the "virtual world" actually often really exists. Therefore, the best definition of virtual reality is probably provided by Lanier:

virtual reality is an immersive, interactive simulation of realistic or imaginary environments.

Immersive has the meaning of the cognitive conviction or feeling of presence, of "being there," surrounded by space and capable of interacting with available objects.

What is needed to provide such a feeling of "being there"? First, a computer generated 3-D "world" is projected with a head-mounted display (or stereo glasses). Different images for the left and the right eyes enable the user to see perspective. As the images are displayed in front of the eyes, the user has a wide viewing angle. Head-tracking systems built into the head-mounted display may be used to define the position of the user's head and to feed back this information to the computer, so that the images change when the user's head is moved. To further interact with the world, the user wears a DataGlove (similar to a joystick) that acts as an input device; the DataGlove appears as a hand in the image of the virtual world. This virtual hand mimics the user's hand movements and moves around in the virtual world or manipulates objects. The DataGlove can also act as an output device to provide force feedback, so that the user also feels an object that he or she has picked up (tactile display). Even more sophisticated complete body suits exist. For an auditory 3-D sensation, stereophonic headphones can be used.

The following provides an overview of how virtual reality is thought to improve the quality of care in medicine.

• *Surgery*

Perhaps the medical domain where we find the most extensive virtual reality applications is surgery. A milestone in this sense was in 1986 when the first gallbladder was removed laparoscopically. In laparoscopic surgery, the surgeon no longer directly sees or touches organs and tissues but watches electronic images and manipulates the organs and tissues with long instruments. Although this event can hardly be described as VR, the success and acceptance of the procedure was a pivotal event. Despite the loss of sensory "feel" and the use of awkward instruments, the advantages of this minimally invasive surgery technique were apparent: an operation without scars, almost no pain, and a quick return home. Since then, a number of improvements were suggested to reduce the disadvantages. To enhance the visual aspect, images can now be presented in 3-D mode, thus decreasing the chance of hand-eye coordination malfunctions. Head-mounted displays improve the interface even further by presenting the images along the normal hand-eye axis. Such initiatives are found in almost all surgical disciplines: for example, laparoscopy, eye ▶

surgery, neurosurgery, and endoscopy. To improve precision, the replacement of the physician, who manipulates the instruments by robotic arms that follow the movements of the physician, is also undertaken. From that, it seems a small step to envision a surgeon doing a procedure in the next city or in a place that is too distant or too dangerous (during military operations, for example). This latter field is also called *teleoperation.*

• Education
A domain where real applications are in use and where VR applications may reap the greatest benefits is in education. Simulators of all sorts (e.g., flight simulators) already exist but VR technology has helped to make them more realistic. VR can provide both a didactic and an experimental tool. A virtual abdomen already exists on which "real" operations can be carried out. The basic idea for these developments is that learning by trial and error is more effective than learning by instruction.
VR applications that aim to produce "rehearsal" models are also under development. Computer programs are fed data from an actual patient, and the physician can plan and rehearse the operation before actually performing it. Such VR planning programs also exist for radiotherapy.

• Psychiatry
Psychiatry is another, maybe surprising, domain for VR applications. VR has already be shown to be successful in the treatment of phobias, where patients undergo a gradual exposure to the stimuli that they fear in a virtual environment. It is thought that VR can also assist in the treatment of obsessive-compulsive disorders and autism and that the technology may provide new insights into schizophrenia.

12

• Rehabilitation medicine
Initiatives are also undertaken to investigate the use of VR in rehabilitation medicine. Wired gloves are being used to aid in the rehabilitation of injuries and as a new kind of prosthesis. Virtual environments have been created for exploration in a wheelchair. In all these circumstances, VR is used to re-empower individuals with disabilities. In addition, the DataGlove has also been used to quantitatively assess movement disorders such as Parkinson's disease.

• Augmented reality
A somewhat different area of virtual reality in health care that is not restricted to a medical subdomain is called *augmented reality.* This is the use of transparent displays worn as glasses on which data can be projected, so that both the real world and a projection of it with a different modality can be viewed at the same time. See-through ultrasound can, for example, allow the physician to view the fetus and the mother at the same time. These types of applications aim at providing the physician with "X-ray eyes."

The application of virtual reality technology is fascinating and rapidly growing. Applications will become more and more immersive. However, the use of VR applications in everyday clinical practice is still thought to be a decade away. At present (1997), computers are still too slow, head-mounted displays are too cumbersome, and tactile feedback systems are too crude to anticipate such systems in the near future. However, VR applications in medical education already exist, and may very soon become widespread in the teaching, training, and testing of medical students.

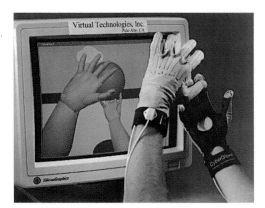

Figure 12.6
Use of two 18-sensor Cybergloves® for the manipulation of objects in virtual reality (Courtesy of Virtual Technologies, Inc.).

12

a receded chin, or of a chin that is too small. Usually, chin corrections require a series of surgical interventions, and it is desirable to have some insight into the effect of the planned corrections on the appearance of the patient's face beforehand. The surgery also involves the dentition to ensure proper occlusion in the final result. Before surgery, video images of the patient's face and X rays of the jaws are taken. These images are merged to produce a new one that shows the relationships between soft tissue, dentition, and jaws. An interactive program makes it possible for the orthodontist and dental surgeon to view the effects of various surgical procedures on the patient's face. The various possibilities are proposed to the patient and discussed. Once the choice has been made, the application provides details about the surgical procedures that will most likely produce the desired result. In fact, these details form the surgical plan. Every patient is made aware of the fact that small deviations from the desired outcome may occur. Most patients are fairly satisfied with this procedure.

Virtual reality is viewed as an important technical development for the education and training of surgeons, for example, for "remote" surgery (see Panel 12.1 and Fig. 12.6). By using three-dimensional cameras a 3-D image can be displayed at a remote site. Specially designed instruments use the information in the image to allow the user to manipulate objects in the image. Immediate visual feedback with respect to the position and movements of the instruments is also provided. The feedback also includes the feeling of pressure, that is, a natural feeling of the degree of resistance when the instruments touch the virtual objects. This technology has also been applied to teach students anatomy. The use of a very large database with images of the human body enables students to "travel" through the intestines, air passages, blood vessels, abdominal cavity, and so forth. Endoscopies and laparoscopies will probably become the first surgical procedures performed remotely.

At present, microsurgery deep in the brain is supported with applications that inform the surgeon about the accurate position and movements of his or her instruments. This is made possible by relating detailed information from computed tomography (**CT**) scans and magnetic resonance imaging (**MRI**) images to certain markings on the patient's skull (see Chapter 9). These markings are obtained through the use of a fixed ring or markers that have been applied on the head. Markers are preferred to a ring, because they allow the surgeon more freedom of movement. As soon as the starting position of the instruments has been related to the markings on the patient's head, the subsequent movements can be followed accurately. This type of application resembles virtual reality in the sense that the surgeon works from a screen, but the difference is that the surgeon manipulates and uses the instruments directly on the patients.

8 Psychiatry

In comparison with other medical specialties, for example, cardiology and hematology, psychiatry uses information technology only marginally. Because there are no strict pathophysiological criteria, many data are collected in conversations with the patient, sometimes in the presence of a partner or a relative. An important

---

PANEL 12.2

Variability in Diagnosing Dementia

Neuropsychiatry plays an important role in the diagnosis of dementia, in which the patient experiences radical changes in behavior as a consequence of mental disorders. Diagnosis of this disorder is also a typical multidisciplinary activity because of the large variety of causes (more than 50) of dementia. This leads to disease classification problems. Considerable differences of opinion even exist, over the meaning of the word "dementia." There is even more disagreement on the causes of dementia and their relative contributions to the incidence of dementia. It is assumed that Alzheimer's disease is responsible for 70 to 80 percent of all cases of dementia. However, at the same time it is still not clear if there is a single unambiguous cause of Alzheimer's disease.

To study the effect of differences in training and specialty, a research project was carried out in which 85 clinicians each diagnosed 10 patients with dementia. The clinicians consisted of neurologists, psychiatrists, general practitioners, nursing home physicians and psychologists. To prevent variability caused by the way that the data were presented, everyone received 10 records with all of the relevant data, and each clinician diagnosed the patients independently. The patients had been selected in such a way that there were clear and less clear cases of dementia among them, as well as some patients without dementia. The patients had been diagnosed beforehand by a team of experts in the field of diagnosing dementia; this team consisted of a neurologist, a psychiatrist, and a psychologist. It was expected that the medical specialty would influence the diagnosis and that the less clear, earlier forms of dementia would especially cause difficulties.

From the results of the research project it became clear that the expectations were justified and that the influence of the medical specialty was large, especially in defining the causes. It appeared that psychiatrists and nursing home physicians particularly limited themselves to the diagnosis of a syndrome, that is, a diagnosis of dementia without any further specification of the possible cause. If a cause was indicated, neurologists had a clear preference for Alzheimer's disease. By contrast, psychiatrists often chose a diagnosis of depression, whereas general practitioners and nursing home physicians often considered medication (intoxication) to be the cause. From the results it became clear that the chance of being diagnosed with Alzheimer's disease is twice as large if a patient is referred to a neurologist than to a psychiatrist.

As far as accuracy in diagnosing dementia is concerned, the situation is not much better. From the results it became clear that the physicians made the correct syndrome diagnosis in 7.5 of 10 cases, that is, they confirmed whether it was a case of dementia. When it came to indicating the causes (etiology), the average dropped to 5.3. In other words: the patient has a 50% chance of receiving the correct diagnosis. Only 4 of the 85 physicians were right for 9 out of 10 cases. When it came to the etiological diagnoses, none was right in all cases and 12 physicians scored less than three correct diagnoses.

part of the diagnostic process consists of describing behavior and experiences in **natural language**, together shaping the patient history. These descriptions are then used to diagnose the patient's disorder. In collecting these descriptions, patient questionnaires and assessment criteria are sometimes used, allowing a considerably less subjective interpretation. In spite of this, the psychiatric examination as well as the interpretation of collected data are very sensitive to subjective influences on the part of the clinician.

The wide range of psychiatric problems adds to the problem of ambiguity; not only is the number of possible causes of behavioral disorders very large but the nature of the disorders also varies considerably. Numerous factors may be influencing the disease, and these may be of social, psychological, pathophysiological, pharmacological, toxicological, or of genetic origin. Besides, these factors often co-occur in different combinations and can also be obscured by somatic diseases. Hence, the psychiatrist needs to have knowl-

edge about a large number of other medical specialties as well. All these factors together make psychiatry a domain with a large semantic information problem: the data are extensive, they come from various disciplines, and they contain a large variety of terms and the use of qualitative observation techniques is obligatory.

The quantity and diversity of medical data that a clinician is supposed to process are generally extremely large. This definitely holds for psychiatry. To illustrate the problems in information processing in psychiatry, Panel 12.2 gives a brief description of research in diagnosing dementia, which illustrates the diagnostic problems even if information processing and available knowledge and experience are used. It became clear from the project reported in Panel 12.2 that even a consensus meeting had little effect on improving the diagnosis. It should be realized that such problems do not exist only in psychiatry; to some extent they also exist in other disciplines of health care.

9 Critical Care

Critical care is a data-intensive environment, and for this reason this area is extremely suitable for extensive use of information technology. Patient monitoring is an important function in these departments. The **diagnostic-therapeutic cycle** mentioned in Chapter 1 is circled many times per hour or even per minute. For instance, in a coronary care unit both the **RR interval** and the ventricular waveshape are processed at every heartbeat. Besides the information produced by monitoring instruments, the critical care nurse and physician must also handle a large amount of information because of their care activities, as well as the data that come from clinical chemistry and imaging facilities.

During the last decade several patient data management systems (**PDMS**s) have become available. These systems are claimed to be the solution to managing the large amount of information produced in critical care.

9.1 Data from Organ Systems

Computerized critical care can be found in areas where invasive function analysis is taking place in real time; in monitoring situations, such as during shock or in coronary, postoperative, perinatal, or neonatal care; during surgery and during hemo**dialysis**; and, in general, in situations in which the effect of an intervention should be carefully watched.

The following body functions or organ systems are monitored:

- the cardiovascular system,
- the respiratory system,
- renal functions,
- the central nervous system, and
- the fluid and electrolyte balances and blood gas levels.

A host of different data originating from the different organ systems may, in principle, be monitored. Most of these data are listed in Table 12.1, where the data have been ordered into three groups:

- variables that are *continuously* monitored,
- data that are *sampled,* and
- data that are *coded.*

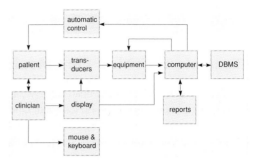

Figure 12.7
Use of computers for patient monitoring.

12

Table 12.1
Type of Data Used for Patient Monitoring in Different ICUs.[a]

Continuous Variables	Sampled Variables	Coded Data	Free text
Cardiac	Temperature	Patient observations	*All other observations or interventions that cannot be measured or coded*
ECG 　Heart rate (HR) 　HR variability 　PVCs	Central Peripheral	Color Pain Position etc.	
Blood pressure 　Arterial/venous 　Pulmonary 　Left/right atrial/ventricular 　Systolic/diastolic 　Per beat/average *Systolic time intervals*	Blood chemistry Hb pH PO_2 PCO_2 etc.	Interventions Infusions, Drugs Defibrillation Artificial ventilation Anesthesia etc.	
Respiratory 　Frequency 　Depth/volume/flow 　Pressure/resistance 　Respiratory gases	Fluid balance Infusions Blood plasma Urine loss		
Neurological *EEG* 　Frequency components 　Amplitudes 　Coherence			

[a] The data have been ordered as continuously available variables, samples, coded data, and free text.

12

PANEL 12.3

Example of Critical Care Monitoring

In some hospitals where open-heart surgery is performed, besides cardiovascular and respiratory parameters, brain function is also followed. One such hospital where patients are continuously monitored during open-heart surgery is the St. Antonius Hospital in Nieuwegein, The Netherlands, a large teaching hospital. During surgery, the staff of the Dept. of Clinical Neurophysiology supervise the monitoring of the brain function. Electroencephalograms (**EEGs**) are derived from the two hemispheres by four EEG leads (at the left side, leads F3-P3 and T3-O1; at the right side, leads F4-P4 and T4-O2; T stands for temporal, O for occipital, P for parietal, and F for frontal). During surgery, four EEGs are processed in real time with respect to their frequency content, from 0 to 20 Hz. Frequency spectra are computed during overlapping time windows of 60 seconds. These spectra are presented as a function of time on a display screen. The surgical team uses these displays to detect abnormal spectra or left-right differences. In addition to the EEGs, other vital parameters are also followed:

- the arterial blood pressure;
- body temperature and the nasopharyngeal temperature;
- the pressure, flow and temperature of the perfusion blood;
- anesthetic agents; and
- biochemical parameters.

Figure 12.8 is an example of an overview of trend parameters that are displayed during surgery. Time runs from the bottom to the top of the display. The following data are displayed in the columns from left to right:

- a vertical line indicating whether anesthetics such as phentanyl or propranolol that may influence the EEG are present,
- the spectra of EEG lead F3-P3 from the left hemisphere (in red),
- the time-averaged amplitudes of the EEGs F3-P3 and F4-P4 (in blue),
- the spectra of the EEG lead F4-P4 from the right hemisphere (in red),
- two temperatures (in degrees Celsius): nasopharyngeal (in yellow) and of the blood during perfusion (in red),
- the arterial blood pressure (i.e., systolic/diastolic in mm Hg) in the arteria radialis (in blue),
- the computed blood flow, required for the perfusion pump (in yellow),
- the measured blood flow, obtained from the perfusion pump (in red),
- a vertical line, indicating whether the heart-lung machine is in operation,
- an auxiliary column for transcranial *Doppler* monitoring of the arteria cerebri media, used during carotid surgery and complex aortic surgery.

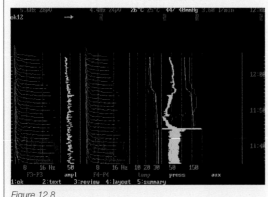

Figure 12.8

Trend plot of parameters acquired during open-heart surgery. Data are obtained from the Department of Neurophysiology of the St. Antonius Hospital, Nieuwegein, The Netherlands (Head: Dr. R.G.A. Ackerstaff; Technical staff: S.J. Hengeveld).

The first two groups of data are collected by monitoring systems. A PDMS contains continuously available variables, samples, coded data, and free text.

Intensive care units (**ICU**s) are equipped with many computerized monitoring systems, which are used for data acquisition and storage, data processing, and the presentation of results, for example, as trend plots. The amount of data to be processed as a function of time is often very large, so that **data reduction** must be carried out before the data and the results can be presented to the user: the nurse or the physician. A typical situation in an ICU is sketched in Fig. 12.7. Patient monitoring is usually applied in life-threatening situations, but monitoring of a medically different type is also applied to special examinations, such as sleep research in neurology and pulmonology or ambulatory monitoring in cardiology.

- To monitor the *cardiovascular function*, signals that are processed include blood pressures as well as the ECG, from which the heart rate and the presence of arrhythmias are computed. **QRS** waveshapes and, especially, **ST-T** segments are analyzed during coronary care monitoring.
- *Respiratory function* is another area for which a large collection of computerized monitoring equipment has been developed. Such systems offer information on respiration rates, volumes, and flows, which are directly or indirectly measured. Respiratory gases are determined by using inspiration or expiration. During surgery, the application of anesthetic gases is monitored as well.
- *Renal function* is monitored by following the electrolyte balance and the clearance of creatinine.
- *Brain function* is followed by carotid flows and pressures, intracranial pressures, and **EEG** parameters.
- The ***fluid balance*** is monitored by measuring drainage, infusions, and urine excretion.
- Blood gas levels and biochemical constituents are measured either on the spot or by the different laboratories involved.

To illustrate perioperative care, Panel 12.3 describes the monitoring during cardiac surgery, in which trends in the patient's condition are computed for several hours.

9.2 Patient Data Management Systems

A **PDMS** resembles an efficient manual ICU record-keeping system. Written ICU bedside flowcharts presenting the monitored data are replaced by a numeric or graphic presentation on a computer screen. Other screens allow the recording of data such as patient demographics, different types of orders, and follow-up notes.

The earliest PDMSs were mainly used to collect and validate vital parameters from monitors and ventilators. This automated charting, which is still an important key feature of today's PDMSs, gives nurses and physicians more time for direct patient care and control, because manual registration of data is no longer necessary. The role of the PDMS is not to replace monitors but rather to centralize the information obtained from different monitors in a more comprehensive fashion. The combination of parameters from different devices (monitors, ventilators, and infusion pumps) gives better insight into the physiological condition of the patient.

At present, PDMS developers pay more attention to the capabilities of PDMSs to support care and to ease multidisciplinary communication. This support is realized by, for example, integrated **protocols** and automated task lists. The system reminds the ICU team of treatments that need to be given at a certain time. The tasks on the list are stipulated by physicians' prescriptions and protocols.

With all the data collected during patient care, the PDMS is a potentially valuable source for information for management and research questions. Information about the patient population, outcome of care in terms of mortality, and information about utilization of human resources, drugs, blood, and blood products is important at the government, hospital management, and department management levels.

12

9.3 Reasons for Computer-Assisted Patient Monitoring

As mentioned above, there are several reasons for using a **PDMS** or computers in general in critical care situations. Some deal with quality of care, and others deal with efficiency. The most important reasons are described below:

• Data acquisition

The ideal frequency for acquiring alphanumeric data, such as observations, during patient monitoring is unknown. In current systems the frequency can vary from as often as every second to every hour, which is the same as that for data recorded manually in paper-based records. In the computer, voluminous amounts of data can be stored, and these data can be easily retrieved and analyzed when necessary.

• Data reduction

Data reduction and presentation of compact overviews in, for example, trend plots are the most important reason for using computers for patient monitoring. Neither nurses nor physicians are able to see gradual changes in data if they are presented in numerical form. Extraction of the most important parameters is also a task done by computers. Most equipment that is used for patient monitoring delivers data in digital form because the instruments digitize the data immediately after acquisition by the transducers.

• Error checking

Patient care in an **ICU** is, first of all, a human activity. Monitoring equipment and computers only offer assistance to such human care of patients. Wherever people work, errors are made. Therefore, another important task of computers is the verification of data for errors, consistency, and completeness.

Although a PDMS does not replace the monitors, it should be the monitors that are equipped with signal validation techniques to recognize artifacts due to mechanical or electrical disturbances from automatic on-line acquisition of the monitored data. The PDMS can support error checking by verifying internal consistency between parameters measured by different devices.

• Information display

In contrast to a paper-based patient record, data in the PDMS are always legible and accessible. Structured, well-presented data related to the care process will give the ICU team a better insight into the patient's condition and will improve treatment.

• Decision support

Continuous decision making is inherent to a critical care environment because of continuous changes in the patient's condition. In life-threatening circumstances, there is not much time to balance all alternatives carefully. Computers may offer support in such situations, for example, by using a model for predicting the outcomes of interventions. Examples are the use of **pharmacokinetic** models or models of the fluid balance. Another example of decision support is the generation of alarms and warnings, for example, in prescribing an incompatible combination of medications to a patient.

• Integration

The integrated presentation of monitoring data from different devices (see Table 12.1) is possible with a PDMS. However, the system is also able to integrate systems from outside the direct ICU area, such as the laboratory system and the hospital information system (see also Chapters 20 and 21). For example, the influence of medication on renal function can be monitored by an integrated presentation of laboratory data, such as the creatinine level, and the administered drug dose, on the medication sheet. Open-system interconnection (**OSI**) and the use of **HL-7** is increasingly promoted for integration (see Chapter 5) of different information sources.

• Ethical and legal aspects

Governments, patient organizations, and health insurance companies increasingly require that proper documentation be kept of all events and interventions in health care. In many countries this is regulated by law (see also Chapters 30 and 34). Most monitoring systems can therefore can generate a full document that may be used for assessment of the quality of care or for medical **auditing** and legal purposes. Access of hospital personnel to the data is limited by function. Most of the data entered, edited, or deleted are tagged with an **electronic signature.**

• Research

Once patient data have been collected in a PDMS, it

12

is also possible to use the data for research purposes. Without computer support this would be impossible. For example, in this way the effect of certain interventions on patient outcome can be investigated. In some countries a national intensive care database has been set up to improve facilities for outcome and performance measurement in ICUs. The PDMS can be used to extract data for these national databases on a continuous basis.

• Efficiency

Several studies have proven that the monitoring computer increases both the quality and the efficiency of care. The former aspect reinforces the latter one and vice versa. The expected time savings obtained by using a PDMS is not realized yet. Automatic data import will save time, but entering a new medication into the bedside paper chart, for example, is much faster than entering it in the PDMS.

10 Radiotherapy

Radiotherapy is a treatment that is used to destroy tumors by using high-energy **X-ray** beams, electrons, and other elementary particles, such as neutrons and protons.

Directly after X rays had been discovered, this type of radiation was used to treat malignancies. However, it took a relatively long time before enough insight was obtained into how **ionizing radiation** may damage biological material.

It was discovered, among other things, that better results could be obtained by dividing the radiation treatment over more than one session.

10.1 Development of Radiotherapy Planning

Until the 1950s, X rays with a maximum energy of 250 **keV** were used. With this type of radiation it was only possible to treat tumors that were located close to the body surface. When the isotope ^{60}Cobalt became available, deeper tumors could be treated. ^{60}Cobalt emits gamma radiation with an energy of 1.2 MeV, equivalent to 4-MeV X rays, and it has a **half-life** of 5.2 years. The situation improved even more after the introduction of **linear accelerators,** which could produce both X rays and electron beams with energies higher than 10 MeV. Higher-energy X rays and electron beams have the advantage of saving the skin, because the

maximum dose is absorbed below the skin, which is caused by the so-called build-up effect. Neutrons have also been used to treat certain tumors. Charged particles like **pions** and ions have also been applied to tumor treatment, but the equipment to produce them is rather expensive. At present, treatment with proton beams is being considered in several countries.

Already in the 1960s computers were used for radiotherapy planning. Panel 12.4 describes the principles of radiotherapy planning. In later years, computer systems were also used to verify the setup of radiation equipment or even to set up the equipment. Apart from these applications, radiotherapy departments also record patient data for administrative and research purposes.

10.2 Treatment Planning

Modern radiation equipment produces beams of X rays, electrons, or gamma radiation. The source of the radiation is located in the head of a **gantry.** The gantry can rotate around the patient, and the head can usually also be rotated with respect to the gantry.

The dimensions of the beam are determined by the dimensions of the tumor. The cross section of the beam must be chosen such that the whole target volume is just covered by the beam. Since this cross section is rectangular, it is sometimes necessary to use blocks of radiation-absorbing material to obstruct part

PANEL 12.4

Principles of Radiotherapy

The aim of radiotherapy is to destroy tumors with the help of high-energy radiation. Use is made of the fact that rapidly multiplying cells, which often occur in tumors, are more sensitive to radiation than the majority of normal cells. The difference in sensitivity, however, is usually not large.

The radiation can be applied from the outside: by means of beams of gamma radiation directed at the tumor and produced by a ^{60}Cobalt source or by means of X rays or electrons that are produced by linear accelerators. It is also possible to introduce radioactive sources inside the body. In this case the therapy is called *brachytherapy,* in which radiation therapy is applied by using radioactive sources positioned near the tumor.

The cross sections of externally applied beams are usually of a rectangular shape, which is accomplished by collimators that absorb the radiation outside the cross section of the beam. The intensity across the beam is uniform but may be modified by inserting wedges into the beam or by using tissue compensators.

When the beam crosses the body tissue, radiation is partly absorbed. Therefore, tissue near the entrance of the beam receives a higher radiation dose than deeper-lying tissues. When the tumor is located inside the body, healthy tissue lying between the radiation source and the tumor will get a higher radiation dose than the tumor itself. The skin or the tissue directly below the incoming beam therefore determines how much radiation can be given because above a certain dose, the healthy tissue will necrotize. For high-energy radiation, the location of the maximum dose is situated below the skin. In this case the skin receives a smaller dose and is relatively saved, which prevents erythema. Whether the dose delivered by the beam is enough to destroy the tumor depends on the depth at which this tumor is located and on the sensitivity of the tumor cells compared to the sensitivity of the healthy tissue cells that are located in front of the tumor.

If one beam is not enough to deliver a high enough radiation dose to the tumor, it is possible to use more beams that are all directed at the tumor at different angles. In this case the summed radiation of the different beams increases the dose delivered to the target volume, whereas the healthy tissues receive the dose from only one of the beams (Fig. 12.11).

To destroy the tumor, it should be irradiated completely. Otherwise, certain tumor cells would survive and the tumor would recur. During treatment planning it must be taken into account that some tissues are more sensitive to radiation than other tissues. Spinal marrow, for example, must be saved, and nerve cells do not regenerate. Therefore, the way in which a patient will be treated must be planned carefully. In short, the goal of treatment planning is to design a treatment in which one or more beams are positioned in such a way that a homogeneous dose is applied to the tumor, while critical organs are saved. Moreover, the treatment should be such that the total dose delivered to the patient is as low as possible, since radiation itself can also induce cancer.

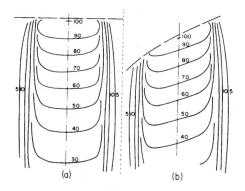

Figure 12.9
Dose distribution in tissue due to a single beam. The lines (iso-dose curves) connect points with the same absorbed dose.
(a) normal incidence.
(b) oblique incidence.

of the beam to obtain a desired cross section.

The dose that is absorbed at each location in the body may be determined in several ways. The easiest way is to measure the *dose distribution* of all possible beam sizes in a tank filled with water. It is known that for high-energy radiation the dose distribution in water is almost equal to that in the body; most tissues absorb an amount of radiation per gram identical to that absorbed by water. Another approach uses a small number of parameters derived from the measured distributions. A computer model is then used to calculate the dose at an arbitrary location within or outside the beam.

When the beam crosses tissues that have a higher or lower density than water, the dose distribution inside the body will differ from the dose distribution measured in water. When the dose distributions obtained in water are used to determine the dose distribution in lung tissue or bone tissue a correction must be made. Corrections also must be made for some oblique incidence of the beam due to body curvature.

The dose distribution measured in water is usually represented graphically by *isodose curves*, that is, lines connecting points that are exposed to an equal amount of radiation. Usually, the isodose curves are computed in planes through the center of the beam and parallel to each side of the beam. As is apparent from Fig. 12.9, the absorbed dose decreases with the depth inside the patient. Information about the isodose curves for all possible beam dimensions is stored in the computer and is used later on during planning of the treatment of individual patients.

To be able to calculate the dose distribution inside the

12

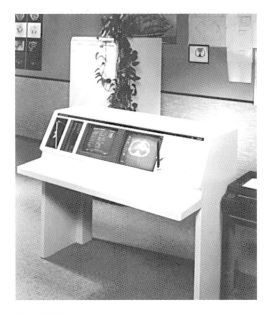

Figure 12.10
Computer system for radiotherapy planning (Philips).

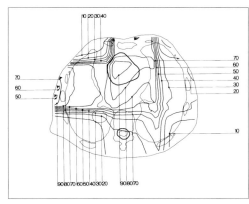

Figure 12.11
Example of a dose distribution inside a patient.

body, at least one cross section through the body, including the tumor, is needed. Such a cross section can be obtained with the help of **CT** or **MRI**. In this cross section the technician is able to outline the tumor, as well as sensitive organs that are in the path of the beams. Then for each beam the size and the angle of incidence will be specified interactively by the technician (Fig. 12.10). When the tumor is irradiated with multiple beams, the system is able to compute the total dose distribution by summing the doses of the various beams at each location in the cross section. The program will make corrections for oblique incident beams. When not only the cross section of the body, but also the density of the tissues in the cross section are available, the computer is also able to correct for differences in density.

The computed dose distributions are presented to the radiotherapist. When this dose distribution is not optimal, it is possible to change the direction of some of the beams, to insert wedges and so forth, and to assess their effects on the dose distribution. An optimal plan is determined interactively (Fig. 12.11). Planning systems that automatically determine the optimal dose distribution by optimizing some target function are also available; in that case a system must take into account a number of constraints that the dose distribution must fulfill, such as a homogeneous dose over the target volume.

With modern radiotherapy planning systems, it is possible to determine the dose distribution in three dimensions. The computations are not very different; again, the program needs information about the location of the isodose curves, now in three dimensions, and more cross sections are also needed. However, the visualization of the results may be different. In addition to providing the dose distribution in one or more cross sections, the results can also be displayed in a three-dimensional way.

10.3 Conformal Radiotherapy

Conformal radiotherapy is a type of radiotherapy in which tumors are irradiated in such a way that the three-dimensional high-dose volume conforms to the shape of the target volume as much as possible. Conformal radiotherapy is used to reduce both the rate of complications from the radiotherapy and the number of local recurrences of the tumor. By rotating the **gantry,** changing the beam shape, and moving the table under computer control, it is possible to obtain a dose distribution that conforms maximally to the shape of the target volume. The beam shape is altered with a so-called multileaf **collimator,** consisting of "leaves" of tungsten that can be moved with respect to each other, thus producing beam cross sections with variable shapes. Each cross section is the sum of small rectangles formed by pairs of leaves.

In conformal radiotherapy the target volume is visualized by means of about 50 to 100 CT scans. The planning program uses this information. It may be clear that conformal radiotherapy needs not only an adequate planning program but also a program that controls the movements of the gantry, the multileaf collimators of the radiation machine, and the table on which the patient is lying.

The planning results in a radiation treatment prescription. In this prescription it is specified how many beams will be used, whether or not wedges will be used, what the dimensions of the beams will be, the angles of the various beams, and the radiation time per beam. The number of irradiations is also recorded. Of course, the radiation prescription will be more complex for conformal radiotherapy than for routine radiotherapy.

The data produced by the planning system (the setup parameters) are transferred to the computer that controls the radiation equipment. These data are used during the complete treatment session. During each session the computer verifies whether the technicians have set up the radiation machine correctly. When deviations larger than some tolerance value occur, the computer will block the treatment. After each irradiation session the cumulated dose is documented.

An accurate determination of the dose distribution is important: the tumor will recur when the dose is too low, whereas necrosis of healthy tissue will develop when the dose is too high. Herring and Compton have shown that a reduction of 10% with respect to the optimal dose will decrease the probability of successful therapy by a factor of 7, whereas the number of cases with necrosis increases noticeably with an increase of 10% with respect to the optimal dose. They conclude that an accuracy of about 5% should be reached to prevent complications.

10.4 Brachytherapy

External radiation beams are not the only forms of radiation used to destroy tumors. It is also possible to introduce radioactive sources into the body at a position close to the tumor or even inside the tumor (hence the name brachytherapy). The sources may be inserted intracavitarily, like in the case of gynecological tumors, or interstitially, for example, the implantation of ^{192}iridium wires, as used in the mamma-saving treatment for mamma carcinoma, or ^{137}Caesium needles implanted in the bladder. Again, it is possible to compute the dose distribution with the help of a planning system.

11 Retrospective Review of Departmental Information Systems

12

The majority of departmental systems have sprouted from local needs and inventiveness. Some have been inspired by practical or potential financial benefit; others are based on a more scientific incentive. Although standardization and data exchangeability are topics that receive global attention, many of the older applications are highly dedicated and specific to the environment in which they are used. Their functions range from pure administration and billing to the creation of research databases, decision support, picture archiving, and image analysis.

The strategies underlying the functions that they provide use old as well as new insights into information technology and domain knowledge. Hence, many of these systems, especially the older ones, cannot easily be used in other environments. However, they have provided valuable experience on which new applications can be based.

Networks, the **Internet,** and message protocols increasingly influence current developments. Therefore, it is likely that recent and new applications will be more easily transferable to locations other than the one where they have been developed. There is a high demand for strategies that are able to interconnect existing systems and that make their contents accessible in an integrated environment in such a way that the end user does not need to know the specifics of the underlying contributing applications. This interconnection could either be done by interchanging messages electronically (e.g., by **HL-7** or **EDI**) or by integration in a network. Such strategies are important, because few institutions can afford full replacement of all existing systems. Furthermore, gradual migration from older to newer applications will always be necessary, because new insights continuously become available.

The main bottleneck of designing widely applicable systems will not be of a technical nature. Personal preferences, departmental habits, lack of standardized nomenclature, and cultural differences will increasingly become bottlenecks for developers. The challenge will be to reconcile the requirements for user acceptance with those for quality assessment, research, and health care planning; in other words, the difficult reconciliation of versatility and uniformity.

Key References

See the Web site for literature references.

13 Clinical Support Systems

1 Introduction

In Chapter 12 we described the role of computers in clinical departments. It is characteristic of these departments that clinicians are directly responsible for patient care. Other departments in the hospital, however, are indirectly involved in patient care. Such departments are sometimes also called *ancillary clinical departments*. In fact, such clinical support departments may deal with and provide service to all other clinical departments. To this group of clinical support departments belong:

- Radiology (see Section 2);
- Physiological function laboratories (Section 3);
- Pathology (Section 4);
- Clinical chemistry (Section 5); and
- Pharmacy (Section 6).

They collect patient data, samples, biosignals, images, and specimens from patients in the outpatient clinic and on hospital wards, perform analyses, and report the results to the responsible physicians and nurses. The clinical support departments take care of data acquisition and validation, storage and retrieval in **database management systems**, reporting, and quality assessment. Reports are generally transmitted electronically (via the hospital network) to the wards. In this chapter we describe the role of computers in such ancillary departments.

2 Radiology Information Systems

The primary function of a radiology department is the acquisition and analysis of radiological images. In radiology departments, radiology information systems (**RIS**s) have been installed, and these perform several functions. The main goal of RISs is to support both the medical and the administrative functions of radiology departments.

A RIS may be a stand-alone system, but it may also be part of a hospital information system (**HIS**) (see Chapters 20 and 21). After the introduction of RISs that emphasized textual information, such departments took greater interest in supporting the **imaging** process.

A number of imaging systems, such as digital **subtraction angiography** (DSA), **computed tomography** (CT), and *magnetic resonance imaging* (MRI), contain computers that generate digital images that must also be viewed at other places in the hospital (see Chapter 9). To support the communication and archiving of these images, **PACS**s (picture archiving and communication systems) (see Chapter 21) were developed. If a PACS is present, it will probably be integrated into the HIS or RIS. The radiologist also needs to be able to access all relevant clinical and administrative data when interpreting the images.

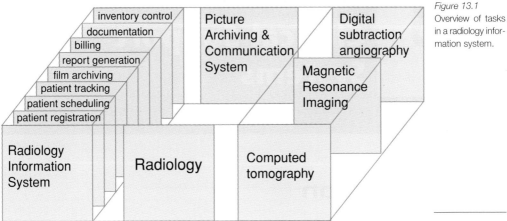

Figure 13.1
Overview of tasks in a radiology information system.

In a radiology department a number of information-processing activities may be discerned (see also Fig. 13.1):

- registration of patients,
- scheduling of patient examinations,
- patient tracking,
- film archiving,
- report generation,
- administration and billing,
- medical documentation,
- inventory control.

Some existing RISs are able to handle almost all of these tasks. If the RIS is a subsystem of an HIS, a number of tasks, for instance, patient registration, will be performed by other subsystems.

The RIS receives orders for examinations, and then the necessary documents are printed and tasks are executed. These include requests for results from previous examinations, checks for duplicate examinations, and so forth. The examination must be scheduled, which also results in a number of tasks: patients, rooms, and personnel must be scheduled, work lists must be printed, and so forth. Also, transport lists must be made for the transportation of patients within the hospital.

After the images have been generated, they are interpreted and the reports are stored in the RIS and reported to the referring physicians, either via a network, **fax** or by paper mail. In practice, a range of computerized reporting facilities is used, ranging from dictated reports with text processing to **speech recognition** systems. The films are archived and occasionally loaned out. A RIS may contain an option that performs the film archiving. When images are stored digitally, this function is taken over by the PACS.

The PACS takes care of the storage and retrieval of digital images, image processing functions, and so forth. Although digital medical imaging equipment is used extensively, at least 80% of the daily workload in radiology departments still concerns screen-film examinations. Computed radiology or digital radiology is now possible via the use of phosphor-plate systems which are replacing the screen-film combination. The resulting digital image is of a quality comparable to that of the screen-film combination. It is possible to analyze analog films as well with the help of laser film digitizers or charged coupled device (**CCD**) digitizers. The films are converted into digital images with a size of, for example, 2,048 x 2,048 **pixels** with 12-bits **grey levels**.

An important part of the PACS is the network by which images are transferred to **workstations** or archive systems. The examinations are reviewed at the display workstation. Current workstations are still not satisfactory for all radiologists: the brightness of the display is eight times less than that of a light box, and the radiologist is used to a rapid display of multiple images. It is not yet clear how many display monitors are needed per viewing station for it to be competitive with the light viewing box.

Digital images are sometimes processed further (see

Chapters 9, 10, and 26). This may be performed at the pixel level, for example, for **contrast enhancement, region-of-interest** selection, or generation of three-dimensional views, but the processing may also concern quantification, such as length, surface, or volume measurements, or **texture** analysis. Finally, it may consist of more complex image processing, such as **image subtraction edge enhancement**, **contour extraction**, or **volumetric displays.**

After being reported, the images are transferred to an on-line archive. After some time, images must be transferred to an intermediate archive, where they are stored for a period of 1 or 2 years. After that period they are stored in a cheaper, long-term archive.

Each type of archive has its own speed requirements, which determine the type of medium on which the images are to be stored. The fastest accessible medium is a magnetic disk. **Optical disks** are somewhat slower but they are able to store more data; worm (write once, read many times) optical disks can store Gbytes of data.

An average image contains about 5 Mbytes. A large hospital may produce 5 Gbytes of images per day. During a radiological reporting session, a mean data flow of about 3 Mbits/s is required, with much higher peak loads. The network must therefore be very fast. For fast retrieval a hierarchical way of storing the images (e.g., fast, intermediate, and long-term storage) is

necessary. **Coaxial cable**-based **local area networks** with effective transfer rates on the order of 400 kbits/s are not fast enough. **Glass fiber** is then required as a transmission medium.

Exchanging image data requires standardization: how are the various archives to be accessed, what types of messages (e.g., images, text, and control data) can be exchanged, and what control commands may be used? All these questions must be addressed to make data exchange between systems of different vendors possible. In an effort to develop a standard by which users of medical imaging equipment could connect viewing systems or other systems to imaging computers, the **DICOM** (Digital Imaging and Communications in Medicine) standard has been defined (see Chapter 34). This standard includes a dictionary of the data elements needed for proper image display and interpretation. DICOM provides standardized formats for images and protocols for electronic communication of images. Digital images are **compressed** so that they can be transmitted faster. Compression is usually expressed as a ratio between the original and the compressed image (e.g., 3:1, 10:1, or 15:1). Certain images can bear much compression without losing **semantic** information. For archiving purposes, data compression without any **syntactic** loss of data needs to be used (in this case, maximum achievable compression ratios are on the order of 3 or 4).

13

3 Function Laboratories

All living organisms are in continuous interaction with the outside world, and they try to find an equilibrium with the outside world to survive. In most instances this equilibrium is maintained by regulatory mechanisms (i.e., by the central nervous system (**CNS**) and the hormonal system). The senses and receptors (e.g., the chemo- and baroreceptors in the circulation), continuously transmit stimuli from outside and inside to the CNS, which maintains the equilibrium via the **sympathetic** and **parasympathetic** system. If the equilibrium is distorted, the CNS attempts to find a new equilibrium. This generally happens within the physiological

range of the biological process (e.g., an increased cardiac output in a situation of physical exercise), but in some cases the biological process enters a pathophysiological state (e.g., **ischemic** symptoms when the coronary arteries are obstructed). In so-called function laboratories (see also Fig. 13.2), also sometimes called *physiological function departments*, these dynamic properties of organs and organ systems are examined. To examine the function of organs or organ systems, data are acquired as a function of time. These data may pertain to:

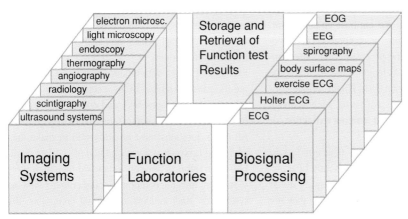

Figure 13.2
Schematic representation of systems operational in different function departments.

- heart and circulation (**electrocardiography, echocardiography, scintigraphy,** and **angiography**),
- the respiratory system (**spirography**),
- the nervous system (**electroencephalography** and **electromyography**),
- the visual control system (**electro-oculography**), and
- the auditory system (**audiography**).

In function analysis and on-line monitoring, large numbers of data flow from the patient to the examining clinician, technician, or nurse through **transducers.** This data flow must be reduced, channeled, and documented, and the computer is the ideal vehicle for this process. The sophistication level of the data acquisition equipment is steadily increasing, since nowadays most **signal-processing** equipment is integrated with microcomputers.

The acquisition of images to obtain insight into the functioning of organs is described in Chapter 9. This section describes the use of **biosignals** for organ function analysis and discusses some applications of the methods described in Chapter 8 (see also Chapter 25). Biosignals offer parameters that support medical decision making and **trend analysis.** This decision making is increasingly based on objective and numerical measurements instead of subjective measurements. Biosignals are examples of objective measurements that may be used as input for interventions (see also Section 5 of Chapter 8). We give some examples below.

3.1 Electrocardiography

On the body surface, the electric field, generated by the cardiac muscle, consists of electric potential maxima and minima that increase and decrease during each cardiac cycle. The recording of these electric potentials as a function of time is called electrocardiography, and the resulting signal is an **ECG**. Theoretically, an infinite number of electrode positions could be used to sample this field. In practice, a restricted number of electrodes is sufficient. The locations of the electrodes for the standard limb leads (leads I, II, and III) were determined by Einthoven, on the basis of his dipole hypothesis for the cardiac electrical field before the physical nature of field generation within the heart had even been discovered. Later, Wilson designed his augmented unipolar leads, aVR, aVL, and aVF, using combinations of the limb leads. The chest leads (leads V1 to V6) are located as close to the heart as possible, in the hope that they would present maximum diagnostic information. This set of 12 leads contains 8 independent leads. Only the electrode positions in **vectorcardiography** have a physical foundation, especially the systems described by Burger in 1946 and by Frank in 1956.

The ECG is composed of a series of events that are normally coupled to each other:

- the **P wave**, generated by the electric **depolarization** field in the atria on command of the sinoauricular (SA) node;

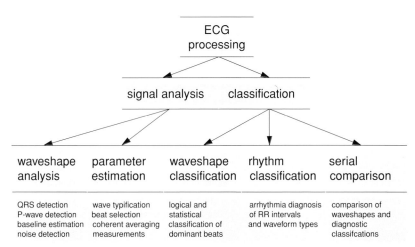

Figure 13.3
Schematic diagram of modular ECG processing.

- the **QRS** complex, generated by the electric field in the ventricles on command of the atrioventricular node (AV); and
- the **ST-T wave,** caused by the **repolarization** in the ventricles. Sometimes a so-called U wave is also discerned, but the electrophysiological origin of this is not fully understood.

In abnormal ECGs, the events generated by the atria and the ventricles might be uncoupled, such as in the absence of SA node activity or in the case of atrial **flutter** or atrial **fibrillation.** In cases in which the ventricles themselves behave abnormally, multifocal intraventricular **extrasystoles** or even fatal ventricular fibrillation is seen.

Interpretation of the ECG can be seen as a chain of processing steps, from the application of the electrodes to the printed document. Because signal entropy tends to increase as a function of processing, signal analysis should start at the **transducer.** It is counterproductive to put much effort in very intricate signal processing and statistical techniques if the transducers are not properly positioned and if the disturbances superimposed on the ECG are unacceptably large, hampering detection, recognition, and classification.

The ECG is a representative example of the processing of biological signals. Its analysis follows roughly the steps outlined in Section 1 of Chapter 8:

1. signal acquisition,
2. signal transformation,
3. computation of signal parameters,
4. **classification** of the signals.

In preparing a system for the processing of biosignals, it is important – as it is for all computer processing problems – to collect all prior knowledge about the biological process and the signals derived from it. In ECG analysis much knowledge is available about the depolarization process, but the repolarization process is less well understood. The following describes some of the prior knowledge that we have and that should be embedded in ECG processing software:

- The ECG is a **quasiperiodic** signal (with a repetition frequency of between 30 and 300 events per minute), but it may also contain **stochastic** components such as atrial flutter or fibrillation or even ventricular fibrillation.
- Generally, it has one dominant waveform, but it may also contain multiform extrasystoles. It also shows aspects of a **point process.**
- The frequency domain of the ECG is defined to be between 0.15 and 150 Hz, with the QRS part comprising the highest frequencies and the P and ST-T parts comprising the lowest.
- Disturbances generated by loose or moving electrodes (e.g., caused by respiration), nearby electrical

13

equipment (50 or 60 Hz, or higher **harmonics**), artificial **pacemaker** pulses, electromyographic signals, and so forth, may be superimposed on the signal.

- The amplitudes of the ECG span a range from approximately -10 to +10 mV, and the smallest waves that are of semantic importance (the Q waves) can be as small as 20 µV or even less.

- ECG analysis has different application areas such as for diagnostic purposes, **serial comparison,** population screening, ambulatory monitoring, coronary and intensive care, or research. Each of these imposes different requirements on the analysis program.

3.2 Modular ECG Processing

The four main ECG processing stages mentioned above can be further split into subtasks. Each task is implemented in a separate software package (a coherent set of computer programs). For ECG analysis this is depicted in Fig. 13.3, which shows a structure of **modular** ECG processing. In Fig. 13.3 we discern first the modular ECG processing system itself, which is split into the following:

1. An input task
   The input module deals with the acquisition of signals from eight or more ECG leads simultaneously. It performs the sampling and temporarily stores the information in computer memory.
2. A signal pattern analysis task
   This pattern analysis can be split into the following subgroups (modules):
   – Signal detection
     Detection of events comprises the computation of the **point processes** that indicate the locations of QRS complexes or P waves of all possible shapes. The estimation and location of noise and disturbances are also done during signal detection.
   – Waveform typification
     Typification of the QRS complexes and ST-T signals according to waveshape is done in separate modules. Here it is important to discriminate between dominant QRS-T complexes and premature or multifocal extrasystoles.
   – Boundary estimation

Finally, **segmentation** or boundary recognition is one for the QRS complex, the T wave, and the P wave (see also Chapter 10). The problem here is to locate the onsets and endpoints of certain waves as accurately as possible to be able to derive features for diagnostic purposes.

3. A classification task
   The classification is subdivided into modules for:
   – Beat selection
     Dominant beats are selected and **coherent averaging** is done (see Chapter 25) preceding waveshape recognition.
   – Parameter estimation
     Temporal and amplitude parameters for all the ECG leads are estimated and relations are computed between parameters in the different leads.
   – Waveform classification
     Classification of waveshape is computed into diagnostic categories such as left ventricular hypertrophy, anterior myocardial infarction, or **left bundle branch block.**
   – Arrhythmia classification
     This makes use of the information contained in the point processes of atrial and ventricular events and waveshape information.
4. An output generation task
   The output module deals with **alphanumeric** and graphical reports and the storage of results on some digital storage device such as a disk.

An ECG processing system as described in Fig. 13.3 is able to interpret the 12-lead ECG as well as the vectorcardiogram. Such software can easily run on present-day personal computers. Figure 13.4 gives an example of a computer-processed ECG and its diagnostic classification. Systems for ECG processing and interpretation are usually integrated with systems for ECG management, which take care of storage and presentation of ECGs recorded at an earlier date, to support **serial comparisons**.

At present, computerized ECG processing is routinely applied in hospitals, in primary care, and for population screening. Systems for ECG processing have undergone international validation, and national agencies and physicians' organizations increasingly require that such systems be assessed.

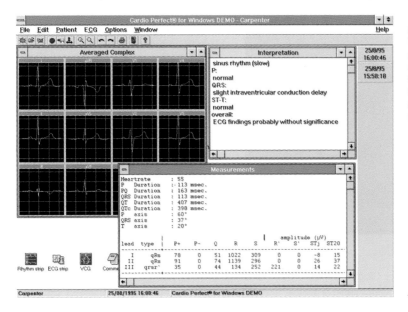

Other versions of systems for ECG analysis are used to process ECGs during physical exercise or for **ambulatory monitoring.** Real-time ECG analysis is applied during cardiac catheterization to detect ST depressions and during patient monitoring (see Section 9 of Chapter 12).

3.3 Spirography

In **spirography,** lung function measurements are obtained, and from these flows, volumes, and pressures can in principle be obtained as a function of time. Instruments for the analysis of spirograms are equipped with processors for signal analysis and data storage. The number of spirograms recorded annually in a hospital is much smaller than the number of ECGs. Besides, the recording of a spirogram takes much more time than recording of an ECG during rest, and cooperation between technician and patient is required to obtain a signal of high quality. The procedure for spirogram analysis is in many respects similar to that for recording an ECG during exercise. Symptoms in patients with chronic obstruction of the airways (e.g., emphysema, asthma, and fibrosis) are in some instances provoked by letting patients inhale an inert gas that contains histamine. The effect on lung function is then compared with the normal situation.

In spirography, the clinician is interested in the lung volume (i.e., the **vital capacity**) and the respiratory flows during forced expiration, both as a function of time. Peak flow and the flow 1 second after the onset of forced expiration are used as parameters for decision making. The flow may be measured directly by a transducer or may be computed by the first derivative of the volume as a function of time. Sometimes, respiratory gases (e.g., the PCO_2) are also measured to obtain further insight into lung function (e.g., by examining during so-called whole-body **plethysmography**). In some instances, the clinician will measure arterial blood gases in combination with spirography during physical exercise.

3.4 Electroencephalography

Electroencephalograms (**EEGs**) are routinely recorded and interpreted in departments of neurology and neurophysiology. Here, too, computers assist in data acquisition, analysis, and storage. The EEG is a typical **stochastic signal** (see Chapter 8) in which the parameters that are of interest cannot readily be seen without processing. Frequency analysis, for instance, is routinely applied to EEGs, for instance, by using a series of parallel **band-pass**

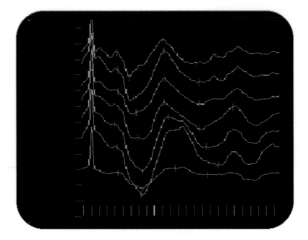

Figure 13.5
Evoked potentials in seven EEG leads resulting from stimulation by light flashes with a frequency of 1.9 flashes per seond. The potentials are the result of the summation of 128 evoked potentials and the interval before the light flash is 10 msec. Data are obtained from the Department of Clinical Neurophysiology of the St. Antonius Hospital, Nieuwegein, The Netherlands (Clinical staff: Dr. E.H.J.F. Boezeman; Technical staff: S.J. Hengeveld).

filters or by **Fourier analysis** (see Chapter 25). Sometimes, the effect on the EEG of a visual or auditory stimulus, called **evoked** potentials, offered to the patient is assessed. Because the EEG itself is a stochastic signal and the effect of an evoked signal is generally very small, **coherent averaging** is applied to increase the **signal-to-noise ratio** (see Chapter 25). Figure 13.5 gives an example of the analysis of evoked potentials. Panel 12.3 on patient monitoring provides an example of real-time EEG **frequency analysis** during cardiac surgery.

4 The Pathology Laboratory

4.1 Diagnosis in the Pathology Laboratory

Pathology plays an important part in diagnosis, and it has two major domains:

1. postmortem diagnosis with the body of a patient, and
2. diagnosis from observations of tissue or separate cells taken from live patients.

The tissue is prepared with paraffin and is sliced into thin sections, which may be colored to make certain tissue structures more visible. Tissue and cells are studied through a microscope. Diagnosis performed by using tissue is called *histology*, whereas diagnosis per-

formed by using separate cells is called *cytology*.

Following surgery, the pathologist often has the last say in a patient's diagnosis and thus has a great influence on the choice of therapy and the prognosis. Although the histopathological diagnosis is reliable in the majority of cases, in some areas of pathology inter- and intra-observer **variability** is relatively high. This is especially undesirable when the differences in therapeutic consequences are large, which is often the case when a potential malignancy is involved. Table 13.1 provides the results of a literature search on diagnostic disagreement in pathology related to tumors. Most discrepancies are related to grading (i.e., the assessment of the degree of malignancy).

Before discussing the potential sources of diagnostic variability, we briefly discuss how pathologists arrive at a diagnosis.

Tissue/stain	Reference	Disagreement (%)
Bladder tumors	Ooms et al. 1983	50
Bone tumors	Sissons 1975	Considerable
Bone marrow	Morley and Blake 1975	0-56
Bowel disease	Dundas et al. 1987	Minor
Breast cancer	Stenkvist et al. 1983	23-40
Cervical cancer	Ringsted et al. 1978	4-58
Colorectal cancer	Thomas et al. 1983	31-44
Endometrium	Baak et al. 1981	25
Gastric cancer	Pagnini and Rugge 1982	4-17
Hydatidiform mole	Javey et al. 1979	45-66
Immunostaining	Muir et al. 1987	10-15
Liver	Garceau 1964	48
Lung tumors	Hansen 1982	10-considerable
Lymphomas	Argyle et al. 1989	20-50
Melanomas	Larsen et al. 1980	30
Muscle fiber	Pool et al. 1979	40
Nervous system	Daumas-Duport et al. 1988	4-19
Esophagus	Reid et al. 1988	13-28
Ovarian tumors	Stalsberg et al. 1988	25-59
Soft tissue sarcoma	Coindre et al. 1986	19-39
Thyroid cancer	Ron et al. 1986	10-15
Urothelial cells	Sherman et al. 1984	Considerable
Various	Penner 1973	4-87

Table 13.1
Disagreement Figures in Pathology Diagnoses.[a]

13

[a] after Baak JPA. *Manual of Quantitative Pathology in Cancer Diagnosis and Prognosis.* Heidelberg: Springer Verlag, 1991:14 (partly cited).

4.2 The Diagnostic Process

When pathologists study histologic or cytologic slides, they will immediately focus on certain features that characterize the type of tissue and will subsequently look for abnormalities. Because of the training that the pathologists have received, they can immediately select areas of interest in the slide and can identify aspects in the tissue that are relevant for the diagnosis. Pathologists may immediately recognize the image and make a diagnosis, but the image may also trigger questions and so they will refer to reference knowledge in the form of books and at-

lases. They will study the slide again to see if the information gathered is sufficient to make a diagnosis. The process is repeated until they feel confident about the diagnosis, or the process is aborted when no solution has been found and the slide is sent to a specific expert.

Pathologists always make reports about their observations. Important steps involve the selection of relevant features, comparison with acquired reference knowledge, verbal expression, and diagnostic classification. If a layperson looks at the slice of tissue through a microscope, he or she may first see the artifacts, like a hair, a crack, or a small tissue fold. For a pathologist, these features may not even enter his or her consciousness. The pathologist's attention will immediately be drawn to the number of lymphocytes or mitoses. This is a highly efficient process in which "noise" is separated from "signal." Yet, there is no guarantee that all signal components are detected: the only things that are interpreted are those within the pathologist's scope of attention.

As has just been indicated, it is the training of pathologists that allows them to make a relevant selection. Reference knowledge, acquired during residency training, case discussions, and literature study, determines not only which features are selected but also how the features are described and, ultimately, how the lesion is diagnosed.

4.3 Potential Sources of Diagnostic Errors

Potential sources for diagnostic errors comprise four main categories: context, optical illusion, random errors, and systematic influences.

- An example of *context* is the clinical question posed to the pathologist. When studying biopsy material in search of parathyroid tissue, the presence of thyroid tissue is not surprising because of the location of the parathyroid glands. However, when the tissue has not been taken close to the thyroid, the presence of thyroid tissue may indicate a metastasis.
- *Optical effects* may cause under- or overestimation of certain features. There is a form of Hodgkin's disease called the *lymphocytic depletion subtype* because there appear to be fewer lymphocytes in this form than in the *mixed cellularity subtype*. Objective counts have shown the opposite. Oddly shaped cells (pleomorphisms) in the depletion type attract so much attention that there seem to be fewer lymphocytes.
- *Random errors* account for much of the intraobserver **variability.** These errors usually involve random shifts due to time of day, fatigue, or previous exposure to similar lesions. Having been confronted with a number of highly malignant cases, a well-differentiated lesion may be diagnosed as borderline. The reverse may also occur.
- *Systematic influences* are related to a pathologist's

reference knowledge. This is first built up during training and is later shaped by study of the literature, case discussions, and clinical experience. Reference knowledge involves how observations are phrased, as well as the criteria used to assign diagnoses. Pathologists may differ at the level of description or at the level of application of diagnostic criteria, or at both levels.

4.4 The Role of Computers in Pathology

As new therapeutic options become available, diagnoses need to be more refined to offer patients optimal treatment. As a result, pathologists and researchers are actively pursuing strategies to minimize diagnostic errors. Computer technology has been applied in several ways to improve consensus in diagnosis. Important target areas are education, research, objectivation of observations, and direct clinical applications.

- Education

Textbooks have some well-known limitations. The three most important ones are as follows:

1. Books are one-dimensional: browsing is only possible by turning pages back and forth.
2. Cost and size limit the publisher to offering only one or at most two pictures of each disease. Atlases contain many pictures but little text.
3. Books are diagnosis oriented, whereas the clinical question is the inverse: from findings to diagnosis.

As computer memory and processing capacity increase rapidly while at the same time costs are reduced, solutions to the limitations mentioned above seem to come within reach. Most common applications involve electronic textbooks and atlases.

Electronic textbooks, when properly indexed, permit different search strategies, such as by organ, by disease, by feature, and by diagnostic technique. Electronic atlases provide access to large sources of reference pictures. The Diagnostic Encyclopedia Workstation for

Table 13.2
Examples of Parameters in Cytometry

Number of mitoses

Size and shape of nuclei

Size and relative position of nucleoli

Chromatin pattern

DNA content and ploidy

Nucleus/cytoplasma ratio

Surface measurements

Absorption of chemical markers

---

ovarian tumors, developed at the Free University of Amsterdam, is one of the earlier systems with full integration of text and images. A similar system is IntelliPath, developed at Stanford University, USA, which is marketed worldwide. Modern electronic atlases often include various degrees of textual information, and the images are sometimes overlaid with arrows and other explanatory markings. These electronic sources of reference knowledge are valuable for pathologists with various levels of experience.

Other computer applications offer questions or quizzes to test pathology knowledge within a variety of domains. In the last few years, simulations of real cases have become available. Such applications allow the pathologist to select areas of interest and ask for certain procedures such as staining with various stains. The trainee will learn about performing differential diagnoses of specimens and the value of certain tests. Such simulations require an extensive set of well-documented cases, including tests of different degrees of relevance. The cases in such a set must be well chosen to be representative of its domain of application. A large case *repository* may also serve for case discussions and seminars and further research (see also the parallel with ECG interpretation, as discussed in Section 3.1 and Panel 15.4 of Chapter 15).

• Research

Pathology is a medical domain that is preeminently suited for research, since the material for observation is of a permanent nature. The researcher can always go back and reevaluate material from the past. Computers are able to help in making the material more easily accessible. **Optical storage devices** allow for the collection of well-documented images, which can then be used for further study. When available in a digitized format, images not only can be studied with the human eye but can also be subjected to image processing (see also Fig. 10.3 in Chapter 10). The resulting parameters can be statistically analyzed. When multicenter studies are involved, it is possible to define study populations on a level more detailed than diagnostic class. Long-term follow-up may provide insight into the histologic responses to certain treatments.

• Making observations objective

An important element involved in the diagnostic errors mentioned above consists of inconsistencies that can be attributed to the fact that results cannot be reproduced. Observations are objective when the same results are obtained, irrespective of time, location, and observer. In other words, objective observations are reproducible observations. Computer programs are examples of functions that perform the same operations every time they are executed. Hence, if certain observations can be performed by computers, the results will inherently be reproducible, although not necessarily correct.

Morphometry involves a set of techniques that support objective measurements of geometric parameters. The term **cytometry** applies to such parameters in cells and tissue. Examples of such parameters are given in Table 13.2.

Nonautomatic, semiautomatic, and automatic types of equipment are available to support measurement of the above-mentioned parameters. An example of a nonautomatic type method is point-counting equipment. This is used to count particles. These particles are easy to detect by human observers, but they are very difficult to detect in an automated fashion. Usually, there is a grid overlaying the histologic image to support systematic counting of certain cell types or mitoses. The size of the grid is known exactly and the observer counts the numbers of cells or other observable entities in a fixed number of squares on the grid. It is a technique routinely used to count various types of blood cells (for leukocyte differentiation), cells in **Papsmears** of cervical mucus, and the concentration of spermatozoa in an ejaculate. Bone marrow and other

13

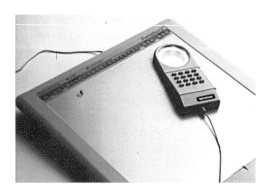

Figure 13.6
Graphic tablet for interactive entry of image features.

biopsy material may be studied in the same way. The equipment also supports measurements of the lengths and surface areas of certain features.

A typical example of semiautomatic equipment is the **graphic tablet** (Fig. 13.6. With the cursor, the user can trace certain areas, such as nuclei, cells, or the surface occupied by a certain type of tissue. The tracings produce coordinates by which the computer program is able to make calculations about size and surface area and to derive parameters such as shape.

Fully automatic techniques include **flow cytometry** and **image processing**. Flow cytometry is used to assess the DNA content in suspensions of nuclei, cells, and chromosomes. The suspension is treated with fluorescent stains, and the flow cytometer measures light intensity. The technique is fast, but it only produces data on quantity, not on tissue structure.

Image processing involves automated feature detection and measurement in digitized images (see Chapter 10). The accuracy of the method highly depends on the quality of the image and on how well the features to be measured can be detected and isolated from the background. In some applications a human observer assists in specifying the areas of interest to the image processor. Although automation of an observation renders it more objective, it does not necessarily mean that it is also more accurate. When the detection of what is to be measured is not precise enough, there will be much contamination noise in the measurements. In other words, the **sensitivity** or **specificity**, or both, may be

low. There is a dilemma between objectivity and noise on the one hand and the expert eye with less reproducibility on the other. The challenge is to combine the strengths of human and computer resources interactively to optimize the results.

• Direct clinical applications

Quantitative techniques serve both research and clinical diagnostic purposes. However, complex and time-consuming measurements on tissue structures are mostly done in a research setting. Although not yet widely used, computer applications help pathologists make diagnoses. Some of the reference systems for education also serve this purpose. A highly indexed electronic textbook or image atlas that can be accessed on the basis of observed features may be of diagnostic help. The initiative in such applications is entirely on the side of the user.

The use of decision-support systems (see Chapter 15) requires much more initiative. They perform tasks that resemble those of a human expert and are therefore sometimes called **expert systems**. The main difference between these expert systems and the reference systems mentioned above is that expert systems have an **inference** engine, which interprets information provided by the user. The pathologist can enter observed features and can obtain a response from the system in the form of differential diagnostic suggestions. After an initial intake of observations, the system is able to produce lists of items that help to confirm or rule out certain diagnoses. A large collection of reference images helps the user to visually evaluate the diagnostic hypotheses as well. Intellipath can also be used for education in the form of case simulation.

Since much of a pathologist's training involves diagnostic reasoning, there is no sharp line between computer applications for clinical practice and education. New developments involve sharing of cases with other pathologists in the form of telepathology. Although it is still expensive, modern network technology is ready for such applications. Also, when storage of images on optical media becomes routine, histologic changes can easily be interpreted in the context of previous slides of the same lesion in the same patient. In addition, comparison with slides of patients with similar lesions will promote more consistent diagnoses.

Nowadays, probably no pathology laboratory is without a computer. However, most applications are for production (i.e., administrative purposes and dictation of reports). Some departments have workstations for education and research. Routine optical or digitized storage is still rare, but the great potential of such means of storage for patient care, in addition to research, will certainly contribute to a rapid increase in its use.

5 Clinical Chemistry and Hematology

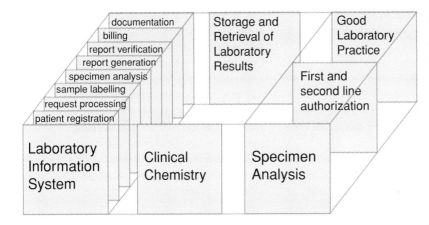

Figure 13.7
Schematic representation of subsystems operational in clinical chemistry.

Clinical chemistry is one of the first areas in health care where computers were introduced to support the entire process from sample collection to final report generation and validation (see Fig. 13.7 for an overview of subsystems). Clinical chemical and hematologic testing are intended to provide the clinician with meaningful information on the chemical and cellular compositions of body fluids and tissues of patients to:

- confirm a suspected diagnosis,
- monitor the effects of treatment,
- exclude or screen for the presence of disease, and
- assess the prognosis once a diagnosis has been made.

The analytical process (or the test request cycle) consists of several stages (see Fig. 13.8):

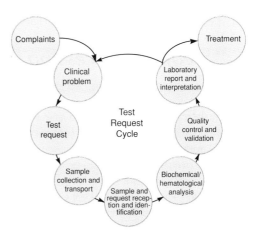

Figure 13.8
Schematic overview of tasks performed by a laboratory information system during a test request cycle.

1. It starts with the translation of the clinical question into a test request.
2. A patient sample is taken, transported to the laboratory, and subjected to one or several preanalytical treatments.
3. In the mean time, the patient data, the sample identification data, and the requested tests are registered or these data are retrieved from, for example, an HIS.
4. The test request cycle proceeds with the distribution of the sample over different analytical stations.
5. This is followed by the actual analysis and is accompanied by analytical quality control (QC) procedures.
6. Next, the results are collected and validated.
7. Finally, the results are interpreted and reported to the clinician.

The clinician will use the obtained test results to answer the original clinical question, which will eventually generate a new clinical question and a new test request (as depicted in the **diagnostic-therapeutic cycle** of Fig. 1.2 in Chapter 1).

Each of these steps is partially or completely supported by automated instruments and computers. In today's laboratories, laboratory information systems take care of almost all administrative procedures, in many cases interfaced on-line with the analytical instruments. The most important functions of such laboratory information systems are described in the following sections.

5.1 Request Processing

The classical way to order a laboratory test for a specific patient is to complete a request form (mark-sense form)on which, in the majority of cases, the test parameters have been preprinted together with the patient identification. In case of **mark-sense forms**, patient information is written in and test requests are indicated on the form by marking the appropriate boxes with a pencil. The form is sent to the laboratory, together with the patient sample. In the laboratory, the test requests are entered into the laboratory information system, either automatically (if it concerns a mark-sense form by an optical mark reader) or manually. Another way of data entry is the use of **OCR**. By using a special scanning instrument (a so called **optical character reader**) with suitable software, even handwritten data can automatically be entered into the system.

If the laboratory information system is linked to an HIS, it will be possible to enter test orders directly into the system through computer terminals at the nursing station by using an order management module of the HIS. The HIS transfers the order to the laboratory system, which awaits specimen arrival in the laboratory. The advantage of the latter approach is that all patient data are automatically entered into the laboratory system, which also generates labels with the patient's name and identification number and the location, date, and time of collection for each individual specimen container. In addition, it is possible to create overviews on request orders for the nursing station, such as pending, collected, delivered, and accepted orders and reported test results.

Test ordering can be organized in different ways. Options are, for instance, requests for individual tests or requests for prearranged s of organ- or disease-specific tests, with or without priority indication. Features such as scheduling a test for a particular time (e.g., for **glucose tolerance** tests) and **deltachecking** the results against the results of earlier test requests to avoid unnecessary repetition may be incorporated in the order management program. The advantages of such an order management program are obvious:

- considerable reduction of administrative effort;
- reducing the chance of misidentification of patients, samples, and request forms; and
- a more efficient use of laboratory services.

After the clinical specimen has been collected, the specimen is transferred to the laboratory reception. After checking its appropriateness for the requested tests, the arrival of the sample in the laboratory is confirmed in the system and a unique identification number is assigned to the sample. This sample number is then linked to the patient identification number and is used to track the sample throughout the complete analysis process.

5.2 Sample Preprocessing

Figure 13.9 gives an example of a bar-coded sample, to be analyzed by a clinical-chemistry analyzer. More and more clinical chemistry analyzers are equipped with sample compartments that contain a **bar code** reader and with sample pipettors with level and clot sensors. This gives them the opportunity to use directly on the analyzer the tube in which the original blood sample was collected and given an identification number in bar code. For hematology analyzers the original whole-blood sample is used; for chemistry analyzers the sample is first centrifuged to separate the serum or plasma from the cell fraction. A physical barrier between cells and serum or plasma is maintained by the silicon gel included in the tube.

Most instruments automatically recognize the specific bar code. If the instrument does not contain a bar code reader of its own, the number can be read by a handheld reader before introducing the sample into the instrument. To avoid errors, the laboratory will try to assign one sample tube to each different analyzer. However, it is unavoidable that a sample sometimes must be divided over one or more daughter tubes. This is a critical phase in terms of mislabeling and mixing up samples. Large laboratories are introducing sample distribution systems in which this process of daughter tube preparation with bar coding is performed automatically on the basis of the test request pattern.

A specific problem is the traceable storage of samples in refrigerators and freezers. Computer programs are indispensable for position assignment and retrieval of a specific sample in sample trays and for registration of sample identification, date of storage, and other relevant information.

5.3 The Preanalytical Phase

One of the most important features of the laboratory information system is to compile the sample identification numbers in groups of tests performed at a specific workstation in the laboratory. Such a compilation is called a *work list* when it is printed on paper. If it is equipped with a bidirectional interface, such a work list can be sent to an analyzer electronically. This uploading enables the instrument to perform the test request pattern for each sample, recognized by its bar code, in random order. Many analyzers choose the test sequence for optimal performance themselves; those analyzers are called random-access analyzers.

5.4 The Analytical Process

The microprocessor built into the analytical instrument usually controls the vital parameters in the functioning of the instrument and alarms the operator when it malfunctions. Test parameters, calibration data, and calibration intervals are introduced, and they are adjustable by the operator. Measurement data are generally printed on paper through a printer output port, and at the same time they are sent to a communications port for electronic data transfer to the laboratory information

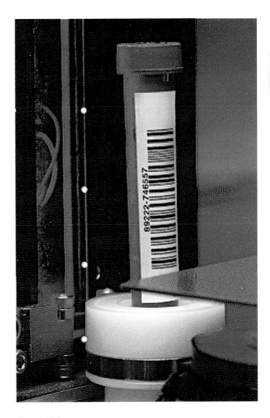

13

Figure 13.9
Sample for a clinical chemistry analyzer that has been bar coded.

system. The results are then put into a temporary buffer accessible only by the operator.

The operator should verify first whether the analytical quality criteria have been met. This process is called the *first-line* **authorization** (see Fig. 13.10). It consists of several steps:

1. A check whether the results for quality control (QC) samples in the same run are within the preset limits. This check can also be executed by the laboratory information system, if it has been programmed to recognize the specific sample numbers of the QC samples in the run, to put the results in a separate file, and to lead the results through a set of rules for QC testing. Generally, the program presents the QC data in so-called Levy-Jennings charts or Youden plots, from which it is easy to follow sequential QC data and to identify specific analytical problems. It is possible to ask the system to fulfill its QC task in the background and to alarm the operator only in case of violation of any of the QC rules.
2. Each individual result is checked for consistency. In case of failing a test the whole series of samples or individual samples are rerun. At this stage it is recommended that an alarm be given if a certain limit is breached. For a small group of tests, the result may be an indication for immediate attention by the requesting clinician. In that case the authorization and reporting procedure should be bypassed by contacting the clinician directly by phone.
3. Test results passing the first-line authorization are transferred to a second buffer, where they wait for the *second-line authorization*. This is a procedure that is performed by a different laboratory worker,

in which the results are checked against each other and against earlier reports of the results for the same parameters (*delta check*). All results exceeding certain preestablished limits are presented on a list and the data are validated either by rerunning the tests, cross-checking the results, or examining the clinical information. At this stage, the systems also signals possible interferences from one component of the sample with the measurement results for another component.
4. When all authorization rules have been passed, the results are sent to the report buffer, from which a hard copy is prepared, or the data are sent electronically to the electronic patient data file. In the majority of laboratories this process of authorization is carried out by experienced senior technologists. One would expect that it is possible to automate such a task, and, indeed, at least one laboratory system that is able to do so is being marketed. This system includes a built-in expert system that verifies laboratory data and clinical information.

A special feature of some laboratory information systems or even automated laboratory instruments is *reflex testing*. This means that the laboratory information system or the analyzer generates new requests on the basis of previously obtained results by following rule-based decision trees. The rules should be established between clinicians and chemists. The advantage is that the clinician is able to start with a limited set of parameters while relying on the self-established rules to select the most appropriate follow-up test for diagnostic testing.

5.5 Reporting

Once the results have been validated, they are ready to be reported to the requesting clinician. This may be done by sending a simple list of analysis data (e.g., sample material, analyte name, kind of quantity name, and numerical value), together with the appropriate units and reference values for the parameters involved. Just as it is possible to use a **knowledge base** at the beginning of the testing cycle to determine which tests or test sequence to follow, it is possible to add interpretations, conclusions, or advice for follow-up inves-

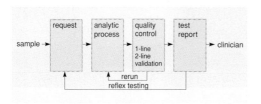

Figure 13.10
The process of first-line authorization in clinical chemistry.

tigations to the test report manually or by using a knowledge base. In practice there are only a few examples of such **knowledge bases** or **expert systems** working routinely as part of a laboratory information system.

In most hospitals, data are stored in a patient-oriented database from which the clinician can retrieve all needed information on a terminal in the ward. The presentation is mostly in the form of a cumulative review, in which measurement results are listed consecutively in order of time and sample type. Many laboratory information systems have the facility to report semivalidated results directly to the ward printer to minimize the reporting time. As mentioned earlier, for a limited set of vital parameters, electronic reporting is bypassed by a direct phone call to the clinician. This is the case when test results indicate a threatening clinical condition.

Because many laboratories also have external clients, electronic mail systems have come into use for fast and cheap reporting of laboratory results. Several communication standards are being used for this type of information exchange, of which **EDIFACT** and **HL-7** are the most popular.

In general, the laboratory information system prepares an electronic message that contains the test results and then sends this message to an electronic mailbox in a specialized and commercially operated computer by direct line or by a public telephone network. The requesting clinician can call this computer and retrieve the mail from the box at a self-chosen moment. In some situations this route may be used in the opposite direction by placing test requests in the laboratory's electronic mailbox.

5.6 Management Information

In a completely computerized laboratory the laboratory information system is able to follow the analytical process step by step, and it is possible to obtain surveys of the progression continuously; at any moment one can see the number of samples that have been received, reported, still being tested, or waiting to be dealt with. For management of the laboratory, it is of great importance that data on sample flow, such as numbers of individual tests per day, week, month, and year can be retrieved from the database on demand. The introduction of a procedure called **good laboratory practice** or any other formal quality system has made it necessary to store all QC data for a long period of time. This requires an elaborate system for dedicated data management, including automatic data storage on backup tapes.

An important aspect of laboratory information systems and their components is the validation of their proper functioning. Since the system is used to process and transport potentially vital information, one must be as sure as possible that no information can get lost or be mutilated in the course of processing[1].

5.7 Electronic Reporting of Clinical Laboratory Test Results

The electronic transfer of laboratory data from an analytical instrument to a computer system and from one computer system to the other, either within or between different institutions, is of utmost importance for the daily practice of health care. It would be of great help if the format in which these data are transferred were standardized. The American Society for Testing and Materials (**ASTM**), and in particular, its Committee E-31 on computerized systems, issued a specification (E 1238) that was the first consensus standard for the consistent transfer of patient identification data, requests and test orders, and clinical observations. The standard was revised in 1994. The standard is also consistent with the more extended Health Level 7 (**HL-7**) standard, which was developed at about the same time. At present, many modern analytical instruments offer data-exchange facilities that use the ASTM standard.

13

---

[1] See the report of the National Committee for Clinical Laboratory Standards (NCCLS) called "Laboratory Instruments and Data Management Systems: Design of Software User Interfaces and Software Systems Validation, Operation and Monitoring" (NCCLS report GP19-P).

The HL-7 standard, the European **Euclides** (European Clinical Laboratory Information Data Exchange Standard) standard, and the ASTM standard primarily describe the format of the data-link layer, but largely leave the contents of the messages free (see also Chapter 34).

A further improvement to standardization would be the introduction of universal names and codes for analytes, units, sample types, test values, or observations and other valuable attributes. Euclides has developed a multiaxial coding system for that purpose. A monoaxial system has been developed under the name of the **LOINC** (Logical Observation Identifier Names and Codes) database. This database contains codes, names, and synonyms for more than 6,300 test observations. To promote its use, it has been made available on the Internet.

6 Hospital Pharmacy

A hospital pharmacy is one of the supporting departments not directly involved in patient care. Like other **ancillary departments**, such as the clinical laboratory and the radiology department, the hospital pharmacy supports the care process by delivering a specific service (i.e., supporting drug therapy, in the broadest sense). The pharmacist in the hospital is responsible for the safe and optimal use of drugs and also for cost-effectiveness in drug therapy. Consequently, the activities in a hospital pharmacy are related to patient care as well as to logistics. Care-related activities include the following:

- keeping records of medication of patients,
- checking prescriptions, and
- providing physicians and nurses with information concerning prescription of drugs and administration.

The logistic activities concern the following:

- purchasing drugs,
- keeping stock,
- manufacturing or compounding drugs, and
- distributing drugs to the wards and patients.

Computer systems have been developed to support the various activities in a hospital pharmacy. Some systems provide integrated support of the main activities, whereas others only partially support specific activities (e.g., systems for stock control, prescription processing, and **pharmacokinetic** dosage calculations).

This section discusses the different aspects of the use of computers in the hospital pharmacy. First, a general description of the processes occurring in a hospital pharmacy is given; this is followed by a more detailed description of the components of hospital pharmacy systems related to the processes that they support. Finally, current trends in hospital pharmacy computing are discussed.

6.1 Processes in Hospital Pharmacy

The processes in a hospital pharmacy can be classified as being related to

1. patient care,
2. **logistics,**
3. manufacturing and compounding, and
4. management.

The *care-related* processes include activities such as

- collecting, processing, and keeping records of prescriptions;
- checking prescriptions for correct dosage, duplicate medications, **drug interactions**, patient allergies, and **contraindications**;
- providing information to clinicians in the form of medication profiles, drug formulary information, and so forth;
- providing information to nurses, (e.g., dispensing lists and instructions about the administering of drugs);

- therapeutic drug monitoring; and
- maintaining a hospital **formulary.**

The *logistic processes* comprise activities such as

- dispensing drugs to be stored on the hospital wards,
- filling medication carts after the prescriptions have been checked,
- inventory control in the pharmacy as well as on the wards, and
- purchasing of drugs (i.e., ordering, receiving, and invoice processing).

From a hospital pharmacy point of view there are two different models of drug distribution:

Model 1   the traditional method of supplying drugs to the ward stock, and
Model 2   patient-oriented drug distribution.

In the traditional method, a standard stock of frequently prescribed drugs is available on a ward. Medications not available in ward stock are requested from the pharmacy. In this model the nurses fill the medication carts. The pharmacy supplies the drugs for the standard ward stock and for the patient-specific stock.
Within patient-oriented drug distribution, the pharmacy is fully responsible for dispensing patient medications. The medication carts are filled in the central or satellite pharmacy and are transported to the ward daily. In this model, the wards have no stock or just a minimal stock of drugs that are used in emergencies only.
The third group of processes are those concerning the *manufacturing and compounding* of drugs and the preparation of drugs. These processes include

- manufacturing of pharmaceutical products, such as infusion fluids and ampoules,
- compounding of, for example, cytostatic drugs and total parenteral nutrition,
- preparation of intravenous drugs, and
- pharmaceutical product analysis.

Finally, there are *management processes,* which are related to general and operational management and quality assurance.

6.2 Computer Applications in the Hospital Pharmacy

Since the early 1970s, many computer applications have been developed to support the hospital pharmacy. These applications can be categorized on levels 1, 2, 3, and 5 in the model of levels of complexity of computer applications in health care mentioned in Chapter 1. Examples are as follows:

- Level 1
  Electronic communication between a hospital pharmacy system and other systems, either in the hospital environment or in the primary care environment or communication with external suppliers.
- Level 2
  Modules for supporting the internal and external **logistics**, keeping stock control, and maintaining the drug file.
- Level 3
  Computation of the drugs used each day or over a certain period (based on dose and frequency) and computation of optimal stock parameters, such as minimum and maximum stock level or order quantity (based on the drugs used or issued).
- Level 5
  Medication surveillance and pharmacotherapeutic drug advice, based on, for example, **pharmacokinetic models** or a **knowledge base**.

The following section contains a survey of the basic functions generally provided by hospital pharmacy systems in supporting daily routine activities of a hospital pharmacy. A complete hospital pharmacy system contains several modules and may therefore be categorized on more than one complexity level. Some systems that support the clinician in decision making while preparing a prescription are linked with the functions of a hospital pharmacy system. Examples of these types of systems are also described.

13

6.3 Basic Functionality

Hospital pharmacy systems have been developed as either stand-alone applications with interfaces to an **HIS** and other clinical applications or as a subsystem integrated in an HIS (see also Chapter 21). Figure 13.11 gives a schematic overview of the tasks performed by a hospital pharmacy system.

In general, a hospital pharmacy system supports either care-related activities or logistics-related activities, or both, including systems for management support. Several currently available systems support both activities. Compounding and manufacturing are usually supported by stand-alone applications within the hospital pharmacy. More specifically, hospital pharmacy systems provide systems to

- process medication orders, including checks for correct dosage, duplicate medications, **drug interactions**, patient allergies, and **contraindications**;
- process ward requests to supply standard ward stock or to issue patient-specific medication that is not available in ward stock;
- process prescriptions for outpatients;
- compound preparations for cytostatic drugs, parenteral nutrition, and so forth;
- support pharmacy management in controlling stock, purchasing stock from external suppliers, and so forth.

On the basis of the patient medication that is entered, pharmacy systems are able to

- print labels, cart-fill lists, and medication dispensing lists, or administrative lists;
- provide clinicians with the current or past medication profile of the patient;
- provide nurses with the necessary information to prepare or administer the medication; and
- provide hospital or pharmacy management with information about pharmacoepidemiology, costs of drug therapy in general or related to prescribing physicians or specialties, adherence to hospital **formulary**, and so forth.

In most situations, pharmacy staff enter medication orders into the system manually, although electronic prescribing is a coming trend. To identify the correct patient or product, **bar codes** may be used in the care process as well as in logistic processes.

In each pharmacy system the file of available drugs is of vital importance. The file should preferably be updated with information from a national drug data bank. Examples of national drug data banks are the ABDA Databank (Germany), the Theriaque Data-bank (France), the KNMP Databank (The Netherlands), or the First Databank (United States). These data banks usually provide:

- general drug information, such as generic name, brand name, strength, package size, and therapeutic class;
- specific information concerning medication surveillance (i.e., drug dosage and interactions, contraindications, etc.);

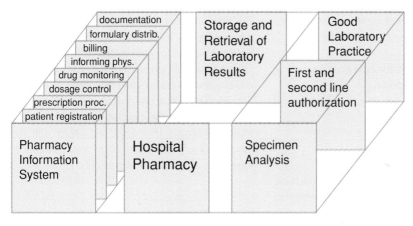

Figure 13.11
Schematic overview of tasks in a hospital pharmacy system.

- information related to the purchasing process (i.e., supplier or manufacturer information, prices, and return conditions); and
- information related to reimbursement and billing.

6.4 Prescription Support

Computer applications for prescription support may be categorized as Level 5 applications as discussed in Chapter 1. They help physicians prescribe the appropriate drugs at the correct dosage, they are able to take account of a patient's allergies or other drug prescriptions, and so forth. Some of the applications provide decision support for complex or possibly dangerous drug therapies.

General prescription support is provided by order entry systems that are part of an HIS such as for the laboratory and radiology. Physicians use such systems also to order medication. During drug order entry, on-line information is available to the physician about the patient's medication profile, the drugs available in the hospital formulary, or about a specific drug (e.g., the common dosage, strengths, and pharmaceutical forms). Some applications also provide on-line alerts related to incorrect dosages, patient allergies, drug interactions, and contraindications. In most hospitals, the use of order entry systems connected to a hospital pharmacy system is still limited, but it will certainly increase in the coming years.

Several applications have been developed for prescription support in specific domains of drug therapy. Some of them, such as pharmacokinetic dosage programs, are widely used in clinical pharmacy practice. These dosage programs give advice on adjusting dosage regimens for drugs with narrow therapeutic margins (e.g., digoxin or aminoglycosides) on the basis of the monitored levels of the drug in blood or serum. Other applications, however, are used in a limited environment, often only in the hospital where they were developed. Examples are decision-support systems for therapy and drug therapy management, such as the **HELP** system and the **ONCOCIN** system for the treatment of oncology patients (see Chapters 15 and 28).

6.5 Current Trends

Studies performed in the 1960s demonstrated high rates of medication errors associated with traditional distribution methods, such as dispensing drugs from floor stock. These results have motivated hospital pharmacists to improve their drug distribution systems systematically. The so-called **unit-dose** drug distribution system, in which drugs are packed and labeled individually, resulted in a reduction of errors compared with the number of errors through use of the traditional system. Nevertheless, drug distribution remains very labor-intensive and prone to error, although hospitals have undertaken various efforts to reduce the numbers of errors.

Since the 1990s, medication management technology has played an increasing role in drug dispensing systems, a development that is stimulated by requirements for cost-containment and efficiency in health care delivery. Medication management technology may be defined as any device or system that helps to

- distribute medication to and from the patient care area (including automated filling of medication carts),
- distribute medication directly to the patient,
- control the inventory, with an interface to a patient record application,
- manage controlled substances, and
- document medication administration.

Current trends in hospital pharmacy automation are related to this technology, resulting in the use of devices for medication distribution and **point-of-care** information systems concerned with medication ordering and administration. Electronic communication between a hospital pharmacy system and other systems inside and outside the hospital is essential.

6.6 Medication Distribution Devices

There are two kinds of medication distribution devices: those based in the patient care unit and those located in the central hospital pharmacy.

Medication distribution devices that are based in the

13

patient care unit usually contain standard ward stock drugs and controlled substances (narcotic drugs) in unit-dose packs. Access to these "vending" machines is controlled, that is, the nurses must identify themselves and the patient(s). When the medication is required, the machine issues only the drugs to be administered to a particular patient. Usually, these machines are linked to a system that maintains the patient's medication profile. These devices are used in some hospitals in the United States and the United Kingdom.

Automated devices located in the hospital pharmacy have been designed to replace or improve the manual process of filling unit-dose carts. For instance, the Baxter ATC-212 system is widely used in the United States and is increasingly used in European countries as well (Fig. 13.12). This device, which is usually linked to a hospital pharmacy system, packages patient-specific unit doses of solid oral medications.

The use of more sophisticated systems such as triaxial **robot**s is still very limited. These robots are equipped with a bar code reader to select **bar-code**d **unit-dose** medications in accordance with a patient-specific medication profile. Such robots are part of a complete system (the *Automated Pharmacy Station*) that also

automates cart filling and verification, as well as restocks returned medications, removes outdated medications, and controls inventory.

So far, none of the currently available devices is able to accommodate all dosage forms, so a manual system is still needed in addition to an automated system. In this respect, there are many parallels with laboratory automation, in which more complex and laborious activities must still be performed manually.

6.7 Use of Point-of-Care Information Systems

Although most of the prescriptions in hospitals are still handwritten, there is growing interest in the use of computer systems for electronic prescription writing. The potential advantages are clear: consistency and efficiency will increase, whereas errors, clinical risks, and waiting times will decrease.

An increasing number of systems provide support to the prescriber by determining which drug and dosage regimen is appropriate for the patient and by performing checks for drug interactions, contraindications, and so forth. For contraindications, however, access to **CPR**s is required. Usually, these kinds of systems provide facilities that can be used to enter and retrieve patient-specific information at the bedside, by using wireless portable terminals.

Point-of-care information systems are usually linked not only to the pharmacy system but also to other departmental systems in the hospital, such as laboratory systems, radiology systems, and dietary systems. In principle, it is possible to construct an electronic patient record system that integrates these data (see Chapter 7). Apart from ordering, medication administration is the other important process that can be supported by **point-of-care system**s. After identifying the patient and the time of administration, the drugs to be administered can be verified by scanning the bar code on the **unit-dose** package. An electronic message to the pharmacy system indicates that the ward stock for that particular drug has decreased.

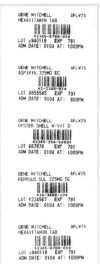

Figure 13.12
Coding in a fully automated drug dispensing system (the Baxter ATC-212 system).

13

6.8 Open Communication

To achieve integrated functionality at the patient's bedside, pharmacy information systems must support open communication facilities. Current interfaces for data interchange include **HL-7** standards, which support: the following:

- admission, discharge, and transfer (ADT) of patients;
- pharmacy orders, either from an HIS or a point-of-care information system;
- medication profiles, that is, pharmacy-encoded orders from or to a pharmacy system to update the patient record; and
- patient record keeping by nurses for ward stock supplies or pharmacy stock supplies.

The ADT interface is widely implemented in many hospitals. The realization of other interfaces is still limited, but the number of interfaces implemented will certainly increase in the near future.

Interchange of data on patient medication at hospital admission and discharge with primary care systems and the systems of retail pharmacists (see Chapter 11) will become increasingly important for ensuring continuity of care. These interfaces will replace manual procedures to provide efficiency and continuity in patient care after admission to and discharge from the hospital.

Key References

See the Web site for literature references.

13

14 Nursing Information Systems

1 Introduction

Nursing is an important link in the chain of patient care because nurses are often identified as both coordinators and providers of patient care. Nurses provide direct care, in which the focus is on individuals who are adjusting to and coping with the consequences of diseases, but nurses also attend to the entire patient, including the patient's psychosocial, somatic, and spiritual needs. This focus on holistic care places large demands on information systems for nurses, because many dimensions of patient care must be visible at the same time. The development of specialized information systems for nurses started in the late 1960s, and the principles regarding the development of nursing support systems have gradually emerged.

In this chapter we describe the development of computer-based information and communication systems that support the nursing discipline. Such systems are usually called nursing information systems. We also define nursing informatics and examine current information systems that support the nursing role.

2 Nursing Informatics

Information systems supporting nursing care cover a range of computer-based applications. These systems include both integrated and stand-alone systems that provide assistance to nurses as they deliver, document, administer, and evaluate nursing care for patients and their relatives. Although the routine use of information systems in nursing is rather new, patient care in nursing has a long history. In the 19th century, Florence Nightingale addressed the question of why nurses should document their observations of the patient. In her opinion, such documentation contributes to the proper care and the healing of the patient. She addressed why nurses should (1) collect data about care systematically and (2) analyze those data statistically. The data that Nightingale collected and analyzed were important for communicating the health status of her patients to other nurses, physicians, other health care workers, and hospital management. In modern times, clinical data derived from the written patient record continue to support clinical decision making, care management and planning, and assessment of the quality of care (see also Chapter 1).

Developers of modern clinical information systems do not focus exclusively on the nursing profession but place attention on the construction of multidisciplinary systems that support a comprehensive electronic patient record. Information systems that contain a broad range of clinical patient data offer support for quality assessment and making improvements in nursing and health care. Hence, the following working definition of **nursing informatics** is proposed to serve as a foundation for the remainder of this chapter:

Nursing informatics is the endeavor of analyzing, modeling, and formalizing how nurses (1) collect and manage data, (2) use data to derive information and knowledge, and (3) make knowledge-based decisions and inferences for multidisciplinary patient care.

Use of this knowledge broadens the scope and enhances the quality of nurses' professional practice. The research methods that are central in nursing informatics focus on:

1. identification of the requirements for computer-based systems,
2. development of models of information and knowledge processing for all aspects of nursing practice,
3. design, implementation, and assessment of information systems for nursing practice, and
4. measurement of the effects of these systems on nursing practice and patient outcomes.

3   Formalizing Nursing Knowledge

There is ongoing emphasis on formalization of nursing knowledge. This process of formalization is an effort to translate nurses' descriptions of patients and clinical observations into standardized frameworks. Many efforts in nursing research concern the development of a common terminology for nursing observations, interventions, and health outcomes, as well as an acceptable system for structuring and classifying them.

A nursing information system consists of computer software and hardware and takes account of the people, organizational structures, and processes that use clinical information for nursing care. A nursing information system may contain both informal (unstructured) and formal (structured) information. As shown in Fig. 14.1, informal information, usually in the form of

narrative text, is very common in nursing practice. Only a small part of this textual information can now be formalized, and only part of this formalized information is suitable for computer processing. This difficulty is attributable in part to lack of a uniform terminology in nursing and to the need for nurses to deal with highly individualized patient problems.

Although it remains difficult to formalize many nursing terms, we describe how nursing information can be structured and used for the development of information systems that support the delivery of patient care and the evaluation of nursing practice.

A particularly difficult issue in formalizing nursing information is the lack of defined methods for creating structured clinical lexicons and clarifying the **semantics** of the terms included in the lexicons. However, researchers in nursing informatics have been able to organize clinical data into discrete types, like those types used in the various steps of the nursing process. The nursing process steps are:

- assessment,
- diagnosis,
- planning,
- intervention, and
- care evaluation.

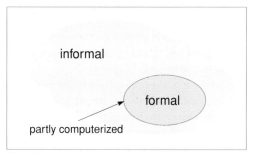

Figure 14.1
The nursing information system in use. Informal information forms the largest part of the system; formal information forms only a small part with a very small part of the formal information currently used for computer support (from Hoy, 1993, with permission).

The distinctions among *data, information,* and *knowledge* noted in Chapter 1 apply equally in the context of nursing, referring to the fact that phenomena of interest to nursing are described at different levels of abstraction:

14

- *Data* can be seen as entities that describe the functional health status of the patient and that have relevance for nurses.
- *Information* represents the clinical view of the nurse: the interpretation of the patient data.
- *Knowledge* is information that is derived by induction and substantiated by scientific methods so that relationships can be identified and verified (see also Fig. 1.1). In nursing, generalizations, clinical views, and interpretations comprise domain knowledge. This knowledge, often based on clinical inferencing, leads to nursing diagnoses and allows nurses to plan interventions and set goals to achieve high-quality outcomes.

This distinction between data, information, and knowledge is congruent with the basic principles of medical informatics, namely, the **syntactic** (data), **semantic** (information), and **pragmatic** (knowledge to be used to make decisions) aspects of information processing (see Chapter 1). The process of nurses' aggregation of data into nursing clinical information and knowledge is little different from that for other clinicians, except that nurses lack a uniform terminology for expressing their more abstract observations.

Knowledge, as in all areas of health care, can be distinguished as either declarative or procedural in nature. Declarative knowledge addresses data, facts, and relationships; procedural knowledge deals with how to do something, such as how to apply a nursing intervention. Nursing knowledge can be categorized as follows:

- *domain knowledge*, comprising facts and relationships about nursing,
- *inferential knowledge*, defining recurring clinical reasoning steps in nursing,
- *task knowledge*, guiding the selection of procedures and activities for proper task performance, and
- *strategic knowledge*, selecting alternative nursing tasks that may be suitable for certain situations.

These distinctions are the same as those used in the knowledge acquisition and design structuring (**KADS**) system for modeling human expertise in general (see Chapter 28, Section 5).

14

4 Multidisciplinary Collaboration

Most nurses work in groups on designated shifts and interact with a variety of clinical colleagues. Consequently, support for multidisciplinary collaboration is an essential requirement of nursing information systems. Such systems must be built collaboratively by using participatory design methods and must then facilitate collaboration among a variety of health care workers within the clinical environment.

In patient care, nurses draw on clinical information from several disciplines. At the bedside, nurses may record and use patient data that are identical to those required by physicians, yet other nursing data are collected as well. Physicians and nurses each may transform data into different clinical abstractions and then use those data to make different diagnostic inferences, care plans, and prognostic predictions. Thus, workers in different clinical disciplines may all use the same data, but for diverse patient-related purposes. The overlap and the distinction in data use are represented in Fig. 14.2.

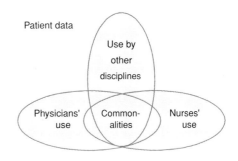

Figure 14.2

A view on the use of patient data, illustrating the multidisciplinary use of patient data.

5 Content of the Clinical Nursing Record

On the basis of the framework provided by the KADS model, there are several implications for information systems that contain a computer-based patient record (CPR):

1. *Domain knowledge* should be represented to offer systematic and uniform ways of referring to nursing clinical events. The absence of formalized data and knowledge hampers the development of **CPRs** (see also Chapters 7 and 29). Conversely, the use of controlled terminology that is too restricted inhibits practitioners from freely expressing their findings and impairs the extent to which a nursing information system is capable of representing the events of clinical practice. Consequently, the search for methods that allow nurses and physicians to describe clinical findings without restriction is an important area of investigation.

2. Support for *clinical inferences* made by nurses is a central area of research. A lack of formalized data and structured domain knowledge hampers the modeling of nursing decisions, which is a prerequisite for the development of clinical decision-support systems.

3. A clinical nursing information system should assist in *task performance*, specifically, care planning. A nurse may not have much time to either plan or document care, but a nurse will still need data and information from the care plan. Standardized and clearly presented nursing terminology, properly automated and with linkages to existing formalized nursing knowledge, may contribute significantly to adequate care planning and task performance. It remains an open question whether information systems will be able to assist in the

14

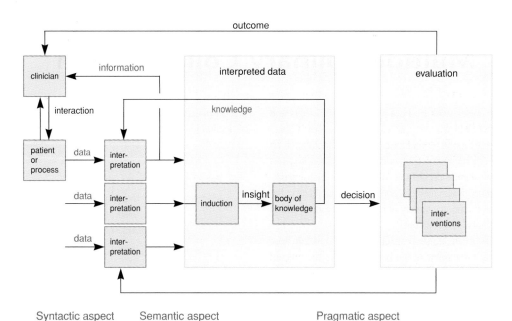

Syntactic aspect   Semantic aspect   Pragmatic aspect

Figure 14.3
Expansion of Fig. 1.1 presented as data and information management to support nursing care.

area of *strategic knowledge*; strategic planning is still ultimately a human activity (as described on Level 6 of Fig. 1.4).

To better understand the important elements of information processing in nursing, Fig. 1.1 has been further expanded by the elements *decisions, interventions,* and *evaluation* in Fig. 14.3. Moreover, these elements can be used to study the clinical content of nursing information systems.

The expansions of the model include the following components:

- *Data interpretation* represents decisions made in clinical practice.
- *Interventions* represent all the activities following the decision making.
- *Evaluation* refers to patient outcomes that result from interventions and includes evaluation of the process itself.
- *Deduction* represents the nursing diagnoses.

The model presented in Fig. 14.3 permits the study of the way that nurses use data to derive information. It also serves as a model for nursing informatics in general; it is a descriptive representation of the data-to-information flow of clinical nursing.

The boundaries of nursing information systems, in the context of systems that support the CPR, are dynamic, but above all, they must allow for the interchange and use of multidisciplinary providers' data, information, and knowledge. Nursing informatics is important for nursing as a discipline. It has the potential to advance clinical nursing knowledge and expand its scientific base. In this way, nursing informatics can contribute to understanding what affects the quality of nursing care.

6 Problems with Paper-Based Records in Nursing

14

In today's information-intensive health care environment, the nursing documentation of patient care takes too much time. Nurses often record the same data in several places in the chart and in administrative tracking lists. This redundancy should not be necessary, given the capabilities of modern computers. Several weaknesses of paper-based records in patient care have been identified (see also Chapters 7 and 29), such as:

- missing data, excessive or redundant data, and lack of decision-making rationale,
- lack of clarity when dealing with different patient problems over a long period of time,
- problems with the accessibility, availability, and retrieval of individual records;
- awkwardness when making changes to a record

and in keeping the record up to date,
- difficulty in evaluating patient outcome on the basis of a poorly organized paper-based record, and
- problems reading the handwriting of care providers.

Because of the explosive growth of clinical knowledge, it is important that relevant knowledge be made available at the point of care and that information be aggregated to allow for the examination of quality of care and of care outcomes. The growth in the complexity of patient care data runs parallel to the excessive growth in requirements for documentation of patient data that need to be made available for multiple providers and for statistical purposes.

7 Levels of Use of Nursing Data

In collecting clinical nursing data at the source (i.e., during direct patient care) data are principally stored only once and may be used many times. The use of data varies, depending on the level where they are used. In Fig. 14.4, the components to the left concern prerequisites, such as unified terminology, forming the basis for the registration of data during nursing care on the first layer. The correct interpretation of these data as information occurs on layers two, three, and four.

7.1 Nursing Minimum Data Set

Nursing is attempting to document nursing care by using standardized terms. These documented data should be represented by using the elements of what has emerged as the nursing minimum data set (**NMDS**), which includes nursing diagnoses, nursing actions or interventions, nursing-sensitive patient outcomes, and the intensity of nursing care. Once the clinical data have been uniformly defined, nursing staff will be able to describe and compare patient problems, procedures performed in caring for patients, the results of care, and the resources required to provide that care across units and agencies. To accomplish these goals, nursing personnel need standardized data formats and a uniform nursing language. Care providers should be allowed to use their own local terminology. They can then use specific translators to convert their descriptions into internationally agreed upon terms. Once nurses can establish basic clinical data at the atomic level, they can generate abstractions of those data using the definitions of the elements in the NMDS, combined with uniform data standards.

The nursing data to be used in clinical information systems have been defined in part by the NMDS. Several early efforts have focused on testing the elements of the NMDS for patient care documentation. Developed as a minimum set of nursing items (or elements) of information with uniform definitions and categories, the NMDS represents nursing's initial attempt to standardize nursing observations and practice so that they are comparable to those from traditional forms of nursing documentation. These nursing care elements include nursing problems and nursing diagnoses, nursing interventions, and nursing outcomes data. These elements have been defined for use in the United States, Belgium, and Australia. Similar projects are under development in

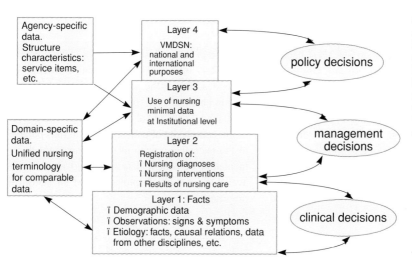

Figure 14.4
A model in which different layers of nursing data are expressed, from atomic-level data, via interpretations and judgments, to management and policy data (adapted from Fig. 14.1; see also Zielstorff et al., 1993).

Name of System	Major Components	Type of Institution	
Omaha System	• Standardized schemes of nursing diagnoses (problems), interventions, and outcomes • Clinical data are used to improve practice, improve administrative oversight, and add to the body of nursing knowledge	Home care agencies, public health clinics, home care, and schools and other ambulatory care settings	Table 14.1 Nursing Support Systems in Use in the United States.
The Automated Community Health Information System (ACHIS)	• Document the daily processes and outcomes of care. • Compose administrative and research agendas: questions such as the nature of client problems, prevention and intervention strategies used in care, and impact of care on outcomes	• Application of the Omaha System • Community health care	
The Hettinger and Brazile System	• System features multiple problem schemes • Well-baby, health maintenance visit and immunization tracking • Asthma, clinical management tool for asthma • Case management, a referral tracking tool • Appointment scheduling	Community health care	
Rural Elder Outreach Program	• Program to track community outreach clients in a program that aims to increase the accessibility of preventive, curative, and health promotion services to rural elderly. The program links formal community-based services, informal community resources, volunteer efforts, and academic resources to strengthen the self-reliance of members of rural communities so that they can care for their elders. • Combination of demographic, encounter, and physical and psychosocial measures data	Community health care	
ComputerLink	• Providing informational and emotional support to home-bound caregivers of patients with Alzheimer's disease • Functional components include a communications area, a decision support module, and an electronic encyclopedia	Community health care	
CareMap	• Care plan system for case management resource overview • Automated bank of nursing diagnoses • Patient outcomes • Intermediate goals and interventions for case types • Critical paths • Continuous quality improvement	All kinds of health care settings	

14

PANEL 14.1

Decision-Support Systems in Nursing

Some of the earliest programs to aid nurse decision making for each step of the nursing process were developed for research purposes, but they were never widely used in clinical settings. Nursing programs that have been developed to assist nurses' decision making have included the following:

- Computer-Aided Nursing Diagnosis and Intervention (CANDI) to assist nurses in formulating nursing diagnoses. A limited validity test for CANDI examined the eight most common nursing diagnoses and tested the extent of agreement between the diagnoses generated by the expert system and those generated by a panel of clinical nursing specialists. Statistically significant agreements between the system and the panel of clinicians could be shown for seven of the eight nursing diagnoses.
- Creighton On-Line Multiple Modular Expert System, which assists nurses in developing care plans.
- Urological Nursing Information System (UNIS), which assists nurses in planning care for incontinent patients.
- CAREPLAN, which is designed to assist nurses in caring for postpartum patients.
- VP-II focuses on deriving nursing problems and is based on patient data for patients with leukemia.
- ACCESs, an ambulatory care expert system consisting of four modules:
  - well-baby (health maintenance visit),
  - asthma (clinical management of asthma),
  - case management (referral tracking), and
  - scheduling (clinic appointments).
  Ongoing verification of the rules and results are under way with this system's implementation, validating its concordance with the reality of clinicians' decisions.
- FLEXPERT, a prototype care plan system about nursing diagnoses and patient symptoms, is in its early stage of development. ▶

---

other countries, including Canada, Denmark, Switzerland, and The Netherlands.

With the use of standardized coding schemes, it should be possible to compare clinical nursing data across different populations, health care settings, geographic areas, and periods of time, as well as to obtain insight into the allocation of nursing resources for patient care. Because the nursing care for a given patient may cross the boundaries of acute care, rehabilitative care, chronic care, or community care, information systems must allow for the collection, retention, and retrieval of those data throughout the entire care continuum. Agency-specific distinctions and structural components (e.g., nursing resources, utilization patterns, occupancy, and care protocols) are needed to place the minimum care data in context. The different types of decisions that are supported by the data from the different layers are illustrated on the right side of Fig. 14.4. When databases containing the NMDS are established, it becomes possible to use these data for several other purposes as well, such as continuous quality assessment, management, and research.

- FLORENCE, another care planning system, is a developmental prototype designed to advise nurses on the identification of nursing diagnoses using case-based and model-based reasoning for care planning.
- ORSS (Operating Room Scheduling System), a recently reported expert system for improving operating room scheduling, is designed to simulate all variables affecting the flow of surgical patients through an institution and develop a surgery schedule.

Generally, evaluative information that contributes to nursing knowledge and that is suitable for increasingly sophisticated developments or improvements in decision-support systems has not been evident from these early decision-support system implementations. With only two exceptions, the pattern of reporting in the published literature about recently developed expert systems continues with little evaluation and with few research-based findings that contribute to advancing the systems or nursing knowledge. A decision-support system for troubleshooting pulmonary artery catheter waveforms has been tested. System users' decision-making skills were assessed before and following system use, as was their satisfaction with the content, accuracy, format, ease of use, and timeliness of the system.

Another system regarding prediction of preterm delivery has been tested. By using extant data it was possible to predict preterm delivery more accurately with the expert system than with manual systems. On the basis of the results obtained with this system it is predicted that future prospective studies with carefully planned and quality-controlled data collection methods should improve the accuracy of predictions in a fully implemented system, resulting in a valid and reliable decision-support system for nurses' assessment of preterm labor risk.

In summary, research on nurses' clinical reasoning and decision making is progressing, albeit at a slow pace. Although many examples of decision-support systems are available in the literature, little knowledge is being generated to guide their inclusion as robust tools in developing information systems. The decision-support systems reported are relatively limited systems that are in the early stages of their development and testing. Most appear to be stand-alone, research-focused implementations that are just being validated. Even the more developed systems still require rigorous evaluation with respect to their support of nurses' clinical reasoning.

14

7.2 Nursing Data

Clinical data for quality assessment and improvement of nursing care can be defined by means of a nursing information system. Figure 14.4 illustrates how patient-specific data, agency-specific data, and domain information and knowledge can be derived from atomic-level clinical data in information systems. Several examples of systems for nurses are provided in Table 14.1. The Omaha System (see Table 14.1), for example, defines standard data elements regarding nursing problems, interventions, and outcomes.

Many conceptual and methodological issues must still be resolved with respect to measurement and evaluation, but the technology for capturing, storing, retrieving, and analyzing nursing outcome data is well within reach. External market forces now demand quality and cost data. Hence, the urgency exists to include atomic-level clinical data about patient status and short- and long-term outcomes in CPRs. Nursing diagnoses, which are just one example of clinical data, could potentially be used to provide an estimate of the complexity of care. Interventions could be used to determine variability in nursing intensity and the amount of nursing care provided.

7.3 Nursing Terminology

The use of standard terminology is an essential component of modern CPRs. Around the world there are several other terminology systems in different stages of development, implementation, and testing. These include the nursing terms in the **Read codes** (see Chapter 6) and a variety of classifications: nursing diagnoses from the North American Nursing Diagnosis Association, interventions from Nursing Intervention Classification and the Omaha System, and many others. An example on the international level is the International Classification for Nursing Practice (**ICNP**), a lexicon for describing nursing events (e.g., nursing diagnoses) and interventions. The ICNP has been derived from several existing classifications and terminologies.

7.4 Nurses' Clinical Reasoning and Judgment

Although the knowledge base of clinical nursing is becoming more mature and explicit with respect to what is needed for nursing information systems, much remains to be accomplished. An important part of designing and developing nursing information systems is understanding how nurses reason and use data. This area still requires much additional research. Although a variety of decision-support systems are reported in the nursing literature, there is a need for more systematic inquiry (see also Panel 14.1).

8   Nursing Information Systems

Early on, discussion focused on how nurses could benefit from information systems and on the influence that such systems would have on patient care. In the 1970s, when early hospital information systems were introduced, attention shifted to gaining more insight into the problems encountered by nurses in the workplace and to the contributions that nurses might make in selecting systems for use. In those early days, nursing was mainly task and process oriented. Thus, only data belonging to explicit stages in the nursing process (assessment, planning, action, and evaluation) could be registered. These general types of systems, were succeeded by some problem-oriented systems and included problem identification and nursing actions. In those systems, the nurse was able to build an individual care plan in a hierarchical database environment. However, retrieval of nursing data still remained a problem.

During this period, research began, and that research is still at the forefront today. Nursing-language systems and **taxonomies**, NMDS, and **classification** systems have become the focus of nursing informatics efforts. This research has led to extensive developments in the field of nursing information systems. It is within this context that questions about the scope, content, and scientific basis of nursing informatics continue to be analyzed. Now the prevailing view is that clinical data should support nursing practice decisions and not merely document nursing tasks. This shift in perspective has helped to define the evolving paradigm from task-oriented systems to future systems. If nursing information systems are to be more than electronic filing cabinets and devices for transmitting information, nurses and designers must create technology that uses the information put into these systems, transform raw data into more useful forms, and propose clinical inferences for the nurse's consideration. These views have resulted in proposals for integrated systems, including integration of *data, presentation,* and *function* (see also Chapter 20).

8.1 What Support Is Needed?

In providing a comprehensive description of nursing information systems, it is necessary to highlight a gradual shift in perspective that is currently under way: from nursing information systems that provide financial and task support for nurses to systems that are focused on clinical data and information as strategic resources for nursing practice. Systems that support nursing should, at the very minimum:

- provide decision support to nurses,
- contribute to advancing nursing knowledge, including defining data of importance to nursing,
- provide information to patients about the care that will be delivered, and
- provide communications facilities such as access to databases that provide nurses with information for delivering the best integrated care that is needed to be able to deliver evidence-based care.

8.2 Systems in Use

Attention should be directed toward transforming existing systems to next-generation systems to support nursing practice. In this evolution, transformation is needed for:

- nursing knowledge bases,
- standard nursing vocabularies and data communications protocols, and
- enhanced professional opportunities for nursing informatics specialists.

Systems that support clinical nursing are available in a variety of health care settings. To get an impression of the spectrum of systems in use, the main components of some of the most widely published systems will be described in a few tables. Table 14.1 provides an overview of community nursing information systems in use in the United States. A second type of system, providing integration of patient data into "virtual" records, provides a better intake and allocation of clients in different health care settings.

In summary, the nursing information systems described here share several common features and illustrate the diversity of care settings in which nurses currently need support in making their clinical decisions and preparing documentation. Some of these systems include clinical data that are useful for supporting nurses' care decisions. Several also are acknowledged for their potential for adding to nursing knowledge. Although they represent stand-alone systems, the nature of their data and system functionality provides an important example of desirable characteristics to be modeled in future systems to support and improve clinical nursing care.

Key References

Brennan PF. Patient satisfaction and normative decision theory. J Am Med Inform Assoc 1995;250-9.

Ozbolt J, Vandewal D, Hannah KJ. eds. *Decision Support Systems in Nursing.* St Louis: CV Mosby, 1990.

Grobe SJ, Pluyter ESP, eds. *Nursing Informatics: An International Overview for Nursing in a Technological Era.* Amsterdam: Elsevier Science, 1994.

See the Web site for further literature references.

14

V
Medical
Knowledge &
Decision Support

Authors of Part V

Chapter 15: Methods for Decision Support
J.H. van Bemmel, Erasmus University Rotterdam; M.A. Musen, Stanford University; R.A. Miller, Vanderbilt University, Nashville; with contribution of A.A.F. van der Maas, University of Nijmegen

Chapter 16: Clinical Decision-support Systems
J. van der Lei, Erasmus University Rotterdam; J.L. Talmon, Maastricht University

Chapter 17: Strategies for Medical Knowledge Acquisition
D.A. Giuse, R.A. Miller, N.B. Giuse, Vanderbilt University, Nashville

Chapter 18: Predictive Tools for Clinical Decision Support
J.D.F. Habbema, E.W. Steyerberg, Erasmus University Rotterdam

15 Methods for Decision Support

1 Introduction

This part of the Handbook describes methods and techniques for the support of decision making in health care. Most of these methods deal with Level 4 of the structured scheme discussed in Chapter 1, primarily involving the *semantic* aspects of the processing of patient data. Data processing for decision making occurs on levels 1 to 5 of Fig. 1.1, as follows:

- data are collected and transmitted at Level 1;
- at Level 2 they are stored into and retrieved from computers;
- the data are processed at Level 3 before entering the decision stage;
- at Level 4, interpretation is done to prepare the final step in the diagnostic-therapeutic cycle, the therapy (i.e., the *pragmatic* aspect), located at Level 5.

A large part of all activities in health care deals with decision making regarding which examinations and tests need to be done or, on the basis of earlier examinations, which further tests need to be ordered. During the first patient visit, complaints and patient history data are collected and a physical examination is done, including simple measurements, such as a blood pressure. If deemed necessary, nonexpensive and noninvasive tests may be ordered, such as a laboratory test. On the basis of the outcomes of these tests, a therapy (e.g., a drug prescription) may be given. If necessary, more complex and more expensive tests are done only when the outcomes of these first examinations, tests, and, sometimes, first treatments are available. All data and interventions are documented in the patient record

(see Chapters 7 and 29).

In short, at many points during patient care, data collection is accompanied by decisions. The chapters in this part of the Handbook deal with two types of decisions:

1. *Decisions related to the diagnosis*, in which computers may assist in diagnosing a disease on the basis of individual patient data, and
2. *Decisions related to the therapy*, in which the best next test or therapy is determined on the basis of the evidence.

The following are examples of the first type, diagnosis-oriented problems:

- What is the probability that this patient has a myocardial infarction, given data in the patient history and the electrocardiogram (*ECG*) results?
- What is the probability that this patient has acute appendicitis, given the signs and symptoms concerning abdominal pain?

The following are examples of the second type, therapy-related problems:

- What is the best therapy for patients at a certain age and with certain risks if an obstruction of more than 90% is seen in the left coronary artery?
- What amount of insulin should be prescribed for a patient during the next 5 days, given the blood sugar levels and the amount of insulin taken during the recent weeks?

- For a patient with hypertension being treated in accordance with a clinical practice guideline, what measures should be implemented when the patient has failed therapy with a particular drug?

For both types of problems we need medical **knowledge**. Only when this knowledge is accurate and complete are we able to develop *decision models* for problems of both types. Once such models are available, decisions may be generated on the basis of individual patient data for both type 1 and type 2 decision problems.

Chapter 16 describes different strategies for diagnosis-oriented decision problems. Chapter 17 addresses the acquisition and maintenance of medical knowledge in **knowledge bases**. Chapter 18 discusses therapy-oriented decision problems. The principle of collecting

reliable patient data for decision making was discussed in Chapters 2 and 6, in anticipation of Chapter 7, on computer-based patient records (**CPR**s).

In the remainder of this introductory chapter to this section of the Handbook, we describe the different types of decision models that are used in decision-support models. We focus on the following elements:

- the forms of medical knowledge (Section 2),
- learning by humans and machine (Section 3),
- decision-support models (Section 4), and
- acceptance of decision-support systems (Section 5).

The four Panels accompanying this chapter discuss some methodological and ethical aspects of medical decision making.

2 The Forms of Medical Knowledge

2.1 Two Types of Knowledge

Two types of knowledge are involved in decision making:

- *Scientific or formal knowledge* (from the medical literature, books, or articles in journals). This type of knowledge deals with **cognition** or **deduction**; that is, one must know and understand principles of biological processes and relationships between pathophysiological conditions and disease symptoms.
- *Experiential knowledge* (as condensed in well-documented patient databases or validated guidelines). This type of knowledge is related to **recognition** or **induction**; that is, a clinician has seen certain symptoms before and recognizes the underlying disease.

In practice, these two types of knowledge are extremes of a continuum of clinical knowledge and are interwoven when clinicians "reason" about the signs and symptoms of a specific patient. In most instances, clinicians have enough knowledge and sufficient patient data are available to make the right decision. Computers

do not need to give support then. Yet, there remain reasons why computers may be required:

1. People sometimes make errors or mistakes (e.g., in routine cases as well as in complex cases).
2. Clinicians cannot keep up with the ever increasing medical knowledge.
3. It is sometimes more efficient to automate decision making when dealing with large numbers of routine decisions (e.g., when many standard laboratory tests must be assessed or when many ECGs must be interpreted).
4. Health care organizations may mandate certain clinical practices both to improve the quality of care and to lower the cost of care.

Computers can store patient data in **databases**. They are also well suited to storing knowledge in **knowledge bases**. Computers require, however, that such knowledge be structured and formalized, similar to data structuring, as discussed in Chapter 4 (database management). Only then can patient data and medical knowledge be used for computer-supported decision making, assisting the knowledge in and the reasoning by human brains.

15

> ## PANEL 15.1
>
> ## Computers, Grandmasters, and Clinicians
>
> Chess is generally considered to be a truly intellectual game. It requires careful observations not only of the pieces on the chessboard but also of one's opponent's past strategy and even of his character. It also requires knowledge of both the rules and risks involved in certain configurations of the pieces on the board (*cognition*) and of the outcomes of many games played before (*recognition*). How the chess grandmaster processes his observations of the game and of his opponent and how he uses the knowledge stored in his brain is largely unknown. Certainly, in-depth analysis of the possible moves that his opponent could make is important, but not decisive. Of possibly greater importance is at least the ability to comprehend the entire game, sometimes expressed as intuition, probably comparable to the clinical intuition of an experienced diagnostician. Seminal studies by De Groot in the 1960s demonstrated that this intuition can be explained by a process known as "information chunking:" With increasing experience, humans are able to make greater and greater abstractions of the arrangements of pieces on the chessboard and to remember the locations of those clusters of pieces with accelerating ease. When most computers are programmed to play chess, their power lies in brute force, that is, in their incredible processing speed and ability to make in-depth predictions about the outcomes of many different future moves. The model that underlies a computer chess program may be powerful, but in many respects it is totally different from the reasoning in the brain of a grandmaster.
>
> How clinicians possessing much knowledge and experience arrive at a final conclusion and decision is largely unknown, even to themselves. The elements or ingredients used to arrive at a decision by both a clinician and a computer may be identical, but the reasoning in the human brain is unknown. How a chess player decides the next best move or how a clinician decides the next best step in the diagnostic process is often not traceable. In science it is called *insight*. The breakthrough in obtaining insight is known in German as an *"Aha! Erlebnis."*
>
> In chess, the rules are known. When making a diagnosis in a complex case, the rules are neither known nor fixed, and the number of "pieces on the board" (the symptoms) may be large and of a totally new kind. Modeling the rules of chess on a computer appears to be feasible; modeling the full scope of medical decision making is only possible to some limited extent.

2.2 Brains Versus Computers

The question is whether computers are able to make the same decisions as experienced clinicians using the same patient data and the same knowledge. In other words, if people are able to store scientific knowledge and clinical experience in their brains, how can we make these two types of knowledge operational in computers? Will the structure of knowledge in human brains be different from the structure of knowledge in computers? Will the data used for decision making by computers be similar to the data used by clinicians when they derive conclusions and make decisions? Regretfully, the key problem here is that, in fact, we do not know *how* people store and use their knowledge: *we do not know which "model" (if any) the human brain uses to solve decision problems.*

However, this is only one of the dilemmas in medical decision making and knowledge processing. An example from a domain outside health care may illustrate this dilemma. In Panel 15.1, solution of decision problems by computers and by human reasoning is compared, using chess as an example. In health care, in addition to areas with strict rules, such as chess, other issues may hamper computer-supported decision making:

- Medical knowledge is ever expanding, but is limited in the human brain;
- Patient data are sometimes only partly available; and
- The problem of a specific patient may be new and unique.

Nevertheless, it is challenging to structure knowledge in a computer in such a way that medical decision problems can be solved, albeit only partly. Chapter 17 describes in more detail how knowledge can be solicited

from the literature and experienced clinicians, and Chapter 28 provides additional insight into the modeling of clinical expertise for representation within computer systems. For now it is sufficient to conclude that computers may assist in solving decision problems, but that they undoubtedly solve problems in a way very different from the way that humans do. Furthermore, computers require formalization and a structured approach to problem solving. This holds for both data and knowledge.

One of the first steps in solving any problem, including a decision problem, is to collect enough and reliable observations and knowledge to solve the problem. In health care this means that signs and symptoms must be collected in the observation stage of the diagnostic-therapeutic cycle (Fig. 1.1), whereupon the decision-making process can be started.

3 Learning by Humans and Machines

Above, we mentioned that for decision making, knowledge is involved in cognition and recognition. *Learning* is done during education and training, and the level of cognition is *tested* during examinations. If the results of this examination are satisfactory, the acquired knowledge may be applied in practice. The two stages, (1) learning and (2) testing, can be observed during both the training of medical students and the training of computers for

decision making. It was already discussed that there are fundamental differences in decision making between humans and machines; nevertheless, the same two stages apply to both. In this section we focus on the first stage, learning, whereas the second stage will be discussed in Section 5, Acceptance of Decision-Support Systems.

First, we focus on the most central issue in all learning processes: the selection of features or symptoms by which we recognize events or diseases.

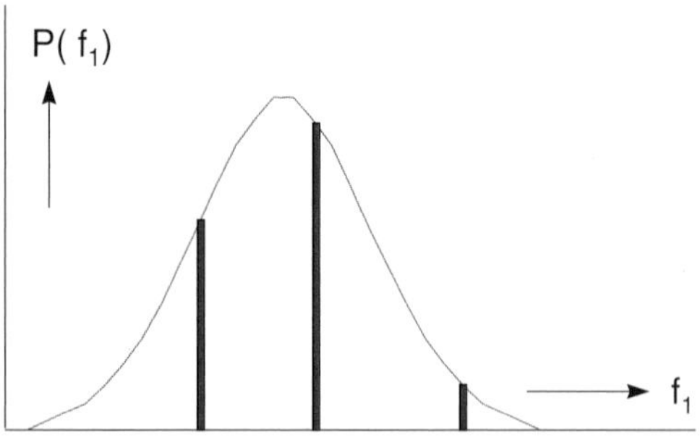

Figure 15.1
Variability in symptoms between patients who possess the same disease. The variability can be expressed in, for example, means and variances.

3.1 Features

- Symptoms versus diseases

To know what signs and symptoms (including results of examinations and tests) belong to a disease, we must be taught, discover it ourselves during research, or acquire empirical associations through experience. However, the fact that we know which symptoms may be seen in disease does not necessarily reveal what disease is present, given the symptoms; the same symptoms may also manifest themselves in some other disease. In general, the first type of relationship (diseases → symptoms) is the result of careful observations during scientific studies and clinical experience and the second type (symptoms → disease) is the task of the practicing clinicians. The same types of relationships apply to decision models in computers. When we "teach" them the forward relationship disease → symptoms, an inverse relationship, symptoms → disease, is required for the decision model to make a decision. In Section 4.1.5 we further elaborate on this inverse relationship when we discuss **Bayes' rule**.

• Variability

Patient symptoms generally show a large **variability** between patients who have the same disease. The symptoms also show variability in the same patient when the disease progresses or the circumstances change. In other words, all symptoms and measurements determined for a population of patients or healthy people may show large variability, which may be expressed in, for example, means and variances (see Fig. 15.1). Symptoms and measurements determined for the same disease category may be correlated and can also be expressed statistically (Fig. 15.2).

• Feature selection

In parallel to the nomenclature used in pattern recognition (see Chapter 27), we often call the signs, symptoms, measurements, and results of diagnostic tests *features* and the computer-supported decision or diagnosis a *classification*. The remainder of this chapter uses this terminology. Decision models can assist in *feature selection*, which is the principal part of training computers for decision support, that is, to determine which signs, symptoms, or measurements are the most important (statistically significant) for discriminating between a healthy or a pathological condition or between different diseases. Without proper features, no computerized decision-support method is able to offer help. The relevant features embody the semantic information of all patient data available in a CPR.

• Features versus decision model

The type of decision model that is chosen is important but if we do not know what features are most relevant, no decision model will provide any help. The decision model may help in selecting the best features, and once we have the best features, the decision model

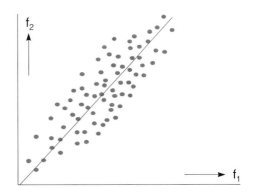

Figure 15.2
Symptoms or measurements, in short: features, determined for the same disease category may be correlated and can also be expressed statistically. In this diagram, observations for features f_1 and f_2 have been plotted.

itself may be optimized (see Fig. 15.3). This is similar to *detection theory*: once we have developed a detector, signals can be better detected (e.g., a signal amidst noise); when we know the properties of the signals, a better detector can be designed (see also Fig. 25.12). When "training" a computer decision model, based on empirical classification, the features of a set of patients with different diseases are entered into the computer (this is called the *training set* or the *learning set*). The

15

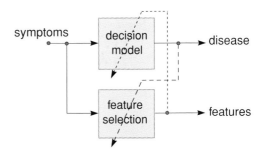

Figure 15.3
A decision model may help in selecting the best features, and once the best features are available, the decision model itself may be optimized. Observe the similarity with detection: once we have a detector, a signal can be better described; when we know the signal, a better detector can be designed (see also Fig. 25.12).

computer can be requested to categorize the patients into different disease groups using the decision model (in pattern recognition this is called *learning*; see Chapter 27). In principle, similar to learning by humans, two types of learning are used by the computer to discern diagnostic categories:

- *supervised learning* and
- *unsupervised learning.*

For the former, a "teacher" is required; for the latter the computer is left alone to find the different diagnostic categories. The following sections address both types of learning.

3.2 Supervised Learning

In supervised learning the researcher (the teacher) tells the computer the disease or health status of each patient in the training set. The computer is then asked to order the features according to discriminatory power (i.e., what is the best feature to discriminate between disease A and disease B, the second best, etc.). Different statistical and other techniques can be

used to arrive at a set of features, ordered according to discriminatory power, some of which are further discussed in Chapter 27. Here, however, it suffices to state that features can generally be ordered in one way or the other but that this does not necessarily always lead to identical results. Ultimately, the "supervisor" determines on the basis of the results of the teaching which features and how many features are to be used in the decision model.

3.3 Unsupervised Learning

In unsupervised learning, the computer is also given the training set of features. However, the "truth" (i.e., information on what disease belongs to which patient) is not known. The computer is then used to discover by what clusters of feature sets the different disease groups can best be characterized. This process is called **clustering** (see Chapter 27).

For instance, if it is known that in the training set only two different disease classes, classes A and B, are present, the computer can be requested to assess whether a certain patient has a higher probability of belonging

15

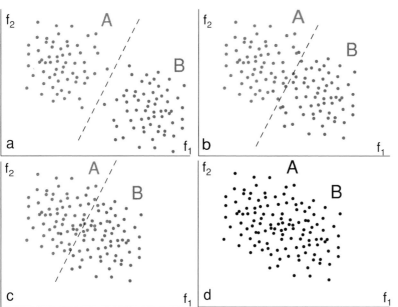

Figure 15.4
Example of a training set that consists of only two classes, classes A and B, and of which only two features, features f_1 and f_2, are known. (a) Clusters A and B are fully separated, which is also indicated by the line between the clusters. (b) The clusters are closer to each other and show some overlap. (c) A considerable overlap is seen between clusters; panel d is identical to panel c, but the labeling of the different elements of clusters A and B has been omitted. Two different clusters can no longer be discerned, and it is clear that unsupervised clustering techniques will also not be able to find a meaningful solution.

to class A or class B. Figure 15.4 provides an example of a training set that consists of only two classes, classes A and B, and of which only two features, features f_1 and f_2, are known. The hypothesis behind a clustering program is that all feature sets of class A are better clustered into cluster A than in cluster B, and vice versa. In Fig. 15.4a clusters A and B are fully separated, which is also indicated by the line between the clusters. In Fig. 15.4b, the clusters are closer to each other and show some overlap, and in Fig. 15.4c, a considerable overlap is seen between clusters. Figure 15.4d is identical to Fig. 15.4c, but the labeling of the different elements of clusters A and B has been omitted. We can

no longer discern two different clusters, and it is clear that unsupervised clustering techniques will also not be able to find a meaningful solution.

Of course, when there is too much overlap between clusters, an unsupervised learning program is no longer able to discern two different clusters, let alone to allocate patients to either one of the clusters. Only supervised learning may then result in a model that classifies at least some of the elements of categories A and B correctly. Chapter 27 discusses different clustering techniques (e.g., nearest-neighbor methods) and provides additional examples of unsupervised learning.

4 Decision-Support Models

The preceding section addressed the most crucial issue in all medical decision making: feature selection. It also briefly described how computers may classify patients with different diseases into different disease categories, which is the next step in developing decision models: "learning" by computers. In this section we introduce different diagnostic decision strategies that may be followed once we know what features to use. In general, the more knowledge we have about patients, symptoms, and the occurrence of diseases in the population, the better decision models we are able to develop.

Diagnostic decision making bears many resemblances to detecting some event amidst a background of other events. The more difficult it is to detect the event or to diagnose the disease, the more effort we must make to

find or diagnose it. For instance, if in a primary care practice some disease seldom occurs, it will be very difficult for the clinician to make the correct diagnosis. For instance, a tropical disease occurs much less frequently in a northern country than in tropical areas: its *prior probability* or *prevalence* is low. Making the correct diagnosis is even more difficult if identical symptoms are also seen in more common diseases. A similar problem in medical decision making is when we deal with "adjacent" diseases that all show more or less similar symptoms, but each of which has a different prognosis or therapy.

Decision-support models in health care can be grouped into different categories (see Fig. 15.5). The main categories are the *quantitative* and the *qualitative* decision-support models:

15

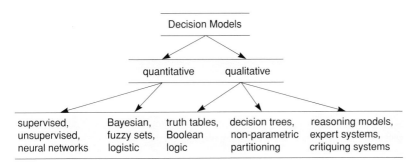

Figure 15.5
Decision-support models in health care can be grouped into different categories. The main categories are the quantitative (statistical) and the qualitative (heuristic) decision-support models, which can also be further split into subcategories.

- The first, quantitative, category is often based on well-defined statistical methods and makes use of training sets of patient data (see Section 3 above); features are primarily selected by using statistical methods and assessing their discriminatory powers. Prior probabilities for the occurrence of diseases are generally incorporated into the statistical models, such as in Bayes' rule (see Section 4.1.5 below).
- The qualitative category uses features that are generally proposed by experts and that are based on clinical studies. The decision-support methods in the qualitative category generally use symbolic reasoning methods, such as "*logical deduction*" which may be best understood in terms of *Boolean logic* (also called combinatorial logic or *symbolic logic*; see Chapter 24). Knowledge-based systems typically are based on qualitative, symbolic reasoning methods.

Combinations of quantitative and qualitative methods are also used to build decision-support models. For example, *Bayesian networks* impose probabilistic models that quantify the strengths of relationships among particular events; in turn, those events may appear in a model that defines particular states of the world and that uses either quantitative (e.g., probabilistic) or qualitative (e.g., symbolic logic) reasoning methods. The models must be properly validated by a test set to ensure the accuracy of their results and to assess their limitations.

4.1 Quantitative Decision-Support Methods

Statistical methods are generally used to test the *probability* of the occurrence of some event (see also Chapter 24). Similarly, statistics are used in a decision-support method to assess the probability of occurrence of a disease. For instance, statistical techniques are used to test whether the probability for "normal" or "healthy" is higher than that for "disease," or whether in *differential diagnoses* the occurrence of disease A is more probable than the occurrence of disease B. In *statistical decision making*, all features (signs, symptoms, measurements, etc.) are generally used *simultaneously*. It should be noted that statistical methods, too, still assume an underlying qualitative model of features and classifications. Before looking at how to use several features simultaneously, we first give a simple example of how to discriminate between healthy and pathological using one feature only. The example is used to illustrate the effect of changing the level of a decision *threshold* and how to assess a decision-support method.

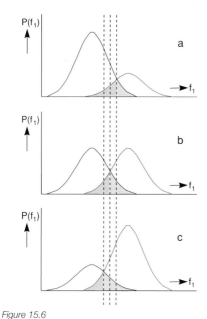

Figure 15.6
Distributions of systolic blood pressures of hypertensive and nonhypertensive people for two hypothetical populations. Distributions for people in a population survey (a), people in primary care (b), and people who visit a cardiac clinic (c) are presented. For all three populations, the two distributions for hypertensive and healthy people show considerable overlap. Decision thresholds are indicated for all three populations. It can be seen that the choice of the decision thresholds is different for each population (indicated by the shaded areas).

4.1.1 One Feature: Single Decision Threshold

Assume we want to discriminate between people with and without hypertension. To do so, we collect the blood pressures of subjects in three different hypothetical populations (see Fig. 15.6):

15

a. a healthy population screened for respiratory or cardiac diseases,

b. a population of patients in primary care who visit their general practitioner for minor complaints, and

c. a population of patients who visit the outpatient clinic of a department of cardiology.

For all people in the three populations it is known whether they have hypertension. The "true" diagnosis of hypertension is ideally determined by taking several systolic and diastolic blood pressure measurements at different times spanning a period of weeks. However, in this example and for the sake of simplicity, we want to use only one systolic blood pressure measurement per subject, although one such measurement is in most instances not enough to make a definite diagnosis of hypertension. This may be caused by a falsely elevated blood pressure due to measurement errors or factors that may raise the patient's blood pressure physiologically (e.g., by stress).

The distributions of the systolic blood pressures of hypertensive and nonhypertensive people for each of the hypothetical populations are presented in Fig. 15.6. For all three populations, the two distributions for hypertensive and healthy people show considerable overlap. Besides, we observe that in the healthy population being screened the distribution of people without hypertension is much larger than that of people with hypertension, that the distributions are about equal in the primary care population, and that in the cardiology population the distribution of healthy people is lower than that of the hypertensive population. Apparently, there are many more people *without* hypertension than

with hypertension in the healthy population being screened, and the reverse applies to the cardiology population. We also see that the mean values and the variances of the nonhypertensive distributions are identical for all three populations. The same applies to the hypertensive populations. (In reality, this is not necessarily so, because hypertensive patients who visit the cardiology clinic could have a more advanced stage of hypertension, and furthermore, the age distributions in all three populations will probably also be different.)

If we were requested to discern between people with hypertension and people without hypertension with the help of some decision model with only one feature (the systolic blood pressure), the easiest way would be to define a *decision threshold*, above which we decide that the person has hypertension and below which we conclude that there is no hypertension. In principle, we are free to choose the decision threshold for each population in the overlapping distributions (see Fig. 15.6, where decision thresholds have been indicated for all three situations). Whatever decision threshold we choose, the resulting decisions would not be error-free. In general, four possible decisions and two types of errors are made (see also Table 15.1):

1. **True positive** (*TP*)
   This is the percentage of people who have hypertension (i.e., who have positively been identified as having the disease) and for whom the decision model decides that they have hypertension. These are all cases of the distribution of hypertensive patients above the decision threshold.

2. **True negative** (*TN*)
   The percentage of people without the disease for whom the decision model has correctly made the same decision.

3. **False positive** (*FP*)
   The percentage of people without the disease, but for whom the decision model wrongly determined that they have the disease.

4. **False negative** (*FN*)
   The percentage of patients who have the disease, but for whom the decision model wrongly made the decision that they have no disease.

Table 15.1
Relationships between True Positive (TP), True Negative (TN), False Positive (FP), and False Negative (FN).

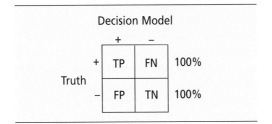

	Decision Model		
	+	−	
Truth +	TP	FN	100%
Truth −	FP	TN	100%

15

Of course, TP + FN = 100% and FP + TN = 100% (see Table 15.1). Sometimes, instead of percentages, the four parameters are expressed as fractions, that is, TP + FN = 1 and FP + TN = 1.

All decision models deal with these four situations or versions of it (see Section 4.1.3). The task of a decision model is to minimize the percentages of errors (FP and FN), given the features, the prior probabilities of the occurrence of the diseases, and the costs involved in either decision.

The effect of the choice of the decision threshold on FP and FN for the three populations is depicted in Fig. 15.6. If we want to minimize the total amount of incorrect decisions, irrespective of the costs involved in making erroneous decisions, it can be seen that the choice of the decision thresholds is different for each

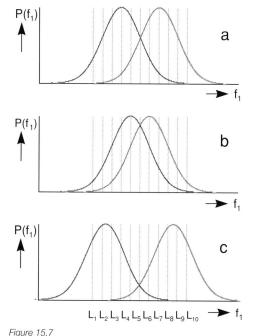

Figure 15.7

In (a) the two distributions of the primary population of Fig. 15.6b are presented, but now with 10 different decision thresholds L_1, L_2, ... L_{10}. For each of these decision thresholds the FP and FN percentages have been computed. These 10 combinations (FP, FN) have been plotted in the ROC curve (a) of Fig. 15.8. In (b) the two distributions are closer together (i.e., more overlap between the distributions) and in (c) the distributions are further apart. This is in Fig. 15.8 reflected in the ROC curves (b) and (c), respectively.

population (indicated by the shaded areas in Fig. 15.6). The effect of the choice of the decision threshold can graphically be seen in a so-called receiver operating characteristic *(ROC)* curve.

4.1.2 Receiver Operating Characteristics

In this section we want to show, by using the same example presented above, that the percentages of FP and FN decisions cannot be minimized independently. In Fig. 15.7a we have therefore taken the two distributions for the primary care population again, but we have now indicated 10 different decision thresholds, thresholds L_1, L_2, ... L_{10}. For each of these decision thresholds the FP and FN percentages have been computed. These 10 combinations (FP, FN) have been plotted in curve a in Fig. 15.8, with FP along the one axis and FN along the other axis. As can be seen from the curve connecting the points, there is a relationship between FP and FN, determined by the two distributions: if FP decreases, FN increases, and vice versa. This graphical representation is called an *ROC curve*. It teaches us that FP and FN cannot be minimized independently. In this example, the ideal point (FP, FN) = (0, 0) cannot be reached.

To show the effect of more or less overlap of the two distributions, we have depicted in curves b and c of Fig. 15.8 the same two hypothetical distributions for hypertensive and healthy subjects in the primary care population, but we have shifted them closer to each other and farther apart, respectively. The effect of more overlapping distributions is seen in ROC curve b in Fig. 15.8, and the effect of less overlap is seen in curve c of Fig. 15.8. The less the distributions overlap, the better the ROC approaches the ideal point of (FP, FN) = (0, 0); the more the distributions overlap, however, the more the ROC approaches the diagonal line that runs from the point (FP, FN) = (100, 0) to the point (FP, FN) = (0, 100). The example shows that the performance of any decision model is primarily determined by the discriminatory power of the features. If features show too much overlap, a different decision threshold does not help. This not only applies to models that operate on one feature but also applies to models that use several features at a time. Therefore, as remarked earlier, the principal task in

15

developing a decision model with an optimal performance is finding the most discriminatory features.

4.1.3   Performance of Decision Models

It has been made clear that the performance of a diagnostic decision-support method should be expressed
by at least two numbers: FP and FN (or their comple-
ments TN and TP, respectively). Preferably, the performance of a decision model should be presented by its
entire ROC curve. In practice, however, we generally
have only two parameters (e.g., FP and FN) for a two-
group decision model (disease A versus disease B or
healthy versus abnormal). The most usual way to
express performance, then, is by a *2 x 2 matrix* (or, in
general, an n x n or an n x m matrix), which is, in fact,
a matrix like that shown in Table 15.1. In Table 15.2
we have rewritten this matrix in a more general form,
and referring to Table 15.2, we now give some further
definitions by which the performance of decision
methods is often expressed:

- The fraction TP = $a/(a + b)$ is the **sensitivity**
- The fraction TN = $d/(c + d)$ is the **specificity**
- The fraction $a/(a + c)$ is the **positive predictive
  value**; and
- The fraction $d/(b + d)$ is the **negative predictive
  value**.

Other well-known parameters can also be expressed in
the numbers *a*, *b*, *c*, and *d*, such as:

Table 15.2
Illustration of Sensitivity, Specificity, and Predictive Value (see
text).

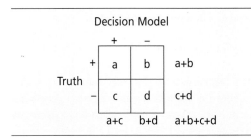

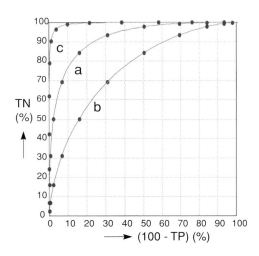

Figure 15.8
ROC curves of the populations of Fig. 15.7, with FP along one
axis and FN (or 1-TP) along the other axis. (See legends of
Fig. 15.7.)

- The *prevalence* of a disease, which is the fraction of
  diseased people in the total population, or
  $(a + b)/(a + b + c + d)$.

Sometimes, the **total performance** *T* of a diagnostic
decision-support method is expressed as the total of
the correct decisions divided by the total number of
decisions, for instance:

$$T = (a + d)/(a + b + c + d). \tag{1}$$

In some instances, total performance *T* is expressed by
the mean of the sum of the fractions TN and TP:

$$T = (TP + TN)/2. \tag{2}$$

This measure runs from 0 to 1. Another measure for
total performance is, for example:

$$T = TP + TN - 1, \tag{3}$$

which runs from -1 to +1. Around the value of *T* equal
to zero, there is hardly any discrimination. We repeat
that the performance of a diagnostic method cannot be
expressed by one number only, as we have seen from

15

the discussion on ROC curves. Having the positive and negative predictive values only is not enough to gain insight into the performance of a decision-support method in any situation without knowing the prevalence of the disease.

4.1.4 Cost and Risks

As discussed in Section 4.1.2, an ROC curve is determined by the distributions of the features and not by the choice of the decision thresholds. The better the features discriminate, the better the method's performance. The specific point that we choose on a given ROC curve does not alter the performance of the method as such. The choice of a certain point on the ROC curve is, as we have seen in the example of the preceding section, related one-to-one with the choice of the location of the decision threshold and, thus, with the choice of some combination of FP and FN. In fact, the three pairs of distributions of the three populations discussed in Fig. 15.6 yield the same ROC curve, but the choice of the thresholds results in three different points on the ROC curve of Fig 15.8 (curve a). Apparently, the choice of such a point is dependent on considerations other than the selection of features and is primarily determined by the *prior probabilities* of the occurrence of diseases in the population, but also by costs and utilities that are the consequence of the choice.

For instance, during population screening finding too many patients with a FP test result for hypertension (a decision threshold which is too low) would possibly result in costs of follow-up examinations that are too high, but too many FN results would make screening senseless. In patient *monitoring*, generating too many false alarms (too many FPs) would lead to less attention from nurses to correct positive alarms. In short, the specific choice of a specific decision threshold depends on:

1. the prior probability of the disease (or the event),
2. the costs involved in FP and FN decisions, and
3. the benefits or *utilities* of making correct decisions.

Costs and utilities are further discussed in Chapter 18. The effect of prior or conditional probabilities on the

probability that a disease is diagnosed by the decision model is beautifully expressed by a rule that was formulated by *Bayes* in 1763.

4.1.5 Bayes' Rule

In describing the **Rule of Bayes**, we use again the simple example of having to discriminate between disease (D) and normal (N). We assume that we know the prevalence of the disease in the population, that is, $(a + b)/(a + b + c + d)$ in Section 4.1.3. This is also called the **prior probability** $p(D)$ of the occurrence of the disease in the population. In our case the prior probability for normal is $p(N)$, with $p(D) + p(N) = 1$. For instance, for the primary care population used for Fig. 15.6, the two prior probabilities were about equal, whereas for the screening population $p(N) > p(D)$ and for the clinical population $p(N) > p(D)$.

In statistical decision-support models, we want to compute the **posterior probability** of the occurrence of the disease on the basis of knowledge of prior probabilities and symptoms S (i.e., the features). This can be expressed by the conditional probability:

$$p(D|S), \tag{4}$$

which is the posterior probability of having the disease D given the symptoms S.

Assume, for instance, that a disease occurs very seldom, for example, with $p(D) = 0.0001$ (1 person in 10,000 has the disease), and that we would like to trace all people who have the disease by population screening. So, if we screened, say, 1 million people, then only 100 would have the disease. In this situation it is tempting not to use any symptoms at all and to say on the basis of the very low prior probability $p(D)$ that nobody has the disease, because this would involve no screening cost at all. The decision method can then be expressed by a very simple formula:

$$p(N) = 1 \text{ and } p(D) = 0. \tag{5}$$

The performance of this "decision-support model" expressed as the total number of correct decisions is impressive: 999,900 of the 1 million decisions are correctly diagnosed. This gives for $T = (a + d)/(a + b + c +$

PANEL 15.2

Bayes' Rule

Before giving an example of Bayes' Rule, a proof of the formula is given.

For sake of simplicity, we assume that disease D is either absent or present. In other words, D indicates that the disease is present, $'D$ indicates that the disease is absent:

$$p(D) + p('D) = 1 \qquad (1)$$

The probability of having D depends on the presence of symptoms. The probability that a patient has symptom S is $p(S)$. The conditional probability that a patient with symptom S has D is $p(D|S)$. The probability that a person has both D and S, therefore, is:

$$p(D \text{ AND } S) = p(S)\, p(D|S). \qquad (2)$$

The same holds for the conditional probability that a patient with symptom S has disease D:

$$p(S \text{ AND } D) = p(D)\, p(S|D), \qquad (3)$$
with $p(D \text{ AND } S) = p(S \text{ AND } D)$

The conditional probability $p(D|S)$ that a patient with symptom S has disease D is what we want to know from diagnostic practice. The conditional probability $p(S|D)$ that patients with disease D have a specific symptom S, and the incidences of diseases, $p(D)$, and of symptoms, $p(S)$, is knowledge that we obtain from clinical experience and epidemiology.

We will now prove that the first probability, $p(D|S)$, can be derived from the latter, $p(S|D)$, with knowledge of the prior probabilities $p(D)$ and $p(S)$.

From Equation 2 we derive:

$$p(D|S) = p(D \text{ AND } S) / p(S). \qquad (4)$$

Combining Equations 4 and 3 yields:

$$p(D|S) = p(S|D)\, p(D) / p(S) \qquad (5)$$

In practice, it is easier to acquire $p(S|'D)$ than $p(S)$.

Therefore, we show that $p(S)$ can be derived from $p(S|'D)$ in case $p(S|D)$ and $p(D)$ are known:

$$p(S) = p(S \text{ AND } D) + p(S \text{ AND } 'D) \qquad (6)$$

Substitution of Equations 2 and 3 in Equation 6 gives:

$$p(S) = p(S|D)\, p(D) + p(S|'D)\, p('D) \qquad (7)$$

Note that $p(D) + p('D) = 1$. By substituting Equation 7 in Equation 5 we find:

$$p(D|S) = p(S|D)\, p(D) / \{p(S|D)\, p(D) + p(S|'D)\, p('D)\} \qquad (8)$$

This is Bayes' Rule or Formula.

Bayes' Rule can also be extended to diagnose multiple diseases, but in that case much more knowledge on occurrences of combinations of diseases and symptoms is needed. In practice, the resulting complexity is reduced by assuming that the occurrence of some disease is independent of the presence of any other disease. The same problem holds for multiple symptoms. Note, however, that the assumption of independence between diseases and between symptoms is only a first estimation. Therefore, in principle Bayes' Rule can be used for a *differential diagnosis* (DD), but then the diseases should be considered to be independent of each other. As a result, for a DD with K diseases D_k $(k = 1, \dots K)$ the following holds:

$$\Sigma_k\, p(D_k) = 1 \qquad (9)$$

Analogous to Equation 7 we can write:

$$p(S) = \Sigma_k\, p(S|D_k)\, p(D_k) \qquad (10)$$

Substituting Equation 10 in Equation 5 we can conclude for disease D_j:

$$p(D_j|S) = p(S|D_j)\, p(S) / \Sigma_k\, p(S|D_k)\, p(D_k) \qquad (11)$$

An example of the use of a version of Bayes' Rule is given in Panel 16.1 of Chapter 16 for the diagnosis of lung diseases by using QMR.

15

d) of Section 4.1.3: $T = 0.9999$. However, although the fraction TN would be 100% (no errors are made), the fraction TP is 0% (all decisions are wrongly FN), resulting in a point at the far end of an ROC curve. This result is very disappointing, which means that by using the prior probabilities of the disease only, we have a bad performance of our decision-support method, although at no cost.

The only way to improve the performance of the diagnostic method is to use not only knowledge about the *occurrence* of the disease but also knowledge about the *symptoms* of the disease. This may, in some instances, result in considerable costs to trace only 100 in 1 million people if the symptoms show much resemblance to symptoms of other diseases or when expensive diagnostic techniques must be applied. This might be a reason to apply no population screening at all.

The *Rule of Bayes* allows us to compute the posterior probability $p(D|S)$ of a disease D, given its prior probability $p(D)$ and knowledge about the conditional probability $p(S|D)$ that symptoms occur in a given disease. In Panel 15.2, Bayes' Rule is derived for the case of either having a disease (D) or being healthy or normal (N). This yields Bayes' Rule for normal versus disease:

$$p(D|S) = \frac{p(D|S)}{p(S|D)p(D) + p(S|N)p(N)} \, p(D). \qquad (6)$$

4.1.6 Multiple Features

Thus far, in Sections 4.1.1 to 4.1.5, we have used examples with one feature or symptom for diagnostic decision problems of two disease categories only. However, the statistical methods that we apply can, in principle, be extended to multiple features and more disease categories. We discussed earlier in this chapter the issue of supervised and unsupervised learning (Sections 2.2 and 2.3) and, therefore, we return to the example sketched in Fig. 15.4, which is essentially a two-dimensional (2-D) illustration of a two-class decision problem.

Similar to the one-dimensional decision problem, where we applied decision thresholds along the feature axis, we can follow the same strategy for two features, usually characterized as a 2-D classification space. In Fig. 15.4a to c we have depicted 2-D decision thresholds (lines) that best separate one class from the other. A typical rule to decide whether some disease is present can, for instance, be expressed by the formula for a straight line in a 2-D *feature space*

$$W_{2\text{-}D} = w_1(f_1 - m_1) + w_2(f_2 - m_2), \qquad (7)$$

in which W is a weighted sum of features with f_1 and f_2 the measured features, m_1 and m_2 their respective mean values, and the values w_1 and w_2 the respective weighting factors. We decide that the disease is present if $W_{2\text{-}D}$ is larger than some threshold value w_0. If we deal with N features f_n ($n = 1, 2, \ldots N$), the formula becomes a hyperplane in an N-dimensional (N-D) feature space:

$$W_{N\text{-}D} = w_1(f_1 - m_1) + w_2(f_2 - m_2) + \ldots + w_N(f_N - m_N), \qquad (8)$$

in which m_n's are mean values and w_n's are weighting factors. We may decide that disease D is present when W (the weighted sum) is larger than some threshold w_0 and that D is absent otherwise. Equation 8 is a very simple form for uncorrelated features. However, when the features are correlated, we use more complex formulas, of which a few are described in Section 3 of Chapter 27.

Also here, the fractions FP and FN can be computed, and when we shift the decision line parallel to the line $W_{2\text{-}D}$ presented in the *scattergrams* of Fig. 15.4, we can compute for the 2-D decision problem ROC curves as well; the same reasoning that we discussed for the one-dimensional case also applies in two or more dimensions. When we do not obtain a decision model with a performance that is high enough, more features can be added, starting with the best-discriminating feature, until no further discrimination is obtained. For the learning set the performance of a diagnostic decision model increases monotonically; for reasons not discussed here, this is not always the case for the test set.

4.1.7 Multiple Diseases

When we deal with more than two diseases that are to be diagnosed, the same rules used for the two-class

15

single-feature decision problem also apply. The only points are that the decision models become more complex and that neither a single pair of performance measures (FP, FN) nor a single ROC curve is sufficient. Sometimes, a way out is to reduce all decisions to two-class decision problems. For instance, if we want to discriminate between diseases A, B, and C, we could test A versus B, A versus C, and B versus C. This is not practical, because after the binary decisions, we need to find a way to decide which one of the three decisions delivers the final decision. Therefore, in statistical methods, we preferably want to develop a method that ranks all diseases according to their probability of being present in a patient. The outcome of this testing can be expressed in a K x L matrix, where K is the number of diseases to be discriminated and L the number of "true" diseases that are present. An example of such a K x L matrix is given in Table 15.3 for the discrimination of

cardiac diseases that can be diagnosed when analyzing ECGs.

4.2 Qualitative Decision-Support Methods

The methods described in the preceding section all have a formal, mathematical basis. Qualitative methods, which may be inspired by or which are perceptions of human reasoning, typically are less formal. Sometimes, people use the expression **heuristic method** to describe problem-solving approaches that perform deductions on symbolic models using logical operations, such as when a decision-support system uses **rule-based** reasoning to conclude a diagnosis based on a case model. However, not all logical deductions performed by knowledge-based systems truly reflect heuristics (i.e., informal rules

Table 15.3
Example of a K x L Matrix for Interpretation Programs of ECGs as discussed in Panel 15.4.

Combined Program Results[a]

Class	N	NL	LVH	RVH	BVH	AMI	IMI	MIX	OTH	VH+MI
NL	382	95.5	0.9	o.4	0.0	1.4	1.6	0.0	0.1	0.0
LVH	183	19.0	69.0	0.5	0.0	4.3	6.9	0.2	0.0	0.0
RVH	55	40.6	6.7	45.8	2.7	1.2	2.1	0.0	0.9	0.0
BVH	53	22.0	54.7	14.5	1.6	5.3	1.9	0.0	0.0	0.0
AMI	170	14.3	2.6	0.6	0.0	80.0	1.8	0.7	0.0	0.0
IMI	273	19.8	2.6	0.2	0.0	0.7	76.7	0.1	0.0	0.0
MIX	73	2.5	4.1	1.6	0.0	51.6	37.4	2.7	0.0	0.0
VH+MI	31	22.6	0.0	0.0	0.0	0.0	0.0	0.0	16.1	61.3

[a] Results of the CSE assessment study (Willems JL, Abreu-Lima C, Arnaud P, van Bemmel JH et al. The diagnostic performance of computer programs for the interpretation of electrocardiograms. New Engl J Med 1991;325:1767-73). Class: true classification; N: number of patient cases in the study; NL: Normal, LVH: left ventricular hypertrophy, RVH: right ventricular hypertrophy, BVH: biventricular hypertrophy, AMI: anterior myocardial infarction, IMI: inferior myocardial infarction, MIX: combined AMI and IMI, OTH: other diagnostic categories, VH+MI: combined ventricular hypertrophy and myocardial infarction.

of thumb). Much of what is represented in a knowledge-based system may be definitional or structural rather than heuristic in nature. Thus, more general terms such as *symbolic method* or *qualitative method* are preferred to the term *heuristic method*.

Symbolic methods may be composed of elementary decision units that, in principle, do not differ from the two-class, single-feature statistical decision problem discussed in Section 4.1 above (see also the discussion of medical logic modules in Section 4.2.2 of Chapter 16) . These elementary decisions test whether some symptom is present or a measurement is larger than some threshold value. In rule-based decision-support methods, the result of such a test, whether some feature value x is larger than a threshold L or whether a symptom is present, can be represented by a Boolean (logical) expression E. The logical value of E can be either TRUE or FALSE (see Chapter 23). For instance, the expression

$$E = "x > L" \qquad (9)$$

is TRUE if the value of the feature x is larger than the threshold L and FALSE otherwise. Some other expression E could be:

$$E = \text{"symptom } S \text{ is present,"} \qquad (10)$$

which is TRUE if the symptom S is present and FALSE otherwise. The expression E, however, can also be more complex and can even form a composed expression involving several symptoms or features and thresholds. Many examples of complex expressions E can be found in health care. An example is the formalism used in the so-called *Minnesota code*. This code is used to classify ECGs in different disease categories and is mainly intended for population screening. The Minnesota code is a mixture of a truth table and a flowchart, with many microdecisions incorporated in sometimes lengthy expressions. An example of Equation 10 in the Minnesota code is:

$$E = \text{"Q/R amplitude ratio} > 1/3 \text{ AND } Q \text{ duration} \\ > 0.03 \text{ s in lead I or V6."} \qquad (11)$$

The value of E can be used to start some other elementary decision unit or to take some action. Therefore, the

most general expression in heuristic reasoning is:

$$\text{IF } E \text{ THEN } [action \ 1] \text{ ELSE } [action \ 2]. \qquad (12)$$

A *logical expression* E can be a simple statement, such as the one in Equation 10, or a more complex one, as in Equation 11; the [*action*] can be either a next or a final decision, or it can be, for example, a request for another test or a different examination. An example of a concrete expression for monitoring potassium levels is given in Panel 16.2 of Chapter 16.

The *sequence* of microdecisions, as in Equation 12, is dependent on knowledge of the disease process, on steps to be taken in the decision-making process, and on the goals of the decision-making process. Generally, three different strategies are followed when making heuristic decisions with computers:

1. use all microdecisions simultaneously (*decision tables* or *truth tables*),
2. use the microdecisions sequentially (*flowcharts* or *decision trees*), and
3. use the microdecisions expressed in situation-action rules (*rule-based* or *qualitative reasoning*).

Below we give examples of all three methods.

4.2.1 Decision Tables

A truth table (more extensively discussed in Chapter 23) takes all logical expressions E_k of the types in Equation 9, 10, or 12 into account at once. A general form of a truth table is:

$$D = E \{E_1, E_2, \ldots E_K\} \qquad (13)$$

A concrete example of a truth table is borrowed from a decision-support method for the classification of some arrhythmias, which uses logical expressions on the presence of waveshapes and the length of *RR intervals* in ECGs. Table 15.4 lists the various logical expressions, and Table 15.5 gives the truth table. The combination of all E_i's in rules 1 to 9 of Table 15.5 consists of the knowledge about the diagnosis of arrhythmias. In principle, a diagnostic decision-support method should assess all the lines (the diagnostic rules) in the truth table (in the case of Table 15.5, all nine rules) before coming to a definite decision.

This knowledge may also be expressed in more comprehensive diagnostic logical expressions, composed of the elementary E_i's (see also Chapter 23). An example is the diagnostic expressions for **nodal rhythm** in Table 15.5, for which the diagnosis is made by rules 3 and 4, so that we may write:

$$D = E_1.E_2.'E_3.'E_5.'E_{12} + E_1.E_2.'E_3.E_5.E_7, \tag{14}$$

where the decimal point stands for the logical operator AND (or for the symbol $\cap$, used in predicate logic), the plus sign stands for the logical operator OR (or $\cup$), and the apostrophe stands for logical negation (or $\neg$) (see Chapter 23).

The different combinations of elementary expressions E_i can also be represented graphically by **Venn diagrams** or **Karnaugh diagrams** (a version of Venn diagrams). These are discussed in Chapter 23. A way of simplifying truth tables is by trying to express the knowledge contained in them by *logical expressions*, as shown in Equation 14. Boolean-algebraic rules may also assist in simplifying complex formulas (this can be done by applying **De Morgan's rules**, see Chapter 23). By applying simple **Boolean algebra** we may write for Equation 14:

$$D = E_1.E_2.'E_3.('E_5.'E_{12} + E_5.E_7). \tag{15}$$

As may be seen from this example, truth tables can easily incorporate decisions on multiple diseases. However, optimization of a truth table is difficult, and only validation of the truth table by an independent test may confirm an acceptable performance.

4.2.2 Flowcharts

Flowcharts use, in principle, the same microdecisions discussed in the preceding section on truth tables. The difference is, however, that more knowledge is contained in the flowchart than in the truth table, because the way that the rules are sequentially assessed is prescribed by the structure of the flowchart. The elementary decision unit of a flowchart is generally depicted as a diamond-shaped figure with one input at the top and two or more outputs at the bottom (see Fig. 15.9). The input is connected to a preceding elementary decision unit, and the outputs are TRUE and FALSE, called **binary decisions** (only one of two decisions is possible). To avoid a possible conflict with the terminology used in Decision Theory (see Chapter 18), in this chapter instead of the term **decision tree**, we use the term *flowchart*.

15

Logical Variable	Logical Expression
E_1	All RR intervals are regular
E_2	All QRS complexes are identical
E_3	QRS durations are longer than 120 msec
E_4	The heart rate is higher than 100 beats/min
E_5	P waves are present
E_6	The heart rate is lower than 40 beats /min
E_7	Negative P in II and positive P in aVR
E_8	No. of P waves / No. of QRS complexes ≤1.1
E_9	No. of P waves / No. of QRS complexes > 1.1
E_{10}	PR intervals regular
E_{11}	PR interval > 200 ms
E_{12}	P waves present in leads other than II and aVR

Table 15.4
Logical Expressions E Used as Elements in the Truth Table for Arrhythmia diagnosis in Table 15.5.

Table 15.5

Truth Table for Arrhythmia Diagnostic Statements D in Which the Logical Expressions E_i of Table 15.4 are Used as Elements for Arrhythmia Diagnosis (after Wartak[a])

rule	E_1	E_2	E_3	E_4	E_5	E_6	E_7	E_8	E_9	E_{10}	E_{11}	E_{12}	Diagnostic expressions D
1	T	T	T	T	F	d	d	d	d	d	d	d	Ventricular tachycardia
2	T	T	T	F	d	T	d	d	d	d	d	d	Idioventricular rhythm
3	T	T	F	d	F	d	d	d	d	d	d	F	Nodal rhythm
4	T	T	F	d	T	d	T	d	d	d	d	d	Nodal rhythm
5	T	T	F	d	T	d	F	T	d	d	d	d	First-degree AV block
6	T	T	F	d	T	d	F	T	d	F	d	d	Wandering pacemaker or Wenckebach or AV dissociation
7	T	T	F	d	T	d	F	F	T	d	d	d	Second-degree AV block
8	T	T	F	d	T	d	F	F	F	d	d	d	Third-degree AV block
9	T	T	d	d	T	F	F	F	T	F	T	F	d	Sinus rhythm

[a] Wartak J. Computer program for pattern recognition of ECGs. Comp Biomed Res 1970;3:344-74.
T stands for TRUE, F stands for FALSE and d stands for "don't care."

15

A flowchart can be considered a decision tree that is upside down, with the root at the top and the branches and the leaves stretching downward. The locations where the microdecisions are made are called the *nodes* of the tree. The tree is crossed on a path from the *root* to one of the end **leaves** where the processing stops with, it is hoped, a correct decision. At the end leaves, similar to the rule expressed in Equation 12, actions take place, such as starting some activity or going to some other flowchart. Flowcharts in decision-support systems bear resemblance to flowcharts in computer programming. Figure 15.9 gives an example of a flowchart, based on the same elementary decisions and logical expressions presented in Table 15.4. The advantage of a flowchart is that it is very efficiently processed (not all combinations of input data must be assessed as in truth tables), but the disadvantage is that the decision-making process is very rigid; once we are on a wrong path in the tree, no return is possible, unless parallel trees are used. Therefore, even more

than for a truth table, a flowchart should be tested extensively before it is applied in practice. A further disadvantage of logically based methods is that training of these decision-support models is difficult. Mathematical formalisms, such as those used for statistical models, do not exist for truth tables and flowcharts.

For flowcharts, there is, however, one method that may assist in building a tree with the help of a learning set, based on user-selected features. This method is called a nonparametric partitioning algorithm (NPPA), and it follows more or less a similar strategy as feature ranking according to the discriminatory power of the features. One well-known NPPA method is the Classification and Regression Trees (*CART*) technique. The NPPA searches for the most discriminating feature and then starts building the first microdecision node at the root of the tree. Then it looks for the next discriminating feature at each of the branches of the first decision node and so forth until all cases in the learning set have been correctly classified. Such a tree is usually far too large to be used in practice, so it must be "pruned;" that is, some of the end branches must be cut off and the user allows for some FP and FN cases. In contrast to statistical classification, one cannot prove that the resulting tree is the best one for the decision problem at hand; its performance should therefore also be assessed by an independent test set.

A diagnostic cycle can also be put in a flowchart. Panel 15.3 presents a flowchart for a general diagnostic process. This process is frequently observed when complex patient cases are reviewed. For instance, **QMR** can be used to implement such a process (see Chapter 16, Section 2.4).

4.2.3 Rule-Based Reasoning

In the preceding two sections we have discussed logical decision-support methods in which the microdecisions were built either into the diagnostic expressions of the truth table or into the nodes of the flowchart. Once changes need to be made in those decision models, for example, when new insight becomes available, in principle the entire method should be scrutinized for changes in the microdecisions. This is why attempts have been made to unbundle the knowledge contained in the microdecisions of the type of the rule in Equation 12 from the structure of the decision model itself. In theory, this modularization makes it far easier to make additions to and changes in the decision method, but in practice it is often a significant problem when the organizing framework that clarifies the relationships among the individual decision units is effectively thrown away (see Chapter 28). Methods in which this unbundling has been realized are known under the name "**rule-based systems**."

The rules in which the knowledge of the type in Equation 12 is contained, form a **knowledge base**, which is similar to a database, but in this case not containing mere data but, rather, logical sentences that describe how possible situations defined by the data for a given case relate to possible conclusions that might be reached about the implications of those data. The microdecisions that were expressed in Equation 14 can also be rewritten as two rules of the type in Equation 12:

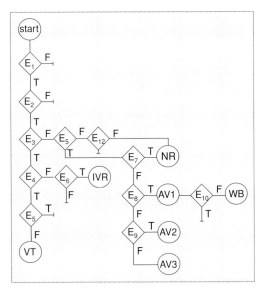

Figure 15.9
Example of a flowchart in the form of a computer program, based on similar elementary decisions and logical expressions as used in Table 15.4.

IF $\{E_1.E_2.'E_3.'E_5.'E_{12}\}$ THEN nodal rhythm or
IF $(E_1.E_2.'E_3.E_5.E_7)$ THEN nodal rhythm,

or as one larger rule based on Equation 15:

IF $\{E_1.E_2.'E_3.('E_5.'E_{12} + E_5.E_7)\}$ THEN nodal rhythm.

Needless to say that here, too, the microdecisions must be firmly based on experience and insight and should be verifiable from a documented database of patient data and the literature. However, it is not always possible to do this (see Chapter 17).

The concept behind heuristic reasoning is that when we possess on the one hand a *patient database* and on the other hand a *knowledge base*, it should be possible to reason about the two and come to a conclusion, originally thought to be similar to what happens in the brain of a trained clinician. (However, essentially we do not know how reasoning is done in the human brain; see Panel 15.1.) Therefore, for this "reasoning" we need a procedure adaptive enough to operate on different patient databases and with different knowledge

15

Flowchart of a Diagnostic Process[1]

Step	Explanation	Examples and Remarks
1	A physician can work only with a limited set of data. Therefore, elementary signs and symptoms are aggregated, that is, combined into "problem groups" (see Section 4.1 of Chapter 7). If clinicians are asked to summarize the case after primary examination, the summary reveals a list of problems (the existence of which can be uncertain).	The following are aggregated to the problem diabetes insipidus: – extreme polyuria – nocturia – polydipsia – urinary specific gravity below 1.003 *Mechanisms of aggregation are recognition and anatomical or pathophysiological association.*
2	Selection of one or two findings as a pivot with the objective of focusing on explaining this pivot.	What can explain the patient's unconsciousness? What can explain his/her acute abdominal pain? *Severity, frequency, and evoking strength (see Chapter 16, Section 2.4) of findings play an important role in choosing a pivot.*
3	A list of diseases that could have caused the pivot is compiled. Compiling the list of possible diseases causing a single symptom is a relatively simple task.	A coin lesion on an X-ray film may be explained by trauma, congenital lesion, malignant or benign tumor, area of infarction or infection.
4	Diseases on the cause list are measured against the findings of the case. So, most of the possible causes of pivot finding can be ruled out, because other findings serve as evidence against it. If the likelihood of a disease falls below some threshold, it is rejected.	Congenital lesions are ruled out on the basis of the history and normal X-ray films in the past. *After ruling out diseases, a differential diagnosis (DD) arises. A DD often is ordered by combining likelihood and prognosis. Panel 16.1 describes supportive QMR functions.*
5	Usually at this point additional tests or procedures are ordered to differentiate between the remaining diseases. Diseases can be compared pairwise in their ability to explain the findings.	The enlarged lymph nodes and spleen suggest the diagnosis of lymphoma and not leukemia. *At this point, often specific and more expensive diagnostic tests are considered to verify or differentiate the diagnosis.*
6	Now the final diagnosis is considered closer: can it explain all the findings of the case? If not, the entire process must be repeated to eventually explain all signs and symptoms.	Lack of abdominal pain by no means excludes the possibility of a dissecting aneurysm. The importance is that asymptomatic dissection does occur.

[1]*After Eddy DM, Clanton CH. The art of diagnosis: solving the clinicopathological exercise. N Engl J Med 1982;306:1263-8.*

bases. This method is called an **inference mechanism** (see Fig. 15.10 for an illustration of the elements required for heuristic reasoning). For inferencing, different strategies exist. These are generally known as **forward reasoning** and **backward reasoning**. In both of these strategies, data on the case about which the system is reasoning cause the inference mechanism to select one or more rules from the knowledge base that can reason about those data; execution of those rules may lead the inference mechanism either to ask the user for more case data or to call up one or more additional rules automatically. Because the inference mechanism causes rules to be invoked one after another, we often refer to the rules in the knowledge base as **production rules**, *because* they "produce" chains of reasoning during problem solving.

We now discuss forward and backward reasoning in more detail.

- Forward reasoning

In *forward reasoning* we start with the *data* selected from the patient database and check in the knowledge base whether there are any production rules that can use the data to make inferences. If so, these rules are executed. The conclusions from these inferences are added to the data set, and then other rules may be triggered if the latter rules depend on the new data that have just been concluded. Therefore, forward reasoning is also called **data-driven reasoning**.

Once no more rules are invoked by the primary data set or by the conclusions from the inferencing process, the program stops. When building decision-support systems that report to clinicians abnormal patient conditions, developers often use forward reasoning to infer clinical abstractions of the primary data to be able to generate sensible reports for the responsible person. For example, a pair of rules in the **Arden syntax** (see Panel 16.2) might include one rule that is triggered if a patient's serum potassium level is below 3.0, placing a flag in the patient database indicating that hypokalemia has been

detected; a second rule, which might be triggered when the notation of hypokalemia is placed in the database, could infer the appropriate hospital staff member to whom a report of hypokalemia should be sent.

- Backward reasoning

In *backward reasoning*, the inference mechanism selects *rules* from the knowledge base and checks whether data are available in the patient database for inferencing. The inference mechanism actually starts with a single rule (the *goal rule*) and then attempts to determine whether the goal rule is true by evaluating each of the premises of the goal rule in light of data known about the case that the rule-based system is analyzing. If there are no case data that suggest whether a given goal rule premise is true, then the backward reasoner determines whether there are any rules in the knowledge base that, if one of these rules were true, would allow the system to conclude that the particular premise of the goal rule also is true. If such rules that might be helpful are available, the system then uses case data to determine whether any of these rules is true. Of course, establishing the truth value of one of these other rules may require the inference mechanism to consider yet other rules in the knowledge base and even more data about the case being evaluated. This **goal-driven reasoning** continues recursively until either the goal rule is proven to be false or until all the premises of the goal rule are known to be true. At any time during the inference process, if not enough data are known, the user may be asked by the backward reasoner to provide more data, if possible. As a consequence of attempting to prove the truth value of the goal rule, the backward reasoner will have invoked many other rules that will have inferred many other conclusions about the case at hand. These conclusions collectively provide answers for the decision problem under consideration.

Some reasoning mechanisms combine both forward and backward reasoning. When we have few data, it is better to start with the data first, because those data can trigger selectively the corresponding rules in the knowledge base. When there are many data about the case at hand, we do not want to trigger a myriad of production rules in a forward-chaining manner; in these settings backward reasoning is much more efficient.

15

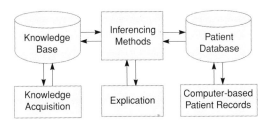

Figure 15.10

Representation of the elements involved in heuristic reasoning. For inferencing, different strategies can be used: forward reasoning and backward reasoning.

4.2.4 Other Elements of Symbolic Reasoning

Although rule-based representations are extremely popular for implementing qualitative approaches to decision support, they are by no means the only ones. For example, since the 1960s, workers in artificial intelligence have experimented with the use of structures known as *semantic networks* and *frames* as a means of representing knowledge.

In frame representations, knowledge is construed as a set of concepts in which each concept has a number of attributes that may take on particular values. For example, a frame for the concept *disease* might have attributes such as name, International Classification of Disease (*ICD*) code, body part affected, standard treatment, and so on. A simple frame for the disease pneumonia might appear as:

Concept:	disease
Name:	pneumonia
ICD code:	481
Body part affected:	lung
Standard treatment:	antibiotic

An inference mechanism known as *inheritance* allows the decision-support system to derive conclusions about certain frames that are related to each other in a hierarchical manner. For example, a frame for pulmonary tuberculosis might appear under the frame given above for pneumonia in some hierarchy. If the pulmonary tuberculosis frame did not explicitly indicate a value for body part affected, the inheritance mechanism would conclude that the value of this attribute for pulmonary tuberculosis should be the same as that for the more general concept of pneumonia, namely, lung.

4.2.5 Knowledge Structuring

As knowledge bases of rules, frames, and other representations grow in size, it becomes increasingly difficult for developers to keep track of what concepts have been represented and of the relationships among them. Considerable work in computer science concerns the development of methods that can help developers in structuring knowledge bases in ways that make them more usable. Such work is discussed in detail in Chapter 28.

4.2.6 Knowledge-Based Systems

A system in which a knowledge base, an inferencing mechanism, and a patient database are discerned is usually called a *knowledge-based system* (Fig. 15.10). In older literature, the term *expert system* is used because such systems contain knowledge from experts and may solve problems in a manner that resembles the reasoning of experts. Characteristic of the knowledge-based system is, as mentioned above, the separation of the case data, the domain knowledge, and the inferencing mechanism. Generally, a knowledge-based system assumes that there is a *knowledge acquisition program* that will be used to build and maintain the knowledge base (see Chapter 17). Knowledge-based systems may also contain an *explanation module* to help justify their recommendations for their users (see Fig. 15.10).

4.2.7 Explanation Support

When nonexperts use a decision-support system that contains expert knowledge, it may happen that the users do not fully understand why the system came to some conclusion. In general, this is one of the problems of using decision-support systems: Should users "blindly" follow the suggestions of the system, or should they still be responsible when they adopt the system's decisions? To assist users in maintaining their own responsibilities, a decision-support system should contain explanation facilities to guide the user on how it came to a specific conclusion. This explanation facility also serves to educate and train inexperienced users.

Most often, decision-support systems report recommendations directly to their users and provide additional justification for their advice via an explanation facility. Sometimes, however, users object to interactions with decision-support systems that require the computer to report to the users how to behave in a particular situation – particularly when the users already feel confident of their planned actions and when the computer may explain its reasoning in rather pedantic terms. Thus, a number of developers have experimented with the construction of *critiquing systems*, which are silent whenever the computer judges the user's planned behavior to be satisfactory given the case data, but which offer a critique of the planned behavior should the user propose to take an action that is not consistent with the decision-support system's knowledge base.

Thus, under normal circumstances, a critiquing system does not offer decision support on its own. On the contrary, the user makes the decisions first, and only under the following two circumstances may the knowledge-based system give advice:

1. Users need decision advice in a situation that is not common to them or just to verify whether their own decisions fall within an allowable range.
2. The user makes a decision that falls out of the range that is considered permissible by the experts who developed and assessed the system. In this case, the system may just alert the user or give a warning, but the system never takes over, nor does it prescribe exactly what decision the user should make.

The use of knowledge-based systems and critiquing systems is further described in Chapter 16; an example of critiquing is given in Panel 16.1.

5 Acceptance of Decision-Support Systems

The clinical support systems that were discussed in the Chapters 11 to 14 of this Handbook are, without doubt, widely accepted, and they are in clinical use almost everywhere. Decision-support systems, however, are not yet in widespread use, with only a few exceptions, and few systems are used at more than one location. Therefore, the relevant question is, what are the criteria for the acceptance of decision-support systems by clinicians? Perhaps the answer lies in the success of the clinical support systems. Several criteria that made the introduction of clinical support systems successful are described below.

- Support of **data acquisition**

Medical imaging systems are successful. They provide clinicians with data that cannot be acquired otherwise. In almost all instances, clinicians draw their diagnostic conclusions directly from the primary imaging data that are processed by computers to give them a better view.

- *Data reduction*

Other successful systems are found in areas where the data stream is too large to be comprehended by the user and so the data must be reduced, transformed, and presented in a comprehensible way. Such systems are seen in operating rooms and intensive care units. Data on organ function are collected in real time by "intelligent" instruments, digitized, stored in computers, and offered in such a way that the treating physician, the anesthetist, or the nurse is able to survey vital parameters immediately. Decision-support systems in these areas are only slowly introduced, mainly with the task of reducing the number of false alarms and increasing the reliability of the primary data that are offered to the users.

- *Data validation*

Laboratory systems are examples of systems that are in high demand when a large number of tests generate a large data stream. Blood and urine samples are analyzed fully automatically, and the results are reported by computers. The laboratory support systems take care of data validation, administration, electronic transport via networks, and computer storage (see Chapter 13). If the clinician is interested in using trends to assess the effect of treatment, the system may also offer support. Decision support is mainly used for data validation and to increase data reliability. Pharmacy systems

15

PANEL 15.4

Validation of Decision-Support Systems

There are legal and ethical reasons why a medical system should not be introduced into clinical practice unless it has been properly evaluated. That it is difficult to evaluate a decision-support system became apparent, for instance, from the early evaluation of the decision-support system *INTERNIST* in 1980. At that time, fewer than a dozen cases were used in its evaluation. The central question in all evaluation studies of medical systems is: What is the objective reference or *"gold standard"* by which the systems should be evaluated? Such objective reference material should preferably be collected in formal studies or by panels of independent experts. Ideally, the reference is material that is not biased by the study itself. However, especially in medicine, this cannot always be avoided: the mere fact that participants of a study are aware that they are taking part in an evaluation study hampers the collection of objective material. It is possible to achieve a certain degree of objectivity by using opinions from a panel or data from independent sources, such as clinical evidence from postmortem evaluations.

Most clinical support systems discussed in Chapters 12 and 13 were assessed by clinical studies. Even then, however, there might remain some doubt on, for instance, the balance between the diagnostic contribution and costs. For example, the continuous growth of laboratory tests, stimulated by the use of automated laboratory support systems, is often questioned.

Evaluation should cover all stages of the development process of a decision-support system. Another important point is that evaluation is a process to be continued after the introduction of a decision-support system into clinical practice, such as in *postmarketing surveillance* studies of drugs. The process of knowledge acquisition should also be part of the assessment. Users, domain experts, and, above all, third, independent parties should be involved in the assessment studies. Only very few decision-support systems in medicine were assessed as extensively as ECG interpretation systems. Therefore, it is relevant to give information on the so-called CSE study (Common Standards for Quantitative Electrocardiography), which was supported by the European Community. The first part of CSE, dealing with the accuracy of waveform recognition in ECG interpretation systems, was completed in 1985. The second stage, on diagnostic interpretation, was completed in 1990[2]. In 1980, at the start of the two-stage evaluation study, about 15 systems for ECG interpretation existed worldwide, and about 6 of these systems were commercially available. In both stages there was the problem of defining an "objective reference." For the first stage this reference consisted of a documented database, reviewed by five cardiologists from five different countries using an adapted *Delphi technique*, which is a feedback method to reduce interobserver variability. In the second study, the diagnostic classifications of about 10 ECG systems were compared with ECG-independent clinical evidence and with the group outcome of the interpretations by eight cardiologists who interpreted 1,220 well-documented ECGs falling into seven main diagnostic categories. The best systems had an overall agreement with the clinical evidence of about 70% and agreement of approximately 80% compared with the combined opinions of the group of cardiologists.

One of the outcomes of the first stage was that several interpretation systems appeared to be much more accurate and stable than others. This sometimes resulted in major changes in the current systems and, in a few cases, even in withdrawal of a system from further evaluation and thus from routine use. ▶

15

The second stage revealed that cardiologists (on average) perform no better than the best systems and that a combination of diagnostic results from different cardiologists is better than the diagnostic results from any individual expert. The latter also applies, however, to the combination of results from interpretation systems.

If all ECG interpretation systems were equally accurate and reliable in the way that they compute diagnostic parameters, it would be possible to use the same diagnostic criteria in all systems. In fact, there is, from a scientific point of view, no reason why the diagnostic criteria for certain application areas would not be identical in all ECG interpretation systems in the world. If verified and universally accepted electrocardiographic criteria were used, this adoption of identical criteria for all systems would have major advantages for the quality of medical care. It would also be more efficient if the collective results of biomedical research were implemented in all systems. Interpretation systems would then only differ in their technical, ergonomic, and economic aspects. Ultimately, the knowledge embedded in such systems should not remain in the hands of research institutions or industry, but it should belong to the medical scientific community as a whole, for instance, controlled by professional organizations of clinicians or by international institutions.

The following are some of the conclusions that can be drawn from the validation of ECG interpretation systems in the CSE study:

1. The development and optimization of decision-support systems takes a long time (for ECG systems, more than 25 years) and requires a large investment in multidisciplinary personnel.
2. The construction, maintenance, and optimization of an interpretation system will be much facilitated if the software is developed in a modular way from the onset and if each software module is evaluated separately, as reflected in the two-stage CSE assessment study.
3. Evaluation of a medical decision-support system should be conducted in a multicenter study, and the principal investigators should not participate in the collection of the patient material and in processing the results from the study (in CSE, a coordinating center did the evaluation).
4. The collection of large validated databases is a prerequisite, but it is expensive and should therefore preferably be done on a multi-institutional scale (independent referees should validate the material).
5. If human experts are involved in the evaluation, an iterative feedback procedure should be built in to reduce interobserver variability (CSE adopted a modified Delphi technique).
6. The data used for the evaluation should be kept secret and should remain in the hands of a coordinating institution to avoid adaptation to the test set (The "truth" behind the CSE database is only known to the coordinating center);

15

A study such as CSE revealed standardization of terminology and parameters for mutual comparison of interpretation results, which is in itself a major accomplishment of an evaluation study. Although a statistical approach to ECG interpretation is mathematically transparent, it has certain shortcomings; one of the most important limitations is that the reasons behind the resulting diagnostic statements would be incomprehensible for most clinicians. Most interpretation systems therefore classify the ECGs by means of heuristic or logical methods or by combinations of several methods.

show the same supporting aspects as laboratory systems, such as the processing of a large stream of drug prescriptions. Decision support is offered for drug-**drug interactions**, checking the dose and duration of treatment with prescribed drugs, and **contraindications**.

It may be clear from the three examples that the systems concerned offer the clinician

1. primary medical data that cannot be obtained otherwise,
2. comprehensive overviews of the data necessary for immediate decision making,
3. administrative support and documentation, storage, and transportation of the data, and
4. processing support for large data streams.

Decision support is primarily used to enhance data reliability.

The question, therefore, is: What extra support could clinicians expect from decision-support systems in addition to the support they already receive from clinical support systems? Furthermore, is there a need for decision support if trained clinicians themselves can see by glancing at the primary data what is wrong with the patient? Are there circumstances in which clinicians are not able to interpret all of these data by themselves, without computer support? Perhaps in the diagnostic-therapeutic cycle the most important task for decision-support systems is enhancement of data reliability.

From publications in the area of decision-support systems, however, it appears that such systems may also offer clinical support other than for data reliability only (as is also apparent from Chapters 16 and 17). For instance, **De Dombal** showed that the use of a decision-support system helped to decrease unnecessary interventions and to reduce perforation rates among patients with appendicitis, as well as to decrease the use of surgical beds. Another area in which decision-support has been fully accepted (for reasons other than only the enhancement of data reliability) is in ECG interpretation. ECG systems are, in a way, comparable to laboratory support systems, but in addition, they are able to deliver a fully interpreted final document which is usually reviewed by the treating clinician (see Panel 15.4).

Decision-support systems are useful when they

- offer guidance to inexperienced users in making complex decisions,
- give support to experienced users in suggesting diagnostic statements in case of routine interpretation of large numbers of cases,
- give assistance to users in making diagnoses in nonroutine cases, and
- integrate critiquing with CPR systems.

In all these cases, decision-support systems may assist in increasing the *quality* of medical decisions. Virtually none of the existing decision-support systems is already used in such a way that data entry, documentation, report generation, the handling of large data streams, and critiquing are fully integrated in routine practice. Decision-support systems, however, not only should be thoroughly evaluated but should also meet legal and ethical criteria. The latter is discussed in the following section.

5.1 Legal and Ethical Aspects of Computer-Assisted Decision-Support Systems

There are a number of legal and ethical concerns related to the use of decision-support programs in clinical practice. In 1985, R.A. Miller (both a medical informatician and a practicing physician), together with two colleagues, a philosopher and a law professor, wrote the paper "Ethical and Legal Issues Related to the Use of Computer Programs in Clinical Medicine."[1] Important legal and ethical issues included privacy, confidentiality, and security (see Chapters 7 and 34), circumstances pertaining to the misuse of computer programs in clinical practice, and the ethical responsi-

---

[1] R.A.Miller, K.F. Schaffner, A. Meisel. Ethical and legal issues related to the use of computer programs in clinical medicine. Ann Intern Med 1985;102:529-36.

bilities of individual and institutional software users. Computers may be misused in clinical practice for a number of reasons:

1. Users may not be qualified from a professional standpoint to use a system safely and efficaciously. For example, a nurse might not recognize when a diagnostic system had made an incorrect diagnosis of a complicated case, whereas a board-certified physician might be less likely to do so. A data-processing clerk might not be qualified enough to abstract from a chart the clinical findings to be run in a decision-support system. A general practitioner might not be competent to run a *robotic* surgical device (due to the chance of complications that might require immediate manual surgical intervention).
2. Users may be qualified to use a system but not trained well enough to understand its strengths and limitations. This includes the often encountered problem of vocabulary mismatch, in which clinician and system mean different things by medical phrases and misinterpret the communication as a result.
3. A program that performs well in isolation may be improperly tied to other systems or a network that provides erroneous or improperly formatted input.
4. Users may use poor judgment in deciding not to use a system when it should be used or in not overriding incorrect system suggestions.

When use of a computer program results in harm to a patient or appears to cause harm, legal remedies are possible. Failure to use a computer program, as well as improper use of a computer program, might lead to legal action on the basis of not upholding the standard of care. In the United States, two aspects of tort law are relevant to people harmed through the use of goods and services: negligence theory and strict product liability. Negligence theory, which governs malpractice actions, relates to the provision of services. Strict product liability relates to injuries caused by defective products.

Negligence theory holds that service providers must uphold the standards of the community for quality and reliability in delivering services; if they do not, they may be found liable in a court of law when injuries or da-

mage occurs. Negligence focuses on whether service providers do "the right thing." So long as appropriate actions were taken, possible adverse outcomes may occur without blame. Patients with acute myocardial infarction admitted to the hospital have a non-zero mortality rate, even under the best system of modern care. So long as reasonably good care is provided to a patient with acute myocardial infarction, the practitioner is not held liable if the patient dies. It is likely that practitioners who use (or fail to use) clinical software systems may themselves be held liable under negligence theory if their actions subsequent to using (or not using) relevant software programs are substandard. Just as with human consultants, clinicians issuing the consultation requests are held liable if their consultants' advice is faulty and they nevertheless follow that advice.

Strict product liability applies when the purchaser of a product is harmed as a result of a defect in that product. For example, if someone purchases a ladder, and while climbing the ladder for the first time, a rung on the ladder breaks (under normal load) and causes the purchaser to fall and have injuries, the manufacturer (and seller) of the ladder may be held responsible under strict product liability. Unlike negligence, which focuses on whether the processes followed were correct, strict product liability focuses on compensation of the innocent injured parties, so long as it can be shown that the product was defective and the defect caused an injury to the purchaser. The standard for strict product liability is absolute perfection: no defects are tolerated when injury occurs. To some extent, fair and honest labeling can partially protect a manufacturer from product liability claims (e.g., warnings to not use a metal ladder near electrical wiring). However, if clinical software programs are viewed by the courts under product liability, the potential exists to substantially stifle software production and distribution, because adverse outcomes commonly occur in clinical practice.

Whether the courts will view clinical software programs as services sold to care providers or as products under strict liability is not yet clear, because there have been few, if any, rulings. At the least, the programs will be treated as services, but licensed practitioners will most likely be held accountable for whatever decisions they make. Since the patient, and not the care provider, is the individual who physically suffers from errors

15

in the clinical process, and the purchasers of clinical software and not the patients are most likely the care providers, it could be argued that strict product liability would not apply.

It may be difficult to demonstrate when a clinical software program is defective, because end-user effects often dominate in how programs perform. Poorly trained users who do not fully understand program capabilities and how to use the program (as well as those who do not understand the input and output vocabularies on a professional level) are far more likely to have poor results in using clinical software programs than are well-trained, well-qualified, expert users. Related ethical questions include whether a vendor should require training to a certain level of competency before allowing users to employ certain programs in clinical practice and whether users are obligated to obtain proper training before employing programs in their practices (just as they should not interpret ECGs or perform gastrointestinal endoscopy without proper training).

Another ethical issue includes the responsibilities of vendors for the academic clinical integrity of knowledge bases embedded in clinical software programs. If a vendor knowingly cuts corners in developing or distributing a medical knowledge base, patients might ultimately suffer. Only well-qualified individuals thoroughly familiar with a program's function should be allowed to build and maintain clinical knowledge bases.

A final concern is the role of institutional and governmental regulations and monitoring of the use of clinical software programs. If governmental agencies aggressively restrict what software programs can be licensed, more harm than good might be done if the programs not licensed improve the baseline quality of care (even though they are not perfect). Local institutions that install complex conglomerations of multiple vendors' products, admixed with locally developed software and networking architectures, have a responsibility to monitor overall clinical software processes for quality and patient safety.

Key References

Berner ES, Bebster GD, Shugerman AA, et al. Performance of computer-based diagnostic systems. N Engl J Med 1994;330:1792-6.

Miller RA, Masarie FE. The demise of the Greek oracle model for medical diagnosis systems. Meth Inform Med 1990;29;1-2.

Shortliffe EH, Buchanan BG, Feigenbaum EA. Knowledge engineering for medical decision making: A review of computer-based clinical decision aids. Proc IEEE 1979;67:1207-24.

(see also Chapters 16,17, and 28.)

See the Web site for further literature references.

15

16 Clinical Decision-Support Systems

1 Introduction

Chapter 15 gave an overview of the different methods that underlie decision-support systems (*DSSs*), but without referring to the specific systems developed in the past and systems that are used for different clinical applications. This chapter therefore describes a representative group of DSSs and sketches the history and the future of such systems. The purpose of this chapter is to provide the reader with a general understanding of clinical DSSs and focuses on how DSSs present themselves to the user. The acquisition and representation of medical knowledge is discussed in Chapter 17.

1.1 History of Systems

The first generation of systems that attempted to aid the clinician in making medical decisions appeared in the late 1950s. These systems were mainly based on methods that used *decision trees* or *truth tables*. Systems based on statistical methods appeared later, followed by *expert systems* much later. Most early systems remained only prototypes.

Researchers developed clinical DSSs for different domains of clinical care. Some systems were intended for narrow, well-defined diagnostic problems in which the clinician had to decide between a limited number of diagnoses. An example of such a system was *De Dombal's* system for acute abdominal pain; this program dealt with 13 different diagnoses for acute abdominal pain and was based on statistical methods. Other DSSs were developed for the interpretation of electrocardiograms (*ECGs*). Other researchers developed systems for much larger domains of clinical care. For example, the system *INTERNIST*, with hundreds of diagnoses, attempted to cover the complete domain of internal medicine.

Thus, clinical DSSs range from small systems for a limited domain (with just a few diagnoses) to very large systems with hundreds of diagnoses and thousands of symptoms.

Clinical DSSs also vary in the type of decisions that they support. Some programs support diagnostic decisions. On the basis of patient data and the results of tests, these systems propose a diagnosis. Other systems may focus on therapeutic decisions. These systems recommend a treatment or aid the clinician in executing a treatment. For instance, systems that help an oncologist execute complex cancer *protocols* belong to this last category.

1.2 Types of Systems

Clinical DSSs vary in how they interact with the user:
- Some systems, such as INTERNIST, require direct *interaction* between the clinician and the system. The clinician initiates a dialogue with the system and provides data to the system by entering the patient's symptoms or by answering questions. Not all systems, however, require that type of interaction with the clinician.
- Some DSSs rely on computers that are interconnected to electronic devices. In some instances a DSS is directly connected to devices that generate the patient data, such as systems that interpret ECGs

(Chapter 15) or to computers that interpret laboratory data (Chapter 13).

- Other DSSs are integrated with computer-based patient records (*CPRs*) (Chapters 7 and 29) and use the data from such records as input. In such settings, receiving decision support does not require the clinician to enter additional data about the patient.

Under the general heading of clinical DSSs, one thus encounters a wide variety of systems that differ in:

- the clinical domain that they address,
- the type of decisions that they support, and
- the method by which the necessary patient data are obtained.

Although numerous systems have been developed, only a few DSSs have progressed beyond the prototype stage and the research laboratory where they were developed to routine use in a clinical setting.

However, clinicians are increasingly encountering routine clinical practice systems that provide decision support. This is particularly true in settings in which DSSs can be directly connected to medical equipment or integrated with CPRs.

In the next section, we first give a definition of the term *clinical decision-support system*. Subsequently, we describe the current impact of DSSs. We then divide DSSs into different categories and discuss some examples of DSSs in each category. Finally, we discuss current trends in the development of DSSs.

2 Definition of Clinical Decision-Support Systems

A number of definitions for clinical DSSs have been proposed. For example, Shortliffe defines a medical DSS as:

any computer program designed to help health professionals make clinical decisions.

The disadvantage of such a broad definition is that it includes any computer system that stores, retrieves, or presents medical data or knowledge. To further specify what we mean by a clinical DSS, we use the definition proposed by Wyatt and Spiegelhalter. In their view, clinical DSSs are:

active knowledge systems which use two or more items of patient data to generate case-specific advice.

This definition captures the main components of a clinical DSS: medical knowledge, patient data, and case-specific advice (see also Chapter 15):

1. *Medical knowledge*. The representation of medical knowledge varies from system to system, as des-

cribed in Chapter 15, which presents different models for representing medical knowledge. For instance, knowledge about a drug could be represented in the form of a **pharmacokinetic model** that describes the behavior of that drug.

2. *Patient data*. The medical knowledge contained in the DSS is used to interpret patient data. For instance, patient characteristics are used to set the parameters for a pharmacokinetic model.

3. *Case-specific advice*. The result of applying medical knowledge to patient data is case-specific advice. For example, applying a pharmacokinetic model to the patient data may result in a suggestion about the dosage of a drug for that particular patient.

This cycle of knowledge is characteristic for clinical DSSs. By this definition, **electronic textbooks** and **World Wide Web** pages are not DSSs.

Clearly, the type of decision support will depend on the type of knowledge represented in the system. A system is directed to a specific group or category of patients or problems. If, for example, the system contains treatment protocols for a particular type of cancer, then only patients with that type of cancer can be supported by the system. Of course, if a system has been built to interpret *ECG*s, it should not be used to interpret *electroencephalograms*. Each clinical DSS is directed to a specific group of patients or problems: the domain of the system.

3 Influence of Decision-Support Systems

Many hundreds of DSSs have been described in the literature. Only a few systems, however, have been subjected to a thorough clinical evaluation. Systems that have undergone evaluation are, for example, systems for the interpretation of ECGs (see Panel 15.4 of Chapter 15) or De Dombal's system for abdominal pain (see Section 3.1 of this chapter). Still fewer systems are in routine use by clinicians. Building systems that are effective in supporting clinicians and that are also accepted by clinicians has proven to be a difficult task (see also Section 5 of Chapter 15). Examples are given from two different areas: the effect of a DSS on the diagnosis of abdominal pain, and the effect of DSSs on patient outcome.

3.1 Abdominal Pain

The DSS for abdominal pain developed by De Dombal helps the clinician in determining the cause of acute abdominal pain. After the physician enters patient data (i.e., the symptoms of the patient) the system gives the probabilities of the possible diagnoses. This system was subjected to an eight-center study involving 250 physicians and 16,737 patients. The authors showed that after the introduction of the system in the clinic, diagnostic accuracy rose from 46 to 65%. The negative laparotomy rate fell by almost half, as did the perforation rate among patients with appendicitis. The observed mortality rate fell by 22%. The authors also demonstrated the extent of the so-called checklist effect: merely introducing forms for recording the signs and symptoms of the patients with acute abdominal pain resulted in a significant improvement; the diagnostic accuracy increased from 46 to 57%.

3.2 Patient Outcome

Johnston and colleagues reviewed the evidence from *controlled trials* on the effects of computer-based DSSs on clinician performance and patient outcomes. The studies reviewed illustrate the wide range of domains of clinical DSSs:

- computer-assisted dosage systems,
- computer-assisted diagnosis systems,
- preventive care reminder systems, and
- computer-aided quality assurance systems.

Two different aspects were investigated:

1. the performance of the clinician and
2. patient outcome.

Improvements of the clinician's performance were demonstrated in three of the four studies involving computer-assisted drug dosage systems. One of the five studies were on computer-assisted diagnosis systems, four of six were on preventive care reminder systems, and seven of nine were on computer-aided quality assurance systems. Only 10 of these studies assessed patient outcome, of which 3 reported significant improvements. The authors concluded that there is strong evidence that some computer-based DSSs may improve clinician performance.

In summary, numerous systems have been developed over the past few decades, but very few of them have left the laboratory environment. Of the few systems that underwent a controlled trial, however, the majority had an impact.

16

4 Categories of Systems

Clinical DSSs can be categorized in different ways. The systems can be divided according to:

- *knowledge representation* (e.g., systems based on *decision trees*, *Bayesian statistics*, or *production rules*),
- *type of decisions* (e.g., systems for diagnosis or therapy), and
- *medical domain* (e.g., systems for general internal medicine or surgery).

From the viewpoint of the clinician, however, systems can be divided into categories on the basis of whether or not the advice was solicited:

- *solicited advice*: systems that provide advice only when they are instructed to do so;
- *unsolicited advice*: systems that provide advice independently of a request from a clinician; and
- *autonomous systems*: systems that monitor incoming patient data and, to a certain extent, take action without human interference.

In Chapter 15 the methods that underlie DSSs have been reviewed. Therefore, we focus on the categorization according to the clinician's viewpoint.

4.1 Solicited Advice

When the clinician takes the initiative to explicitly consult a DSS, we speak of *solicited advice*. The clinician decides that a certain case warrants the use of a DSS. A number of systems, some of which are commercially available, are intended to address broad domains, such as the entire field of internal medicine. In the following section, we use *QMR* ("Quick Medical Reference") as an illustration of a system that provides solicited advice in a broad domain. The QMR system is a commercial descendant of the system INTERNIST.

4.1.1 Characteristics

In most instances, solicited-advice systems are stand-alone systems. The user evokes the system and a dialogue is started. The system asks the user for input, for example, through input forms in which several items are requested or through some kind of question-answer sequence in which the questions asked often depend on the answers to previous questions. Whenever the system has obtained the required information, advice will be provided. Often, the user can ask the system for an explanation of why the advice was given and why certain questions were asked.

These systems often give the clinicians some control over the reasoning performed by the DSS. The clinician is able to steer the system in a certain direction. For example, the clinician may have a diagnosis in mind, but wonders whether all the symptoms are explained by that diagnosis. The system is then able to critique the diagnosis proposed by the clinician. In this situation, the clinician enters the suspected diagnosis, together with the symptoms. The system subsequently points out to the clinician those symptoms that are not explained by the proposed diagnosis.

For some of these domains, the system may require little or no additional interaction with the clinician. The computerized analysis of ECGs can be viewed as solicited advice when the user has the option of either making a strip-chart recording of the ECG or requesting the same recording to be accompanied by an interpretation by a DSS. In modern recording equipment the interpretation software is often included in the recording system. The user is able to decide whether, in addition to recording the ECG, an interpretation by the system is wanted.

4.1.2 Example: QMR

QMR, a program that assists the user in the diagnostic process, contains information on more than 600 diseases and more than 4,500 clinical findings. The clinical findings are grouped into the following categories:

- past medical history,
- symptoms of current illness,
- findings on physical examinations,
- simple, inexpensive laboratory tests,

- moderately expensive and/or invasive laboratory tests, and
- very expensive and/or invasive laboratory tests.

For each disease, the knowledge base in QMR contains a list of the clinical findings that are required for decision making. For example, the list of clinical findings for "malignant melanoma (nonocular)" comprises 57 different findings; among these are:

- hair color at age 5 red or blond,
- anorexia,
- skin lesions of variegated color,
- increased serum calcium level,
- skin biopsy indicating malignant melanoma, and
- lymph node biopsy indicating malignant neoplasm.

The relation between a clinical finding and a disease varies; some findings are often present in a given disease, whereas others are only rarely observed in patients suffering from that disease. In addition, some findings are very common (such as cough) and can be observed in many different diseases, whereas other findings may be very specific for a given disease (observing that finding makes it very likely that the patient has that disease). In QMR the relationship between diseases and findings is characterized by two parameters: the **evoking strength** and the **frequency**. Both evoking strength and frequency are coded as numbers ranging from 0 to 5.

The evoking strength indicates how strong the finding suggests the presence of the disease. An evoking strength of 5 indicates that if the finding is observed the disease is almost certainly present. The evoking strength may be considered a subjective kind of the positive predictive value of a symptom, that is, the **conditional probability** of a disease given a finding (i.e., the probability $p(D|S)$, as mentioned in Chapter 15, Section 4.1.5) (see also Table 16.1).

A finding that strongly indicates the presence of a disease, however, may not always be present. The **frequency** is a measure of how often a finding is found in a given disease, comparable to $p(S|D)$ in Section 4.1.5 of Chapter 15. A frequency of 5 indicates that nearly all patients with the disease show that finding. The frequency value can thus be seen as a subjective measure for the **sensitivity** of the finding (see Table 16.2).

For the example of malignant melanoma (nonocular) given above, the evoking strengths and frequencies are defined as presented in Table 16.3. These numbers in Table 16.3 indicate, for example, that red or blond hair

Evoking Strength	Description
0	Nonspecific item
1	Item minimally suggests the presence of the disease
2	Item mildly suggests the presence of the disease
3	Item moderately suggests the presence of the disease
4	Item strongly suggests the presence of the disease
5	Item always suggests the presence of the disease

Table 16.1
Descriptions of Evoking Strength Values.

16

Frequency	Description
1	Item seen rarely in patients with the disease
2	Item seen in a large minority of patients with the disease
3	Item seen in about one half of the patients with the disease
4	Item seen in a majority of patients with the disease
5	Item seen in essentially all patients with the disease

Table 16.2
Descriptions of Frequency Values.

Finding	Evoking Strength	Frequency
Hair color at age 5 red or blond	0	3
Anorexia	0	2
Skin lesions, variegated color	2	4
Increased serum calcium level	1	1
Skin biopsy specimen indicating malignant melanoma	4	4
Lymph node biopsy specimen indicating malignant neoplasm	2	2

Table 16.3
Evoking Strengths and Frequencies of Findings for *Malignant Melanoma*.

Findings Potentially Supporting Hypotheses . . .
Past Medical History . . .
    Alcohol Ingestion Heavy Recent Hx[a]
    Foreign Body Aspiration Hx
    Pneumonia Acute Recent Hx
    Pneumothorax Treatment For Tuberculosis Hx
    Tuberculosis Contact Hx
    Tuberculosis Hx
Findings on Physical Examination . . .
Simple, Inexpensive Laboratory Tests . . .
    Chest X-Ray Lung Field(s) Abnormal
    Chest X-Ray Lymph Node(s) Calcified
    Chest X-Ray Mediastinal Shift
    Chest X-Ray Pleural Thickening Laminar
    Tuberculin Skin Test Positive
    White blood count 14,000 to 30,000
Moderately Expensive and/or Invasive Lab Tests . . .
Very Expensive and/or Invasive Laboratory Tests . . .
Related Diseases Potentially Supporting Hypotheses . . .
    Closely Related Supporting Diagnoses . . .
    Moderately Related Supporting Diagnoses . . .
    Remotely Related Supporting Diagnoses . . .
    Symptoms of Current Illness . . .
Findings on Physical Examination . . .
Simple, Inexpensive Laboratory Tests . . .
Moderately Expensive and/or Invasive lab Tests . . .
Very Expensive and/or Invasive Laboratory Tests . . .

Table 16.4
List of Possible Findings in the Hypotheses *Pulmonary Abscess* and *Tuberculosis Chronic Pulmonary*.[a]

[a] Headings ending with . . . indicate that they contain a number of items that the user may display or suppress by clicking on the sentence.

[a] "Hx" denotes "history of."

315	Pleural Malignant Mesothelioma
307	Pulmonary Lymphoma
283	Histoplasmosis Chronic Pulmonary
283	Pulmonary Asbestosis
274	Pulmonary Abscess
274	Tuberculosis Chronic Pulmonary
271	Blastomycosis Chronic Pulmonary
265	Lymphomatoid Granulomatosis
265	Pulmonary Infarction
260	Bronchoalveolar Cell Carcinoma
256	Pulmonary Silicosis Chronic
254	Pulmonary Malignant Neoplasm Secondary (Lymphogenous Type)
253	Pulmonary Atypical Mycobacterial Infection
253	Pulmonary Malignant Neoplasm Secondary (Hematogenous Type)
253	Pulmonary Nocardiosis
247	Pulmonary Alveolar Proteinosis
244	Bronchogenic Carcinoma Squamous Cell Type

Table 16.5
Possible Diagnoses after Entering New Findings.

Past Medical History . . .
    2 4 Asbestos Exposure Hx[b]
    0 4 Sex Male
    0 4 Weight Loss Gtr Than 10 Percent
Symptoms of Current Illness . . .
    1 4 Dyspnea Exertional
    1 3 Chest Pain Lateral Exacerbation with Breathing
    1 3 Dyspnea at Rest
    1 3 Chest Pain Lateral Sharp
Findings on Physical Examination . . .
    1 4 Chest Percussion Dull Localized
    0 4 Lung(s) Percussion and/or Auscultation Abnormal
    1 3 Breath Sound(s) Decreased Localized
    1 3 Fremitus Tactile Decreased Localized
    1 3 Chest Movement Asymmetrical
Simple, Inexpensive Laboratory Tests . . .
    3 3 Chest X-Ray Pleural Mass or Nodular Thickening
Moderately Expensive and/or Invasive Laboratory Tests . . .
    2 4 Pleura Biopsy Malignant Neoplasm
    0 4 Pleural Fluid Obtained by Thoracentesis
    1 3 Lung(s) Forced Vital Capacity Decreased
    2 3 Pleural Fluid Malignant Neoplastic Cell(s)

Table 16.6
Findings that, when Absent, Rule out *Pleural Malignant Mesothelioma*.[a]

16

[a] *Note the high values for the frequency.*
[b] *The first number is evoking strength and the second number is frequency.*

STRONGLY SUGGESTS (66-96%) presence of . . .

    4 4 Pleura Biopsy Mesothelioma

MODERATELY SUGGESTS (36-65%) presence of . . .

    3 3 Chest X-Ray Pleural Mass or Nodular Thickening

MILDLY SUGGESTS (6-35%) presence of . . .

    2 4 Asbestos Exposure Hx

    2 4 Pleura Biopsy Malignant Neoplasm

    2 3 Pleural Fluid Malignant Neoplastic Cell(s)

Table 16.7
Findings to Rule in Pleural Malignant Mesothelioma.

at the age of 5 is seen in about half of the patients with malignant melanoma, but that having red or blond hair at the age of 5 is nonspecific. On the other hand, finding malignant melanoma in a skin biopsy is seen in the majority of the patients with malignant melanoma and strongly suggests the presence of the disease.

In addition, diseases can be associated with other diseases in several ways. First, a disease may cause another disease. Second, the given disease predisposes an individual to another disease.

How the evoking strengths, frequencies, and links are used to rank possible diagnoses is based on the methods developed for the INTERNIST system. The

approach for combining evoking strengths and frequencies is heuristic. A concrete example of how to diagnose the disease of a particular patient is given in Panel 16.1, including Tables 16.4 to 16.9.

One of the strengths of QMR is its flexibility. It is able to answer a number of relevant questions in a diagnostic session. Furthermore, it can be used as a kind of textbook that can be used to find information about disease profiles, as in medical textbooks. The advantage over a textbook is that it is interactive. It also has the findings as entries: given an entry, the system is able to provide a list of diagnoses in which this finding occurs. QMR also has its weak points. The reasoning heavily

Disease Causes . . .

    1 4 Pleural Effusion Exudative

    1 2 Cardiac Neoplasm Secondary

    1 2 Hepatic Neoplasm Secondary

    1 2 Pulmonary Malignant Neoplasm Secondary (Hematogenous Type)

    1 1 Chylous Ascites

    1 1 Cerebral Neoplasm Single Parietal

    1 1 Pleural Effusion Transudative

    1 1 Bone Neoplasm Secondary

    1 1 Antidiuretic Hormone Inappropriate Secretion Syndrome (Siadh)

    1 1 Pulmonary Malignant Neoplasm Secondary (Lymphogenous Type)

    1 1 Brain Neoplasm Secondary Multiple

Disease Predisposes to . . .

    1 3 Hypertrophic Osteoarthropathy

Disease is Predisposed to by . . .

    2 2 Pulmonary Asbestosis

Table 16.8
Disease-Associated Disorders for Pleural Malignant Mesothelioma.

Critique Diagnosis: Pleural Malignant Mesothelioma

Findings Consistent with the Diagnosis . . .

0 3 Age 26 to 55
1 4 Dyspnea Exertional
0 4 Sex Male
3 3 Chest X-Ray Pleural Mass or Nodular Thickening
1 3 Chest Movement Asymmetrical
1 3 Dyspnea at Rest
1 3 Chest Pain Lateral Dull Aching
1 3 Fremitus Tactile Decreased Localized
0 3 Tachypnea
1 2 Chest X-Ray Lung Field(s) Abnormal
1 2 Pleural Friction Rub
1 2 Finger(s) Clubbed
1 2 Rales Localized
0 2 Tachycardia
1 1 Sputum Blood Streaked

Findings NOT Consistent with the Diagnosis . . .

0 0 Chest X-Ray Diffuse Nodular Density(ies) Noncalcified
0 0 Cough Chronic Productive Hx

USEFUL Questions Regarding the Diagnosis . . .

4 4 ?Pleura Biopsy Mesothelioma
2 4 ?Asbestos Exposure Hx
2 4 ?Pleura Biopsy Malignant Neoplasm
2 3 ?Pleural Fluid Malignant Neoplastic Cell(s)
1 4 ?Chest Percussion Dull Localized
0 4 ?Pleural Fluid Obtained by Thoracentesis
0 4 ?Weight Loss Gtr Than 10 Percent

Potentially Interesting Related Diagnoses . . .

Contains Problem Area #1 Pulmonary Asbestosis...

82 Pulmonary Asbestosis
80 Pleural Effusion Exudative

Table 16.9
Critique of QMR on Pleural Malignant Mesothelioma *for the Case Discussed in the Example.*

16

depends on the evoking strengths and frequencies for the various findings. The numbers stored will not transfer well from one site to another. An example is the disease profile for acquired immune deficiency syndrome (AIDS), which according to the frequencies is a disease that occurs among homosexual males (see Table 16.10). However, in large cities or in parts of Africa, females are at an even greater risk because of differences in culture and sexual behaviors. So, the use of QMR in an area with a setting of the evoking strengths and frequencies of rural areas will in some countries or cities lead to inaccurate decision support. In addition,

---

PANEL 16.1

Diagnosing Diseases in QMR

When QMR is used to obtain assistance for the diagnosis of a particular case, the system asks for two basic data: the age and the gender of the patient. Next, the user may enter a number of items of the patient's past history and current symptoms.

Suppose we have a *54-year-old male*[1] who visits a pulmonologist because of *chronic productive cough*. Recently, his *sputum* had a *streak of blood*. Furthermore, he experiences a *dull lateral chest pain*. He also has *dyspnea at rest* that *increases during exercise*.[2]

With this list of information from the history, QMR is already able to provide a (long) list of what are called "potentially interesting diagnoses"; in our example, Bronchitis Chronic (simple) and Tuberculosis Chronic Pulmonary are at the top of the list.

The physical examination reveals *tachypnea* and *tachycardia*. We also see *clubbed fingers*. When these findings are entered in QMR, the list of potential diagnoses is now headed by Pulmonary Abscess and Tuberculosis Chronic Pulmonary; Bronchitis has moved far down the list.

Further examination shows that the *chest movement is asymmetrical, localized rales, pleural friction rub,* and a *localized decrease of the fremitus.* When these findings are entered, QMR still suggests 35 potentially interesting diagnoses. The following are the top five:

1. Pulmonary Abscess,
2. Tuberculosis Chronic Pulmonary,
3. Histoplasmosis Chronic Pulmonary,
4. Pulmonary Asbestosis,
5. Pulmonary Atypical Mycobacterial Infection.

Thus far, we have entered findings and requested from QMR a ranked list of possible diagnoses. The clinician, however, has the opportunity to focus QMR on a subset of these diagnoses. For example, the user can ask QMR to discriminate between two diagnoses by selecting these two diagnoses and instruct the system to discriminate between these two. QMR will then generate a list of findings that discriminate between the selected diagnoses. In our example, we select Pulmonary Abscess and Tuberculosis Chronic Pulmonary. QMR subsequently lists 39 findings of possible interest (see Table 16.4).

Among the simple, inexpensive tests is a chest X-ray that yields some discrimination. When we look at the X-ray we observe *noncalcified diffuse nodular densities* in *both lung fields,* which are considered to be abnormal. Furthermore, we discover a *pleural mass* or *nodular thickening.* We enter these findings in QMR. Now the list of potentially interesting diagnoses is reduced to ▶

---

the description of AIDS in Table 16.10 is dated because the presentation of the disease has changed significantly in recent years; the disease profile in Table 16.10 does not reflect these changes. Although the producers of QMR warn that the knowledge base is incomplete and that some diseases may be erroneously suggested, it is essential that users have a full understanding of these limitations of QMR.

17 (see Table 16.5). Before each hypothesis, the system gives a score that indicates the degree to which the diagnosis is supported by the findings, taking into account the prior probability. Note the major change in the top five diagnoses.

From here, QMR provides various options to continue reducing the *differential diagnosis*. One option is to ask QMR to remove diagnoses from the differential diagnosis. On the basis of the frequency parameter the system will then generate a list of findings with which one can rule out a diagnosis from the differential list. For example, ruling out Pleural Malignant Mesothelioma can be done by checking the findings as seen in Table 16.6.

Another option is to rule in a diagnosis (Table 16.7). Here one is looking at findings that have a high evoking strength; that is, when the finding occurs, the disorder is likely to be present. Although in the rule-out situation one would like to have inexpensive tests, in the rule-in situation it is the evoking strength of the test that is important.

For example, for Pleural Malignant Mesothelioma, QMR notes that a biopsy of the pleura showing mesothelioma strongly suggests the diagnosis (evoking strength = 4, frequency = 4). Exposure to asbestos in the past is only mildly suggestive, although this finding is noted for a majority of patients with pleural malignant mesothelioma (evoking strength = 2, frequency = 4) and, hence, may be used to rule out the disease.

Another option that may guide the user in following the proper treatment and follow-up of the patient are the links between the diseases covered by QMR (Table 16.8). Eleven different diseases can be caused by pleural malignant mesothelioma, with exudative pleural effusion being the most frequent one. There is also a list of diseases to which pleural malignant mesothelioma predisposes an individual, as well as a list of diseases that predispose an individual to pleural malignant mesothelioma (e.g., pulmonary asbestosis).

A possible problem that one may encounter is that not all findings are covered by the most likely disease. When a diagnosis is selected, QMR can provide a critique for that diagnosis, consisting of a listing of the findings that are consistent with the diagnosis, as well as the findings that are not consistent (such as the noncalcified nodular densities on the X-ray and the productive chronic cough in the patient history, as in our case for the diagnosis pleural malignant mesothelioma). The system provides a list of useful questions for ruling in or ruling out the diagnosis that was entered. QMR supports entry of positive and negative findings, in this case by selecting from this suggested list (Table 16.9). The system also provides a list of potentially interesting related diagnoses that can be supportive of the diagnoses under critique.

16

---

[1] *We denote items that were entered in QMR in italics. Only parts of the words must be entered. For example "cou chr prod" is sufficient to get the item cough chronic productive Hx (with "Hx" denoting "history of").*

[2] *Here we must be careful. There are two issues at stake: "dyspnea at rest" and "dyspnea increasing at exertion." When we combine the two in one string, we get another result: "chest pain paroxysmal increasing in duration and/or severity recent Hx." Thus, one becomes dependent on the different terms that QMR uses. On the other hand, entering only "dyspnea" gives a list of options from which one can select.*

4.2 Unsolicited Advice

Systems that provide unsolicited advice do not require the initiative of the clinician to generate advice. These systems rely on available patient data (e.g., data from a laboratory system or from a CPR), and they will generate advice independently of a request from the clinician.

Is associated with 110 Finding(s) arranged:

1. In textbook order: history, symptoms, signs, laboratory tests
2. By frequency

Past Medical History . . .

    0 4 Sex Male

    2 4 Homosexuality Male

    0 4 Age 26 to 55

    0 4 Weight Loss Gtr Than 10 Percent

    1 2 Pharyngitis Recent Hx

    2 2 Drug Abuse Hx

    0 2 Age 16 To 25

    2 2 Herpes Zoster Hx

    0 2 Age Gtr Than 55

    1 2 Drug Hypersensitivity Hx

    0 2 Sex Female

    0 2 Residence or Travel Tropical or Semitropical Hx

    1 2 Hepatitis Acute Hx

    0 2 Sexual Partner(s) Number Gtr Than Five Hx

    1 1 Transfusion(s) Blood Multiple Hx

    1 1 Blood Product(s) Administration Multiple Hx

Symptoms of Current Illness . . .

Findings on Physical Examination . . .

Simple, Inexpensive Laboratory Tests . . .

Moderately Expensive and/or Invasive Laboratory Tests . . .

Very Expensive and/or Invasive Laboratory Tests . . .

Table 16.10
Part of the Disease Profile for AIDS.

4.2.1 Characteristics

Typically, systems that provide unsolicited advice are clinical DSSs that are integrated with CPR systems (see also Chapters 7 and 29). The clinical DSS evaluates patient data as they become available. The CARE system, developed by McDonald, is an early example of the use of CPR data to review treatment. The *CARE* syntax allows the user to write rules that *remind* the clinician of diagnoses or problems that might otherwise be overlooked. A set of rules was developed, and the impact of the rules on the delivery of care was demonstrated. Typically, these rules use simple ***Boolean logic*** (see Chapter 15), and they cause a fixed paragraph of text to be reported as a standard response to a definite or potential abnormality.

A limiting factor is the amount of patient data that are available to the DSS. If, for example, only a prescription is available from the CPR system, then the DSS can only verify whether the prescribed dosage is within the range between the minimal and the maximal dosage. If the age and the weight of the patient are also known, then the dosage could be corrected for age and weight. If additional data are available (such as the patient's previous responses to the drug), a pharmacokinetic model may even be used to verify the prescribed dosage. In general, when more information becomes available in a CPR system, a DSS will, in principle, be able to generate more specific advice.

In this situation, the clinician does not specifically ask for advice; the advice can be viewed as a by-product of routine data management activities. Therefore, a goal and a challenge is to avoid, despite the limited data available, generating an excessive amount of advice, particularly because *false-positive* advice or incorrect alerts may generate antagonistic responses. Consequently, for systems that generate unsolicited advice, a high *predictive value* (see Chapter 15, Section 4.1.3) is of great importance. The dilemma is that increasing the *sensitivity* of the advice will likely decrease the predictive value, because the amount of false-positive advice will increase (see Chapter 15, Section 4.1.2).

A reason for the generation of false-positive advice may be that the system failed to determine correctly the diagnostic and treatment goals of the clinician on the basis of the data in the patient record. Knowledge of those goals is essential for inferring the appropriateness of a clinician's actions. Patient records contain both data describing the patient's state (e.g., the results of laboratory tests) and data describing the objectives of the treating clinician (e.g., a list of treatment goals). The patient record, however, is primarily a record of *actions performed* (see Chapters 7 and 29); it records what the clinician did rather than why the clinician did it. A clinician often does not label a particular prescription "for the treatment of bronchitis" and does not necessarily label diagnostic tests "to exclude disease X." Moreover, a clinician does not document in the patient record all actions taken or all decisions made. The absence of coded data in the patient record that can allow the computer to ascertain the intentions of the treating clinician represents a fundamental obstacle for systems that should generate unsolicited advice (reminders, alerts, or critiques). As a result, systems may provide advice that is inappropriate, because the reasoning of the clinician has been misinterpreted

4.2.2 Example: Arden Syntax

Several systems that review treatment by using data from CPRs have been developed. Researchers acknowledged the difficulties that they faced in sharing knowledge among similar review systems. The purpose of the so-called *Arden syntax* is to allow sharing of medical

knowledge across review systems. To facilitate sharing, the Arden syntax identifies separately the local, institution-specific implementation issues (such as accessing patient data) and the shared procedural knowledge that transcends institutions. The Arden syntax is aimed at knowledge bases that can be viewed as distinct, independent modules. It allows users to construct *medical logic modules* (**MLMs**); each MLM encodes a discrete segment of medical knowledge. The MLMs built with the Arden syntax should therefore be viewed as independent microdecision units (see also Chapter 15, Section 4.2). Using the Arden syntax, the clinician is able to write rules that will generate alerts or reminders. An example of the creation of an MLM in the Arden syntax is given in Panel 16.2.

4.3 Autonomous Systems

When solicited and unsolicited advice systems are used, it are still physicians and nurses who decide on how to act on the provided advice (see also the issue of responsibility, which is briefly discussed in Chapter 15, Section 4.2.3). When the advice is directly applied by the system, however, we speak of *autonomous systems*. Prototypes of autonomous systems have been developed in the domains of anesthesia, ventilator control, and drug delivery. These systems measure certain parameters at regular times and then decide whether the current treatment needs to be adapted. When a change is indicated, the system will adapt the setting of, for example, the infusion pump or the ventilator, to bring the observed parameters within the target range. A risk of autonomous systems is that, in addition to the condition of the patient as a cause of abnormal parameter values, failure of equipment or transducers may also cause faulty parameters. These systems therefore need additional knowledge to make their decisions, for example, information on the shape of a blood pressure signal to accommodate signal validation.

The development of autonomous systems has triggered a discussion on whether DSSs are to be considered a service or a device. In the United States this distinction is particularly relevant, because the safety requirements for a device are much stricter than those for a service.

16

PANEL 16.2

Rules in the Arden Syntax

The *Arden syntax* supports the generation of rules for alerts or reminders. This Panel provides an example of how to write rules in the Arden syntax that monitor potassium levels in patients treated with a thiazide diuretic.

Thiazide diuretics may cause a decrease in potassium levels. If the serum potassium level decreases during a treatment with a thiazide diuretic, the clinician wishes to receive a warning indicating the diuretic as a possible cause. In addition, when starting treatment with thiazides, the clinician wants a baseline measurement of the serum potassium level.

In the example, only the medical logic of the medical logic modules (*MLMs*) is defined; other slots in the MLM, such as *author* and *maintenance,* are omitted. Braces are used in the Arden syntax to identify institution-specific components of the MLM (such as queries to a patient database). To detect a low potassium level and to identify thiazides as a possible cause, the following MLM is created:

```
DATA:
    POTAS-STORAGE := event {serum potassium}
    POTAS := LAST {serum potassium}
    THIAZIDE-US E := {current prescription for thiazides}
EVOKE:
    POTAS-STORAGE
LOGIC:
    IF POTAS < 3 THEN CONCLUDE TRUE
    ELSE CONCLUDE FALSE
ACTION:
    SEND "Patient is hypokalemic. This condition could be caused by thiazides."
```

This MLM will be executed each time that a serum potassium level is stored in the database (the EVOKE slot). The patient data required are the last serum potassium value and whether the patient uses thiazide diuretics (the DATA slot). If the last potassium level is less than 3 (the LOGIC slot), an alert is sent to the clinician (the ACTION slot). The following statements specify that the potassium level must be measured when treatment with a thiazide is initiated:

```
DATA:
    THIAZIDE-START := event {start of prescription for thiazides}
    POTAS := LAST {serum potassium}
EVOKE:
    THIAZIDE-START
LOGIC:
    IF POTAS OCCURRED WITHIN 2 MONTHS PRECEDING NOW THEN CONCLUDE FALSE
    ELSE CONCLUDE TRUE
ACTION:
    SEND "When starting a treatment with thiazides, obtain a baseline measurement of the potassium level."
```

This MLM will be executed each time a patient is started on thiazide diuretics (the EVOKE slot). The patient data required involve the last serum potassium value (the DATA slot). If the last potassium value is older than 2 months (the LOGIC slot), an alert is sent to the clinician (the ACTION slot).

5 Current Trends

In discussions about computer-based DSSs, a recurring theme is that thus far these systems have failed to gain widespread acceptance by clinicians. The ultimate goal of developing DSSs is, of course, that they be used by clinicians. One of the characteristics of our technological era, however, seems to be that developments may take decades to mature. The development of CPRs constitutes an example of decades of research that has not yet resulted in systems that are in widespread use. In a number of countries, however, a rapid dissemination of CPRs has already been accomplished (see Chapters 7, 11, and 29). In The Netherlands, for example, general practitioners are replacing paper-based records with CPRs. The same holds for the United Kingdom and some Scandinavian countries.

We need to refrain from making the issue of present utilization the sole indicator of success of DSSs; actual utilization is often the final phase of a long process. It is important, however, to understand why clinical DSSs have a low frequency of utilization; each failed attempt contains valuable lessons.

It seems that two major *paradigms* were governing initial research on DSSs:

1. The notion that expertise could be extracted from medical experts by the experts developing DSSs (generally called **knowledge engineers**); the underlying assumption was that the medical expert was able to articulate his or her expertise in such a way that the knowledge engineer could cast that expertise in the formalism of a decision model.

2. Once the knowledge was cast in a system, the expertise would be available in a consultation-style interaction with the nonexpert. The nonexpert would then have the expertise of the expert readily available in the form of an "**expert system**."

In retrospect, both *paradigms* are no longer valid. The role of the expert as the sole or dominant source of medical knowledge has been abandoned. There are several reasons for this:

1. Initial ideas about how to represent knowledge were too simple; for example, the notion of **production rules** as "independent chunks of knowledge" was both a poor model of human expertise and a poor model for implementing complex systems.

2. The intra- and interobserver **variabilities** of medical expertise have been known for decades; different experts will judge identical situations differently, and the same expert often judges a situation differently when facing the same situation a second time (see also the remarks in Chapter 15 on human recognition). The consequences of this inter- and intraobserver variability, however, were largely ignored when systems were built.

3. Medical practice is only in part scientific, but primarily based on empirical evidence. Although, ideally, treatments are based on scientific data, in reality many decisions are made in the absence of scientific data. Medical decisions can often be understood only in the environment or context in which they were made.

4. Research has shown that the explanation given by experts about how a decision was made does often not reflect the actual reasoning in making that decision, a phenomenon known as "the paradox of expertise."

The paradigm of making the expertise available in a consultation-style interaction with the system has also been largely abandoned. This also holds for systems that were originally stand alone systems, such as QMR. Although a valid paradigm for research, it was insufficient in a practical setting. The intellect of the user was largely ignored in this approach; this prompted Miller to state that DSSs should not be "*Greek Oracles*" from which users solicit advice (see Sections 2.1 and 2.2 of Chapter 17). In addition, DSSs were often not integrated with other systems; as a result, all patient data had to be entered by the clinician. Many researchers have identified this failure to integrate systems as one of the causes of the low acceptability of these systems.

16

As old paradigms are discarded, new ones emerge. Two complementary paradigms are emerging in the area of clinical DSSs:

- First, those who develop systems for actual use increasingly focus on the environment and setting in which medical decisions are made. That is, the DSS's emphasis shifted from casting medical knowledge in some formalism to enabling clinicians and other health care professionals to improve the delivery of care and to improve communication and interaction. As a result, it will be increasingly difficult to separate the DSS from the environment in which it is embedded. This trend is emerging in many ways: electrocardiographs incorporate software that interprets the ECG recording, CPRs generate unsolicited advice or critiques, systems that support treatment protocols are interwoven with patient records, and so forth.
- The second change involves the *modeling* of medical knowledge and how to apply it to different settings. The emphasis will be on modeling medical knowledge as it emerges from research, as it is transferred between clinicians, and as it is taught to students. This is more than a subtle change when compared to the notion of modeling the knowledge of a specific expert or group of experts. Many early

expert systems with a focus on individual expertise did not attempt to document the source of the knowledge in, for example, references to the medical literature. When medical knowledge, however, becomes the subject of modeling, the justification of that knowledge should be part and parcel of the models.

Key References

Middleton B, Detmer WM, Musen MA. Diagnostic decision support. In: Osheroff JE, ed. *Computers in Clinical Practice: Managing Patients, Information, and Communication.* Philadelphia: American College of Physicians, 1995:59-75.

Miller RA, Pople HE, Myers JD. Internist-1: An experimental computer-based diagnostic consultant for general internal medicine. N Engl Med 1982;307:468-76.

Miller PL. *Expert Critiquing Systems: Practice-Based Medical Consultation by Computer.* New York NY: Springer-Verlag, 1986.

See the Web site for further literature references.

17 Strategies for Medical Knowledge Acquisition

1 Introduction

This chapter describes the inner core of a symbolic decision-support system (**DSS**): the knowledge base (**KB**) that contains all the knowledge and experience to be invoked by a reasoning program to produce advice that supports a decision. The quality of an advice generated by a DSS depends heavily on the availability of high-quality medical knowledge, as represented in the KB. This chapter deals with problems related to acquiring such knowledge and gives an overview of developments that can be used to reach that goal. The topics covered include:

- information needs (clinical questions related to patient care) and problem solving,
- types and examples of medical KBs,
- problems of medical KB maintenance,
- delivery of medical KBs to clinical practice and
- evaluation of medical KBs.

A medical KB is here defined as:

a systematically organized collection of medical knowledge that is accessible electronically and interpretable by the computer.

A medical KB usually:

- includes a lexicon (vocabulary of allowed terms) and
- specifies relationships between terms in the lexicon.

For example, in a diagnostic KB, terms might include patient findings (e.g., fever or pleural friction rub), disease names (e.g., nephrolithiasis or lupus cerebritis) and diagnostic procedure names (e.g., abdominal auscultation or chest *computed tomography*).

1.1 Sources of Medical Knowledge

Medical knowledge is, generally, retrievable from:

- the medical literature (documented knowledge) and
- experts in a specific domain (clinical experience).

However, neither current medical literature nor experience from experts is expressed in a form that is accessible electronically. Therefore, mechanisms must be developed to facilitate the collection and electronic dissemination of medical knowledge. Such mechanisms, however, go beyond the current standard of printed journals or the way that experts transfer their experience from one person to another. One such mechanism is the creation of KBs, which can potentially provide physicians and other health care workers with instantaneous access to large bodies of information. Knowledge from the medical literature must then be expressed in the terminology of the KB and methods must be designed to acquire knowledge from experts.

1.2 Distribution of Medical Knowledge

Starting in the mid-1970s, a growing number of KBs have been developed in the health sciences. Such KBs often include combinations of:

- literature data (from journal articles and textbooks) and
- factual data (e.g., guided by experts and derived from well-documented patient cases).

Large KBs under active development have the potential for becoming national and international repositories of medical knowledge. For example, the American Board of Family Practice has proposed to develop a knowledge base of all of family medicine that can serve both as a reference for standard general practice and that also can be the basis for a computer-based recertification examination for all family physicians in the United States.

2 Information Needs and Problem Solving

The goal of medical KB construction and maintenance is to address one or more clinical information needs and to solve specific problems experienced by health care practitioners or researchers. The context for medical KB development should therefore be well-founded in research on real-world health care information needs and in the theory and practice of human problem solving. A model for DSSs and medical KB usage should include:

- a problem description,
- a method of solving the problem,
- the intended user community and
- the anticipated assets that the user and the system bring to bear in solving a problem.

People and particularly experienced clinicians, are capable of reasoning with incomplete and imprecise information and they often make clinical judgments even at a time when they have unfulfilled information needs. As was demonstrated by Covell, Uman and Manning, clinicians are often unable to identify prospectively the information sources they should use during clinical practice. A fair number of information needs go unmet in the setting of a busy practice. Data generated by Williamson and colleagues suggest that unmet information needs may compromise care.

Information needs in an academic health center were identified and classified by Osheroff and colleagues during the practice of patient care, using participant observation, a standard anthropological technique. They identified three components of comprehensive information needs:

1. currently satisfied information needs (information recognized as relevant and already known to the clinician),
2. consciously recognized information needs (information recognized as important, but not known by the clinician) and
3. unrecognized information needs (information important for the clinician to solve a problem at hand, but not recognized as such by the clinician).

They noted the difficulty that humans and machines have in tailoring general medical knowledge to specific clinical cases. The dilemma is that there may be a wealth of information in a patient record and also a large medical literature describing causes of the patient's problems, but it is problematic to quickly and efficiently reconcile the patient data with the available knowledge. Timpka and colleagues have analyzed information needs arising in the clinical setting by videotaping clinician-patient encounters and subsequently debriefing the clinicians to determine the reasons for their actions as they were recorded by the camera. They verified that a considerable number of information needs go unmet.

The key question is whether the unmet information needs would substantially alter the *quality of care* delivered. In many instances, there is more than one solution to a clinical problem. In other words, the solution of the clinical problem is not always unambiguous. For instance, it may be acceptable to give the second-best therapy if the patient is likely to respond anyway. Clinical experience often plays a key role in selecting one solution from many possible ones. Therefore, developers of DSSs and their underlying medical KBs must take into account the considerable knowledge and intelligence that the human user can contribute to a medical DSS.

2.1 Decision-Support Systems as Greek Oracles

In the early years of developing DSSs and medical KBs, researchers hoped to be able to realize systems that could support or even replace human decision making, not fully realizing the incompleteness of patient data and medical knowledge, the unrecognized information needs of clinicians and the ambiguous character of medical decision making (see also Section 4.2 of Chapter 16). Perhaps such researchers had the idea in mind to develop a medical version of the Greek Oracle, to which problems could be posed and from which answers could be obtained (albeit not always unambiguous answers).

Having gained more basic insight into computer-based decision support in health care, developers abandoned the Greek Oracle model by the early 1990s. Over the years, several DSSs evolved along the way of this better insight into usable medical DSSs. For example, the style of diagnostic consultation in the original 1974 *INTERNIST-I* program viewed the clinician as unable to solve a diagnostic problem. The model assumed that the clinician would transfer all patient history informa-

tion, physical examination findings and laboratory data to the INTERNIST-I diagnostic consultant program. After patient data entry, the clinician's subsequent role was that of a passive observer, answering "yes" or "no" to questions generated by INTERNIST-I. Ultimately, the omniscient Greek Oracle (i.e., the consultant program) was supposed to provide the correct diagnoses and their probabilities of occurrence and to explain its reasoning.

2.2 Shortcomings of Decision-Support Systems

There were fatal flaws in the Greek Oracle model. A clinician cannot convey his or her complete understanding of a patient case to a computer program. One can never assume that a computer program "knows" all that needs to be known about the individual patient case, no matter how much time and effort it takes to enter data into the computer. On the contrary, a clinician who evaluates the patient's problems must be considered the primary source of information about the patient during the entire course of any computer-based consultation. In addition, the highly skilled health care practitioner who understands the patient as a person possesses the most important knowledge and experience to be employed during a consultation. Besides, only the practitioner – and not the computer – bears responsibility for the medical decisions and the care given to the patient. The user should intellectually control the process of computer-based consultation, in a way, in a manner similar to a pilot controlling a complex aircraft.

The training and experience of anticipated system users must be taken into consideration in DSS and medical KB development. Experts reason more efficiently than novices in diagnostic settings, because they possess a greater store of compiled knowledge and experience, a more seasoned knowledge of pathophysiology and a broader array of strategic approaches. DSSs should, at best, behave as novices in patient care.

17

3 Categories of Decision-Support Systems and Medical Knowledge Bases

At present, modeling of medical knowledge appears to be an inexact science. Past and present DSSs incorporate imperfect models of the incompletely understood and exceptionally complex processes of medical diagnosis, therapy and prognosis. Although computers are able to perform a number of impressive tasks fast and accurately, there is one task that computers cannot do well, if at all. This task is to synthesize or deduce medical knowledge either from basic principles or from poorly organized patient databases (see also Fig. 1.1). Medically useful computer programs, whether intended for education or for clinical decision making, must obtain their medical KBs externally, that is, from humans, either directly from experts or indirectly from scientific studies reported in the literature. A medical computer program can only be as good – or as bad – as its underlying medical KB.

3.1 Types of Decision-Support Systems

In a review of reasoning strategies employed by early DSS systems, Shortliffe and colleagues identified the following classes of DSS systems (we list some examples that are partly discussed in Chapter 16):

- Clinical *algorithms*
  Example: rules that determine the generation of warnings or alarms in patient monitoring (see also Section 2 of Chapter 12 and Chapters 15 and 16).
- Clinical databases that include analytical functions
  example: a database of drugs containing rules for *drug-drug interactions* (see also Chapter 13).
- Mathematical pathophysiological models
  Example: pharmacokinetic models to compute the effect of drug infusions (see also Chapter 13).
- *Pattern recognition* systems

Example: the *classification* of white blood cells according to type (e.g., neutrophils, eosinophils, leukocytes) (see Chapter 9).
- *Bayesian* statistical systems
  Example: the classification of *ECGs* by statistical decision algorithms (see Chapter 12).
- *Decision-analytical* systems
  Example: computation of risk involved in surgical interventions (see Chapter 18).
- *Symbolic reasoning* or "expert" systems
  Example: the *INTERNIST-I/QMR* system to diagnose cases in internal medicine (see also Panel 16.1 of Chapter 16).

Symbolic reasoning or knowledge-based systems can further be categorized according to their underlying *inferencing* methods. The oldest forms of knowledge-based systems include *rule-based* systems, *frame-based* systems and ad-hoc *heuristic systems* that run as consultation programs. *Critiquing* models (see Chapter 15) offered an advance over the traditional consultation system, by providing decision support only when the user requests it or when the program deems that advice is particularly needed. In recent years, there has been increased interest in the use of *Bayesian belief networks* (which overcome the limitations of ad hoc schemes for representation of uncertainty) and in non-symbolic approaches, such as artificial *neural networks* – which are particularly well suited to perform multivariate classification tasks when there may be strong interaction affects among the input variables. As discussed in Chapter 28, current work on symbolic knowledge-based systems emphasizes principled architectures that allow developers to map explicit domain descriptions (ontologies) onto the data requirements of domain-independent, reusable, problem-solving methods.

The spectrum of knowledge contained in medical KBs parallels that contained in DSSs. Some medical KBs are

17

developed primarily as repositories of medical knowledge (examples include *MEDLINE*, *PDQ*, INTERNIST-I/QMR and *repositories* of patient cases). Such systems are often based on the medical literature and expert opinions, combined in a manner that can be replicated at sites remote from the original site of creation of the KB. Other KBs are developed more directly to support implementation of a specific system (such as training sets for artificial *neural networks* or rule bases for production systems). Simple *branching logic* programs require an in-depth understanding of the domain at hand and may be based on the opinions of a small number of experts.

3.2 Quality of Data Underlying Knowledge Bases

The usefulness of decision-support systems depends on a number of factors, including the quality of the data that are input into the system in the first place, the ability of the end-user to believe in and to interpret the results and the manner in which users interact with the system. Despite all these complexities there is no question that the value of any DSS will be constrained by the domain knowledge that is represented in the underlying system.

3.2.1 Patient Data Repositories

Although not knowledge-based systems, large databases have long been used as vehicles for decision support. Overcoming biases in data collection is essential before such systems can be used to aid prospective decision making. For example, for patient data *repositories*, such as the Duke Cardiovascular Diseases Databank, entry criteria and concise definitions of the patients' clinical parameters to be collected, have carefully been defined and they often represent the level of rigor present in controlled *clinical trials*. The utility of such repositories for diagnosis, therapy selection and prognosis is substantial, because patients can be matched with groups of similar other patients with a high degree of confidence. However, patient databases based on large health insurance data sets or on semi-controlled entry of patient parameters into a clinically

useful medical information system are less reliable than patient data repositories, because there are significant problems with definitional issues (e.g., does the patient really have the diagnosis stated in the patient record when uniform criteria for diagnosis have not been applied?) and completeness of data collection (e.g., the patient diagnosis and therapy involve arbitrary selection of some but not all possible interventions as part of a workup or follow-up).

3.2.2 Statistics for Bayesian Systems

The KBs required for Bayesian systems consist of probabilities, but there are few areas of medicine where controlled trials yield such information with more than one significant digit. In reviewing the medical literature related to diagnoses over the past two decades, it has been found that probabilistic information for diagnoses, in aggregate, has a resolution of about one part in five (i.e., plus or minus 10%). Humans are notoriously inaccurate sources of probabilistic information and when medical experts are relied upon as the source of probabilistic information for Bayesian systems or *Bayesian belief networks*, inaccuracies may become problematic. Developers of Bayes' networks argue, however, that probabilisitic inference based on biased, subjective probabilities is far superior to reasoning under uncertainty in the absence of *any probabilistic information at all*. They point to the potential use of sensitivity analysis to help users identify situations when a Bayesian system's conclusions are clearly off the mark and maintain that subjective probabilities based on an experts' analysis of a particular situation may be much more valuable than would be data from controlled experiments that could never capture the nuances of the circumstances at hand.

3.2.3 Training Artificial Neural Networks

Equally difficult is the accumulation of a large number of adequately characterized real patient cases to be used as the training set for an artificial neural network. Often, the best sources of data for such systems are the data sets collected for randomized controlled trials, or cases from patient repositories. The problem is that

17

such training sets create is **case mix**: Entry criteria for studies often exclude representative samples of healthy individuals and neural nets trained on **skewed data** sets may not behave appropriately in a general clinical setting. Of course, the use of representative training sets is an important issue for all **multivariate** classifiers, including systems based on more traditional, statistical pattern-recognition techniques (see Chapter 27).

3.2.4   Maintenance of Knowledge Bases

As KBs grow in number and size, it becomes essential to establish processes that can ensure their consistency and accuracy. Many KBs are constructed in an ad-hoc fashion and standards for the systematic validation of their contents do not yet exist. The development of reliable methods that can be used to build and maintain large collections of data is vital for the future of medical KBs and medical practice. Large-scale KBs cannot be assembled and maintained by a single individual; instead, they should be built through a collaborative effort. Once a project has created and tested its KB representation format and developmental methods and has demonstrated the clinical and educational utility of its KB, groups of individuals from diverse geographic sites (possibly at the level of professional societies) should be able to contribute to the project's KB construction and maintenance.

4   Medical Knowledge Bases and Medical Knowledge Acquisition

Development of real-world diagnostic systems involves a constant balancing of theory (model complexity) and practicality (the ability to construct and maintain adequate medical databases or KBs, as well as the ability to create systems that respond to users' needs in an acceptably short time interval). In theory we understand how to develop systems that take into account gradations of symptoms, the degree of uncertainty in the patient or the clinician regarding a finding, the severity of each illness under consideration, the pathophysiological mechanisms of disease, or the time course of illnesses. However, it is not yet practical to build such broad-based systems for patient care. Early system developers faced such constraints, yet made far-reaching discoveries.

The collection of the knowledge contained in the KBs resembles that for other activities in health care in which knowledge is brought together. Several of these activities are reviewed in the following sections.

4.1 Practice Guidelines

Some of the problems in KB construction are analogous to those found in other information-gathering activities within medicine. One close analogy is the establishment of regional or national practice guidelines for medical practice. Various organizations use different methods to develop practice guidelines, such as:

- combinations of formal or informal reviews of the literature,
- expert review panels and consensus meetings,
- consultations with local experts, and
- early publication in medical journals to stimulate discussion.

To date, no objective evaluation of the effectiveness of the various methods has been conducted.

4.2 Meta Analysis

Another analogous activity is **meta-analysis**. This is a discipline, whose broadest definition is

a discipline that critically reviews and statistically combines the results of previous research.

By meta-analysis one attempts to draw conclusions by combining different studies (usually randomized clinical trials) reported in the medical literature. Although the activity of combining different results is so important in medicine as to be ubiquitous, it is usually conducted in an information and error-prone fashion. Meta-analysis provides useful guidelines to improve the activity and avoid the classic pitfalls that beset the informal approach. The reproducibility of meta-analysis techniques has been reviewed by Chalmers and colleagues, who presented useful guidelines for achieving more standardized meta-analyses.

4.3 Quality of Knowledge Sources

Another activity that is important for the creation of medical KBs that are based on the medical literature is the evaluation of the quality of different sources. The everincreasing volume of published medical knowledge is creating considerable interest in measures of the relative quality of the literature. Such measures could be used, for example, to locate the most relevant references for a specific medical question. Quality measures that operate at the level of entire articles, however, may be too imprecise. Several articles, for example, present authoritative descriptions of the results of a diagnostic procedure, but only cursory descriptions of the physical signs associated with a particular disease. Research in knowledge acquisition deals with a variety of practical and theoretical issues, ranging from knowledge representation to the verification of the completeness and correctness of a KB. Knowledge acquisition in medicine has become an important research area in its own right.

4.4 Two Knowledge Sources

Knowledge acquisition in medicine has taken diverse forms, but in general it can be divided into two categories according to the source of medical knowledge:

1. In the first category, knowledge is obtained from clinical experts, either following the classic interaction between a system analyst and a clinical expert or by allowing the expert to interact directly with the KB by using a knowledge-editing program.
2. In the second category, knowledge is obtained primarily from the published medical literature, generally by clinicians who conduct extensive reviews of the published material about a certain topic. As previously noted, the field of meta-analysis has followed this latter path.

Independent of the methodology, the construction of high-quality medical KBs entails large investments in time and effort. For instance, more than 35 person-years of effort have been devoted to building and maintaining the QMR KB; developers of *ILIAD* estimate that more than 50,000 hours of effort have gone into developing its KB. Identical efforts are reported in the field of computer-assisted ECG interpretation.

4.5 Tools for Knowledge Acquisition

The traditional methodology, requiring intense cooperation between a computer expert and a medical expert, created a severe bottleneck because the two experts had to reach a common understanding before progress could be made. The response to this problem has been to allow medical experts to create KBs directly, without computer experts as intermediaries. The resulting programs are often called *knowledge-based editors* (*KBEs*).

Despite intense research, few KBEs have been used in the sustained construction of large-scale KBs; most are limited by their inability to modify and maintain a KB over a period of years. Musen and colleagues have pioneered the development of knowledge acquisition tools for medical protocols that contain detailed models of the types and uses of knowledge in each application domain, but for the most part, these methods have not yet been used by the developers of more general medical KBs. Creating tools that fully support large-scale KB construction has been and continues to be one of the main goals of the research of the authors of this chapter.

17

A limitation of present-day KBEs is that they do little to help clinicians to locate and process the relevant knowledge, an activity that typically dominates knowledge acquisition time. Each new disease profile created for the *QMR* KB, for example, requires an average of 10 to 20 days of full-time effort to analyze the medical literature. To reduce the effort related to knowledge acquisition, future systems should help clinicians locate the relevant information. Automated or semiautomated text analysis systems that quickly locate the portions of medical articles that are most likely to contain relevant information could prove to be a valuable tool in this regard. Creating such systems, however, is very complicated, both because of technical difficulties and because of the difficult problem of vocabulary mapping.

As a direct function of the desire to process medical texts electronically, interest in different aspects of the vocabulary mapping problem has grown considerably in recent years. Research includes the ability to browse existing controlled vocabularies to look for best matches, expressing problem lists and using controlled vocabularies as the structuring mechanism through which users can input terms they would otherwise have expressed in natural language.

Over the years a number of research systems have explored different strategies and different philosophies for knowledge acquisition. In Panels 17.1 to 17.4 some different key themes are presented, exemplified by various systems.

5 Trends in Knowledge Acquisition

The examples presented in Panels 17.1 to 17.4 indicate the wide array of possible strategies for knowledge acquisition. Despite the differences, some general lessons can be drawn:

• Creation of expert systems by domain experts
One of the clear trends has been toward removing the "analyst" (earlier: the *knowledge engineer*) from the knowledge acquisition process, enabling domain experts to create and edit KBs directly.
• High-level representation
A second, related theme is the gradual, but obvious move away from the internal representation (e.g., production rules and backward chaining) to more abstract representation including domain-level concepts (e.g., disorders, test results and pathogens). Clearly, this shift is necessary if medical domain experts are to be able to manipulate KBs directly.
• Better user interfaces
Another trend has been toward easier to use point-and-click interfaces; this is shown by all modern systems, such as *OPAL* and *QMR-KAT.*
• Use of natural language
Finally, there is continued hope for some form of natural language processing, which was relatively primitive

in early systems such as TEIRESIAS (see Panel 17.1). Unfortunately, however, the current state of the art in natural language processing is far from the ability to support natural, unrestricted text input. Clearly, if natural language processing were to mature rapidly, it would open up huge potential opportunities for knowledge acquisition.

Other important themes that have emerged more recently are toward the collaborative creation of KBs and toward ways to ensure that the knowledge acquisition process itself is reproducible. For medical KB construction to become reproducible, several requirements must be met:

• The purpose of the KB must be explicitly stated;
• The components of the KB must be carefully defined;
• Reliable sources of information must be available;
• Methods for resolving conflicts must be applied when the information from separate sources differs; and
• The procedures for reviewing, testing, and updating the KB contents must be clearly delineated, tested over time and revised on the basis of performance with actual patient cases.

17

PANEL 17.1

TEIRESIAS

The system *TEIRESIAS*, developed by Davis, was developed as an experimental knowledge acquisition system for the rule-based expert system *MYCIN*. TEIRESIAS was among the first systems to introduce explicitly the notion of computer-assisted knowledge acquisition, that is, the use of computer programs to help experts enter new knowledge. The system used a debugging context to guide knowledge acquisition by assuming that the expert was repairing a diagnostic problem by attempting to find the rule (or rules) responsible for the incorrect behavior. Use of a specific context has the advantage of simplifying the task of the system considerably, although it does not lend itself well to situations in which entirely new knowledge needs to be added to a KB.

The system also discerned between knowledge and meta-knowledge. The former provides the medical content needed by an expert system for sound medical reasoning. The latter is used to control and guide the expert system's progress toward its goals, choosing the most appropriate strategy. Meta-knowledge was expressed in TEIRESIAS as "rule models," which were compact descriptions of the structure, organization, or content of a group of related rules. Davis realized that meta-knowledge could be useful in guiding the knowledge acquisition process itself, guiding the KBE to assume that the new rules entered by the system's user were consonant with previously entered rules, requiring the medical expert to understand the underlying production rules and their behavior; as such, this strategy would not be suitable for medical experts who lack a precise understanding of the control strategy used by *backward-chaining* expert systems (see Chapter 15).

Successful collaboration on medical KB construction requires that individual contributions be of consistently high quality, regardless of who creates them. The ability to replicate, in a scientific manner, KB construction is thus an important determinant of the quality and viability of any KB. Panel 17.5 describes a study of a collaborative effort to obtain reliable medical knowledge. Other issues for future KB construction are listed in the following sections.

5.1 Reproducibility

Objective evaluations of the reproducibility of KB construction have important consequences for the future of computer-based medical applications. Such applications require KBs containing precise descriptions of the relevant medical facts. So far, lack of documented reproducibility in the construction of certain medical KBs may have hindered their widespread diffusion. If reproducibility for a given KB can be shown, however, different groups of qualified individuals may be able to collaborate toward the construction and maintenance of that medical KB. Computer-based medical consultant systems and national and international medical KBs that use such reproducible KBs would then become feasible and would have lasting value as tools for the timely dissemination of current and reliable information.

5.2 Textual Sources

One recurring theme for KB acquisition research is the use of textual materials as sources of knowledge. More and more interest is now evident in the use of on-line full-text medical material to facilitate knowledge acquisition.

17

PANEL **17.2**

OPAL

OPAL is an interactive, graphical knowledge acquisition system for the cancer therapy management program ONCOCIN. OPAL recognizes that few medical experts can be expected to have substantial computer science backgrounds. Rather than taking an approach similar to the one in TEIRESIAS, therefore, OPAL attempts to require only knowledge of the medical domain of the experts that use it. In addition, the system uses intuitive point-and-click form-filling interfaces that mimic closely the paper forms that are already familiar to oncologists. When necessary, procedural knowledge (the equivalent of a short program) is also specified graphically via a *flowchart*-like visual programming language that supports conditions and loops.

Strong assumptions about the domain (protocol design for oncology) make it possible for OPAL to perform effectively. The system generates an expert system that uses a fixed problem-solving model (skeletal plan refinement) and is tailored for the ONCOCIN framework. Musen showed that, using OPAL, oncologists could generate working expert systems (that is, versions of ONCOCIN customized to manage specific oncology protocols) in only a fraction of the time that it would have taken with conventional knowledge acquisition methodologies involving expert-knowledge engineer interactions.

This interest is based on the expectation that more and more full-text material will be available electronically. availability of full on-line text will enable future semiautomatic or automatic extraction of information.

5.3 Electronic Journals

On-line abstracts available from *AIDSLINE* and MEDLINE are generally inadequate for medical KB construction. However, certain commercially available bibliographic retrieval systems (e.g., CD-PLUS/BRS Colleague and Dialog) and several specialty-specific CD-ROM vendors already distribute full-text articles and books. In some cases, entire families of journals are becoming available on-line. For instance, the full text of the *New England Journal of Medicine*, complete with Figures, is available electronically. Textbooks are also becoming increasingly available. An increasing number of "electronic journals," such as *the Online Journal of Current Clinical Trials* (OJCCT), are published exclusively in electronic form and the text of more traditional journals such as *Science* and the *New England Journal of Medicine* are readily available on the **World Wide Web**. This trend toward increasing

5.4 Free-Text Analysis

Research on the computer-based analysis of medical texts has been carried out over the past three decades. Much current research is devoted to the extraction of specific medical concepts from free text. The semantics of medical concepts are typically expressed either by mapping expressions directly into terms in a controlled vocabulary or by using intermediate representations. Intermediate representations are often based on research on knowledge representation, much of which was influenced by the desire to encode the semantic knowledge contained in natural language (and not necessarily medical) texts. **Conceptual graphs** are a popular, logic-based representation language that has been used in several text-processing research projects in medicine. Frame-like representations of medical ontologies have been used in machine-translation research to act as the *interlingua* between two natural languages and in

PANEL 17.3

PROTÉGÉ-I

After the completion of OPAL, Musen undertook a new research effort to generalize the results of that project in a way that would be applicable to a number of related knowledge-based systems. The resulting system, PROTÉGÉ-I, can be described as a high-level tool that generates knowledge acquisition tools similar to those generated by OPAL (which itself generates specialized knowledge-based systems). The domain of the generated knowledge-based systems is clinical trials, similar to that of OPAL. PROTÉGÉ-I itself, however, is domain independent and can be used for other, related knowledge acquisition tasks. The system achieves much of its generality by adopting an externalized representation (e.g., information entered by the user is stored externally in a *relational database*) and an explicit model of how different slots in a form can communicate with each other. PROTÉGÉ-I achieves good levels of performance by being restricted to a specific problem-solving model-skeletal plan refinement, which not surprisingly, is the model supported by ONCOCIN. (Subsequent work in Musen's laboratory has resulted in a successor to PROTÉGÉ-I that can generate knowledge-based systems that incorporate arbitrary reusable problem-solving methods; see Chapter 28).

The highly abstract nature of PROTÉGÉ-I enables it to achieve remarkable reductions in the time to create a new expert system. Consider, for example, that adding a new cancer protocol to ONCOCIN by using the conventional knowledge acquisition method required several weeks or even months (a *systems analyst* had to be intimately involved). OPAL allowed an oncology specialist to enter a complete protocol in just a few hours; however, changing ONCOCIN to work on a different task would have required several months of programming time. With PROTÉGÉ-I, however, a system like OPAL may be generated. As a feasibility demonstration, Musen also showed that PROTÉGÉ-I could be used to generate a knowledge-based editor for a different domain (clinical trials for antihypertensive drugs) for which the same problem-solving method was appropriate.

medical informatics research to act as the interlingua between two or more controlled medical vocabularies. Based on this considerable interest and level of activity, it is to be expected that the next 5 to 10 years will see the advent of practical, large-scale KB construction methods that increasingly rely on textual analysis as a key source of data and knowledge.

5.5 Prestored Bibliographic Search Logic

A related aspect of knowledge acquisition is the use of prestored search logic as a mechanism for accessing new medical information as it gets published. This mechanism can facilitate finding the most appropriate texts to be used as described above. This idea has already been used in the past, to a limited extent, for routine knowledge maintenance tasks, using the *MeSH* search logic (see Chapter 6) that is stored with each QMR disease description. Their goal, however, was to locate bibliographic references, because on-line texts were not available at that time. *NLM* already supports a service known as Selective Dissemination of Information (*SDI* services). SDI services allow user-defined searches to be run automatically every month on an NLM database and send the results of the search to the user for manual examination. There will be

17

PANEL 17.4

INTERNIST-I/QMR

The knowledge acquisition methodology for the *INTERNIST-I/QMR* knowledge base was originally developed by Myers in the early 1970s and has been used continuously for nearly three decades. Philosophically, this strategy is based on the idea that the published medical literature is, in the aggregate, the most reliable available source of medical knowledge. This strategy places less emphasis on an individual expert's opinion than on other knowledge acquisition strategies.

For each new disease profile, the following steps are followed:

1. A volunteer selects a disease or clinical syndrome not yet described in the INTERNIST-I/QMR knowledge base.
2. The volunteer conducts a comprehensive survey of the medical literature on the diagnosis of the disorder. Textbooks are first examined, and then the volunteer reviews an average of 50 to 100 journal articles from the literature regarding diagnosis of the disorder. One to 2 weeks of full-time effort are usually required. The goal of the literature review is to create a list of the clinical abnormalities (findings) that have been reliably and verifiably reported to occur in patients with the given illness.
3. Medical experts specializing in the diagnosis and care of patients with the disorder are consulted to clarify problems encountered during literature review and to supplement the information obtained by literature review.
4. The net result of literature review and consultation with experts is the creation of a disease profile, a list containing an average of 85 findings per disease (range, 25 to 250 findings per disease). In addition to the findings in a disease profile, "linked diagnoses" are identified. Linked diagnoses are those conditions that predispose an individual to the development ▶

17

increasing research activity in this area, dictated in part by the converging interests of organizations such as NLM and medical KB builders.

5.6 Knowledge Base Maintenance

KB maintenance is critical to the continued clinical validity of a DSS. Yet, it is hard to judge when new medical knowledge becomes an established "fact." The first reports of new clinical discoveries in highly regarded medical journals must await confirmation by other groups over time before their content can be added to a medical KB. KB construction must be a scientifically reproducible process that can be accomplished by qualified individuals at any site. If the process of KB construction is highly dependent on a single individual or can only be carried out at a single institution, then the survival of that system over time is in jeopardy. Although much of the excitement generated by computer-based decision-support systems lies in the computer algorithms and interfaces, the long-term value and viability of a system depend on the quality, accuracy and timeliness of its KB.

of the disease under consideration, are causally related to the disease, occur more often than chance in association with the disease, or temporally precede the development of the disease.

5. After a draft of the disease profile has been compiled by literature review and consultation with experts, members of the INTERNIST-I/QMR project team review the profile in a seminar led by the senior clinician.

6. Once a final consensus about the new profile has been achieved, the profile is added to the KB.

7. The new profile is first tested by presenting the system with a "classic" case of a patient with the disease, constructed from a standard textbook description. The system rarely has difficulty concluding the correct diagnosis.

8. The profile is subsequently tested with more difficult CPC (clinicopathological conference) cases.

9. Every 2 to 3 years, the entire series of "classic" cases is again analyzed, to make certain that changes in the KB (made since the original case analyses) have not adversely affected performance with actual cases. Previously run CPC cases are also intermittently reviewed and examined.

In recent years, the methodology described above was augmented with the creation of *QMR-KAT*, a graphical knowledge-based editor program that is specifically tailored to support the creation and maintenance of QMR disease profiles. In addition to allowing creation and editing of disease profiles by using an intuitive interface, QMR-KAT embeds considerable knowledge about the structure and relationships of the QMR knowledge base. It is thus able to perform sophisticated error and consistency checks while the user is working on a profile, preventing a large class of errors and giving helpful warnings to the clinician when some newly entered information could result in an inconsistency. (See Chapter 28 for a discussion of how a tool like QMR-KAT can be created automatically.)

6 Delivery of Medical Knowledge Bases for Clinical Use

17

The use of lexical matching techniques and other straightforward methodologies to achieve impressive levels of diagnostic performance raises a philosophical issue of interest to all DSS developers. Given that no approach to computer-based medical decision support is adequate for all situations, how much reasoning power and how detailed a representation of medical knowledge are enough? Is it adequate to use textual information sources and perform lexical matching between loosely worded summaries of the clinical situation (using synonym mapping), simply to produce a list of possible courses of action for the intelligent and knowledgeable clinician to consider? Or is it necessary to develop extremely detailed and labor-consuming databases and KBs that go far beyond the knowledge of the average clinician to provide assistance in the majority of challenging cases? Although it is a tautology that common things are common, few, if

---

PANEL **17.5**

Interauthor Agreement on KB Construction

It has been shown that medical KB construction can be scientifically reproducible, at least under certain circumstances. A study conducted by the original QMR research team provided a systematic evaluation of interauthor agreement among clinically active clinicians who were asked to consult the medical literature to extract precise diagnostic information for use in a medical KB. The study revealed considerable agreement among the participants.

Despite the number of articles used in the study (a set of 109 articles was given to each profiler) and despite being allowed to consult local experts and medical textbooks, participants used a relatively small number of findings in their disease profiles. Of 4,350 existing QMR findings, the participants used only a total of 252 distinct findings to describe the clinical manifestations of acute perinephric abscess, showing that a relatively small set of findings was sufficient to describe all the diagnostic information found in the articles. The seven participants' selection of findings associated with the disease was significantly different from chance. All participants agreed in their choices 78 times more often than predicted by pure chance; all but one participant agreed 9.8 times more often. Even though six of the participating clinicians had never created a QMR disease profile, their choices showed considerable agreement among themselves and with the choices of an experienced profiler.

---

any, detailed analyses have been carried out to examine the clinical challenges that generalists and specialists encounter or the level of sophistication required to address the majority of such problems. Important research on clinical DSS effectiveness will have to continue and to be extended to answer those questions.

Another critical issue for the success of large-scale, generic DSSs is their environment. Paradoxically, small, limited "niche" systems will be adopted and used by the focused community for which they are intended, although physicians in general medical practice, for whom the large-scale systems are intended, may not need diagnostic assistance on a frequent enough basis to justify the purchase of one or more such systems. Therefore, it is common wisdom that DSSs are most likely to succeed if they can be integrated into a clinical environment so that patient data capture is already performed by automated laboratory or medical information systems. In such an environment, the clinician

will not have to enter all of a patient's data manually to obtain a diagnostic consultation.

However, it is not straightforward to transfer the information about a patient from a medical information system to a diagnostic consultation system. If several dozen arterial blood gas measurements were made during a patient's admission, which one(s) should be transferred to a knowledge-based consultation system: the mean, the extremes, or the value typical for a given time in a patient's illness? Should all findings or only those findings relevant to the patient's current illness be transferred to the consultation system? How should such information about relevance be represented in a KB? How should such questions be answered with a medical KB?

Answers to these questions must be determined by careful studies before one can expect to obtain patient consultations routinely and automatically within the context of a medical information system.

7 Evaluation of Medical Knowledge Bases

Elements of a critical area relevant to all DSS systems are validation, evaluation, and ongoing quality assurance. The medical informatics and clinical communities have not yet fully determined what a proper evaluation of a DSS should entail, although much past and present work has been devoted to this topic.

An issue of *Methods of Information in Medicine* (January 1993) contained a series of editorials on the current state of evaluations of DSS technology. The staged approach to system evaluation proposed by Stead and colleagues summarizes current thinking about this difficult problem. It is clear that a system cannot be validated for use at a single point in time. Just as practicing clinicians in many countries are required to take recertification examinations, it will be necessary to recertify DSSs to document that their performance is up-to-date and as reliable as in the past.

Staged evaluation of knowledge-based systems will require examination of KB elements for validity as facts per se, and KB maintainers will need to keep the KB updated and of appropriate depth and breadth. Because there will always be more detail in the medical literature and in the knowledge of subspecialist experts, the intended scope and relevance of a medical KB to a stated purpose (that is, its form of decision support) are important. A key challenge in the NLM's *UMLS* Information Sources Map project is how to categorize the relevance of a KB or DSS to particular categories of tasks. In a world with ever increasing numbers of electronically available knowledge sources, selecting the best sources with information about a particular problem will be as important as the content of the individual resources themselves.

A strategy for staged evaluation of a knowledge-based system would first look at KB elements for completeness, consistency and relevance to stated objectives. System performance with retrospective, anecdotal cases should be evaluated in an informal manner to determine if the system performance is likely to place patients at increased risk of harm or inappropriate care. Next, careful evaluations with retrospective data should be conducted, preferably by individuals not involved in system construction, maintenance, and marketing. It is important to distinguish between KB-related defects in system performance and algorithm-related flaws in performance. Indeed, it is critical for medical KB maintenance to have as many forms of constructive feedback as possible.

Evaluations of DSSs must be considered in their clinical context. Two KBs are always brought to bear in a computer-based DSS consultation: that of the system and that of the user. The goal is to improve the performance of both the user and the computer over their performance in their native (unassisted) states. The unit of intervention for evaluation studies becomes more complicated for this reason; it must be viewed as human plus machine, not simply the machine analyzing cases in isolation.

17

8 Conclusion

High-quality KBs may eventually become nationally and internationally shared repositories of knowledge that can be used by:

1. diverse groups doing research and development in medical informatics,

2. medical practitioners who require authoritative reference sources, and

3. medical DSSs which require such knowledge as the foundation for clinical decision making.

Medical KBs may eventually combine the ease of

computer-based access and updating with the thoroughness of the published medical literature. They may also provide structured access to the medical literature by indicating which references are most relevant to particular aspects of a given disease.

Widespread distribution of medical KBs could revolutionize the dissemination of medical information, in the manner that the invention of the printing press revolutionized the distribution of books. By editorially reviewing what we know about individual topics in medicine (i.e., by summarizing the peer-reviewed literature and experts' opinions), by placing that knowledge in a format that can be processed by a computer and by documenting how we know what we know (i.e., by providing relevant references), we can overcome the limitations of current print technologies. In an electronic medical KB, all terms can be cross-indexed with one another and dynamically rearranged. The same set of findings that have been reported to occur in patients with a given disorder (disease description) can be presented in multiple ways. The disease description might be sorted for one person to show how patients usually present with the disease (i.e., the most common findings of the disease would be shown first), displayed for another person to show the best tests to be performed to confirm the diagnosis (that is, sorted by descending positive predictive value), or displayed for a third person to indicate common textbook order (history, physical examination, and laboratory results).

The dissemination of knowledge-based systems in medicine has the potential to create stronger ties between academia and clinical practice. The written comments that authors of medical textbooks now receive cannot readily be incorporated into those textbooks, because the interval between textbook revisions is usually several years. However, practicing clinicians can provide valuable feedback regarding medical KBs. Clinicians can identify findings or conditions that they believe are either missing or inappropriately present in medical KBs. Suggestions from the community can be reviewed by the academics maintaining medical KBs and KB updates containing any necessary corrections can be issued electronically.

Key References

Musen, MA. An overview of knowledge acquisition. In: David JM, Krivine JP, Simmons R, eds. *Second Generation Expert Systems.* Berlin: Springer-Verlag, 1993:415-38.

See the Web site for further literature references.

17

18 Predictive Tools for Clinical Decision Support

1 Introduction

Clinicians must continuously make decisions on what diagnostic procedures they should perform and on what therapeutic actions they should take. These decisions are taken with the ultimate aim of improving the patient's prognosis. However, decision making in clinical practice is complicated by uncertainty in many aspects. This includes the diagnosis of the disease of a patient, the best therapy for treating the disease, and the prognosis of the patient given the diagnosis and the therapy. Prediction of diagnostic or therapeutic outcomes may guide this decision making and thus comes may guide this decision making and thus

improve the patient's prognosis. Decision-support tools may provide predictions by using clinical information in a systematic way. These predictions may support clinicians in their decision-making processes. The methods to be discussed in this chapter deal with the management of the clinical care process, assisted by tools that predict the patient's future condition. These methods are an extension of the diagnostic and therapeutic decision-support methods described in Chapters 15 to 17.

2 Development of Predictive Tools

Development of a predictive tool usually involves several steps (see Table 18.1):

1. In the first step, the clinical problem and its specific characteristics must be examined. The decisions must be described clearly, including the potential role of the decision-support tool.
2. Second, a desired clinical outcome that the clinician considers central for decision making and that is thus important to predict must be indicated. Examples of clinical outcomes may include diagnostic categories, such as benign or malignant disease, or treatment outcomes, such as short-term mortality, long-term mortality, complications, or relapse of disease.
3. The third step is determination of the clinical char-

acteristics that might be used as **predictors** of the clinical outcome. These clinical characteristics may include quite diverse features, depending on the particular clinical problem. In oncology, for instance, the extent of disease is often a predictive sign for survival. In many other patient groups, survival will be related to the age of the patient, as well as to indicators of coexisting diseases (comorbidities).

4. Furthermore, the relation between the predictors and the clinical outcome must be quantified. The quantification may be provided by expert clinicians who possess the required clinical knowledge. More often, a data set is used that contains patient records containing the values of both the predictors and the outcome. This data set may be analyzed by statistical tech-

18

Step	Interpretation
Decision	Timing and type; role of the predictive tool
Outcome	Diagnosis; treatment outcome
Predictors	Clinical characteristics related to the outcome
Quantification	Relating predictors to the outcome (expert opinion, regression analysis)
Data set	Data file with patient records containing predictors and the outcome
Presentation	Show results in a readily applicable way (with or without a computer system)

Table 18.1
Overview of the Six Main Steps in the Development of Predictive Tools.

niques (e.g., forms of *regression analysis*) to quantify the relation between predictors and the outcome.

5. Finally, the predictive tool must be presented in a readily applicable way to the decision-making clinician. This presentation does not necessarily include a computer, although a computer is often useful in the development of the tool. Presentations with and without a computer are discussed separately in the following.

Each of these development steps should be validated to guarantee the reliability and accuracy of the predictive tool. The effects of the predictive tool on clinicians and their patients should also be assessed. This evaluation is vital for convincing potential users of the benefits of the predictive tools.

Section 3.1 of Chapter 16 described the decision-support system (*DSS*) of *De Dombal* for the diagnosis of acute abdominal pain. The role of this diagnostic DSS was to support the clinician in making the right diagnosis, so that treatment decisions could be based on this diagnosis to improve the prognosis of the patient. Treatment decisions included, for example, whether acute surgery had to be performed.

Over the past decades, many predictive systems have been developed. These systems have been based on *Bayes'* theorem (see Chapter 15) and on other statistical methods such as *logistic regression* (see Chapter 24). *Neural networks* and supervised *pattern recognition* methods (see Chapter 27) have also been used. In the following section we discuss some decision-support tools that do not necessarily require a computer for presentation.

3 Decision Support with Simple Predictive Tools

Simple predictive tools may be based on different types of analyses. We first focus on predictive tools that are based on a statistical analysis of a clinical data set that contains the outcome of interest and a number of predictors preferably for a large number of patients. Thereafter, we describe decision-support tools that are based on the results of decision analysis.

3.1 Prediction Rules Based on Statistical Analysis

The calculations involved in statistical analysis often require the use of a computer. The results of the analysis may be presented as a clinical prediction rule, which does not require the use of a computer system. The statistical analysis is often a form of regression analysis. The exact type of regression analysis depends on the type of outcome. For continuous outcomes, such as a blood pressure, linear *regression analysis* can be applied. For dichotomous outcomes, such as short-term mortality, *logistic regression* is often used. For *dichotomous* outcomes occurring over time, such as long-term mortality, failure-time analysis (e.g., *Cox's proportional hazards regression analysis*; see Chapter 24) may be used. Details on these regression techniques can be found in statistics textbooks. General guidelines for the evaluation of prediction rules have been formulated. These guidelines include the following:

- a clear definition of outcome and predictive variables,
- a proper description of the patient population and the study site to allow clinicians a comparison with their population,
- a description of the mathematical technique that is used,
- the availability of the accuracy or the misclassification rate of the rule, and
- the effects of the use of the prediction rule on patient care.

More specific aspects of the statistical model-building process are discussed in the following sections that describe four main steps:

1. selection of variables,
2. estimation of regression coefficients,
3. evaluation of model performance, and
4. presentation of model results (Table 18.2).

Step	Interpretation
Selection	Selection of variables, interaction terms, and classifications for inclusion in the regression model
Estimation	Estimation of regression coefficients
Evaluation	Assessment of discriminative ability and goodness-of-fit
Presentation	Table or graphical display of model results

Table 18.2
Main Steps in the Development of a Prediction Rule by Regression Analysis Techniques.

18

3.1.1   Selection of Variables

The selection of variables that can be used as predictors is a complex issue in statistical modeling. Often, many potentially predictive patient characteristics may be available (possibly 50 to 200), and it may seem both impractical and unnecessary to use all these available characteristics in the predictive tool.

The method most frequently applied to selecting a limited number of predictors is *stepwise selection*. This method automatically selects variables on the basis of the amount of variance (or related measures such as the *log-likelihood*). Stepwise selection may be applied in a forward, a backward, or a combined backward-forward way. The usual *significance level* for the selection of a variable in the model is 5%, which is identical to the significance level commonly used for hypothesis testing. When forward stepwise selection is applied, variables with a *p-value* below 5% may be selected and the variable with the lowest *p*-value is selected first. After one or more steps, none of the remaining variables will have *p*-values below 5% and the selection is considered complete.

Advantages of the stepwise selection method are that it leads to a limited number of variables in a predictive model and that it is widely available in most standard statistical computer packages. The method also corresponds nicely to the concept that once a limited number of variables is included in the model, the remaining variables add hardly any extra predictive information.

The fundamental problem of stepwise selection is, however, that the regression coefficients are overestimated. This *bias* is caused by the fact that coefficients that are more extreme are more likely to be selected than coefficients that are less extreme, since larger coefficients are associated with lower *p*-values.

A second, related, problem is that of the *statistical power* of a stepwise selection procedure. We define statistical power here as the probability that a predictor is selected if the predictor has, in fact, predictive value. The power for selection of a predictor with moderate predictive value is low, especially in small data sets, since the predictor will often, by chance, have a regression coefficient that is too small to be selected. These problems with stepwise selection are especially pronounced in studies with relatively small sample sizes.

Alternative selection strategies have been proposed to overcome the problems of stepwise selection. An obvious option is to limit the number of potential predictors to be assessed in the data set under study. This can be achieved, for example, by critically reviewing the plausibility of the predictive value of the candidate variables by using clinical knowledge of the disease or related diseases. Empirical evidence from other studies may also be used in the selection process.

3.1.2   Estimation of Regression Coefficients

Once the predictors for the outcome are selected, regression coefficients must be estimated (Table 18.2). A proper estimation requires a data set of high quality, which means that the data must be complete and accurate. Also, the larger the data set, the smaller the uncertainty around the estimated regression coefficients and the more precise the predictions.

3.1.3   Evaluation of Model Performance

Next, an impression of the quality of the statistical model is required. Discriminative ability refers to the ability of the model to distinguish between patients with and patients without the outcome. Goodness-of-fit refers to the characteristic that the predictions correspond to the actually observed outcomes. If the predictions are probability estimates, an estimate of, e.g., 70% should correspond to the observation that 70 of 100 patients for whom a certain outcome was predicted actually had that outcome.

3.1.4   Presentation of Model Results

The final step includes the presentation of the results of the statistical model in such a way that clinicians are able to apply the model as a predictive tool. Application should be very easy, requiring no more than paper and pencil. If the number of predictors is limited and no continuous predictors are used, one can construct a simple table showing the predictions for all combinations of the predictors. An alternative presentation is a score chart that lists the predictors, their possible values, and their corresponding scores, in which scores are based on the statistically estimated regression coefficients. Two examples of such score charts are given in Panels 18.1 and 18.2.

PANEL 18.1

Prediction of Histology in the Decision to Resect in Testicular Cancer

Our first example of the development of a simple predictive tool is the decision to perform surgery in the treatment of patients with testicular cancer[1].

Patients with a nonseminomatous tumor in one of the testicles are usually treated with hemi-castration to remove the testicle with the primary tumor. The primary tumor may have caused spread of the disease through the body as metastases.

Metastases most commonly arise in the abdominal lymph nodes. If metastases are present, cis-platin-based chemotherapy is administered, usually in four courses. After completion of the courses of chemotherapy, remnants of the initial metastases called *residual masses*, may remain. Residual masses may essentially contain a totally benign histology or residual tumor. In the case of a benign histology , resection is unnecessary; the patient is exposed to the surgical risks but no benefit is achieved. In contrast, surgical resection is indicated for the residual tumor to prevent growth of the residual mass and spread of the disease to new metastatic sites.

The clinical dilemma for the treating oncologist and urological surgeon is whether these residual masses must be removed by surgery. The alternative to surgery is observation of the mass at regular intervals during follow-up. Further treatment can then follow if growth occurs or new metastases appear, but the patient's prognosis is poor in this situation. Obviously, the choice for surgery or observation depends on the likelihood of a benign histology or tumor in the residual mass. In patients with a high likelihood of benign tissue, observation is preferred, whereas patients with a high likelihood of residual tumor should undergo resection.

Now that we have described the clinical decision and the relevant clinical outcome to support the decision, we will continue with the other steps in the development of a predictive tool (See ▶

Table 18.3
Characteristics of Three Examples of Predictive Tools.

Step	Testicular Cancer	Fertility Problems	Risky Heart Valves
Decision	Surgery	Further diagnostic workup and therapy	Surgery
Outcome	Histological diagnosis	Spontaneous pregnancy	Survival time
Predictors	Six characteristics	Six characteristics	Two key characteristics
Data set	International, from six centers (n = 544)	two studies (n = 996 and n = 751)	Generated by previous model; follow-up study (n = 2,303)
Quantification	Logistic regression	Cox's regression + extension of age effect	None
Presentation	Score chart	Score chart	Graph

18

Table 18.4

Prognostic Score Chart to Estimate the Probability of Benign Tissue (Necrosis) in Residual Retroperitoneal Masses.

Predictor	Value of Predictor and Score	Score
Primary tumor histology	Teratomanegative +9	....
Prechemotherapy markers		
AFP	Normal AFP +9	....
HCG	Normal HCG +8	....
LDH/normal value[b]	0.6 0.8 1.0 1.5 2.0 3.0 4.5 −5 −2 0 +4 +7 +11 +15	....
Postchemotherapy mass size		
Transversal diameter (mm)[b]	2[a] 5 10 20 30 50 100 −4 −6 −9 −13 −16 −20 −28	....
Shrinkage 100 · (presize minus postsize) / presize[b]	−50 0 50 75 100 −7 0 +7 +11 +15	....
Constant		− 10 +
Sum Score (add)		....

[a] If no mass is detectable on the postchemotherapy CT scan, a size of 2 mm is assumed.
[b] Continuous variables; scores for intermediate values can be estimated with linear interpolation.

Table 18.3). To predict the finding of a benign histology at resection, cooperation was sought with several international centers to gather a sufficient number of patients for statistical analysis. The international data set eventually consisted of 544 patients from six centers. The clinically relevant outcome was the histology at resection (benign in 245 (45%) patients; tumor in 299 (55%) patients). Six predictors were identified from studies in the literature (996 patients). The predictive value of these predictors was confirmed in the international data set. Logistic regression analysis was used to quantify the relation between the predictors and the outcome. In logistic regression, the 0 to 1 scale of a binary outcome is transformed to a continuous scale by the logit transformation:

logit (*outcome*) = log{odds (*outcome*)} = log{*p*(*outcome*)/[1 minus *p*(*outcome*)]},

where *p*(*outcome*) denotes the probability of the outcome. The original regression equation was as follows:

▶

log(odds(*necrosis*)) = − 0.978 + 0.858 · *teratoma negative* + 0.870 · *AFP normal* + 0.761 · *HCG normal* + 0.969 · ln(LDH_{st}) − 0.283 · Sqrt(*postsize*) + 0.0147 · *shrinkage*.

The number -0.978 is the intercept of the equation, and the other numbers are the logistic regression coefficients for the predictors. The *predictor* teratoma negative indicates whether the primary tumor contains teratoma elements (1 if true, 0 if false), the predictors *AFP normal* and *HCG normal* indicate whether the prechemotherapy blood levels of the tumor markers alpha-fetoprotein (AFP) or human chorionic gonadotropin (HCG) were normal (1 if true, 0 if false). Another tumor marker, lactate dehydrogenase (LDH), was standardized by division by the upper limit of the normal value range and transformed by taking the natural logarithm (ln). The variable *postsize* indicates the postchemotherapy residual mass size (expressed in millimeters, with square root (Sqrt) transformation), and *shrinkage* indicates the reduction in mass diameter (expressed as percent).

A score chart was used to facilitate the practical application of this regression model. The regression coefficients were multiplied by 10 and rounded off to integers. For example, the regression coefficient of the variable teratoma negative was 0.858, resulting in a score of +9. This score chart is shown in Table 18.4.

Table 18.4 can readily be used to calculate the probability of benign tissue (necrosis) for individual patients. The value of each predictor has a corresponding score in the chart. The scores for each predictor are added, resulting in a sum score, which corresponds to a probability, according to a logistic transformation (Fig. 18.1).

Decision making on resection may be supported by this predictive tool, since some patients could be identified to have a very low likelihood and others could be identified to have a very high likelihood of benign tissue. A difficulty remains on the choice of a cutoff value for the probability of benign tissue to distinguish low-risk from high-risk patients. A comparison with currently used selection strategies suggests that reasonable **cutoff** values are 70 or 80%, which implies that patients with a probability of benign tissue of more than 80% are observed, whereas patients with a probability of lower than 70% undergo resection. For patients with probabilities of between 70 and 80%, no clear preference exists for either resection or observation. Note that it remains the responsibility of the treating clinician to decide on the exact cutoff value for the probability and on the subsequent treatment.

Clinical experience with application of this predictive tool is limited thus far. Further confirmation of the validity of the statistical analysis underlying the score chart may help to convince clinicians of the usefulness of this tool.

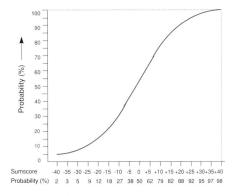

Figure 18.1

Predicted probabilities corresponding to the sum scores calculated with the prognostic score chart (Table 18.1). For example, a sum score of +15 corresponds to a probability of 82%.

18

Prediction of Spontaneous Pregnancy Chances in Fertility Medicine

A simple predictive tool was developed in the field of fertility medicine to predict the chance that couples who seem to be infertile will conceive spontaneously. These couples present to fertility clinics and routinely undergo various diagnostic tests. Once the results of these standard diagnostic tests are known, the couples are counseled on further actions. If the chance of conceiving spontaneously is high, treatment may safely be postponed. On the contrary, if test results and other characteristics are unfavorable, the chance of conceiving spontaneously is low and the couple must be informed about this. The couple's decision may vary from accepting a childless life to requesting fertility treatment, for example, in vitro fertilization or donor insemination. Predicting the chance that the couple will conceive spontaneously is obviously important in this decision-making process.

The relevant clinical outcome is the occurrence of spontaneous pregnancy. For practical purposes, the predicted pregnancy rate at 1 year was chosen. Potential predictors included characteristics from history and physical examination of both the woman and the man, semen analysis, postcoital test, and sperm penetration meter test. The predictive value of these characteristics was determined in a data set consisting of 996 couples, among whom 215 pregnancies occurred within one year. The relation between the predictors and the outcome was quantified by a *Cox regression model*. This model can be used to estimate the probability of spontaneous pregnancy for couples with various combinations of predictive characteristics. The model accounts for differences in follow-up between couples and adjusts for the correlations between predictors. The most important predictors were selected by using a forward stepwise procedure. As explained in Section 3.1.1, this selection strategy may have caused a bias toward regression coefficients that are too large. This bias will be limited since the number of patients with the outcome is relatively large (215 pregnancies).

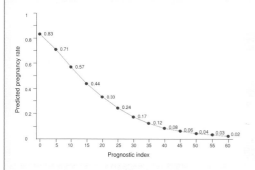

The eventual model is presented as a score chart to estimate the probability of spontaneous pregnancy within 1 year (Table 18.5). The effect of the woman's age was estimated from a combination of two data sources. The first data set (996 couples) came from a time when the large majority of the women had not yet passed the age of 35 years. Therefore, no reliable estimates could be made for women older than age 35. The second data set included 751 women attending a fertility clinic for artificial insemination, among whom 6% of the women were older than 35 years of age. The effect of age on fertility was estimated from this data set, which enabled the extension of the age range to 40 years in ▶

Figure 18.2

Relation between the prognostic index in Table 18.5 and the predicted pregnancy rate at 1 year.

the model presented in Table 18.5. Table 18.5 can readily be used to calculate the probability that an individual couple will conceive spontaneously. The value of each predictor has a corresponding score in the chart. The scores for each predictor are added in a prognostic index, which corresponds to a probability, as calculated by the Cox regression model (Fig. 18.2). This predictive tool distinguished couples who had a wide range of probabilities of conceiving spontaneously. About 10% of the couples had a predicted spontaneous pregnancy rate of greater than 50%, and 43% had a rate lower than 20%. Decision making may be based on this tool, but the choice remains the responsibility of the individual couples. This predictive tool has frequently been applied in fertility counseling. Especially in the contemporary situation in which many diagnostic and therapeutic options are available, and medical advice is often sought after only a short period of unwanted childlessness, information on the probability of spontaneous pregnancy is considered highly valuable.

Predictor	Infertility score
Age of female (years)	
21 to 25	0
26 to 31	2
32 to 34	4
35 to 37	10
38 to 40	16
Duration of infertility (years)	
1	0
2	2
3 to 4	4
5 to 6	8
≥ 7	12
Female infertility	
Secondary	0
Primary	7
Fertility problems in male's family	
No	0
Yes	5
Post-coitum test	
Progressive	0
Nonprogressive	10
Negative	20
Motility (%)	
≥ 60	0
40 - 59	3
20 - 39	7
0 - 19	10
Prognostic index (encircle relevant scores and add)	

Table 18.5
Score Chart to Estimate the Probability of Spontaneous Pregnancy in Subfertile Couples within one Year.

18

Prediction of Survival Time in the Decision to Replace a Risky Heart Valve

This decision problem concerns patients with artificial heart valves with an increased risk of mechanical failure. This problem is specific for Björk-Shiley convexoconcave (BScc) heart valves. The BScc valve was developed in the early 1970s and was implanted in about 86,000 patients worldwide. In 1986 the valve was withdrawn from the market after repeated reports of mechanical failure, which led to acute mortality in most patients. In 1997, over 30,000 patients were still living with a BScc valve.

The clinical dilemma for the treating cardiologist and the cardiothoracic surgeon is whether BScc valves should be replaced by another valve to avert the risk of mechanical failure. In this dilemma, we must weigh the short-term risk of surgery against the cumulative long-term risk of mechanical failure. Conceptually, the short-term risk of surgery is relatively easy to consider, although individual risk estimates may require the inclusion of several risk factors. The cumulative long-term risk is difficult to assess. First, the patient may die before mechanical failure occurs; this is not unlikely in older patients. Also, large numbers of subgroups with different mechanical failure risks have been distinguished, which makes the dilemma even more complex for the treating clinicians.

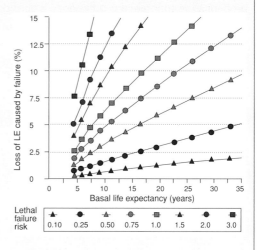

Figure 18.3
Loss of life expectancy (LE) for several lethal failure risks in relation to basal life expectancy.

As a relevant clinical outcome, we may think of the life expectancy of the patient with replacement compared to that of a patient who is observed only. The treatment option resulting in a higher life expectancy is the preferable one. Life expectancy is defined as the area under the survival curve for a cohort of patients. In a decision-analysis model, survival curves can be constructed for hypothetical cohorts. For each subsequent year, the proportion of patients alive is then calculated until all patients have died. The sum of these proportions is the life expectancy. Taking the general Dutch population as an example, the life expectancy of newborn males is 74 years and that of newborn females 80 years (calculated with the 1990-1994 mortality figures).

In the BScc problem, we can distinguish three life expectancies:

1. basal life expectancy: life expectancy of patients with an artificial heart valve without the mechanical fracture risk (equal to life expectancy after successful replacement); ▶

18

2. life expectancy with replacement: basal life expectancy multiplied by the probability of surviving surgery; and
3. life expectancy with observation: life expectancy with inclusion of the mechanical failure risk and the associated acute mortality.

Predictors for these three life expectancies were included in a decision-analysis model. Basal life expectancy depended on age, gender, and the position of the valve (aortic or mitral), according to a follow-up study of 2,303 patients with BScc valves in The Netherlands. For the life expectancy with replacement, surgical mortality must be estimated. In a study of 2,246 patients undergoing reoperation on a heart valve, surgical risk was around 5% on average, but depended on age and several clinical characteristics. Life expectancy with observation requires estimates of mechanical failure risk and acute mortality. According to a recent analysis, the mechanical failure risk depends on several valve characteristics, such as aortic or mitral valve position, size of the valve, 60° or 70° opening angle, and production characteristics, such as date of welding and the welder of the valve. The acute mortality may be estimated as 51% for mitral valve failures and 86% for aortic valve failures. These figures are based on data for limited numbers of subjects: 42 mechanical failures in the follow-up study of 2,303 patients with BScc valves.

The essential weighing in this problem is between the expected loss of life expectancy by the surgical risk and the expected loss by the cumulative mechanical failure risk. The predictive tool should show this weighing as directly as possible. This is achieved by a graph that shows the loss of life expectancy due to mechanical failure for several combinations of the failure risks and basal life expectancy (Fig. 18.3). A lethal failure risk must be used in this graph, which is simply the multiplication of the mechanical failure risk by its associated acute mortality. For example, the lethal failure risk is 0.5% per year for a BScc mitral valve with a mechanical failure risk of 1.0% per year (51% · 1.0% = 0.5%). The core of this presentation of the predictive tool is that the percent loss of life expectancy caused by failure (shown vertically) can directly be compared to the surgical risk of replacement, because a certain percentage of surgical mortality implies the same percentage in loss of life expectancy. Thus, the lines in Fig. 18.3 can also be read as *threshold* lines for which the life expectancies with observation and replacement are equal.

This predictive tool can be used to evaluate individual patients with fixed estimates of surgical mortality, basal life expectancy, and lethal failure risk. There may be considerable uncertainty about the true values of these three quantities. The effect of variation in estimates on the preferred course of action is usually called *sensitivity analysis*. The predictive tool can easily be used for such a sensitivity analysis, since variations in the three essential estimates can directly be incorporated. If the lethal failure risk is very low, for example <0.05% per year, the preference for observation will be strong and variation in the other estimates over plausible ranges will not influence the preference. On the other hand, if the loss of life expectancy with surgery is practically equal to the cumulative loss caused by failure, variations in the estimates may have a substantial effect on the preference.

Limitations of the tool are caused by the type of outcome considered, that is, life expectancy. This measure only considers whether the patient was alive or not; it does not consider the health status of the patient. After both elective replacement and acute failure, the patient may survive with permanent morbidity, especially neurological damage. Also, replacement is ▶

18

associated with a hospital stay of several weeks, with a subsequent period of reconvalescense taking several months. Furthermore, the risk of replacement is a short-term risk, in contrast to the long-term risk of mechanical failure. Most patients are risk averse and attach more value to nearby years than to years in the distant future. This implies that replacement would be less attractive. Cost calculations also show that replacement is more expensive than observation. Therefore, replacement should be performed only if a clear advantage over observation is expected.

The original decision-analysis model has been applied to individual patients in The Netherlands. Some patients underwent surgery, following the recommendation of the model. No clinical experience is thus far available with the predictive tool presented in Fig. 18.3.

1 Steyerberg EW, Keizer HJ, Fosså SD, et al. Prediction of residual retroperitoneal mass histology following chemotherapy for metastatic nonseminomatous germ cell tumor: multivariate analysis of individual patient data from 6 study groups. J Clin Oncol 1995; 13: 1177-87.
2 Eimers JM, Te Velde ER, Gerritse R, Vogelzang ET, Looman CWN, Habbema JDF. The prediction of the chance to conceive in subfertile couples. Fertil Steril 61:44-52; 1994. Van Noord-Zaadstra BM, Looman CWN, Alsbach H, Habbema JDF, Te Velde ER, Karbaat J. Delaying childbearing: effect of age on fecundity and outcome of pregnancy. BMJ 1991; 302: 1361-5.
3 Van der Meulen JHP, Steyerberg EW, Van der Graaf Y, Van Herwerden LA, Verbaan CJ, Defauw JJAMT, Habbema JDF. Age thresholds for prophylactic replacement of Björk-Shiley convexo-concave heart valves: A clinical and economic evaluation. Circulation 1993; 88: 156-64.
4 Steyerberg EW, van der Meulen JHP, van Herwerden LA, Habbema JDF. Prophylactic replacement of Björk-Shiley concave valves: an easy-to-use tool for decision support. Heart 1996; 76: 264-8.

3.2 Tools Based on Decision Analysis

Decision-support tools may also be based on the results of a decision analysis. A decision analysis aims to support the clinician and the patient by an explicit and quantitative consideration of relevant aspects of a decision problem. Several stages can be distinguished:
- First, the clinical problem must be defined in a decision tree.
- Next, quantitative estimates are required for the probabilities and relative value judgments (utilities) of the diagnostic and therapeutic outcomes.
- Computations must be performed to determine the preferred choice.
- Finally, the results of the analysis must be presented in a clinically useful way.

The example in Panel 18.3 illustrates a decision analysis. We focus on the presentation of the key results as a simple predictive tool.

18

4 Evaluation and Conclusions

In short, we have discussed the development of predictive tools for decision support with two kinds of presentations: one with a computer system and one with paper and pencil. The latter form of presentation is illustrated with three examples:

- The first example (Panel 18.1) concerns decision making on surgery in testicular cancer patients. The predictive tool helps to integrate clinical information about individual patients for the prediction of a totally benign tissue, the presence of which makes surgery superfluous. With this tool, it remains up to the treating clinician to decide on the level of certainty on benign tissue that is required to preclude surgery (e.g., 70 or 80%).

- The second example (Panel 18.2) illustrates the same principle: clinical information is integrated for a quantitative prediction, but the consequences of the predictions for clinical actions, such as diagnostic testing, are left to the subfertile couple in discussions with their treating clinician.
- The third example (Panel 18.3) shows that a simple tool can be developed to show the key elements of a complex decision analysis, in this case, the weighing of a short-term mortality risk against a long-term mortality risk.

The future will show whether these simple predictive tools will become more frequently used in clinical practice than more extensive computer systems. With any decision-support tool, however, a user-friendly presentation is of paramount importance.

Key References

Altman DG. *Practical Statistics for Medical Research.* London: Chapman and Hall, 1991.

Habbema JDF, Bossuyt PMM, Dippel DWJ, Marshall S, Hilden J. Analysing clinical decision analyses. Stat Med 1990;9:1229-42.

Pauker SG, Kassirer JP. Decision Analysis. N Engl J Med 1987;316:250-8.

Weinstein MC, Fineberg HV. *Clinical Decision Analysis.* Philadelphia, PA: Saunders, 1980.

See the Web site for further literature references.

18

VI

Institutional Information Systems

Authors of Part VI

Chapter 19: Health Care Modeling for Information Systems Development
A.J. ten Hoopen, A.A.F. van der Maas, University of Nijmegen; J.C. Helder, Erasmus University Rotterdam

Chapter 20: Hospital Information Systems: Clinical Use
P.D. Clayton, Columbia University, New York; E.M. van Mulligen, Erasmus University Rotterdam

Chapter 21: Hospital Information Systems; Technical Choices
H. Lodder, A.R. Bakker, University of Leiden; J.H.M. Zwetsloot, University of Amsterdam

Chapter 22: Health Information Resources
C. Zeelenberg, TNO Prevention and Health, Leiden

1 Introduction

This chapter is in part complementary to Chapters 11 to 14 on clinical information systems and offers at the same time an introduction to Chapters 20 to 22. It describes *models* of public health and health care that support the development of *information systems*. Such models are mostly in the form of a schema with explanatory text, but they are also in the form of formal text.

They describe processes and entities or objects in a particular area of interest. A model with a lower level of abstraction approaches the description of an information system, and relationships may take the form of sources, sinks, and connecting flows. This chapter first describes the structure of models of public health. It then elaborates on the planning and modeling of information systems for large, complex organizations.

2 Public Health and Health Care

Politicians are confronted with the problem of how to allocate to competing goals scarce resources for improving the health of the population. Usually, most of the resources are spent before a critical appraisal of the various health care options has been made; the distribution of resources may not be based on thorough discussions of goals and alternative ways of distributing resources and their possible impacts. Possible reasons for this are that

- health care has a complex organizational structure, and
- it is difficult to estimate which measures will have a maximal influence on health.

Therefore, it is hard to predict the effects on the population of changes in resource allocation or in the organization of health care.

2.1 Public Health

The World Health Organization (*WHO*) defines **health** as follows:

Health is a state of complete physical, mental and social well-being, and not merely the absence of disease or infirmity.

This is a positively oriented definition because it centers on well-being. It is also a broad definition because it includes mental and social well-being and does not define health only in terms of diseases or infirmities.

To make the concept of health operational, the term **health status** is used here as a condition that can be described in objective and measurable quantities and that can be attributed to individuals and populations.

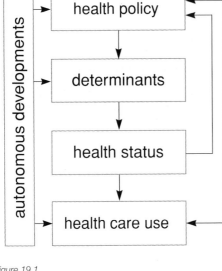

Figure 19.1
Conceptual model of public health.

The term **public health** is not only a neutral description of the health status of a population as a whole or of subgroups. Public health also comprises:

the science and art of preventing disease, prolonging life, and promoting health through organized efforts of society.

During the last three decades many countries have felt the need for a fundamental, critical reappraisal of their health policies. All countries follow to some extent the ideas originated by Lalonde[1]. Two analytic approaches led to the identification of factors influencing health:

1. The first one considers history and follows the variety of events and developments that have had an effect on mortality and morbidity. McKeown[2] remarked that because of *behavioral change* in past centuries, the level of health was greatly influenced

by improvement in income, security, and education. Progress in protection from public health hazards was achieved by, for example, a healthier physical environment (*environmental influence*).

2. The second approach examines the nature and underlying causes of present mortality and morbidity. For instance, from age- and cause-specific mortality data it can be concluded that self-imposed risks and the environment are the principal factors in each of the five major causes of death between ages 1 and 70, and unless the environment is changed and the self-imposed risks are reduced, death rates will not be lowered significantly.

2.2 Conceptual Model of Public Health

A **conceptual model** describes the main concepts (objects) and their relationships of a domain from a certain point of view. Each concept or object can be considered in more detail. The relationships are not necessarily of a causal nature. The model of public health presented here serves a number of goals:

• It defines concepts in the field of public health to create a common reference for discussions and the development of ideas.
• It defines the domain for health policy makers.
• It explains the relationships between the various elements that influence health.
• It gives measurable and objectifiable quantities, for example, for health status.
• It provides a framework for further extension of the models, such as for mathematical modeling or for building information systems.

A conceptual model of public health, as originally devised for the Dutch Public Health Status and Forecast Document[3], contains elements of previously published models. It is shown in its basic form in Fig.

---

[1] Lalonde M. A New Perspective on the Health of Canadians (Working document). Ministry of Supply and Services of Canada in the International Year of Disabled persons, 1981.
[2] Mckeown T. The Role of Medicine: Dream, Mirage or Nemesis. London: Nuffield Provincial Hospital Trust, 1976.

[3] Ruwaard D, Hoogenveen RT, Verkleij H, Kromhout D, Casparie AF, Veen EA van der. Forecasting the number of diabetic patients in The Netherlands in 2005. Am J Public Health 1993;83(7):989-95.

19.1. The model shows that health status is influenced by factors called **determinants**. Health policy influences health status indirectly via determinants such as· lifestyle or the health care system. Health status also contributes to the direction of health policy. In turn, health status influences the use of health care, which is also subject to the effects of health policy. This entire process is influenced by autonomous developments such as economic developments. We discuss the different terms of the conceptual model in Panels 19.1 and 19.2. One object, however, has intentionally been left out: the financing of health care. Although in many countries payers of health care do not pay only for medical care, they also try to influence the determinants. The diversity of the various economic policies in health care, however, prohibits the development of a detailed model that can be applied to all countries.

The next necessary step in developing a "rational" health policy is to analyze which of the factors mentioned above is causing health problems and which can, at the same time, be associated with a measure that could help solve the problem. A classic example that can be used to illustrate this are the health effects of traffic accidents. Although the health care system

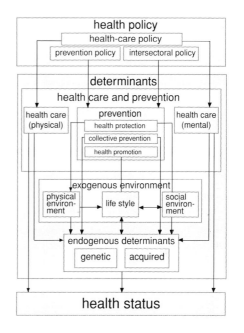

Figure 19.2
Interaction between various determinants.

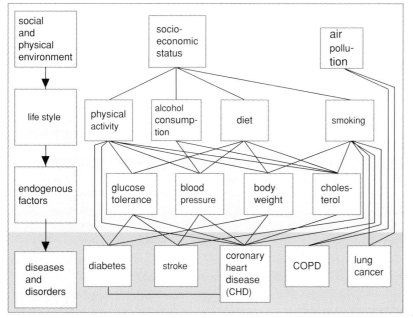

Figure 19.3
Determinants of diabetes, stroke, coronary heart disease (CHD), chronic obstructive pulmonary disease (COPD), and lung cancer.

19

has no effect on the number of people who die *during* an accident, it may try to keep people alive *after* the accident by organizing efficient transportation to the hospital and subsequent optimal treatment. However, the health care system's ability to repair the injuries are limited, because the human body (bones, organs, tissues) generally cannot cope with the large quantities of energy to which it is exposed in the short time of the accident. Various body parts can easily get damaged beyond repair. These given biological characteristics can hardly be changed.

It must further be noted that, paradoxically, to a certain extent health care ultimately even contributes negatively to health: the number of years that people live with disabilities increases by keeping seriously injured people alive, offering them only a disabled, independent state of living. ***Prevention policies*** and ***intersectoral policies*** are important in preventing accidents and reducing the negative health effects of accidents. Influencing lifestyle or behavior can definitely be a factor in preventing accidents by improving driver training programs and instituting speed limits. However, more important are adaptations to our environment, that is, safety measures (such as seat belts, helmets, and technical improvements to vehicles and roads).

In a way, assessing the effects of causal factors of traffic accidents is not much different from assessing factors that influence ***ischemic heart disease*** or lung cancer. In this assessment, not only political questions but also ethical issues must be considered, such as the value of added years to the life of a person if these years are burdened with disease or are severely restricted by disabilities.

Figure 19.2 provides the major interactions between various determinants. As an illustration of the complex network underlying this general scheme, Fig. 19.3 indicates the pattern of associations of determinants of coronary heart disease (***CHD***), diabetes, stroke, chronic obstructive lung disease, and lung cancer. In this "causal network," a particular disease is associated with more than one determinant, and it is clear that the determinants influence each other. For CHD, this results in a complex picture of interacting determinants (both endogenous and lifestyle factors), with direct influences, such as smoking, and indirect ones, such as diet. The other diseases are in part associated with the same determinants as CHD.

A schematic representation of all the relevant patterns of determinants for the diseases with the highest prevalences (insofar as such information is already available) would be extremely complex. Figure 19.3 does not indicate the influences of prevention and the effects of medical care.

2.3 Health Care

It is not yet possible to give a conceptual model of health care that is sufficiently detailed, consistent, and all embracing to be useful in the context of this chapter. There is agreement on a global functional level, but all national health care systems have different subfunctions and organizational patterns. At the lowest level, all health care organizations have unique differences with idiosyncracies that affect their behavior. Attempts to develop more detailed functional decompositions for parts of the cure and care functions will be presented in Section 4. Although it is impossible to present an all embracing model, it is of importance that clear objectives of the purpose of health care be formulated and elaborated into explicit strategies.

The primary activities of organizations in the domain of public health and health care can be divided into four main functions:

1. health promotion and prevention,
2. early detection and follow-up,
3. cure, and
4. care and palliation.

These four areas mirror the questions that policy makers may have for every major health problem, such as:

- Can we really *prevent* negative health effects by some intervention aimed at the determinants or induce positive health effects by some other measure?
- If a disease is not fully preventable, to what extent can we organize *early detection* to prevent the need for a costly cure of the disease?
- Do we have means and facilities for *cure* when this is indicated and needed?
- For those who have to live with a disability or restriction or for those who face some incurable disease, can *suffering* be relieved and adequate *care* be given?

Health Status

Health status can be described in objectifiable and measurable quantities: "health status indicators" or simply "indicators." An indicator is defined here as a measurable quantity that elucidates a particular aspect of health status. Figure 19.4 shows the interrelated indicators of health status within a four-layered structure that is increasingly integrated from top to bottom:

- Disease-specific indicators. These are indicators that are defined from a diagnostic point of view, for example, in terms of the International Classification of Diseases (*ICD*, see Chapter 6). They include, for example, incidence and prevalence figures for specific diseases.
- Mortality, a consequence of diseases, disorders, or external causes. Data on age-specific mortality rates can be used to compute life expectancy at specific ages.
- Indicators of physical, mental, and social functioning. These include indicators such as the prevalence of disabilities or handicaps (according to the *ICIDH* classification; see Chapter 6), measures of aspects of the quality of life, including the ability to work, and measures of mental well-being. To some extent, such measures are independent of the prevalence of a disease: health may be perceived as bad even in the absence of disease. This layer can also accommodate some of the social consequences of diseases such as the use of medical facilities and disability.
- Compound (integrated) health measures or indices. Here, information on health in terms of disability or a quality-of-life measure is integrated with information on mortality (or, more specifically, life expectancy or premature mortality) to give a single overall measure, that is, "health expectancy." Measures of this kind can integrate both the length and the quality of life.

This layered data structure indicates that data can be analyzed to answer questions such as the following: How much of health expectancy is determined by specific functional disabilities or deficiencies in the quality of life? What percentage of mortality is determined by disease *a*, *b* or *c*? How much of a reduced quality of life is determined by disease *d*, *e*, or *f*? Behind this is the question: How much of disease *d* is the result of determinants *g*, *h*, or *i*?

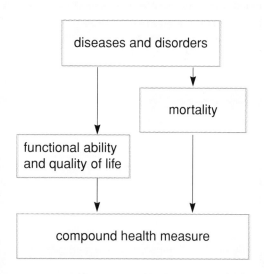

Figure 19.4
Interrelated indicators of health status.

PANEL 19.2

Determinants, Health Policy, Health Care, and Autonomous Developments

Determinants
A determinant is defined as a factor that has an effect on health status. This implies that there is more than a statistical association between factor *x* and health effect *y*, although in most cases it is not a question of a simple cause-effect relationship, but is one of a not completely known complex of causal relationships. We distinguish various groups of determinants:

- biological or endogenous factors,
- exogenous factors, which encompass physical environment, lifestyle, and social environment, and
- prevention and health care, which is a determinant of health, but which also occurs as a separate item in the conceptual model.

In the model, the effects of the health care system (as a determinant) are separated from the use of health care (see section Use of Health Care below). The distinction between endogenous and exogenous arises because of the interaction between an individual's **attributes** and the influence of environmental factors. These *endogenous* and *exogenous determinants* can be influenced by the health care system (cure and care) and prevention. Many endogenous determinants have both genetic and acquired components (e.g., stature, blood pressure, and personal psychological attributes).
Health care affects endogenous determinants or acts directly on the state of health itself (e.g., by surgery). Within the "prevention" block, collective prevention acts above all on endogenous determinants (e.g., the effect of vaccination on the immune system), *health protection* primarily acts on the physical environment (e.g., safety of food and clean air) and on the social environment (e.g., working conditions), and *health promotion* acts mainly on lifestyle (information and education).

Health Policy
Health policy in the broadest sense is characterized here as the actions of governments and others aimed at maintaining and improving the population's state of health. When looking more closely at health policy in the model, a distinction can be made between health care policy, *prevention* policy, and *intersectoral health policy*. ▶

19

At least two other issues emerging in health policy should be mentioned:

1. The first is a constantly growing interest in cost-containment in health care.
2. The second is the call for quality improvement.

This has resulted in various regulations for recertification of health care professionals and in a type of health care delivery system that presents itself as **evidence-based medicine**. The latter means that there should be scientific proof that a given type of care (e.g., early detection and follow-up) or a selected treatment is effective.
Almost any health policy aimed at establishing more

- Health care policy comprises the organization of diagnostics, treatment, nursing, and cure and care. Broadly speaking, it covers activities aimed at people who already have health problems.
- Prevention policy is geared to measures and activities whose purpose is to prevent health problems from occurring or deteriorating. It may involve collective measures to prevent specific diseases (vaccination and screening programs), measures to promote health (health information and education), and measures to improve safety (health protection, e.g., regulations on the safety of food).
- The term *intersectoral policy* is used to describe a health-related policy that lies outside the official public health sphere, but that still involves the prevention of damage to health. Examples are traffic safety policy, building regulations for houses, employment policy, and agricultural policy.

Health policy works by influencing determinants (Fig. 19.2). The health care provided is affected by health care policy, whereas prevention is determined both by the prevention policy of a ministry or department of health and by intersectoral policy for which other ministries and departments are responsible.

Use of Health Care
We have already discussed health care in the section on determinants, where we included the effect of medical interventions on health status in the model. The separate reference here to the use of health care is mainly intended to highlight the use of health care as a consequence of ill health and the resulting economic aspects of medical care.

Autonomous Developments
Finally, the model considers a group of autonomous developments, such as:
- developments in medical technology,
- sociocultural changes, for example, in the demand of care,
- the effect of economic developments on spending choices and levels of service, and
- demographic developments, for example, the age composition of a population or the immigration rate.

These developments are at the macro level and are considered to fall beyond the scope of health policy. However, they affect determinants of health, policy making, and the use of medical care.

effective health care induces changes in the structure of health care. Tasks will be reconsidered or embedded in different organizational structures. Almost every change in a health care system also affects the information systems that support health care.

In short, clear objectives, explicit policies, and coherent plans are needed to achieve the objectives of the health care system as a whole and information systems in particular. In this section on the structure of health care, reasoning was top-down from the viewpoint of, for example, the government, which must formulate policies and implement them to achieve better health for a country. For this general management process, information is needed. Therefore, information systems supporting policy and

19

decision making, policy implementation, and evaluation must be developed.

In establishing information systems to support policy makers, two main problems are usually encountered:

1. There is a "fuzzy," not yet well-defined set of information needs of policy makers in developing, implementing, and evaluating their health policies. The basic questions appear to be what are the determinants of health in detail (on a level that is ready for intervention) and which are valid and sensitive health indicators.
2. There is a patchwork of information sources that easily matches in complexity the patchwork called "health care" (for some of these information resources, see Chapter 22). The only way out of this complexity is to use some top-down reference framework for health and its relations with the rest of society, such as the one developed in Panels 19.1 and 19.2. This conceptual framework should bring clarity to the picture of all the information that is needed, after which a clear strategy can be formulated to transform the patchwork into a coherent set of information systems.

The information analysis conducted along with the first systematic attempt to evaluate and forecast health on a national level produced the following results[4]:

"The assessment of the future Health of the Nation contains uncertainties, mainly caused by lack of data and by unpredictable developments in the sociocultural, economical, and medico-technical areas. Uncertainties in the sketch of the current situation are caused by the unavailability of data about many diseases and disorders, other health indicators and health determinants on the level of the population as a whole. Uncertainties about projections up to 2010 are also a consequence of the lack of data on trends in the recent past. This holds for data about disease trends and other health indicators, but also for many determinants. Mortality data are exceptions. In addition, certain developments which are difficult to predict may have an influence, such as the sudden appearance of unknown or locally restricted (infectious) diseases (e.g., HIV or the Ebola virus), an increase in socioeconomic differences as a result of social or economic developments, increased immigration, or breakthroughs in medical technology. The identified gaps in information and knowledge can be overcome by monitoring, by biomedical and epidemiological research, by health services research, and by the development of simulation models."

3 Models for Information System Development

The preceding section indicated that to rationalize a complex development, explicit conceptual models are needed. This holds for health policy development in organizations, such as hospitals (Chapters 20 and 21) and primary health care centers (Chapter 11). It also holds for the development of computer applications.

3.1 Nolan's Growth Model

Information systems, and especially computer-based information systems, impose changes on an organization. Organizations follow several stages in their growth toward a situation in which information systems are fully integrated in the organization. The basic growth model of Nolan[5] consists of four phases (Table 19.1):

---

[4] *Citation from: Ruwaard D, Kramers PGN, Van den Berg Jeths A, Achterberg PW, eds.* Public Health Status and Forecasts. The Health Status of the Dutch Population over the Period 1950-2010. *The Hague: SDU Publ, 1994.*

[5] *Nolan RL. Managing the crises in data processing. Harvard Business Review 1979;March-April:115-26.*

19

Stage	Description	
Initiation	Early use of computers by small numbers of users to meet basic organizational needs. Decentralized control and minimal planning.	*Table 19.1* Basic Stages of the Growth Model of Nolan.
Expansion or contagion	Experimentation with and adoption of computers by many users. Proliferation of applications. Crisis caused by rapid rise in costs.	
Formalization or control	Organizational controls established to contain growth in use and apply cost-effectiveness criteria. Centralization. Control often prevents attainment of potential benefits.	
Maturity or integration	Integration of applications. Controls adjusted. Planning is well established. Alignment of information systems to organization.	

1. Initiation,
2. Expansion or contagion,
3. Formalization or control, and
4. Maturity or integration.

Nolan observed that most organizations pass these four stages one by one, and that the transformation into the formalization and maturity stages especially requires explicit interventions by the general management of the organization. The growth into maturity often implies a redesign of the entire organizational structure, including the information systems. An in-depth comprehensive view on the use of data by all activities in the organization is then needed to be able to effectively integrate applications. These stages have originally been observed in introducing large information systems. The same growth model is applicable to the introduction of personal computers in organizations and, perhaps, also to the introduction of *Internet* applications. Even the introduction of copiers or facsimile equipment showed the same pattern, but on a smaller scale.

Thorough planning of information systems for an organization is of utmost importance for growth into the last stage, which can be divided into plans on the strategic, tactical, and operational levels:

1. *Strategic planning*

The objectives and strategies for implementation of the information systems are derived from the core business of the organization. For example, a health care organization that is oriented toward curing patients of disease and that plans to extend its activities by screening patients for the early detection of diseases will have to extend its information systems to support such activities as the identification of the population at risk, the selection of candidates for screening, call and recall of candidates in line with the screening program procedures, and organization of follow-up for patients found to have a disease. It will be clear that the organization then must reconsider its existing objectives and strategies for its actual information systems if these support only cure-oriented activities.

2. *Architectural planning*

All required subsystems and their interconnections are described in an overall information systems architecture or a blueprint of system modules. This should include an analysis to estimate how each subsystem contributes to the goals of the information system. One of the approaches to developing an architecture uses the so-called *create-use matrix*, which describes the relation between activities or processes in a busi-

19

ness and its relevant objects (data entities). This matrix describes for all activities or processes (the rows of the matrix) the allowed operations, such as create, use, delete, and so on, on data entities (the columns). By reordering the rows and columns of the matrix in such a way that –ideally – the matrix can be decomposed into a number of submatrices, candidate information systems can be identified.

3. *Planning of projects*

The development of subsystems or changes in existing systems must be carefully planned within a finite period of time. Decisions on budget and personnel allocations must be made, and priorities in relation to other, competing projects must be set (see also Chapter 35 on project management).

3.2 Cascade Model for System Development

Figure 19.5 presents the main steps in the system development process up to the introduction of a newly built system into the organization. This schema can be refined (decomposed) for some of the steps. Moreover, some steps may be combined for a development method or given somewhat different names. The

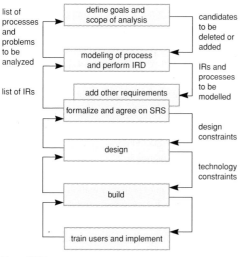

Figure 19.5
Part of the steps in the software development process.

schema can also be extended in a variety of ways. One might add boxes representing "support and maintenance" and "evaluation of system use." The latter can result in a reconsideration of the original goals, as stated by the activity represented by the box at top of Fig. 19.5. This may initiate a new system's development cycle. The entire information system's "life cycle" is represented by these kinds of extensions. By so doing, the typical cascade structure may be transformed into a three-dimensional spiraling picture, depicting the influence that a system has on the organization when a new development cycle is initiated on a *higher* level.

To speed up the whole process of system development, a **prototype** of the system is sometimes built rapidly so that the users can gain experience with the system in reality. This experience is then used to refine or clarify user requirements. Important characteristics of any approach to system development are the following:

- The division of the development process into phases, to make the whole process manageable;
- The sequential structure of the process, which implies that a next step is driven by the results of the previous one and, more important, the quality of the results of a next step depends heavily on the quality of the preceding steps;
- Problems with input in a step can be resolved only by giving feedback to the preceding steps, which may cause delay in the overall throughput; and
- By going from top to bottom in Fig. 19.5, decisions shift from domain-related to information-technology (**IT**) related. In principle, technical design- and IT-related decisions should not be taken in the beginning of system development, because technical decisions taken too early generally restrict the solution of problems at subsequent steps.

3.3 Business Modeling

Business modeling takes place on the highest level of Fig. 19.5. In general, a *business* is composed of several processes. A process is a related group of activities that create results in a stepwise manner. This process requires contributions by people ("agents"), information, and other resources and has well-defined starting

19

and end points. Sometimes, a single activity may be considered a separate process.

A **business model** is a concise, well-structured, semi-formal description of the processes that are essential to the business. It should support the understanding and analysis of how operational activities work or should work. It should be the starting point for the realization of changes in the organization.

The model starts with a few fairly simple concepts, uses decomposition for subproblems, and leaves out all aspects that are irrelevant for the anticipated use of the model. It should be able to offer easy-to-understand and comprehensive overviews. Formalization of the model and the use of well-defined symbols are required to let all people involved have the same understanding of the business model. Modeling the processes in an organization in sufficient detail is the only way to structure the requirements for the information system that must support these processes.

In short, the reasons for business modeling are:

1. To obtain a comprehensive view of essential details and to avoid irrelevant and confusing details;
2. To document the core of the business so that it is equally understood by both the potential users and the developers of information systems, as well as by the managers and end users who are responsible for the organizational change and who have requested the introduction of new or redesigned information systems; and
3. To break apart the complex infrastructure of health care delivery to support discussions with all people involved at all operational levels, for example, by interviews, to determine their information needs. This is the main approach that gives some assurance of the quality and completeness of the inventory of information needs, and it is the best starting point when designing information systems.

3.4 Modeling Clinical Practice

Some examples borrowed from health care will illustrate the foregoing general remarks on business modeling. The National Health Service (NHS)

Information Management Center in the United Kingdom developed a model that comprises the view of clinicians on the process of health care delivery. In this model, the clinical process is shaped by three basic activities (see also the stages in Chapter 1):

1. observing,
2. planning, and
3. plan implementation.

How clinicians learn from their own work (in the framework of the clinical process) is represented by including an activity outside the clinical process called *learning*. This activity is initiated by the results produced by the clinical process, and it is hoped that it results in improved knowledge and skills (see also the inductive process depicted in Fig. 1.1). Knowledge and skills drive the clinical process. This model of the clinical process can be refined further by iteration between clinical activities and improved knowledge and skills, resulting in, for instance, protocols or clinical practice guidelines.

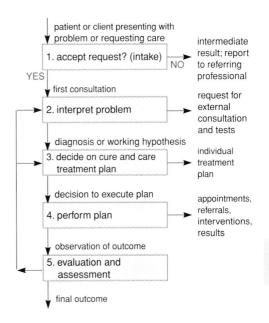

19

Figure 19.6
Basic steps in a primary health care process.

The clinical process starts with observing when there is a patient demand and when resources and knowledge and skills are available. Incorporation of processes such as education and training or medical research that have an important impact on knowledge and skills and processes such as managerial control and general business management are omitted from this model because there was no immediate use of the model anticipated with respect to those activities.

Figure 19.6 presents an example of a care-delivering process. It is the result from task analysis of primary care centers in The Netherlands and is based on interviews with health care professionals in about 25 primary care centers. The model serves as a common ground for discussion between professionals and information analysts. Incorporation of the decisions to be made enables the generation of protocols and guidelines for primary health care to be improved.

3.5 Modeling Public Health Surveillance

Public health *surveillance* (*PHS*) is an activity that monitors changes in the health status of the population to prepare interventional measures (see also Section 2.4 of Chapter 22). PHS heavily depends on an ongoing and systematic collection, analysis, and interpretation of health data that are essential to planning, implementing and evaluating public health practices and is closely integrated with the timely dissemination of these data to those who need to know. The main goal of PHS is the timely detection of significant changes in the space and time patterns of diseases in the population and the dissemination of information to the responsible authorities or health care professionals. The dissemination of health statistics should be timely to be effective. For example, it is important to be informed about relatively small local outbreaks of infectious diseases that have a large impact, such as tuberculosis. In developing information systems to support PHS, one should be aware of the distinctions between PHS and epidemiological research. Depending on the nature of the diseases to be monitored and the structure of the specific health care system, there are several potential sources of health data for reporting · health statistics, from general practitioners, laboratories,

and hospitals to local health authorities and many others. To improve the quality of data, it is necessary to combine data from different sources for a structured description of the myriad of information services that have emerged throughout the various health care systems that exist throughout the world (see Chapter 22). This process of merging data is called *record linkage*. Problems of case identification and privacy problems sometimes arise. Feedback of health statistics to the providers of the data has a positive effect on the motivation of the providers and increases the quality and completeness of the data. Therefore, it improves the quality of the PHS network.

A PHS process (also considered part of the health care business) can be characterized by:

1. the observation and recording of phenomena at distributed locations;
2. the periodic transfer of data to a central database;
3. the analysis and assessment of the quality and completeness of the data, error checking, computation of incidences, trends, comparison of the results with thresholds for notification, and matching of the results with those from predictive models;
4. the interpretation of the results of the analysis and the comparison of the results with those from other surveillance systems;
5. the determination of interventions or measures to be taken; and
6. the diffusion of information to responsible authorities to initiate the actual intervention.

PHS is an ongoing activity, so the effects of interventions and new disturbances will be detected by the cyclic nature of the process.

3.6 Reference Models in Health Care

Reference models have been developed for, among other things, *business processes* (see the Section 3.3 on Business Modeling above), *information requirements* of processes (see below in this section), and *data structures* and *information systems* (for an example of the latter from primary health care, see Sections 3.2 and 4 of Chapter 11). Reference models represent the best avail-

19

able knowledge, based on the experiences of other organizations, needed by an organization to support, for example, an information requirement determination (*IRD*) study (see Section 4.1 of this chapter). The main presumption to applying reference models is that it is more economical to *share* the knowledge in a reference model than to reinvent it. In the case of an IRD study, reference business and information models can greatly reduce the analyst's effort in grasping the essential views of both the processes and information needs required to prepare the interviews, as described in Section 4.1.

Reference models are, however, seldom applicable in a straightforward manner. They are generic; that is, they are valid for parts of the reality of a business and must be *instantiated* and sometimes enlarged to fit the peculiarities of the concrete organization: the hospital at A, the public health department at B, the nursing home at C, and so forth.

Reference models are used for at least two purposes:

1. to describe what *should be* done, is available, should happen, and so on. This description of the desired or standard situation is therefore *normative* by nature, and

2. to shape the description of the current situation to allow for a first comparison with the desired situation. Note that, in general, this comparison is the first step in establishing a migration path from the current to the desired situation.

The examples from health care given below will clarify these two main purposes. Experience with developing and applying certain types of these reference models has been gained in both the United Kingdom's **NHS** and the Dutch health care system for more than a decade. The remainder of this section is mainly devoted to that experience.

3.6.1 Common Basic Specification

The Common Basic Specification (CBS) in the United Kingdom's NHS emerged in about 1990. It is initially based on the earlier experience in the United States that successful database applications almost all depend on agreement on a common corporate-wide data model (see Chapter 4). This NHS-wide entity-rela-

tionship data model (see Chapter 4) was developed and published by the NHS in 1986 and 1987. Since it summarizes the best available knowledge on the subject, it is the *standard* or *reference* for anyone in the United Kingdom who wants to reflect on the subject.

This **entity-relationship** model (Chapter 4) , however, is primarily a **database** developer's tool. The extension of the NHS data model into a common framework for both the health care and IT worlds needed in some way to complement the data model with a recognizable structure depicting actual health care activities and relating health care and IT in a systematic way. The first version of CBS thus contains a tree structure of activities, which was the result of a decomposition process that starts with maintenance and improvement of the health of the population as the top-level activity. The decomposition process then uses a very simple generic process model, the so-called **activity quartet**, *enable-plan-do-evaluate*, borrowed from a general system development method. Its rationale is that any work that must be done on any level of abstraction and of any kind by some professional in a business must first be *enabled* (authorized, resources allocated), then be *planned* (scheduled, appointments made), actually be *done* (executed or in part executed by someone else), and finally, be *evaluated*, monitored, interpreted, and reported. An example from the level just below the top activity, consists of:

> MAINTAIN BASIC DATA
> PLAN SERVICES
> ENABLE SERVICE DELIVERY
> → DELIVER SERVICES
> MONITOR SERVICES

The compound activity DELIVER SERVICES is further decomposed into:

> CANCEL SERVICE ACTIVITY
> PROGRESS SERVICE DELIVERY
> MONITOR SERVICE ACTIVITY
> PLAN SERVICE DELIVERY
> → PERFORM SERVICE ACTIONS
> SCHEDULE SERVICE DELIVERY

19

The activity PERFORM SERVICE ACTIONS is an example of a *leaf* activity (on this level); that is, it is not further decomposed. The description of a leaf activity includes its use of entities from the data model.

Among the strong points of CBS are the very detailed level of the data model (e.g., more than 250 entity types are distinguished), as well as both its elegance and simplicity and its all-embracing scope of the activity structure. It very efficiently offered the knowledge and experience gained in the NHS in the preceding decade for whoever needed it.

The model also has its weak points. The tree structure of business activities is not considered sufficiently close to the daily practice of all kinds of processes in health care for which computer applications must be developed. This very close relation is crucial in communicating with health care professionals about what they really need from the applications.

Certain adaptations are made for specific health care sectors, such as public health and primary care (by general practitioners). Special modeling efforts are devoted to a central issue in health care: the *clinical process* (see Section 3.4).

3.6.2 Orders and Acts

An important adaptation of CBS took place when developers of CBS combined their efforts with those of a European Union-funded project called *RICHE (Réseau d'Information et de Communication Hospitalier Européen)*. The classical "*act management*" concept adopted within this project was incorporated in the next versions of CBS. An act is considered to be any activity undertaken for the benefit of a patient (see also Chapter 29). Examples of acts are:

- a consultation,
- a visit,
- a laboratory test,
- the laboratory test-associated sampling operation,
- drug administration, or
- meal taking.

The key model of the act management concept is that there is someone in the role of *requester* (e.g., a physician, nurse, or the patient) who issues an *order* to per-

form some act and there is someone in the role of *performer* who receives the request to execute that act at some point in space and time and subsequently *communicates* back what has happened (replies and reports), that is, *results*. The dynamics of "acts" are reflected by the states that an act can be in: requested, accepted, and so forth.

This is, in fact, not different from the approach used in the development (starting in the United States in as early as 1966) of a number of hospital information systems (*HISs*) in which *all* orders issued by any professional contributing to the primary process of patient care delivery are directly entered into the kernel of the HIS (see also Chapters 20 and 21), thus preventing common problems and associated errors of circulating handwritten documents: an *order and result communication management* module. Besides various functions to manage the results in an orderly fashion, this type of system has another important feature that makes it popular with end users. This is the *order set* concept. This allows users to issue prepackaged groups of orders applicable to a specific diagnosis or to a specific time period within a period of care (e.g., admissions or postoperative orders). Users can further define their personal or departmental sets of orders to fit seamlessly into their needs as specialists or to reflect and enforce departmental policies and guidelines.

3.6.3 Hospital Information Model

The *Hospital Information Model (HIM)* was developed in the early 1980s by the Dutch National Hospital Institute. The goals of the project that produced HIM were:

- to establish a *common reference* to be used in the assessment of proposals for the development of information systems submitted by different hospitals or hospital groups;
- to determine *overlap* and "*white spots*" describing the information needs of hospital processes that were or were not (yet) covered by those system development proposals;
- to identify the map of necessary information *flows* between care-delivering processes and other processes, such as for supporting a better architectural design of information systems; and
- to achieve *better quality* in IRD at affordable costs

19

PANEL 19.3

Example of Activities, Information Needs, and Relations in the HIM

FUNCTIONAL ENTITY: Admission and Nursing

DESCRIPTION: The selection of patients to be admitted from the waiting list, making arrangements for urgent admissions, and considering the departmental capacities and availability of resources (staff, rooms, supplies, etc.) and the medical, social and functional urgencies of admission per patient (on the waiting list)

INFORMATION NEED

---

* Number of patients on waiting list per clinician and per category of urgency

* Medical, patient, and resource-oriented data per patient on the waiting list

* Number of nonoccupied beds with bed-condition per department

* Number of nonoccupied beds per clinician

* Planned number of beds to be released with bed-condition per clinician by date of release

* Capacity/resource data of diagnostic and treatment departments

* Capacity/resource data of nursing departments

* Planned appointments per admission candidate

* State of outpatient diagnostic and treatment procedures per planned admission candidate

* Canceled planned admissions per clinician

* Admission capacity per clinician

* Methods for admission planning

---

by defining a common (or generic) model for information requirements to be used by various hospitals as a sound basis for their local adaptations.

The attempt to describe information flows at some level of detail was inspired by attempts in the early 1970s to look at the underlying information flow structure of a company in general. To describe the information flows in some detail for a hospital appeared to be too complex, given the manual tools available at that time.

The HIM describes for all activities in a hospital a list of the information needs required to perform those activities. The overall structure of the HIM is based on a simple model of a business and its supporting information systems and is depicted in Fig. 19.7.

Note that activities that are performed identically at various places in the organization are described only once in the HIM. Activities concerning admission, discharge, and transfer (**ADT**) are generic and may therefore be performed at various locations throughout the

19

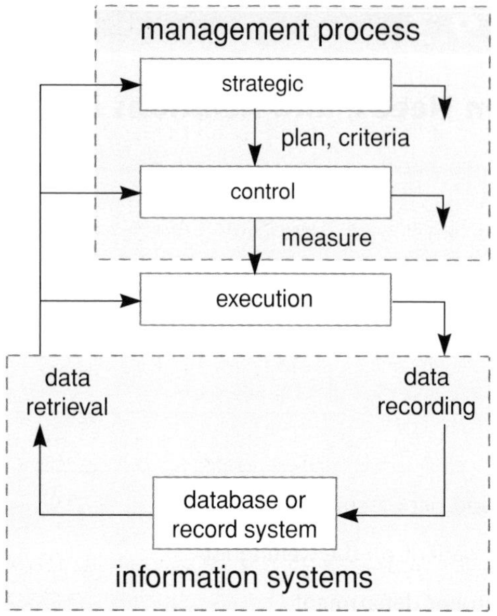

Figure 19.7
Overview of processes described in HIM.

hospital, but they are described only once in the HIM. This means that a reference model such as the HIM must be specialized (instantiated) to the specific organization where it is applied.

Panel 19.3 describes an example of how the activities, information needs, and data structures in the HIM are related (see also Fig. 19.7). It contains an example of the primary hospital activities as distinguished in the HIM. These primary activities are grouped in generic primary hospital functions (see also Section 2 of Chapter 21):

- professional activities of clinicians,
- diagnostics and treatment activities, and
- admission and nursing.

The other supporting functions distinguished in the HIM are:

- general organizational structure and procedures, **EDP**, etc.;
- hotel function;
- financial aspects;
- material aspects;

- personnel;
- technical aspects, such as maintenance;
- training; and
- scientific research.

The last two functions apply primarily to teaching and university hospitals.

The complete set of data groups (entity types) and their relations form the data model of the HIM. The HIM encompasses only 58 data groups because large groups of data items were clustered. For example, the entity type "patient" consists of three groups of attributes, one with identification items, one with financial and regulatory items, and one with medical items. Each attribute type must be defined unambiguously by some classification scheme or measurement method (see Chapter 6). This defines the *common body of terminology* for the organization type for which the reference model is developed. It also defines the scope for the **data dictionary** for the information systems supporting all processes.

3.7 Development of Reference Models

There are striking and perhaps even confusing differences between the examples of reference models given above. These differences are partly caused by the different historical backgrounds, the different starting points, and the different objectives of the projects that produced them.

These differences can be grouped around four basic questions that should, in fact, have been answered before developing these generic models:

1. How should the domain (health care) be described and how should it be modeled, given the use at which it is aimed? What elements are contained in a process description, how are they linked to each other, which functional aspects are dealt with, and on what concepts (task description, value chain, product, or transaction flow) is the process structure based?
2. How are information requirements determined, represented, and related both to the domain description or model and to the data model? How

does the domain description influence the results of IRD, how is data processing described, and which *meta-model* should be used to represent the data structure: Should it be some **entity-relationship** kind of model, or should it be **object oriented**?

3. What is the "right" level of abstraction or genericiness for these types of generic tools? Depending on the nature of the application, at least two levels are required: (a) a business systems planning process, requiring a broader insight into the relation of processes and data, and (b) an information system or application development process.

4. What guidelines and training are needed to use these models? What experience should users of these models have to be able to use them efficiently and effectively?

As long as we have no clear answers to these questions, it will not be easy to compare the contents or to judge the quality of these reference models or to harmonize and improve the way in which they are developed. The core of the matter is that we do not know what their common root or common *meta-model* should be. All that can be said at this moment is that these reference models are the product of a process that uses both **induction**, that is, where we abstract from business-specific examples of models, and **deduction**, that is, when we apply theory. An example of the latter is that, if some execution activity is to be initiated and controlled or managed in general, this results in an interaction between the activity and the management process. From this, on a theoretical basis, some kinds of information needs for both sides in the interaction can be deduced:

- The execution activity needs an explicit input (stimulation or request) to change its state, and it needs to know how to produce some result; that is, it needs a way of "working."

- The management process at least needs to be informed (for subsequent actions or decisions) of both the results produced and the changed state.

Table 19.2
Examples of Entity Type Descriptions for the Shared-Care Process.

Request for Assessment

#Patient	The patient involved
#Care provider	The care provider who puts the problem of this patient forward to the team meeting
Reason	The reasons for assessing/submitting to the team meeting
Date	The date of the meeting in which the patient is discussed
Result	The result of the assessment

Management Plan

#Patient	The patient for whom the management plan has been formulated
Goal	The goal to be attained by care delivery as described in this management plan
Date	The date the management plan was decided to be final
Disciplines	The disciplines/processes to be involved on the basis of patient's problems
Care arrangements	The collection of instructions and agreements on contents and time management of the care delivered by the involved disciplines/processes
Coordinator	The person who is responsible for coordinating care delivery
Evaluation items	Aspects of care delivery that must be discussed in progress evaluation meetings with the disciplines involved
Frequency of evaluation	The frequency of evaluating the progress in meetings of the disciplines involved

19

These examples of theoretically deduced kinds of information needs can be used to enforce minimal consistency in developing a detailed reference information model for a given domain. This, in fact, obeys a fundamental principle of modeling. Much research still must be done on these principles and their applications.

3.8 Application of Reference Models

Throughout the preceding text, several ways of using reference models have been mentioned or suggested. Both the CBS- and the HIM-type models have been complemented by manuals supporting various kinds of uses. In The Netherlands, the HIM has been the precursor for many other models, such as models for physiotherapeutic care and psychiatric hospitals. The use of these models can form a starting point for system development, such as:

- information system planning and architectural design,
- systematic documentation and evaluation of existing information services, and
- information system development.

Reference models also support standardization in the areas of both terminology and information interchange:

- identifying the messages to support effective information exchange, and
- defining a common body of terminology and thereby facilitating standardization.

Reference models also influence the organizational development of the domains for which they refer to, that is, the redesign of tasks, jobs, and business processes.

4 Information Requirements Determination

This section deals with how to obtain information about the structure of the domain necessary to make a model of processes, the information requirements of the processes, and the relationships between processes and infromation requirements.

Before starting the process of actually building an information system (designing and developing the software), one must be sure about what information this system should deliver, in which way, and to whom; in short, what are the system requirements? If one reviews evaluation studies of information systems, one invariably finds that the reasons for failure upon the introduction of the system or the reason for exceeding the development budgets are that the information requirements determination stage had been insufficient or underestimated. This means that certain requirements are still too vague or even incorrect and are therefore misinterpreted by the system designers and builders. Our basic statement is

therefore that doing an extensive **IRD** is neither redundant nor simple and is extremely important.

4.1 Essential Issues in IRD

Both future users and systems analysts or developers should be well aware of a number of essential points and problems regarding IRD.

1. There is a major difference between doing a real analysis of the information needs of the users of an information system to be developed and just defining the data to be recorded, including the retrieval that has been used for years in some system, possibly a manual system. The latter is called *data analysis* and must be clearly distinguished from IRD. Galliers[6] stated, in this

respect, that "data analysis is a very useful tool for efficient database design. It is much less useful as a means of identifying information requirements (especially where these are "fuzzy" and unstructured), or in allowing different viewpoints to be taken into consideration. Too often based on an analysis of current situations, data analysis – in the extreme case – is a great way of encapsulating organizational ineffectiveness in the resulting database."

2. Davis's classical work on IRD[7] starts with distinguishing four major reasons why it is difficult to obtain a correct and complete set of requirements:

   - the constraints on humans as information processors and problem solvers,
   - the variety and complexity of information requirements,
   - the complex patterns of interactions among users and analysts in defining requirements, and
   - an unwillingness or incapability of some users to provide requirements (for political or behavioral reasons).

3. Apart from distinguishing the levels in an organization on which requirements must be determined (organizational, database system, and application levels), Davis stresses the importance of using a well-chosen, explicit strategy (and subsequent methods) in IRD. His four strategies are:

   - just plain *asking about* the requirements,
   - straightforward *derivation* of the requirements from an existing information system,
   - *synthesizing* the requirements from characteristics of the system to be developed, that is, from the work processes of the future users, and
   - *discovering* the requirements from experimentation with an evolving information system, that is, discovering from *prototyping*.

The first two strategies generally have limited application possibilities if the domain in which the information system is to be used is still not very well known or if there are problems with existing information systems. The last strategy sometimes seems to be an alternative to the third one, but one must be careful not to use it as the last resort if the third strategy results in too many complications and seems to be too time-consuming. One might encounter one of the gross failures of informatics, that is, that it is both "quick" *and* "dirty."

It is interesting to compare the way that systems' analysts acquire and handle the knowledge that they need with the way that knowledge is acquired for **decision-support systems** (Chapter 17). The main differences seem to be that that knowledge acquisition for decision-support systems extensively uses and explicitly makes reference to the literature. Both areas have in common the fact that experts should be interrogated to extract the necessary knowledge.

On top of all these problems in determining a correct and complete set of requirements, the analyst must deal with the intricacies of a particular domain, in our case, health care. In health care, one often has no other choice than to use Davis's third strategy, especially if one must determine the information requirements for a system that has to support the "core business," that is, the actual delivery of care by the primary care processes. As stated in Chapter 21, the development of subsystems that support the care processes has only very recently been done systematically. It is now the central issue in many development projects.

4.2 IRD in Health Care

The process of performing requirements engineering is still an area of active investigation by computer scientists. The method sketched below is a practical model for requirements engineering for health care applications.

To achieve a set of requirements that is as complete and correct as possible given the problems described above, interviews with key informants from the health care domain should be organized. These interviews can be followed by group sessions to try to achieve consensus on the results, that is, correctness and completeness of the requirements. The selection of key

6 *Galliers RD, ed.* Information Analysis: Selected readings. *New York: Addison-Wesley, 1987*
7 *Davis GB, Olson MH.* Management Information Systems. Conceptual Foundations, Structure and Development *(2nd ed). New York: McGraw-Hill, 1984.*

19

informants and the structure of the interview (including training of the interviewers) should aim at optimizing the completeness and correctness in IRD, mentioned by Davis (see Section 4.1). Three general points concerning IRD, obtained from interviews in a Dutch health care setting, have been identified as follows:

1. The most crucial point is that the analysts should have acquired sufficient knowledge of the terminology used by professionals and on the structure of the process to be analyzed. This means that considerable effort must be put in modeling the process, as described earlier in the sections on business modeling. An interview protocol that supports the synthesis work of analysts must be developed. It functions as a checklist (to raise the same complete range of items and questions in each interview) and as a decomposition tool to keep discussions in interviews sufficiently focused and manageable.

2. Key informants should be selected among professionals who:
   - are qualified for at least 5 years for the particular job under investigation,
   - have substantial experience in replacing colleagues,
   - are involved in training novices,
   - have a clear opinion on why they do the job the way they do it (expressed, e.g., by participation in job description committees or publishing in professional journals),
   - have no special or heavy interest in IT (informants' answers should not be technology driven but should be domain expertise driven), and
   - are regarded as very busy in their job and cannot be missed from daily practice, even not for an interview.

3. To minimize bias for each job type that is distinguished, about three to five key informants must be selected, possibly adding a few informants from other departments or organizations performing the same process and function. They act as a source that can reflect on the results that are obtained. Practical experience in interviewing reflects the "law of diminishing returns:" after three to five interviews, using the same checklist of standard questions (see

item 1 above), the results of another interview add only marginally to the set of requirements.

Since the preparatory work for the IRD interviews contains process-modeling activities, a preparatory interview round with key informants (for which the same selection criteria stated earlier hold) is often needed before the IRD interviews proper. In this round, abstract or generic process models are made more specific and are refined.

Some examples taken from the process of shared care in primary health care centers illustrate this. For the whole process, but also for each step within the process, the analyst must ask systematically what is the specific terminology used by the professionals. For example, if in some center for primary health care "collaborative care," "teamwork," or "case management" is used instead of "shared care," the analyst should first check the extent to which the used terms cover the same concept and then stick to the preferred term of the key informants. The same should be done for the naming of steps or separate activities. Note that this can lead to a revision of the terminology and the actual structuring in separate steps of the process description and definitions that have been developed so far in the analysis. Next, for the whole process and for each step, the most important types of questions are:

- What result (added value for the object of care) is required, how is this result recorded if it is to be used afterward (for what activity, by whom, and what is the purpose of recording)?
- What input is needed, that is, what event initiates the activity or process, and what information is needed?

An analyst should always be able to determine at least a triggering event, some use of data, and possibly, a single result of a step. This is needed to integrate the results of the interview into a consistent description in which for every information item it is evident how and why the information is needed or used. For example, the shared care process in centers for primary care in The Netherlands only deals with patients who are on the patient list of one of the general practitioners of the center. So, if another professional is proposing a patient for shared care, at least the name of this patient's general practitioner must be known. Another example is that the analyst should be familiar with the existence of professional guidelines for certain types of problems (e.g., chronic obstructive lung disease in children or home care for terminally ill individuals). For validity reasons, these guidelines usually contain explicit inclusion criteria. This means that in some step of the shared care process, information about patient characteristics is needed to be able to judge the applicability of the guideline. If this information need is not denoted by some key informant, the analyst has the task to use this a priori knowledge to discuss the information.

Key References

Martin J, Leben J. *Strategic Information Planning Methodologies* (2nd ed). Englewood Cliffs: Prentice Hall, 1989.

Davis GB, Olson MH. *Management Information Systems. Conceptual Foundations, Structure and Development* (2nd ed). New York: McGraw-Hill, 1984.
Lalonde M. A new perspective on the health of the Canadians. Ottawa, 1974.

Davis AM. *Software Requirements. Objects, Functions, States* (rev. ed.). Englewood Cliffs, NJ: Prentice Hall, 1993.

See the Web site for further literature references.

19

20 Hospital Information Systems: Clinical Use

1 Introduction

For three decades (1960-1990) the primary use of computers in hospitals in the United States was to ease the task of reimbursement for care rendered and to automate reporting of results for high-volume, time-critical tests such as clinical laboratory procedures. Typically, these applications ran on a single computer and users interacted via *"dumb" terminals*. Hospitals were regarded as independent organizations and revenue centers that could pass the costs on to third-party payers.

Beginning in the mid-1980s, however, dramatic health care policy and technology changes in the United States generated correspondingly broad changes in computer applications in hospitals. In contrast to previous conventions, hospitals were no longer reimbursed on a fee-for-service basis for many patients but, instead, received incentives to reduce costs. Hospitals in the United States are now seen as cost centers in the health care delivery system. Technology architectures are changing from centrally controlled local mainframes to network-based global application servers and networks of personal computers (*PCs*) and *workstations*. Today, administrators and health care providers can access libraries of information resources and a longitudinal patient record, in addition to the needed administrative and managerial applications. In addition, several of the leading hospitals use computer-based logic rules to alert care providers when standards of care are not being achieved. Such systems reduce costs and improve the quality of care. Although certain management functions remain hospital centered, *clinical information systems* must now cover a spectrum of patient activities within the ambulatory and inpatient areas.

Computers are a means to an end and not an end in themselves. In a health care setting, they should be used whenever it is possible to reduce costs or errors or to improve the speed with which patient care can be delivered. Computer applications can also reduce the cost of controlling the allocation of resources or achieving standards of quality. In this chapter we review the use of computers in the hospital setting and describe applications and information architectures that have been used to improve hospital operation and management as well as patient care.

2 The Historic Development of Hospital Information Systems

Hospitals were originally places where supportive care could be administered more economically than in the home. Physicians could see many patients quickly, there was around-the-clock support in an emergency, and nurses could serve more than one patient simultaneously. Stays were typically lengthy and costs were primarily for room, board, and nursing care.

With the improvements in sterile techniques, antibiotics, anesthesia, surgical procedures, and intensive care units (*ICUs*), hospitals became a focus for expensive procedures and heroic efforts to prolong life. These innovations caused the cost of hospital care to rise sharply, and many large US employers spread the risk by offering insurance coverage. Soon, health insurance coverage for most hospital care for employees and their families was regarded as an expected fringe benefit by employees. In 1965, all elderly Americans were guaranteed insurance coverage for hospital stays through the *Medicare* program. Until recently, the economics of the hospital business were based on fee-for-service or cost-based reimbursement. The more procedures a patient received or the longer the patient stayed, the more the hospital was reimbursed.

Naturally, a very cost-effective use of computers in such an environment would be to ensure that all possible charges be collected and that billing and accounts receivable be automated. Such automation would improve accuracy as well as save personnel effort compared to those achieved through manual processes. Because of this reimbursement focus, several characteristic aspects of hospital systems evolved. These are explained in the following sections.

2.1 Admission and Discharge

The data for each patient were focused on a patient's encounter with the system. Most systems did not easily link multiple encounters for a single patient into a longitudinal record. In fact, the individual medical record number was often subordinate to the financially important encounter billing number. A fundamental application was the Patient Admit/Discharge/Transfer (*ADT*) module. This module collected insurance and *demographic* information and formed the basis (since per-diem charges were room based) for a hospital census application. The census application could, in turn, be used to direct visitors, phone calls, housekeeping, phlebotomy teams, and so forth.

2.2 Order Entry

Desired data were usually not collected by a health care professional at the point of service. Physicians, nurses, therapists, and others wrote progress notes, vital signs, and orders into the paper-based patient record. Dictated reports were transcribed on typewriters and placed in the patient chart. For the purpose of efficiency, error avoidance, and reimbursement purposes, a ward clerk would enter the requests for diagnostic tests and diagnostic or therapeutic procedures in the computer-based *order-entry* application. One of the primary purposes of order entry was to enhance the charge capture function in the hospital. The patient also benefited from the order-entry system, because each request was rapidly communicated to the appropriate *ancillary* system in a standardized manner. The chances of omission were reduced, although in some instances the ward clerk might misread the physician's handwriting. A nurse or a physician would generally sign off on the transcribed orders to certify an accurate rendition.

Additional computer-based applications such as surgery scheduling evolved to improve efficiency, enhance utilization, and increase the accuracy of charge capture. For example, customized "case carts" were defined for each surgical procedure that a particular surgeon might perform. After a patient and procedure were scheduled, a list of surgical supplies and instruments for the procedure would be generated. A cart containing those supplies was wheeled into the operating room. Not only would the surgeon have all desired supplies readily available, but the hospital could properly bill for every packet of suture that was used. These systems functioned primarily to support the billing process, not to support clinicians.

2.3 Results Review

Generally, "results review functionality" was coupled with the order-entry application. These types of applications benefit the hospital and the health care providers. Clinical laboratory computer systems were probably the first health care applications to be developed on stand-alone *minicomputers*. The high volume of laboratory tests, the limited number of types of tests, the need for accurate linkage between test results and patients, and the desire to review test results immediately and in a variety of settings all combined to create significant advantages for laboratory automation (see Section 5 of Chapter 13). These results were sent back to the central order-entry, results review application through specially programmed, one-of-a-kind (laboratory vendor A or order-entry vendor B) interfaces that were originally **batch** oriented. Later, these interfaces transmitted data in real time. On the basis of the success of clinical laboratory automation, many hospitals also moved on to the use of computers for pharmacy and radiology management and results reporting applications (see Chapter 13). Again, the advantages were: the hospital accurately captured the resources used and health care providers could see test results or medication lists for hospital patients, even if the paper-based record was not readily available.

2.4 Stand-Alone Applications

In contrast to ADT and order-entry applications (which are primarily administrative), several stand-alone appli-

cations that were specifically designed to improve either the efficiency or the quality of patient care were developed. These systems (e.g., *catheterization* laboratory, *ICU*, pulmonary function testing, *electrocardiogram interpretation*, and *nuclear imaging*; see Chapters 12, 13 and 9) were typically offered as stand-alone applications that did not run as part of the hospital information system offered by major vendors. These applications often involved signal processing and thus required high-speed *analog-to-digital conversion* and the buffer controls of a dedicated machine. One view is that these systems came about to aid state-of-the-art research in medicine, and hence, their scope was narrow.

2.5 Storage Facilities

Because computer memory and disk storage were relatively expensive, the patient information was generally stored on magnetic tape shortly after the patient was discharged and the billing was completed. Of course, hospitals also used administrative systems not restricted to the health care business: payroll, human resources, general ledger, accounts payable, materials management, and budgeting.

3 Advanced Clinical Information Systems

The historical synopsis presented above generally represents the state of hospital computing in the United States and elsewhere from 1960 to 1990. However, a few U.S. hospitals and commercial firms can be singled out for developing clinical information systems that were primarily patient focused: the hospitals Beth Israel Hospital in Boston, Massachusetts; the Brigham and Women's Hospital, also in Boston; the LDS Hospital in Salt Lake City, Utah; and the Regenstrief Institute in Indianapolis, Indiana, and the commercial firms HDS (Ulticare Product) and Phamis. In Europe, patient-focused information systems are exemplified by the systems at the University Cantonal

Hospital in Geneva, Switzerland; the University Hospital Gasthuisberg in Leuven, Belgium; and the University Hospital in Leiden, The Netherlands (see also Chapter 21). The Kommunedata system (Denmark) exemplifies the patient-focused European commercial approach. The development of most of these systems started in the late 1960s or early 1970s. These systems integrated the wide variety of clinical applications within a *monolithic* architecture. By monolithic, we mean that the patient and provider context is preserved as the user switches between applications (see also Chapter 21).

The various applications use common databases of

20

code and structured terminology and run on a central host or hosts with a common operating system. This architecture provides a common user interface, development environment, and back-end database. The main drawback to this approach, which applies not only to these groups that developed patient-focused applications but also to almost all vendors of the traditional hospital information systems, is the requirement that most or all applications be developed within the monolithic environment. As new development environments emerge, all previous applications must be upgraded.

3.1 Policy and Technology Change

By the mid-1980s, the technical and policy environment changed rapidly. The first change reflected the reimbursement policy of the U.S. federal government. Technological change involved the emergence of PCs (and *word processing*) and *networks*.

The U.S. federal government had seen unabated growth (see Fig. 1.4 in Chapter 1) in costs for health care for the elderly (Medicare) since it agreed to pay the hospital costs for that group. In an attempt to stem that growth, the government began to reimburse the hospitals according to the particular type of illness or procedure that the patient had, regardless of how many days the patient stayed in the hospital or how many diagnostic tests or procedures that the patient received. The federal reimbursement for each patient depended on the diagnosis-related group (*DRG*) approach (see Chapters 6 and 21), which the patient assigned to a DRG by coders in the hospital's medical records department. This assignment was based on retrospective analysis of the data available in the paper-based patient record. Thus, hospitals in the United States immediately focused on computer-based coding assistance and DRG grouping applications.

Small changes in the patient's coded status can have a significant impact on reimbursement. When a patient is admitted for an acute exacerbation of asthma, it is imperative to document not only whether this is a status asthmaticus but also whether the patient has chronic obstructive pulmonary disease (*COPD*) with asth-

ma. For example, say a 67-year-old female Medicare recipient is admitted to the hospital for asthma, but it is not stated as being status asthmaticus. The DRG assigned for this diagnosis is 097, with an average payment of $4,531. However, if the patient has COPD with asthma, the assigned DRG would be 088, with an average reimbursement of $7,455. Therefore, when a patient is admitted with asthma, for the hospital to assign the correct DRG and receive accurate reimbursement, it is important to document COPD when it is present.

In some states, such as New York, all patients (not just the elderly) were reimbursed according to the DRG payment scheme. Before this change in reimbursement policy, if a hospital performed an additional radiological examination, the hospital earned more money. After the change, if the hospital performed the extra examination, it incurred the technician and film charges and received no additional reimbursement. For the first time, this policy gave hospitals an incentive to limit expenditures on behalf of a sick patient. Up to that point in time, these reimbursement changes addressed only hospital charges. The patient did not have an incentive to limit expenditures if he or she was covered by traditional insurance (reasonable and customary charges were paid), and the clinician was paid additional compensation if he or she delivered more care.

In this new environment, hospitals suddenly began to cut costs. To see where the hospital was spending money, the data from the existing charge capture systems were pooled into what became known as *management information systems* and *decision-support systems*. The terms are confusing, because it can refer to the executive as the recipient of the decision support. As we shall see, the terms can also be applied to the health care provider as the one who benefits from a system that generates alerts, reminders, and suggestions.

In any case, a management information system is used to aggregate the charge data for populations of patients so that a hospital executive can tell whether the hospital is making or losing money on patients with a particular DRG classification. The executive can also see if the hospital makes or loses money for each individual clinician who admits patients.

20

In this sense, the existing order-entry and billing systems continued to provide value to the hospital, but one major category of applications suffered a setback: nurse charting and bedside systems. In the hospitals that used these systems, nurses entered information such as *vital signs* and medication administration directly into the computer at the bedside. The end product was an all-electronic nursing note. Although various investigators showed that the record of care was more accurate and complete, it was not easy to demonstrate that such systems saved money or substantially affected patient outcome. In any event, a totally electronic record was never actually achieved because clinicians continued to write in the patient's paper-based chart. Clinicians generally resisted the use of automated systems because the *user interface* was not efficient for them (see also Chapter 31). In most instances the nurses' electronic shift report was also printed and added to the chart. For reasons that we will explain, we expect that these nursing documentation applications will see a resurgence in the near future as care plans and *critical pathways* become standard hospital fare.

3.2 Today's Hospital Systems Environment

The use of management information systems (as well as studies by health economists) showed that resource consumption for patients with similar illnesses varied widely from clinician to clinician, from hospital to hospital, and from region to region. The most coarse measure of resource consumption was length of stay. When hospital administrators saw the variance, they began to realize that in many cases the length of time that a patient stayed in the hospital could be cut substantially. This push, which initially did not require heavy computer support, led to two major issues: hospital occupancy rates and questions about compromised quality of care.

When people tried to determine whether a patient was being discharged so rapidly that the patient's care was compromised, they found that there were very limited data that could be used to answer such questions. Because most hospital systems did not have coded data about anything but laboratory tests and medications, it was difficult to measure outcomes. Did a patient receive better treatment and receive a better outcome at a major academic medical center than at a community hospital?

The answers to this type of question lie in truckloads of mostly handwritten, paper-based notes. Decades of collecting episodic data, primarily for generating patient bills, had not generated enough information to show whether a new mother should stay in the hospital 1 day or 2 weeks. Many hospitals could not measure their true postoperative wound infection rate or the number of adverse drug events. To add balance to the argument about the need for clinical information, it is also noteworthy that it is difficult to look at long-term outcomes when the technology of the therapies changes rapidly.

The decreasing bed occupancy rate (which occurred because lengths of stay were cut for the same numbers of patient admissions) also stimulated hospitals to seek outcomes data because they began to compete with one another for patients to fill the beds. The only competitive metric other than price is patient outcome. (Most payers will not pay a significant premium for friendly service.)

In any case, it was difficult to compare one hospital's data to those of another hospital. The U.S. government's Health Care Financing Agency and some states that mandated reporting ended up with the best databases, which could be used to compare hospitals' and clinicians' relative performance. Using data obtained by mandated reporting regulations, New York State has been able to publish death rate-by-surgeon information for patients undergoing coronary artery bypass surgery.

Because of the clamor by the clinicians and hospitals that did not fare well in these comparisons, it was necessary to adjust those gross mortality rates by "severity of illness." Most hospital information systems cannot generate such information without resorting to manual extraction of the data from the patients' charts. Since the DRG classification is determined in the same manner, administrators are now seeing an economic incentive to invest in clinical information systems that acquire patient-based clinical information at the point of care. Additionally, there are two other incentives:

20

- the ability to generate alerts, suggestions, and reminders and
- the ability to encourage the provider to follow a "critical pathway" in deciding how to best care for the patient and to track the compliance with those standards.

These concepts will be addressed later in this chapter. The major disincentive is the need for clinicians to enter data into the computer.

In summary, the 1990s has seen major shifts from administrative hospital information systems to systems that are used by physicians, nurses, and other health care providers as part of the process of delivering health care (i.e., *clinical information systems*). The motivation for investing in these systems is now economic. Physicians, nurses, and other health care providers must be encouraged at the point of service to help the hospital manage the allocation of resources. The group at the Regenstrief Institute showed a reduction of 12.6% in hospital charges by use of such a system.

An organization gets better outcomes data and providers receive immediate alerts when standards of care (from a quality and cost perspective) are not being achieved. Perhaps most importantly, by giving the clinician a system that gives him or her substantial value, the clinician becomes dependent on the use of the clinical information system. The administrator may thus gain some level of control over clinician behavior as the clinician writes orders to allocate resources. From an administrative perspective, this sort of control is desirable because, in the absence of guidance, a highly autonomous group of individuals allocates resources according to the best judgment of the group. Individual judgment may or may not be at odds with established standards of care. Given existing variance in practice patterns, there is ample room for some improvement in human performance.

In short, the computer lowers the cost of guidance without totally removing clinician autonomy. Previous generations of hospital information systems that focused entirely on charge capture ignored the ultimate source of resource allocation: the individual clinician. The next generation of information systems permits direct measurement and flexible control over the allocation of resources by practitioners.

Given the clinicians' long-standing tradition of autonomy and the historical difficulty in making computer data entry palatable to clinicians, the practical success of clinical information systems is still questionable. What are the critical elements that will motivate clinicians other than residents in training to enter orders (resource allocation) and progress notes (critical pathways, care plans, etc.) into the computer instead of writing them on paper or dictating them for transcription?

There are several reasons that physicians, nurses, and other caregivers will use well-designed clinical information systems:

1. Data presentation

   Presentation of data about the patient in an organized, comprehensive manner with instant access any time, anywhere to data that are needed to care for a patient. Such information would include immunization history, drug allergies, status of preventive measures, laboratory and other test results, specialist's referral reports, problem lists, visit notes, discharge summaries, surgical procedures, and images. Reliable, accurate, well-organized information will definitely help the physician, his or her staff, nurses, and health care workers save time and reduce errors. The challenge is to gather enough of this information in an electronic format to make it the main *repository* of desirable patient information. It is certainly easier to organize and present the data in the electronic version than asking someone to flip through a paper-based chart. *Confidentiality* issues must be addressed in a manner different from that when dealing with paper-based records, which can be at only one place at a time. However, it appears that those issues can be adequately addressed (see Chapter 33). Not all data need to be entered by professionals. Information that is not immediately needed to determine if standards of care are being achieved could still be dictated and transcribed in a timely manner (e.g., a discharge summary). Promising technologies such as handheld *writing tablets* and *voice recognition* (see Chapter 7) are gradually becoming acceptable from a performance standpoint.

2. Knowledge

Highly convenient availability of immediate, highly cogent sources of *additional expertise or knowledge* as part of the system. The use of **MED-LINE**-based literature searches has been warmly embraced by caregivers (see Chapter 6). Several investigators concluded that clinicians wished that they had additional information during one-third of their patients' office visits. The explosion of information resources on the World Wide Web (**Internet**) promises the desired content. The challenge is to filter the information and present only that which the user is most likely to desire when caring for a particular patient with a unique set of problems and challenges. Promising prototypes of such work are beginning to be used, although research in this area will likely require another decade before "knowbots" or "mediators" are able to automate this process. It is likely that such files will be based on the demonstrated expertise of the provider as well as the condition of the patient.

3. Communication

Communication with colleagues and patients. **E-mail** is a wonderful way to leave a note to a colleague who is covering a patient for the weekend. **Video teleconferencing** is just beginning to pay demonstrated dividends. Nowadays, it is technically possible to hear a previously dictated radiologist's opinion about a patchy infiltrate while seeing her move a cursor on the image. Integrating such sources of information into the clinical information system will clearly improve a clinician's ability to get an instant interpretation of an X-ray image of a patient in the ICU.

4. Alerts, reminders, and suggestions

Automated generation of *alerts, reminders, and suggestions* when standards of care are not being achieved. All of the previous three benefits can be achieved to some degree with paper-based patient charts, books, and telephones or letters; the computer primarily increases the efficiency and convenience of achieving those ends. The mechanism for achieving real-time quality control, however, can realistically be achieved only in an electronic environment. The use of manual oversight to encourage compliance is prohibitively expensive, and obtrusive and is subject to the same human foibles that one is seeking to avoid. **Second opinions** are mandated by insurance companies for some big-ticket examinations or interventions, but the manual approach does not match with the myriad hourly tasks and decisions that can improve the quality and efficiency of care.

In the case of automated reminders and alerts, the computer adds real additional value. Most clinicians make mistakes infrequently. When their decisions are in accord with established standards of practice, the care providers are generally unaware that their actions are being critiqued by the computer. It is only when there is a deviation that a message is delivered to the clinician.

The most exciting aspect of the computer-based decision-making capability is the ability to structure a critical pathway as a series of rules that will respond independently whenever certain criteria are satisfied. By this approach, it is not required that a patient be followed by a branching protocol that loses significance when unexpected events take place. Rules from three or four different protocols or pathways could generate simultaneous and valid suggestions if the patient's clinical condition warrants such suggestions. Clinicians and administrators can choose to focus on the important parts of a critical pathway rather than requiring that every aspect of a patient's care be addressed.

Automatically generated alerts, suggestions, or warnings can also be used to generate lists of pending crucial tasks (see Fig. 21.1) that are specifically germane because the patient's clinical data satisfy logical criteria. This dynamically generated task list based on the patient's condition is a totally different approach to care plans than a one-size-fits-all flowchart (whether it is paper based or electronic). The research groups at Beth Israel Hospital, Brigham and Women's Hospital, LDS Hospital, Columbia-Presbyterian Medical Center, and Regenstrief Institute in the United States have demonstrated that computer-generated messages have the ability to

20

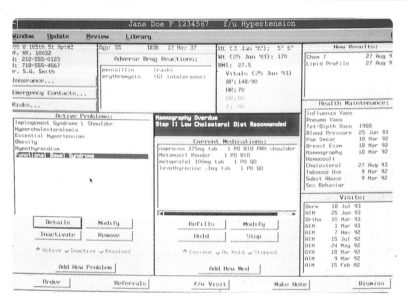

Figure 20.1
A mock-up of a screen for integrating critical pathway and care plan messages with the results review function in a clinical information system. Medical logic modules contain the logic of the pathway and are evaluated to present pending and expected tasks as well as to alert the clinician when tasks are not completed in a timely manner.

alter provider behavior. From a hospital executive level, adherence to the critical pathway gives a two-fold benefit: the patient is treated in an efficient and cost-effective manner, and standards of quality are maintained. Discharging sick patients prematurely may save the hospital money, but there must be built-in safeguards for quality of care that counteract the new motivations to cut costs.

3.3 Technical Aspects of Current Hospital Information Systems

To accomplish the economically motivated patient care goals described above, it is likely that clinical information systems will be created by interfacing and integrating many disparate applications. These applications will not all come from a single vendor or run on a single computer. A hospital must create an *information architecture* that is not based on the offerings of a single vendor. The basic architecture should depend on a network of desktop computers that can run application programs based within any of multiple application hosts also connected to the network. These applications can be run in *"terminal emulation"* mode or as *client-server applications*. The front-end work-

station may require scripting and log-on facilities so that connection to the back-end application is seamless as far as the end user is concerned. This architecture is a powerful reason for the dramatic increase in the use of World Wide Web facilities.

Of particular importance at the desktop level is heterogeneity. One should assume that users will want access, whether on site or remote, from workstations with various types of operating systems (*Windows* 95, Macintosh, Windows NT, *UNIX*). Multiple presentation modes on that local machine must be supported; IBM 3270 emulation, DEC VT100 emulation, Microsoft Windows, X-Windows, and *World Wide Web browsers* are all viable candidates.

The network architecture should allow for secure transmission of data and the use of *passwords*. Further elements of the network architecture include a *repository* (long-term patient database), *protocols* for sending messages between various sources of information (e.g., *TCP/IP* and *HL-7*), a dictionary that translates information representation (terms or codes) between various applications, and an interface engine (database interface) that receives messages and queries and routes them to the correct destination(s).

This architecture is presented in Fig. 21.2. A patient is registered by using a hospital *ADT* application or a local departmental application (e.g., ophthalmology or obstetrics). The admitting program must query an

20

enterprise-wide patient index to determine whether to assign a new unique patient identifier (patient record number). The demographic data are broadcast in the HL-7 format to other systems (laboratory, pharmacy, billing) that want or need to know about all patients in the system (a local copy of the patient index).

Each of the multiple local applications (clinical laboratory, urology, anesthesia, ICU, etc.) also may have a local copy of the patient data needed to run that application. Each of these domain-specific applications may receive data (in HL-7 format) from the central system via subscribed broadcast or patient-specific query. In turn, each application sends its collected information (again, using the HL-7 format) to the enterprise repository.

Work is proceeding to improve standards for interchanging data between applications. In addition to HL-7, which is becoming ubiquitous in the United States, **EDI-FACT** is common in Europe. Other emerging data exchange standards include **CEN/TC251** (PT004), **IEEE/MEDIX, ANSI, NCPDP,** and **DICOM** (see Chapter 34). These are higher-level standards than **CORBA** (Common Object Request Broker Architecture), or **OLE** (Microsoft). The repository must be flexible, scaleable, and extensible so that new data types can be conveniently added to the repository.

Another requirement is a minimal response time for data queries at both the server and the network levels. For reasons associated with the automated decision-making capability, the response time to queries for data is an extremely important criterion. To optimize patient-specific queries, many institutions create additional research databases that are optimized for cross-patient (population) queries. Some of these research databases are under the control of local administrators in individual departments. The research databases are populated via subscription to the interface engine-database interface.

The role of the dictionary is to map the terms or codes used in the various applications into a common representation. This mapping is typically accomplished as data flow through the interface engine. The architectural advantages of this approach are multiple. Data may be collected in any interfaced application. Those data are communicated to the longitudinal patient database, which is logically centralized but which can be physically distributed. Any application can access

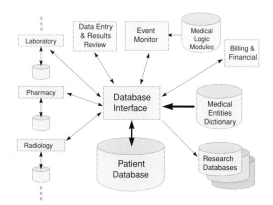

Figure 20.2
Architecture for a clinical information system. Communication between the modules is based on standardized protocols. This architecture lets applications from multiple developers coexist. Integration takes place at the database level, and some integration can also occur at the application level. A single results review application can present data from disparate sources by accessing the patient database.

data collected by other applications. It is not required that the user applications be constrained to reflect monolithic hardware or software conventions. In a multihospital chain, there might be multiple results and review or data-entry programs, but each such application can get the data as long as it uses the standard interface protocols.

Many feel that this architecture was initially articulated by Simborg, who originally felt that the integration could be accomplished at the workstation rather than at the database. Most groups now realize that a **repository** that is separate from any particular application has performance and longevity benefits. In fact, multiple repositories can exist simultaneously. Queries received by the interface engine are translated into database access modules (or objects). This library of modules could be rewritten to query the new database, and the existing application programs would not realize that they were getting data from a different source.

The European **CEN/TC251** committee (see Chapter 34) is working to abstract the architecture presented in Fig. 21.2. This reference architecture would allow for the development of components that could be used

20

together in a plug-and-play fashion while achieving the same level of integration afforded by the monolithic systems. Systems integrators would be able to purchase various components from various vendors and have competing versions of specific components from which to choose. Accomplishment of these far-reaching goals would allow developers to pool their efforts to develop information systems and dramatically shrink the time that is currently required to construct clinical information systems.

Integrating patient data from multiple sources may be the only alternative (as opposed to a homogeneous monolithic approach) in an era of mergers and consolidations of health care facilities. Piping data to a logically central **hub** also enables the automated decision making to function. As each packet of data is stored in the repository, the event monitor looks into its **knowledge base** to see if there are any rules involved in evaluating the new data. Additional data required by the logic are also retrieved from the database. If the criteria are satisfied, an appropriate message is generated. This alert or suggestion can be displayed as part of a results review screen or can actively be transmitted by opening a process on a multitasking workstation, by e-mail, by an autodial beeper, or by **fax**.

How does one obtain such a hospital information system? In previous environments, one selected a **turnkey** vendor. In today's environment, one must develop in-house integration expertise or hire a systems integrator. There is a need to develop a resource pool to manage the disparate systems. This pool will have a mix of skills far different from those needed when dealing with a system from a single vendor. There are several commercial sources for the systems components, interface engines, and repositories. HL-7 is a rapidly maturing standard; in some cases (clinical laboratory and demographics) the format is extensively specified. In other cases, one simply uses the HL-7 header as an envelope to enclose information that must be **parsed** by a data access module.

Dictionaries are beginning to emerge as a result of the leadership at the U.S. National Library of Medicine and the National Health Service in the United Kingdom. The National Library of Medicine fostered an approach in which medical entities can be related by **semantic** and hierarchical links and qualified by local and global **attributes**. The lists of entities for inclusion in the dictionary are quite comprehensive for the clinical laboratory and pharmacy domains. **SNOMED ICD**, **Read code**, and **DICOM** (see Chapter 6) are vocabularies that remain to be integrated into the appropriately modeled semantic structure. Comprehensive coverage within the dictionary is not needed to begin storing data. One can create dictionary content as additional applications are added. However, robust, institution-independent tools and skills for editing, managing, and merging the dictionaries are not yet available.

From a technological standpoint, there are several steps to be followed as one implements a clinical information system:

1. Establish a network of desktop and host machines.
2. Avoid proprietary protocols.
3. Implement e-mail.
4. Select fundamental hospital applications (registration, billing, clinical laboratory, radiology, pharmacy, results review, and order entry) that can send and receive HL-7 messages.
5. Implement a repository.
6. Use an interface engine to route data messages between various applications.
7. Establish a data dictionary for defining the content of the patient record in a coded format.
8. Establish a front-end scripting environment for the workstations that allows for seamless access to any of the applications. With a Web browser, **Perl**, and **Java**, it is becoming easier to create such an environment.
9. Add information resources (MEDLINE, pharmacy handbooks, procedure manuals, etc.).
10. Encourage domain- or department-specific applications.
11. Implement a decision-making application.
12. Facilitate clinician-based order entry.

4 The Future of Hospital Information Systems

By the time that the technological steps described above are completed, the next round of the health care revolution will have occurred. Hospitals in the USA will no longer be reimbursed according to the fixed DRG rate but will bid to health care payers to provide care for the patient at a negotiated price. This will reward the cost-efficient hospitals, but payers and patients will demand evidence of quality. It may finally be possible to measure patient outcomes in a meaningful way. Programs to analyze the clinical data will become available.

The final twist involves emerging motivations to keep the patient out of the hospital entirely. In the previous model, clinicians and hospitals earned money when the patient was sick. Insurers could raise premiums to cover the costs of care. The trend now is to pay providers a certain fee to care for a population whether they are sick or healthy (capitation). In the emerging capitated environment, providers would make money if they can keep patients out of the hospital. This may mean that the information system will be extended into the home. At the very least, the hospital data would be interfaced into the information system of a vertically integrated health care provider.

In the past, hospitals have taken the initiative in building information systems because they had a critical mass of financial resources and a financial benefit to be gained. It was also the fact that hospitals could pass the costs of their information systems onto the payers. In the new environment, the deployment of information systems will need to be financially justified to an extent never before encountered. Hospitals have more incentive than ever to reduce costs. Information systems must contribute to the efficiency and quality of care in an economically meaningful way. The only problem with this scenario is that the cost savings are likely to come from the computer-based decision-making applications. There needs to be a critical mass of clinician use and acceptance before it is cost-effective.

The noteworthy clinical information systems referenced in this chapter have all taken 15 to 25 years to reach the point where they can demonstrate that payback. On the basis of the experience at Columbia-Presbyterian Medical Center, the use of the distributed, interfaced architecture may cut that time by a factor of 3. However, 5 to 8 years is still a long time to wait for payback. If the *reference* architecture being investigated in Europe bears fruit, the time cut may be further shortened.

In the future it is likely that there will not be only hospital information systems located in hospitals. It appears that these systems will become nodes that feed a ***longitudinal patient record*** controlled by a vertically integrated health care provider. These systems will be built of modular components that are integrated across multiple settings (including the home) in which the patient receives care. Computer-generated real-time critiquing will be the value-added capability that will justify investments in information systems. This automated decision-making capability will enable health care organizations to control resource utilization and to maintain or improve quality by implementing logical criteria contained in critical pathways, practice guidelines, and care plans. If our systems can accomplish these goals, we can finally obtain the systems foreseen more than three decades earlier.

Key References

McDonald CJ, Blevins L, Tierney WM. Regenstrief Medical Records. MD Computing 1988;5:34-7.

Simborg DW, Networking and medical information system. J of Med Systems 1984;8:43-7.

See the Web site for further literature references.

20

21 Hospital Information Systems: Technical Choices

1 Introduction

As noted in Chapter 20, the functioning of a complex organization such as a hospital, with its many departments, mainly depends on the availability of data. Data may concern patient care on the one hand and the functioning of the hospital on the other. Therefore, a distinction should be made between patient-oriented and hospital-oriented data. Over the years, patient-oriented data have changed considerably both in nature and in number, because diagnostic and therapeutic possibilities are continuously expanding and clinical specializations have continuously increased. The hospital organization also continuously changes in character and requirements for operational data are growing (see also Chapter 20). Examples of such changes are:

- the hospital reimbursement system that evolved from a fee-for-service system to a fixed-budget system, bringing along the need for hospitals to better control the costs of medical care and to be more market oriented, and
- the increasing interest in quality of care.

These changes force hospitals to rely increasingly on computer-based information systems. The only way to collect, store, process, communicate, and present large quantities of data in a way that fits the user requirements is with computers. The user may be a nurse who enters or retrieves patient data, the head of a clinical department who is planning the provision of care for the following week, or a member of the hospital board who uses the system for management support. These requirements can largely be met by a hospital information system (**HIS**). The following are particular functions of an HIS:

1. support of day-to-day activities,
2. support of the planning and organization of these day-to-day activities,
3. support of the control and correction of planned activities and their costs, in view of agreements on medical and financial policies (this is usually called *management control*), and
4. support of clinical research through use of the HIS database, which is particularly important for university hospitals.

The means by which HISs can meet these requirements are varied and in many ways depend on a variety of technical and organizational factors. In this chapter these factors are explored in some depth.

The concept of an HIS and how it can support the activities on operational, tactical, and, to a lesser degree, strategic levels are discussed in Section 2. Section 3 describes how different architectures may be used to realize an HIS. The fact that integration is one of the most important notions in any discussion about an HIS will be considered later in this chapter in Section 4. In Section 5, two different European hospital information systems are described to provide a clearer explanation of notions introduced in preceding sections. Section 6 describes two aspects of an HIS that collide with each other: accessibility of relevant data on the one hand and data protection measures on the other hand. In

---

PANEL 21.1

The Role of an HIS in Clinical Epidemiological Research

An HIS database can be used for clinical research in three different ways:

* to select and compose a *trial group* (i.e., use the HIS as a sampling tool),
* to collect patient data that are used in the trial (i.e., use the HIS as a data collection tool), and
* to register data especially collected for the purpose of the research (i.e., use the HIS as a registration tool).

Using an HIS as sampling tool

In experimental studies the assignment of patients to a trial group is generally determined by the *protocol* of the experiment. In these situations an HIS will not play a part in the selection of patients. However, for exploratory studies a trial group will be established according to one or more selection criteria. Such a criterion can be some action, a diagnosis, or a treatment. Usually, patients will be selected by using an existing database, because the complete trial population will then immediately be available. If a clinical researcher is not able to use an HIS, the only remaining possibility is to spend time in the medical records archive searching for records of, for instance, patients with lung carcinoma.

Therefore, it is very important that a clinical researcher has at his or her disposal a patient population that can be used as a *sampling frame*. The selection of a patient population for research purposes puts great demands on the completeness and the reliability of the data (see Chapter 2).

Using an HIS for data collection

Once a trial population has been established, part of the data relevant for the research can possibly be sampled via the HIS. This applies both to experimental and to exploratory studies. Specific laboratory reports or X-ray reports, for instance, can often be extracted from an HIS. This prevents much unnecessary administrative work. Incompleteness and inaccuracy automatically become apparent, since not only the data but also the patient number can be used as a selection criterion.

Using an HIS as registration tool

If the HIS contains the facility to design input screens and to store data efficiently, it can be used to register data that are specially collected in the context of a research project. Use of the HIS as a registration tool assists the researcher with professional data management. The HIS also offers the researcher an infrastructure for data entry. It permits the registration of data at the time and place where they originate. For statistical processing the data will often be transferred to a *PC* or some other computer. ▶

Using an HIS for selecting a trial population

A clinical researcher is dependent on the availability of sampling frames (e.g., an existing large database), especially when setting up an observational research study. Advantages of sampling frames are the relatively large number of cases that are practically instantly available and the possibilities for *longitudinal* observation. Selecting patients from a sampling frame is done by applying one or more selection criteria to the data in the database.

Before making a selection, the researchers feel rather confident that the selected population is representative of the entire group of patients who suffer from a certain disease or who have undergone some intervention. The completeness and reliability of the data selected must also be checked carefully.

How can we verify whether the data for a trial population are complete, reliable, and representative? This can be done by verifying how the data were collected at the source. The starting point should be the medical actions concerning the patient population to be selected, along with the corresponding administrative procedures. Questions to be asked are, for instance, the following:

* *What were the functions of the data registration?*
   This determines data completeness, that is, whether all patients belonging to the trial population were included in the registration (e.g., patients having undergone a renal biopsy). For instance, if the registration is essential for day-to-day patient care, the registration will generally be complete.

* *Which data were incidentally or always registered?*
   The fact that the user's instructions state that an item must be entered is insufficient to guarantee that the data are always indeed entered. One must check whether entering the data is necessary for day-to-day patient care or for, for example, authorization or reporting. Only if this is the case can it be assumed that the data will always be entered.

* *Which definitions apply to data and concepts?*
   The definition of the data or concepts in a registration cannot always be derived from the name of the data. To assess the usability of a registration for the selection of a trial population one should not only be aware of the definitions and descriptions of data and concepts, as given in the documentation of the data registration, but one should also know exactly what the researcher means by data and concepts to be used in a trial. Examples of concepts that are often interpreted in different ways are the terms complication and readmission.

* *Which classification and coding systems have been used?*
   It is important to know whether the classification or coding system consists of mutually exclusive categories. If this is not the case, it will be possible to use several codes for the same concept. The extent of detail can also result in the use of several codes.

21

Section 7 the role of the HIS for management support is elaborated and Panel 21.1 provides an illustration of the use of data in an HIS to support research. The chapter concludes by indicating future HIS developments, of which the outlines are now becoming visible.

2 The HIS Concept

The function of an HIS is to support hospital activities on operational, tactical, and strategic levels. To cite Collen:

The goal of an HIS is to use computers and communication equipment to collect, store, process, retrieve, and communicate patient care and administrative information for all hospital-affiliated activities and to satisfy the functional requirements of all authorized users.

Another characterization of an HIS is:

An information system for the benefit of a hospital, in which data are coherently stored in a database, from where they are put at the disposal of authorized users at the place and at the time the data are required, in a format adapted to the specific needs of the user.

In general, the following are aims of such an HIS:

1. more efficient use of the restricted resources available for patient care,
2. qualitative improvement of the service to the patient,
3. support of research, and
4. support of teaching.

The last two apply especially to university hospitals. To meet the requirements listed above, an HIS should at least contain the following:

1. a facility for the storage of data (i.e., a *database*),
2. facilities to enter data into the database and to retrieve or edit the data (i.e., *applications*),
3. *data communication* facilities, and
4. facilities that enable the user to use the system (i.e., *terminals* or *workstations*).

A database (Chapter 4) may be considered a logically structured set of data in which data are stored for the benefit of various applications. The applications form the bridge between the database and the user. A widely implemented HIS easily contains several dozen applications.

Until now we did not discuss which applications an information system should contain to be allowed to carry the label "HIS." This simply originates from the fact that there is no unanimity about the scope of an HIS or, to phrase it differently, which hospital functions an HIS should support and to what extent they should be automated.

A distinction can be made between functions that are specific for some clinical department (see Chapter 12) and functions that support processes in more than one department (Chapter 13). The discussion concerning the scope of an HIS especially concerns applications that are specific for one department only. Applications that are commonly used throughout the hospital, such as patient registration or billing, are generally considered to belong to an HIS, but this opinion does not hold for applications for specific departments, such as laboratory automation (see Section 5 of Chapter 13) or radiology file-room management (Section 1 of Chapter 13).

As an example of two extreme views, we will discuss the concept of an HIS, which, in principle, supports all functions in an integrated way, and a *kernel HIS*, which only supports common hospital applications. In practice, most situations will lie somewhere between these two extremes.

The distinction described above implies that applications considered to belong to an HIS are related to hospital functions. A frame of reference describing all hospital functions developed in The Netherlands, is the Hospital Information Model (*HIM*, see also Chapter 19). The HIM comprises the following *functional entities*:

21

Table 21.1
Structure of Different Subsystems in a Hospital Information System.

Patient is Central		Hospital is Central	
Diagnostics and Treatment	*Registration Support of Medical Activities*	*Technical and Housekeeping Management*	*Finance*
• Patient identification and registration • Laboratories • Radiology • Picture information systems	• Support of diagnostics and therapy • Registration of diagnoses	• Energy control • Food supply • Planning of technical maintenance • Housekeeping maintenance	• Administration of medical actions • Administration of authorizations • In- and outpatient billing
	Admission and Nursing	*Miscellaneous*	*Resources Management*
	• Admission planning and waiting list management • Registration of locations of inpatients • Support of nursing activities	• Management information system • Exchange with national registrations • Other external information exchange	• Purchasing administration • Stock keeping and purchasing • Loan administration
			Personnel
			• Personnel administration • Administration

21

1. professional activities of clinicians,
2. diagnosis and therapy,
3. admission and nursing,
4. registration of medical activities,
5. finance and billing,
6. resources management,
7. personnel,
8. technical aspects such as maintenance, and
9. miscellaneous aspects, such as management information, education and research, and external information exchange.

Table 21.1 gives a few examples of corresponding hospital functions the last eight functional entities. A complicating factor in this discussion is that a useful HIS *reference model* describing the dividing lines between HIS applications is lacking. Until there is such a reference model, it is up to the supplier of the application whether, for instance, a laboratory system will contain functions for order entry, for reporting, or for financial processing, in addition to the essential laboratory functions of such a system.

An alternative way to describe the scope of an HIS,

thereby detailing the functions of an HIS, is to consider the various types of medical data that are supported and the possibilities to process them. The following is a general categorization of the medical data stored in computers (see also Chapter 2):

1. Structured data
   - numbers,
   - measurements (e.g., in the form of biosignals and images), or
   - coded data.
2. Unstructured data
   - free text as data that are entered into a computer, or
   - free text as dictated medical reports.

The earliest HISs were necessarily restricted to the processing of structured data only. Nowadays, it is at least technically possible to realize an HIS that conforms to one of the conclusions of an international meeting on HISs:

In principle an HIS should contain all aspects of information management of a hospital, including pictures and management information.

Finally, it is becoming more and more difficult to point out the geographical boundaries of an HIS, because of the increasing possibilities for communicating with information systems outside the hospital.

3 Architectures of an HIS

This section describes various architectures that have been proposed to shape the HIS concept as discussed in Section 2. The most common distinction between architectures is:

- monolithic systems,
- evolutionary systems, and
- distributed systems.

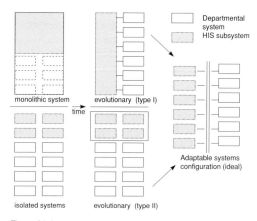

Figure 21.1
Development of HIS architectures along two possible paths. A rectangle denotes an application; for the sake of clarity all databases have been omitted.

Theoretically, the choice of a particular architecture is not related to the functionality offered to the user. However, the choice of a particular architecture does have consequences for the development and maintenance of an HIS. The characteristics, disadvantages, and advantages of various **architectures** are briefly discussed by using Fig. 21.1, in which the two directions in which the development of an HIS apparently takes place have been outlined.

In Fig. 21.1a the starting point is a **monolithic** system, the structure of which is determined from the beginning and in which all hospital functions have been positioned in a more or less integrated way. In contrast, Fig. 21.1b starts with a set of isolated applications that are partly specific for a department and partly more broadly applicable. It depicts more or less the situation as it used to exist in the United States, although examples of both ways of development can be found in many countries.

In the following, we use the word **composable** instead of the word **distributed** to indicate that, in composing an HIS, flexibility has priority; the fact that an HIS be distributed is only one aspect. If we put the various types of architectures in their own time frames, it becomes immediately obvious that each architecture can only be based on what is technically possible and what is organizationally feasible at the moment of origin. For example, the opportunity of migrating to a composable system became possible only when network facilities and communication standards became available at the end of the 1980s. The availability of networking facilities, however, does not mean that all operational systems should follow or will follow the outlined path of migration. In practice, when a hospital chooses to invest in a new HIS architecture, there is often a negative component (i.e., users having considerable problems with the current system) and a positive component (e.g., the advantages of the new system are manifest). Anyhow, for the current situation as well as for the required situation, different aspects such as flexibility, performance, **cost-benefit** aspects, and user-friendliness should be thoroughly considered before making such a choice, because the choice of the system often has far-reaching organizational consequences.

3.1 Isolated Applications

The situation in which all applications are separately developed and applied can, in fact, not be called an architecture. In many cases, the monolithic architecture was preceded by a period of time when there were only stand-alone applications. The only advantage of this situation, namely, that a head of a department can buy his or her own system, bypassing any hospital policy, does not outweigh the disadvantages, such as diversification and the impossibility of using the data or functions of other systems. The consequences of these disadvantages are that there is no coherent presentation of patient data to the user, duplication of functions and data, inconsistency of data, a security that is rarely warranted, and continuity that is seldom guaranteed.

3.2 Monolithic Systems

Monolithic HISs have been constructed on the basis of a *holistic* approach, that is, from the idea that, in principle, it is preferable to arrange the systems so that all hospital functions are supported from one

overall perspective. Not only the implementation of all applications into one computer system but also the development of software and the choice of standards and of peripheral equipment are determined as much as possible by that perspective. It is important to realize that these systems originated at a time when personal computers and network facilities, taken for granted nowadays, were in the distant future. The advantages of this holistic approach are especially that system development can be well managed and that applications can be optimally integrated (see also Section 4). Drawbacks observed in the earliest systems were a lack of flexibility and the fact that external applications could not, or could hardly be linked to the system because of the closed character of these systems.

3.3 Evolutionary Systems—Type I

If its functionality and number of users are constantly increasing, an HIS that is completely based on the monolithic architecture will run out of control at some point. This could well be the most important reason for the appearance of an architecture that circumvented some of the drawbacks mentioned for the monolithic architecture while preserving the overall perspective: evolutionary architecture type I, as we call it here. Such an architecture became possible when the state of the technology had advanced far enough. By linking applications for local processing to the central system as separate *modules*, the architecture becomes more flexible and easier to extend.

3.4 Evolutionary Systems—Type II

The evolutionary system type II is a logical subsequent step to arrive at a form of integration of separate applications. These applications are sometimes far along in their development and functioning well. In most cases, applications that are important at several locations in the hospital are installed on a central system,

21

whereas the applications with mainly local importance are linked to that central system as modules. Data to be used at several locations are generally consolidated in a data repository, where they are accessible within their context. In general, the evolutionary systems mentioned here, types I and II, are more alike than different.

3.5 Composable Systems

HIS suppliers who select the type I path and those who chose the type II path are setting a trend in the direction of composable systems, which is made possible by current technology. In the ideal situation, an architecture is characterized by optimal flexibility, in which the HIS can be composed of applications from different HIS suppliers. These applications may be running on different *platforms* that communicate with each other and with the database via standards. The following are examples of present communication standards (see Chapter 5):

- *TCP/IP*, a communication protocol;
- *CORBA*, for systems integration;
- *SQL*, communication with the database;
- *HL-7*, internal communication; or
- *EDIFACT*, external communication.

Since most standards are not stable yet and since the HIS reference model mentioned before is still lacking, the ideal situation outlined above still lies in the future.

In the framework of a composable architecture, the *client-server* model deserves to be mentioned. In a client-server model, the components database, application logic, and user interface are partitioned between clients and servers. This means that users can utilize applications that run on another computer (i.e., the *application server*) via their own workstation; these applications communicate with a database that can be implemented on a separate computer, a *database server*. However, we want to emphasize here that even when using the most advanced models, including those based on a so-called *middleware* concept, successful communication between systems is only possible when there are agreements about the logical concepts, the data definitions, and the division of functions, as well as coordination of the communication standards to be used. This condition is generally difficult to fulfill.

Section 2.3 indicated that the availability of an HIS reference model would clarify the demarcations of HIS applications, from which hospitals as well as HIS suppliers could benefit. A similar need exists for a reference architecture of an HIS, with which each hospital will be able to assemble an HIS adapted to its own situation and to its established information policy. Initiatives attempting to create a reference architecture have been extremely slow, which is partly caused by the complexity of the subject. A common reference architecture in combination with standardized interfaces would form the basis for an HIS generation in which *portability* (i.e., transferability of software to other platforms) and *interoperability* (i.e., ability to approach data and functions from another platform) are the keywords.

It was mentioned in Section 2 that there are different opinions about the functionality that an HIS should have, regardless of the underlying architecture. According to one opinion, only those functions that are applied in the whole hospital belong to an HIS; all other functions should be linked to that HIS as modules. According to another, extreme, opinion all applications used in a hospital should be integrated within one HIS including, for example, systems used for picture archiving and communications (*PACS*; see Section 5 and Section 2 of Chapter 13) and *document management*. The next section discusses the notion of *integration* which means much more than that there is a relationship between the parts of the system that will be assembled together.

4 Integration Between HIS Applications

From the user's point of view, at least three types of integration can be distinguished:

- *Data integration.* This means that data registered in one application are available to another application, if necessary and provided that it is not conflicting with confidentiality. This prevents repeated recording of the same data and reduces the risk of mistakes.
- *Presentation integration* implies that data from various applications are presented to the user in an adequate and consistent way. Especially for dynamically changing data, this is not self-evident.
- *Functional integration* means that functions of different applications are available to the qualified user within one user environment.

The term *complete integration* may be used when all three types of integration are jointly realized. Another distinction that is technically oriented can be made by looking at the way in which integration is realized. We mention two possible means:

1. *By means of a direct link*
   Applications communicate with each other and with the database through direct procedure calls or function calls. The interfaces of the applications have been put in so-called application programming interfaces (*APIs*). This is a common and effective way of integration, especially for monolithic systems, in which all applications, usually from the same supplier, are implemented in the same computer system. It is possible to realize complete integration by this means.
2. *By means of message exchange*
   Applications communicate with each other and with the database by exchanging messages. It is of essential importance that there is a good communication infrastructure, which ensures that in all cases messages are correctly delivered to the addressees in the proper sequence and that standard **message protocols** (see below and Chapters 5 and 34) are used. If both requirements have been met and if there is agreement on the **semantics** of the messages to be transmitted, then all applications supporting the

message protocol will, in principle, be able to communicate with each other, irrespective of their physical location and of the supplier of the application. It is possible to realize perfect data integration in this way, but more complex types of integration will hardly be possible, if they are possible at all.

4.1 Standards for Message Exchange

21

Communication between sender and receiver completely depends on the use of messages for which both sides agree on **syntax** and **semantics**. In other words, integration between two systems is possible only when both systems support the same message standard. A disadvantage is that until now there have been various standards (see also Chapters 5, 9, and 34). Below we mention the most important ones.

- EDIFACT and HL-7

For the health care sector as a whole, two standards are available:

1. EDIFACT messages, which are generally used for communication with systems outside the own organization, and
2. the HL-7 standard, which is generally used for communication within the own organization.

The EDIFACT (Electronic Data Interchange for Administration, Commerce, and Transport) standard, originating from systems for international trade, is a set of agreements on the setting up of messages and on the use of segments and fields. An example of such a message is the laboratory report sent from a hospital to a GP (see Chapter 11). The HL-7 (Health Level Seven) standard, which originated in the United States, not only contains a syntax to compose messages but also allows for the definition of so-called **trigger events**, on the basis of which messages are sent to the various applications. Examples of trigger events are the admission of a patient, a placement of a laboratory order, or transfer of a patient to another department.

- DICOM

The **DICOM** (Digital Imaging and Communication in Medicine) standard has especially been developed for the exchange of image information by the American College of Radiology/ National Electrical Manufacturers Association. For the non-image information within the message, the DICOM approach is comparable to that of HL-7. Communication of image information often occurs within a PACS, which should ideally be linked to the HIS or be an integral part of it.

- ASTM and EUCLIDES

The American Society of Testing and Materials (**ASTM**) standards and the **EUCLIDES** standard, which is the result of a European collaboration, should also be mentioned. They are specifically intended for the exchange of laboratory orders and reports.

- ASN/1

The **ASN/1** notation, developed by the International Standards Organization (**ISO**) and the Consultative Committee of the International Telegraph and Telephone (CCITT) is a meta-standard for providing a general mechanism for defining standards by presenting a syntax in an abstract way from which message-handling programs can be generated.

4.2 Integration and the Multivendor Aspect

The standards described above indicate that there are two ways to integrate stand-alone applications with an HIS. We want to emphasize that integration is not an aim in itself, but that the purpose is to enhance the efficiency and the practical value of the HIS; in other words: the whole is more than the sum of its parts. However, both the use of a direct link and the exchange of standardized messages have advantages and disadvantages. Considering all the pros and cons, the choice seems to be between the possibility of complete integration and greater flexibility in assembling the various HIS components. An attractive option for hospitals might be to obtain applications that need strong mutual integration all from one vendor who will be able to provide this required degree of integration, but to link to the HIS those applications that need a lesser degree of integration; for instance, they can be linked via HL-7. For these applications it is possible to select the best supplier for each application. However, it remains a choice between incomparable items (i.e., incomparable in terms of degree of integration and flexibility).

Chapter 32 provides a survey of cost-benefit analyses on which the choice of the HISs discussed here can be based.

5 Operational HISs

This section describes two operational European HISs to show how earlier choices with respect to scope, architecture, and integration work out in practice. Both HISs, the **Hiscom** HIS and the **Diogene** HIS, meet the criterion that is perhaps most important for an HIS, but that, unfortunately, can only be determined after it is in place, namely, that it has proven itself in practice. This proof refers to the reliability and to the availability of the system (i.e., it must be reliably available 24 hours a day, 7 days a week) as

well as to the flexibility with which the system can be adapted to the continuously changing requirements of the users.

5.1 Hiscom HIS

The HIS of Hiscom (Leiden, The Netherlands) is used by most Dutch university hospitals and a large number of general hospitals and psychiatric hospitals. The

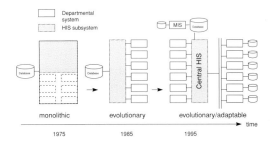

Figure 21.2
Development of the Hiscom HIS architecture (Leiden, The Netherlands) between 1975 and 1995.

Hiscom HIS is considered to be a complete system with a high level of integration. It is an example of a system that from the beginning has actually gone through the steps in the development of an HIS architecture mentioned above, using technology that is functionally relevant for the users of the system.

Figure 21.2 depicts this development in time. The current architecture is indicated in Fig. 21.2 by "evolutionary/composable," to indicate that for optimal integration and performance a combination of both architectures is preferable. Departmental systems and external systems from other suppliers are able to communicate with the central HIS via the network, using standard protocols and messages (e.g., HL-7). If required, all forms of integration mentioned above (i.e., data integration, presentation integration, and function integration) are possible for Hiscom applications that have been directly linked to the central HIS. A communication *engine* can be used to connect Hiscom to departmental systems of other suppliers.

The Hiscom HIS is based on one logically central database in which medical as well as administrative and logistic data are stored. It concerns current as well as historic data. The registration of data supporting the primary process of the hospital was already given priority at the first stage of development of the system. Thus, the functions of central medical support departments, such as laboratories, the pharmacy, or the radiology department, were assisted early on. The more than 80 applications render support to a large number of hospital functions, focusing on the patient as well as on the hospital facilities. Examples of applications that since the late 1980s are considered to belong to the HIS functionality are:

- nursing support by individualized nursing plans,
- a picture information system (PACS), and
- a management information system (*MIS*) (see Section 7).

Proceeding from this principle, Hiscom has been participating in research on PACS to realize a satisfactory integration with the kernel HIS. The MIS has a direct link to the HIS database, ensuring that each report made by the MIS is based on actual, reliable, and consistent information.

To comply with the very strict requirements for availability posed to an operational HIS – hospital operations never stop – all central equipment of the Hiscom HIS has been duplicated. In case of an emergency or for maintenance, it is possible to switch over to the standby system immediately, often without the users even realizing it. In this way, the realized level of availability is 99.7%.

An example of open communication between the Hiscom HIS and the outside world are the developments in the area of *EDI* (Electronic Data Interchange), which have resulted, for instance, in communication with *GPs*, health insurance companies, health services of companies, and suppliers.

5.2 Diogene HIS

The Diogene HIS, which has been developed and is still under development in Geneva, Switzerland, can be considered an example of a successful HIS that was also started as a monolithic system (see Fig. 21.3). In its present form it can be regarded as a composable system. Contrary to the Hiscom HIS, it did not develop in an evolutionary way, but after Diogene I the development of Diogene II was in fact started anew. Diogene was started in 1971 as a project with, as its basic concept, a complete HIS without barriers between administrative and medical applications. The official start of Diogene I, as it was baptized, was in 1978. It operated on a *mainframe* computer. With its homemade database management system (*DBMS*), its many applica-

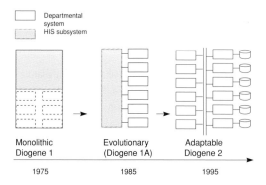

Departmental
system
HIS subsystem

Monolithic	Evolutionary	Adaptable
Diogene 1	(Diogene 1A)	Diogene 2
1975	1985	1995

Figure 21.3
Development of the Diogene HIS architecture (Geneva, Switzerland) from 1978 to 1995. Initially, no central repository was applied, but this was changed later on. The development did not proceed in an evolutionary way; in fact, after Diogene I the development was started anew in Diogene II.

21

tions, and its starlike network, it was the correct answer to the requirements of a large hospital in the 1970s.

By the mid-1980s it was recognized that the increasing use of the system as well as the new technological possibilities required a new system architecture, with the following as its most important characteristics:

- a *relational DBMS,*
- a multicomputer system,
- an efficient network, and
- portable applications to decrease dependence on the hardware supplier.

As an intermediate step in the migration of a monolithic system to a composable system, an initial decen-

tralization of functionality occurred from the central mainframe computer, where most of the functionality remained, toward a number of satellite computers. The communication between satellite computers (*UNIX* machines) and the central system was based on an *Ethernet* network using the de facto standard *TCP/IP.* Communication with the outside world was performed by an electronic *mailbox.*

The client-server concept, which means a separation of database, applications, and user interface, has been applied to realize the step from an evolutionary system to a composable system. The applications were distributed on servers that had been installed in each department. Each user had an *X-terminal,* a PC with *X-emulation,* or a UNIX workstation with *X-Motif* as its graphical user interface.

The migration towards a client-server architecture requires particular attention to the choice of standards and procedures, since there exists a large variety of machines, and they can communicate with each other only by means of recognized standards. The management of the large number of processors that are connected to the network is only possible when from the beginning a distinct hierarchy or segmentation has been applied to organize the locations, the names, and the addresses of the machines. In a large hospital such as the University Hospital of Geneva, many dozens of processors were involved. The management of the various software versions (several applications on an application server) requires clear installation procedures. The largest problem to be solved in the migration from Diogene I to Diogene II appeared to be the choice of management tools in a distributed environment, and not the choice of optimal communication standards or of the operating system and the DBMS.

6 Accessibility and Data Protection

As mentioned in the introduction, the accessibility of relevant data on the one hand and measures for *data protection* on the other hand are in conflict. Each threshold that has been put up to ensure that HIS users have access only to the data to which they have been aut-

horized access, is an obstruction when data must be promptly available in an emergency situation (see Chapter 33).

This section briefly discusses the measures required to protect the aspects of *accessibility, availability,* and quality of data and programs. Each of the data protection measures, whether it concerns the access regulations to the HIS or the assurance that a **backup** of the database is regularly made, is a combination of measures in the area of hardware and software, along with the corresponding procedures. For backups of the database, for instance, equipment must be present and available so that a copy can physically be made and retained. The same holds for software that is able to control and check the equipment and for procedures that ensure that the backup is performed at fixed times, including holidays, when the operator is ill, and so forth.

In the most clear-cut situation the principle of the access regulations to the HIS consists of the following steps: identification of the user by a **password** or a card, a check whether the user is authorized to perform certain functions and to receive certain data and, finally, a check on the relation of the user to the specific patient. In emergency situations specific users are allowed to use their "burglar competence." The system asks for the reason of the "burglary" and reports it, for instance, to the medical records officer or to the director of patient care.

Chapter 32 considers in detail data protection and legal regulations with respect to data.

7 Management Control

Efforts to restrain the increase in health expenditures have led to greater demands on the management's control of a hospital. Budgetary restrictions may imply great changes in the management function in hospitals. In the past, the number of admissions, outpatient visits, and diagnostic and therapeutic actions were often the parameters determining the income of a hospital. Now, most of the time there exists no direct relationship between the number of actions during the treatment of a patient and the income of a hospital. This implies that all workers in the hospital, medical specialists included, will have to be more conscious of costs to prevent spending more than is allowed for in the budget. For this purpose good insight into the costs connected with treatments and actions is necessary. Since the charges for care hardly agree with the real costs, the cost of medical actions must be calculated. This requires that financial data (e.g., material and personnel costs) be linked to the actions performed in the care process. Subsequently, insight into the costs of

treatment per patient or patient group can be obtained by determining the type of actions per patient or patient group. Apart from budgeting, the increased marketing orientation and attention to the quality of care, in which the patient is central, influence the way in which care processes are managed and controlled. During the last few years the organizational structure of a hospital has been changing from being more *function oriented,* in which each professional group has its own department or service, toward a more *process-oriented* structure, in which the professional groups in a hospital are grouped around the care process for specific groups of patients. A process-oriented organization structure combined with decentralization of authorities offers better opportunities for a patient-oriented approach and for cost-containment.

The changes mentioned above have led to an increasing demand for information to answer questions such as "What do we produce?" and "What does it cost?"

8 Trends

This section indicated some trends that will determine the future of HISs. In many cases these trends appear

to be related to trends in health care and information technology, for instance, increasing influence of health care insurers, increasing attention to quality and efficiency of care, diversification of HIS subsystems, and networking. Panel 21.1 illustrates the use of patient data in an HIS for epidemiological research.

8.1 Support of Patient Care

- CPRs

Data that are generated and registered in the patient care process (i.e., during examinations, treatments, and nursing) are the basis for almost all other processes in a hospital. In addition to the data obtained directly from the patient, the data obtained from *ancillary* diagnostic departments also belong to this category. With the present technology it is possible to introduce computer-based patient records (*CPRs*) containing all patient data (see descriptions of CPRs in Chapters 7, 11, 12, and 29).

- Nursing

An important development is the support of *nursing* care (see Chapter 14), in which four stages are discerned:

1. establishing the type of patient care,
2. setting up a care plan,
3. the care itself, and
4. evaluating the care given.

Applications have been developed to support this labor-intensive process, in which an individual nursing care plan is outlined for each patient, possibly based on a "standard" nursing care plan. In a nursing plan the need for care is registered in combination with the goals to be reached and the necessary nursing interventions.

- Order Entry

A third development in supporting the care process is *order management*. In an order management system both requests for and results of, for instance, nursing actions, an X-ray, or an operation can be entered at the clinical workstation. A characteristic of an order

management system is that the physicians or nurses must enter the orders themselves and the results are automatically entered into the medical or nursing record. The requested activity is registered in the system and can be traced by the user. With a well-functioning order entry system, the care process information improves in quality and is more easily and quickly accessible. In addition, the numbers of individuals involved in the chain of oral and written communications will decrease.

8.2 Workstations and Bedside Terminals

It can be expected that HIS terminals will gradually be replaced by "intelligent" workstations, in which graphical user interface data are presented in a coherent manner and data input is supported for, for example, drug prescriptions, progress notes, or order entry. Another development that deserves to be mentioned are so-called *bedside terminals*, through which physicians and nurses are able to enter data into the system at the time and place where these data originate: at the patient's bedside. It is obvious that the application of such *point-of-care systems* will enhance the quality and availability of data.

Key References

Bakker AR, Ehlers CT, Bryant JR, Hammond WE, eds. *Hospital Information Systems: Scope-Design-Architecture*. Amsterdam: North Holland Publ Comp, 1992.

Hammond WE, Bakker AR, and Ball MJ, eds. *Information Systems with Fading Boundaries*. Amsterdam: Elsevier, 1995.

Prokosch HU, Dudeck J, eds. *Hospital Information Systems: Design and Development Characteristics; Impact and Future Architecture*. Amsterdam: Elsevier, 1995.

See the Web site for further literature references.

22 Health Information Resources

1 Introduction

Health information resources (*HIRs*) comprise all aspects of data collection, storage, analysis, presentation, and communication in the field of *public health*. It includes:

- health care information networks,
- public health,
- occupational health care (*OHC*),
- registries, including tissue banks and blood banks, and
- surveillance, including *vigilance* and epidemiological monitoring.

HIRs cover approximately the *exogenous* and *endogenous determinants* shown in Fig. 19.4. HIRs provide the information structure for population-based health care, defined as the nonclinical services of health and public health. The importance of the field can be gauged from the estimate made by the U.S. Public Health Service that, although 10% of early deaths in the United States can be prevented by medical treatment, population-based approaches have the potential to prevent 70% of premature deaths.

An important difference between HIRs and systems for clinical use (see Chapters 11 to 14, 20, and 21) is that HIRs are less directed toward the functioning of a specific health care organization. In most cases their goal is the acquisition, storage, analysis, and presentation of large amounts of data about healthy people or patients. Since the target of HIRs is not the individual person but the population, their records can be presented anonymously in most cases. Characteristic of HIRs are the large number of records, the fact that the data may be related to a large geographical area, and the diversity of purposes.

Health Information Resources are important for various consumers. These include policy makers; health care inspectorates; health care professionals and researchers; the pharmaceutical, medical device, and bioengineering industries; and the media. There would be no HIRs without health care consumers (patients, home care consumers, company employees, and the general public). Some HIRs are international or supranational (registries, information resources, and tissue banks), and others are national or are even restricted to a workplace (OHC). HIRs form a wide and heterogeneous field whose basic units are:

- the administrative system, providing day-to-day management (home care, screening and prevention, and OHC);
- the registry, the basic information resource for research and policy support; and
- the surveillance system, including vigilance and epidemiological monitoring.

Almost all forms of general-purpose computer hardware are used, such as *handheld computers* (home care and OHC), *mainframes* (information facilities and public health), stand-alone personal computers (*PCs*), *local area networks*, *wide area networks*, or *Internet* servers and clients. *Databases* range from simple card-index structures to *data warehouses* and *geographic information systems*. Applications range from query systems through disease incidence monitoring to scheduling of home care aides, tissue and blood bank management, pharmacovigilance (see Section 3.6), and integrated national health care systems.

This chapter provides a brief overview of the field, starting with an examination of the general characteristics and common aspects in Section 2. This is followed by looking at a variety of HIR domains in Section 3. Section 4 summarizes prevailing trends and looks at new directions.

2 HIR Characteristics and Features

A wide range of hardware and software is used for HIRs, with a large installed base of **legacy systems**, even including largely manual ones. The specific medical informatics aspects of HIRs relate more to the type of data handled and the associated questions of accuracy and privacy than to the software engineering techniques used. The following points are common to a majority of HIRs, but they cannot be considered universally applicable.

2.1 System Characteristics

Health Information Resources are built around a **database** or, more commonly, multiple linked or stand-alone databases that are generally characterized by a small amount of data per basic record and large to very large numbers of records. According to the purpose of the registration, basic records may be person oriented such as to patients, inhabitants, home care clients, donors, or care providers, but basic records may also be oriented in other directions, such as to device model or serial number, chemical substance, bacterial or parasite strain or sample, drug prescription, tissue sample, organ, or blood unit.

In general, records are for a large population obtained over a long period of time, and there are usually many **instances** of each record. Most HIRs incorporate internal communication only (dial-up messaging, local or wide area network, and **intranet**), external communication only (dial-up facility and **Internet** presence), or both internal and external communication.

System security and data privacy are serious concerns in most HIRs, where not only the patient data but also those of the care provider may be accessible. Unless the HIR is specifically patient oriented (such as a phenylketonuria-monitoring program), the data are often partially or completely anonymous, although a key to the data may be retained at some level of the information provider organizations. The areas where standards applicable to HIRs are found are shown in Panel 22.1 (see also Chapter 34 for a discussion of standards in medical informatics).

2.2 Data Acquisition

Data acquisition for HIRs generally uses techniques applicable to the usually textual data that are collected. Many of the HIR data are initially collected on forms. These forms are then entered into the HIR manually, via **off-line batch** with later correction, **on-line** with validation, by on-line registration (e.g., for timing care sessions), or by **optical reading**. Some data are coded for identification, for example, with a **bar code** (for sample recognition and document handling), magnetic strip (for personnel and client registration), or **chip card**.

In practice, many of the data input into an HIR are derived from other computer systems. Cost-efficient schemes concentrate on *"capture at source,"* whereby the system handling the original data (e.g., hospital information system, home care support, general practice, or pharmacy) transmits the required data typically by using electronic data interchange at appropriate intervals or on demand. Capture at source is not without problems: in some important areas, especially

---

PANEL 22.1

Standards Applicable to Health Information Resources

The principal types of standards applicable to HIRs are as follows:

- medical aspects such as diagnostic and intervention coding (e.g., *Unified Medical Language System*, see Chapter 6);
- medical informatics aspects (*CEN/TC251* standards, see Chapter 34), including *information system architecture*, message exchange, and message notation;
- technical aspects such as communication protocols (e.g., *TCP-IP*, see Chapter 5), languages (e.g., *hypertext markup language*), *bar code* specifications (e.g., *EAN 128*);
- safety aspects, usually determined by agencies such as the *International Standards Organization* or the U.S. *Food and Drug Administration* (FDA);
- communications aspects, such as standards for information exchange (e.g., *EDIFACT* specifications, see Chapter 5);
- security and *privacy* aspects, usually set by national legislation (see Chapter 33);
- digital signatures; and
- database aspects such as minimum data sets (e.g., *International Agency for Cancer Research* and *WHO* specifications) (see Chapter 4).

A discussion of standards applicable to health care can be found in Chapter 34

22

---

disease surveillance, it has proved to be difficult to achieve a level of data quality and completeness that can compete with the traditional manual systems.

2.3 Data Storage

HIRs are founded on database technology. Most of them, except those for legacy systems, use standard *relational databases* with *SQL* queries (see Chapter 4). Read-mostly (information) systems may add features (specialized *indexing* and search techniques) to improve access. The following is generally more relevant to HIRs than to other areas of medical informatics applications.

- Record linkage

Record linkage is an essential aspect of integrating existing systems, combining data from two or more databases for studies, checking overlap between data from different agencies, and building a *data warehouse*.

Linking personal records accurately is difficult, even when adequate data are present; it is extremely hard when the data are anonymous, as in most registries and surveillance systems. Some countries have personal numbers that can be used for linkage (e.g., the Social Security number in the United States and the New Zealand on-line National Index), although privacy considerations reduce their use. Zip or postal codes can be used when linking data to geographical databases (see Section 2.4). Public key *cryptographic* techniques may also be applied in secure file linkage.

- Duplicate Records

Duplicate records are the occurrence of more than one record, for instance, for the same patient, which should be combined. This is an issue in all registration systems, and much research has been directed toward reducing their incidence. Strategies depend on the available data, the source(s) of specific items and its expected reliability, susceptibility to change, possibilities of cross-checking, and the existence of some form of universal identifier in the country concerned. The Dutch Cancer Registry uses a "nearness index" based on matching fields (gender, date of birth, first four letters of last name) to link their own data to other databases. Internally, they use more fields because duplicate records are commonly caused by registration errors and change of address. *TECN* has developed a biological patient identification code for those on European transplant waiting lists who have had human leukocyte antigen (*HLA*) matching.

- Missing Data

Missing data are an inherent problem in all health care databases, which affects registries and surveillance systems. Software techniques, such as multiple imputation, may be applied if it is known that there are missing items and if records are essentially complete, making it possible to carry out valid statistical analyses. It is possible to verify the correctness of the method applied by simulation. Such procedures are not applicable to voluntary reporting systems (see the section on *postmarketing surveillance* below).

2.4 Geographical Information Systems

Geographical information systems (*GIS*s) manage geographically referenced data. They generally provide:

- data management (acquisition, storage, and maintenance),
- analysis (statistical and spatial modeling), and
- data presentation (mapping and other graphics).

GISs are useful tools for health care, particularly for epidemiological research and health resource planning. A GIS can be used to organize any health information that includes an explicit geographical component; at the simplest level this may consist of the organization of data entry by using a map or street plan rather than typing addresses and then running a check program.

A GIS is made up of two databases that are more or less closely integrated. The *spatial database* contains locational data, usually in the form of digital coordinates or vectors, which describe the spatial features of the region concerned. For a health care application these might be points (e.g., hospitals and general practitioner (GP) practices), lines (e.g., roads and rivers), or polygons (e.g., administrative regions, catchment areas, and bodies of water). Applications usually contain several sets of locational data, known as layers or overlays, for example, environmental data, health care services, educational services, public transport, housing, emergency services, epidemiological data, or data from registries. Each layer may be present in several instances, for example, showing changes over time.

The *attribute database* stores all data describing the spatial features for each layer: names, rates, values, scores, and so forth. These data are usually stored in a relational database and are presented via a **spreadsheet** or a query-driven user interface. The database management software has the usual facilities for searching, sorting, and selecting data on the basis of feature attributes, for example, selecting and ordering alphabetically the names of all hospitals with more than 500 beds. However, the strength of a GIS lies in its ability to select data on the basis of spatial features. The same selection could be made with the limitation that they be within 100 meters of a river, less than 5 kilometers from a railway station, and not on a major road. In a single retrieval, data may be combined from different layers and weightings may be applied to different layers.

Essential to a GIS is the ability to import map data from external digital sources or directly by scanning a map and tracing the features. The latter is a time-consuming and difficult job, but today it is usually possible to avoid this, because many resources supply digital map data of different kinds. The GIS also supports all normal database functions (enter, edit, and list) for the attribute data. GISs usually have support for special data entry devices, such as a global positioning system (*GPS*) or *remote sensing*, and for address or telephone number checking (using commercially available databases).

Output facilities center on mapmaking and map display with tools that also support high-quality printing (*PostScript, plotter,* and film). Many applications of GISs in health care are concerned with either the relation between environmental factors and health conditions or the planning of health care facilities. Panel 22.2 provides two examples of such applications.

PANEL 22.2

Examples of Projects using a GIS

The following *GIS* applications highlight some of the advantages and difficulties found in applying GISs in health-related research.

Projecting Demand for Psychiatric Services is a New Zealand case study exploring the feasibility of using a GIS to project the demand for psychiatric services in the Waikato Region. *Supermap*, a demographic GIS distributed by Statistics New Zealand, was used to project areas of potentially high demand for psychiatric services. Comprehensive census data on psychiatric issues were not available, so data from mental health surveys in the region, which showed the relationship of three types of mental illness to such factors as ethnicity, gender, age, and socioeconomic background, were combined with the demographic information. Standardized scores of vulnerability (*Z scores*, a normal distribution statistic) were calculated by using ethnic and socioeconomic factors similar to those in the surveys, and the regional scores were converted to a scale of vulnerability and demand for psychiatric services. Supermap was used to analyze the data and visualize the likely patterns of demand, as well as to investigate the problems of access to facilities and the impact of a planned hospital closure. The authors suggest that the findings will need testing over several time intervals and that porting to a more powerful GIS platform (such as *ARC/INFO*) would be indicated for advanced mapping and facilities management, for example, for optimizing the distribution of clinics, equipment, and personnel.

The *Russian Environment and Health Mapping Project* is a research project that is using the Strategic Environmental Distributed Active Archive Resource (*SEDAAR*) to explore the impact of environmental problems on the health of the Russian population. Data from the Environmental and Health Atlas of Russia were loaded into ARC/INFO, the GIS on which SEDAAR is based. The research project investigates the possibility of a correlation between the spread of ^{137}Cs and the health of the population. The project conclusions indicate difficulties in executing the project, points that are relevant to setting up any such work:

- The Atlas contained data from various sources; determining the lineage and integrity of the data was complicated and not always possible.
- The ^{137}Cs data showed a coarseness of granularity and a lack of precise location (this probably obscured the impact of environmental factors).
- SEDAAR maps were insufficiently detailed and scaled too small to show political borders accurately.
- Additional (discrete) layers of detail were needed (e.g., locations of nuclear plants, industrial plants, and various types of pollutants).
- Health data were too coarse and were not attached to exact geographic locations.
- Performing map digitization and performing GIS-based manipulations in ARC/INFO were difficult for novices.

The project shows the feasibility, but also the difficulty and time involved, for a novice to set up and use a GIS to analyze environmental health issues.

22

22

PANEL 22.3

Data Mining and Knowledge Discovery in Databases

The techniques of data mining (*DM*) and knowledge discovery in databases (KDD) were originally developed to process corporate sales and production data, but they are equally relevant to the parameters of health care. The techniques are usually applied to "scrubbed" data in a data warehouse or data mart, although certain techniques are able to use knowledge representation tools to logically describe databases. DM refers to the basic tools used to extract patterns from the data, whereas KDD is often used to describe the process of applying the tools to extract knowledge from the original raw data. DM and KDD tools are:

- bottom-up (the tool is let loose on the data and proceeds unattended) or
- top-down (analyst-controlled, interactive, and hypothesis-testing), although some experts do not consider this true DM;

and they may be:

- general-purpose (e.g., *OLAP*) or
- tailored to the application.

There are four basic data mining operations, each of which is supported by a variety of techniques:

- predictive model creation: supervised induction,
- link analysis: association discovery and sequence discovery,
- database segmentation: clustering methods, and
- deviation detection: statistical techniques.

Most automated DM techniques are based on artificial intelligence methods and employ a *training set* (to generate the hypothesis) and a *test set*. *Neural networks* have also been applied to deduce patterns in this way.

2.5 Data Warehouses

Two discordant concepts pervade many HIRs: system integration and data distribution. A third aspect is the large installed base of legacy systems. HIRs (specifically, OHC, registries, and health information networks) are generally characterized by large amounts of data from various sources and by the need to use these data as efficiently as possible to extract information for policy decisions. An information technology architecture that tries to address these concerns is the data warehouse (*DW*).

The DW, also called an information warehouse, is a subject-oriented, integrated central data storage facility which is read mostly. "Scrubbed" data, that is, data that have been cleaned up to remove duplicate records and inconsistent coding and to standardize name and address formats, are imported periodically from the contributing systems, which are usually highly diverse as to hardware, software, and structure.

The DW is designed to input, store, and search a large amount of related data. These data are derived from multiple sources; therefore, the DW provides a single, consistent interface to data derived from various sources. It has specialized and powerful tools supporting management decision making and, often most important, user queries and user reporting. In its classical form, it is implemented in a high-performance processor, acting as a network server. It provides a framework for *data mining* (see Panel 22.3).

A number of problems are associated with DW technology. The design is extremely important, if the desired flexibility of data retrieval and investigation is to be attained. Implementing and using a DW leads to finding "holes," that is, data that have not been recorded, and errors in the system. The process of inventorying, extracting, scrubbing, and loading the data is a major part (up to 80%) of the work involved. The maintenance of a DW is itself a nontrivial task, involving update frequency, update speed, maintenance of data integrity, outdated data, and support for changing contributing databases. These factors mean that the investment can be extremely high. A thorough *cost-benefit* analysis (see Chapter 32) should be carried out in advance.

Data warehouses have been used in health care for several purposes. A few examples are:

- patient activity costing, determining the impact of funding changes (Alberta Health),
- extending the life of legacy systems at a commercial multihospital, multipractice organization (Promina Health Systems),
- providing access to data from incompatible, previously isolated systems (Piedmont Hospital),
- extracting utilization reports and speeding up provision of statistics and patient data (Tufts Health Plans HMO), and
- extract billing patterns and audit medical providers (Washington State Department of Labor and Industries).

2.6 Data Analysis and Retrieval

Searching is an important aspect of many HIRs. Search speed is a common source of user dissatisfaction, and attention must be paid to search strategies. Tailored indexing techniques may be needed (see Chapter 4). Specialized statistics are used in many HIRs. System design must include support for the type required, for multiple mathematical models if appropriate, and for basic data investigation (descriptive statistics).

3 Health Information Resource Domains

3.1 Health Information Networks

Health information networks (*HINs*) are implemented at a national or regional level:

- to identify, link, store, retrieve and transmit health care files in a secure setting between many systems and health care providers that are geographically distributed and that vary as to equipment and functionality;

- to improve internal (local and wide area networks) and external (usually Internet) communications in the health care region (*electronic mail* is implemented if it is not already generally available);
- to reduce paperwork by filling in forms with data that are already machine readable (e.g., by automatic data extraction and transmission to appropriate registries), as well as reduce other overhead tasks; and
- to improve quality and to reduce costs,

PANEL 22.4

Media and Electronic Publishing Formats

Electronic publications may be found on:

- *diskette*,
- *CD-ROM* (particularly for large volumes of information),
- the *Internet* (World Wide Web, and *FTP* download sites),
- *electronic mail* systems,
- *bulletin boards* and other dial-in facilities,
- *intranets* and other internal information networks, and
- *magnetic tape* (various types, increasingly uncommon except in *legacy* systems)

These publications are usually encountered in one of the following formats (the list is not exhaustive, but it covers the most popular ones, and it is worthy to note that only standard generalized markup language (*SGML*) and *ASCII* are formal standards):

- Hypertext markup language (*HTML*), the language of the World Wide Web, is the most widely used and accepted.
- Portable Document Format (*PDF* files for *Adobe Acrobat*) is used extensively for publishing complex hypertext documents to be read on multiple platforms.
  Readers are available for most common personal computer and workstation operating systems; *PostScript*, a page description language, is a simpler alternative to PDF (in practical situations only for hard-copy printing).
- *Word processor* documents are often supplied if the document is undergoing frequent revisions.
- Microsoft HELP is a proprietary hypertext file format, for which readers exist for Windows and Macintosh.
  It is the format most commonly found on diskette or CD-ROM distributions.
- Lotus Notes (*groupware* for internal networks, it also interfaces to HTML) is a proprietary format that is not available on all platforms, but that is often encountered within organizations.
- Microsoft *Powerpoint* (for downloadable slideshows) is limited to Windows and Macintosh.
- Plain *ASCII* (seven-bit, with no extensions).
  Unformatted ASCII text is the most widely understood of all machine-readable formats. Virtually all systems still operational are able to read this file type.
- *SGML*, the source language of HTML, is the least widely used, but it is a standard in the publishing world.

There are a number of guidelines and initiatives for the *architecture* of HINs, such as the *CEN/TC251* pre-standard (see Chapter 34). HINs vary considerably in architecture, target group, data stored, and facilities provided. *Integrated health care networks* couple together existing, fragmented legacy systems for administering and registering all forms of health care within an area. Long-term goals include provision of common interfaces for the user and standard facilities for searching, retrieval, and reporting, whereby DW (see Section 2.5 and Panel 22.3) and GIS techniques play a role.

An *index of health care consumers,* such as the New Zealand National Index, incorporates data from older systems, but is implemented as a central resource providing an unique identification of an individual. It is accessible on-line and has both extensive searching capabilities and the ability to handle *aliases.*

This may be extended to carry a summary of a medical history (allergies, interventions, immunizations, etc.). Many services (such as risk factor and allergy notification) can be based on such a resource.

In the United States, Information Networks for Public Health Officials have been initiated by the federal Centers for Disease Control and Prevention to improve information access, communication (external and internal), and efficiency for public health practitioners. The Arizona Health Information Network is an effort to share computing resources, expertise, and health care information across the state. HINs have also been set up by major commercial or nonprofit health care provider organizations. HINs are generally set up as part of a drive to contain costs and improve efficiency in health care. Tools for ongoing quality assessment, quality and cost control, and cost-benefit analyses should be made an integral part of the system.

3.2 Public Health Information Resources

Information resources for public health may be maintained by a governmental body (state, county or province, a municipality; or a national health department), by a care provider organization, by a professional body

or charitable institution, or by a commercial firm. Information is provided for health care professionals, health care researchers, and health care consumers.

The information (reports, statistics, guidelines, and summaries) is distributed by printed reports, but these are usually backed up by some form of on-line resource:

- *bulletin board* (limited or general access),
- electronic mail,
- on-line (subscription) service (such as the *TOXNET* service of the National Library of Medicine in the United States),
- electronic publications (see Panel 22.4),
- an information kiosk (in a town hall, library, or other public building), and
- a *World Wide Web* site.

Information resources intended for the general public, usually through information kiosks, require a simple interface that is based on an easily grasped metaphor clearly relating to the type of help given. Such resources are often designed to help the consumer find his or her way through the bewildering maze of social security and support, to assist in the equally complex maze of health care providers, and to point the way toward services (blood banks and donor registries) that need volunteers, supplying additional background (e.g., donor experiences and stories of those who have been helped) and lowering the threshold for the potential volunteer.

Another important type of information resource is that provided primarily for health care professionals and researchers by international bodies such as the World Health Organization (*WHO*). Panel 22.5 lists a small sample of such resources, and Panel 22.6 describes an example of an on-line information resource, the Chemical Abstracts Service (*CAS*) Registry.

3.3 Administrative Systems

- Home care support

Home Care support systems are primarily administrative systems supporting alarm centers, telecare (intelligent alarms), or home care workers (nurses, aides, and therapists). *Alarm centers* are primarily for emergency

22

22

PANEL 22.5

Electronically Available Information Resources

Many international, national, commercial, and nonprofit organizations host on-line or otherwise electronically available information resources: on the Internet (World Wide Web) and on bulletin boards and other dial-up facilities or by using other methods of electronic publishing (diskette, magnetic tape, CD-ROM). The following lists a small sample of the relevant organizations, along with a few of the resources that each hosts, to give an idea of the types of resource and their providers.

*World Health Organization (WHO) Statistical Information System (**WHOSIS**).*
WHOSIS has many resources, among which are the following:
• G7 Global Health Care Project,
• International Classification of Impairments, Disabilities, and Handicaps (*ICIDH*), and
• WHO databases, e.g., the Mortality Database (cause of death statistics by country, age, gender, year, and cause of death).

*International Agency for Cancer Research (**IARC**)*
IARC coordinates and conducts research into the causes of human cancer and develops scientific strategies for cancer control. IARC is the permanent secretariat of the International Association of Cancer Registries and European Network of Cancer Registries.

*Bone Marrow Donors Worldwide (**BMDW**)*
BMDW coordinates 40 donor registries (volunteer bone marrow donors and cord blood units) from 28 countries and:
• provides general information (how to become a donor, addresses of donor registries, the HLA system, and statistics on participating registries) and
• distributes donor data and has a match program and an on-line match program (by a secure protocol).

*National Center for Infectious Diseases (**NCID**), Centers for Disease Control and Prevention (**CDC**)*

Emerging Infectious Diseases, a peer-reviewed journal published by CDC, is accessible by various electronic means.

Morbidity and Mortality Weekly Report, CDC

Malaria Database, maintained by the Department of Microbiology, Monash University, and the Walter and Eliza Hall Institute of Medical Research, is funded by *UNDP/World Bank*/WHO Special Programme for Research and Training in Tropical Diseases. It is an information resource for scientists working in malaria research. Malaria genome information and malaria strain and isolate information are freely available and there is a malaria discussion group.

Chemical Abstracts Service
Panel 22.6 describes this resource and gives an example of a search.

National Cancer Institute's Cooperative Breast Cancer Tissue Registry
This registry is an on-line database providing access to and selections from a large collection of breast cancer tissue specimens available for research. Tissue sections are prepared to meet requirements of individual research protocols. Applications are reviewed.

PANEL 22.6

The Chemical Abstracts Service Registry

The *CAS* Registry is an important, internationally accessible on-line information resource. The Registry is a chemical structure and dictionary database containing records on unique substances identified by CAS.

- Records contain many types of data, including names, polymer class terms, citations, ring analysis data, structure diagrams, and molecular formulas, all of which are searchable.
- There were more than 15 million records in 1996;
- Coverage is from 1957 to date for all types of chemical substances described in the literature, including alloys, biosequences, coordination compounds, minerals, mixtures, polymers, and salts;
- Sources are GenBank and the CAS Registry System, which identifies new substances from sources such as journal articles, patents, conference proceedings, and regulatory lists.
- The records are indexed by the CAS Registry Number for that substance. CAS Registry Numbers are unique identifiers for chemical compounds. Records contain CAS Registry Numbers for all the substances that have been indexed by CAS from a particular document.
- Each record contains all information on one substance.

22

---

care. The main functions of such systems are to automatically display client details and history when calls arrive, register the call and the response, call relevant care providers, and display the type of emergency and the reason for an alarm when telecare is supported.

Home care agencies (in the United States, home health agencies) also schedule care provider time; allocate resources, possibly on the basis of the care needs predicted from past history; and report time, activities, and costs to the central organization. Common to all home care support systems is the need to track costs and productivity and to coordinate care. Health care organizations controlling home care (often municipal or regional health departments) require detailed reporting. The administrative overhead of time and activity reporting subsumes a considerable proportion of available resources. Home care support systems must be engineered toward improving the efficiency of care (see Panel 22.7).

- Screening and Prevention

Screening and prevention are closely linked both in purpose and in administration; screening may be con-

sidered secondary prevention. The primary computer use is for administration: Selection, registration, notification of clients, and facilities are often hosted by a larger resource, such as municipal health care or OHC, which manages the facility. Informatics aspects are in general those common to any registration and follow-up system with emphasis on quality.

The National Child Health System in the United Kingdom is a nationwide information system for screening and prevention within a specific target group; it has been operational since 1972 and has been extensively documented. Research in screening and prevention forms part of epidemiology. Many surveillance systems (see Section 2.4) are concerned with prevention, which is also an important aspect of many OHC systems.

- Occupational Health Care Systems

The objectives of OHC services are to prevent work-related disease, to promote and maintain employees' health and working ability, and to restore working ability to those with a diminished working ability. Thus, OHC systems must provide a wide range of services.

22

Home Care Systems Using Handheld Computers

To increase efficiency and reduce the administrative overhead, commercially available packages for home care organizations often use handheld computers or personal digital assistants (*PDAs*) for data capture. In a typical example, the handheld computer is set up from a host personal computer at the base. On arrival at each client's home the care worker is able to display basic client details:

- *demographics*,
- GP,
- contact history for last 6 months,
- treatment details and special instructions,
- drug administration schedule, and
- notes (of care workers, colleagues, and GPs).

The care worker can update any or all of these data on departure, with the handheld computer timing the visit. On return to base the records in the handheld computer and the host computer system are reconciled and the client records are updated. In turn, the host system extracts care worker, client, and activity data for transmission to a regional or national home care registry. A bonus for the care worker is the ability to make use of other functions provided by the handheld computer: client schedules, to-do lists, phone and address lists, and information files (e.g., drug interactions). If the handheld computer or PDA has an integral modem, reconciling can be done before the care worker departs, ensuring that any last-minute instructions can be carried out or changes of schedule can quickly be passed on.

The primary functions are to:
- document the health records of employees, record the degree of health-related absenteeism and employee exposure to potential health hazards, and document compliance with safety measures;
- determine whether measures are necessary to improve working ability or reduce health-related absenteeism; and
- provide statistics, incident reports and other information needed to comply with safety and other legislation.

OHC systems may also include:
- health screening administration,
- support for prevention programs, and
- surveillance systems to detect sudden increases in potentially work-related accidents or disease (see Section 3.4).

OHC departments may also be concerned with occupational hygiene, ergonomics, and research.

3.4 Registries

The *registry* is the basic information resource for research and policy support (see also Chapter 6). A very old definition (15th century) of registry is that it is a collection of records, particularly records of a legal, parliamentary, or public character, in which regular entry is made of particulars or details of any kind that are considered of sufficient importance to be exactly and formally recorded. The definition is as applicable today as it was in the 15th century, although in health care the term is usually restricted to those registries that are maintained on electronic media and relate to a single topic.

Registries are the most important forms of HIRs, often acting both as an independent information resource and as part of another, larger entity. They are primarily used for epidemiological studies and other health care research, surveillance (see below), reference, policy support, resource allocation, and financial planning. The following are typical aspects of registries:

- They are maintained regionally or nationally; where large numbers are needed, as for donor and transplant registries (see Chapter 12), they are maintained internationally.
- They behave as a node in a hierarchy: recording data abstracted at a lower level, publishing the information, and passing an abstract to a higher level.
- They are frequently mandatory (enforced by legislation).
- They are concerned with privacy; where human data (patient, care provider, and client data) are involved, the data are usually anonymous to preserve confidentiality.

Particular points to consider in operating a registry are the use of national and international standards, record linkage, and duplicate record checking (see Section 2.3). The inclusion of sufficient **demographic** information for research purposes often conflicts with privacy regulations and may affect data collection for both disease (patient) and intervention (patient and clinician) registries.

Registries come in many forms, and they may roughly be grouped by their principal recording unit or purpose. The following is a small subset of the applications commonly encountered. *Patient registries* are of various types:

- *disease registries* relating to the occurrence of a specific disease (e.g., cystic fibrosis) or class of diseases (e.g., cancer);
- *intervention registries* relating to a specific intervention (e.g., hip replacement surgery);
- *transplant registries* relating to those in need of an organ or tissue transplant;
- *congenital malformation registries* that are part of congenital malformation surveillance;
- *immunization registries* that are used in disease prevention programs; and

- *implanted device registries* relating a patient to a specific device (model or serial number), of which *pacemaker registries* are the most widespread.

Disease and *intervention registries* are systematic collections of data relating to the incidence of the disease or disease group or the performance of an intervention within one or more defined geographical areas. They are primarily used for epidemiological studies, policy support, resource allocation, and planning. Depending on the additional information recorded, disease registry data may also play an important role in controlling the quality of care. Data may be derived from a single source or set of sources (pathology laboratories and surgical departments) or from multiple sources (other registries, laboratories, hospital records, and GPs). The degree of coverage (the monitoring of which is important) will depend on whether the registry is mandatory (backed by legislation) or voluntary.

Donor registries are a special case, because they are registries of privacy-sensitive data which cannot be completely made anonymous. Donor registries resemble the donor lists of blood banks, since they concern living people willing to donate in their lifetimes. Detailed data (e.g., HLA type), must be recorded, and for genetic, immunological, and economic reasons, no country alone has the resources to build a national donor registry of sufficient size, which has led to international cooperation in the field to the extent that, for example, more than half the unrelated bone marrow transplants between unrelated individuals in Europe have been performed with the donor and patient originating from different countries (see Chapter 12). On-line facilities for matching may be offered if secure access can be guaranteed.

Location registries are registries that primarily provide specific information about individual entities and that can be used to locate further information or the entity itself. Access is often limited to research scientists, who may need to provide a protocol to the registry. Issues are security of access, search facilities, data reliability, data accuracy, and data completeness. Examples are tissue registries such as the National Cancer Institute's Cooperative Breast Cancer Tissue Registry (see Panel 22.5), and the CAS registry (see Panel 22.6).

22

Medical device registries are the result of legislation requiring registration, certification, tracking, and post-marketing surveillance (see below) of medical devices. Notified bodies are responsible for certification, and they maintain their own device registration. A public registry is commonly maintained by a separate non-profit organization. The registry will contain details of all medical devices allowed on the relevant market, for example, within the European Union or North America: manufacturer(s), suppliers, model types, series and numbers, certification details, alerts (from the literature and from warnings issued by national watchdog groups), and device use, characteristics, and features. Such a registry typically publishes an abstract of its database electronically (on *CD-ROM* with periodic updates or as a dial-in service) by subscription. There are many other types of registries, some of which are described in the next section. If locational information is included (as in patient registries) data from one or more registries may be combined with geographical data in a GIS (see Section 2.4 and Panel 22.2) for research and planning.

3.5 Health Surveillance and Vigilance

Health surveillance involves collection of ongoing routine data to examine the extent of disease, to follow trends, and to detect changes in disease occurrence. The terms *surveillance* and *vigilance* are not clearly differentiated by all writers, but pharmaco-vigilance has been defined as "all methods of assessment and prevention of adverse drug reactions," with surveillance being one aspect. The term *vigilance system* is also extended to monitoring medical devices. Surveillance, vigilance, and epidemiological monitoring together form a complex field that is only superficially discussed here.

Surveillance systems operate in many areas, the principal ones being infectious disease monitoring, congenital malformations, postmarketing surveillance (drugs, medical devices, and antibiotic-resistant bacterial strains, as well as other forms of resistance and other microorganisms). Surveillance systems may make use of GIS techniques to examine the patterns of disease incidence or spread. In surveillance and vigilance systems, data acquisition is an extremely important aspect. Vital to a reliable operation are accuracy, timeliness, and completeness (not feasible in voluntary reporting). This makes the idea of capture at the source attractive, but in practice, it generally does not achieve the same levels of data quality and completeness as nonautomatic methods do. For epidemic monitoring (e.g., influenza) the use of a small but geographically well distributed set of highly motivated "*sentinel GP*s" has proven reliable. Whether for voluntary or mandatory reporting, the form filling and data transmission may be implemented in the GP's local system. Further important aspects of surveillance and vigilance systems are:

- the type of mathematical *model* used, which must be a good match to observed patterns and frequencies,
- estimation of *missing data* (see Section 2.3.), and
- statistics for alerting health care providers and policy makers (e.g., to the possibility of a significant. adverse side effect in pharmaco-vigilance or to give an early warning of a coming epidemic in infectious disease monitoring).

The statistics used are based on the mathematical models applied to the incidence of usually rare events in a long time series. Techniques are specialized and are outside the scope of this chapter.

Congenital malformation monitoring is a highly developed area of surveillance initiated after the thalidomide (Softenon) disaster in the 1960s. Thalidomide was insufficiently tested and the lack of monitoring prohibited the timely recognition that it caused severe congenital malformations. National registries report congenital malformations to the WHO.

Antibiotic resistance surveillance is important because with the widespread use of antibiotics, particularly in animal husbandry and often as a prophylactic in humans and animals, many microorganisms are developing resistance to single or even multiple drugs. Vigilance systems also monitor the patterns of spread of resistant strains of bacteria, as well as resistance in parasites such as those causing malaria, bilharzia, and trypanosomiasis.

- Postmarketing surveillance

Postmarketing surveillance (PMS) covers a wider area than surveillance as such (it may include all forms of verification of the alerts hypothesized), but it is a term that is commonly applied to voluntary or mandatory systems for registering and monitoring side effects and malfunctions. PMS systems provide alert signals (the smoke detector function) that are then analyzed or complemented by further studies. PMS is primarily used for adverse drug side effects, medical implants, and medical devices. In most countries *PMS of drugs* is based on voluntary reporting by GPs, pharmacists, and other care providers. The most important items that are registered are:

- suspected drug (active constituents), dosage, and duration of therapy;
- side effect(s) observed;
- clinical diagnosis or indication; and
- patient demographic data.

Registration based on voluntary reporting is biased, incomplete, and unrepresentative; in addition, the total exposure is not always available. Mathematical models and specialized statistical techniques have been developed to generate useful hypotheses about previously unrecorded adverse drug reactions from such data.

PMS of medical devices is linked to medical device registration. The U.S. Food and Drug Administration (**FDA**) rules on certification of medical equipment, in particular, for implantable devices (artificial organs, pacemakers, stents, etc.), which had to be registered with FDA; this registration was also mandated by various other national regulatory bodies. Lifetime tracking of individual devices is sometimes mandated, requiring patient registration as well as device registration.

3.6 Organ, Tissue, and Blood Banks

Blood bank automation has a long history and is usually subject to both special legislation and a degree of direct governmental control. Reference to the relevant national requirements is mandatory. Systems use automatic identification for tracking; in fact, coding of blood units was one of the earliest applications of **bar code** technology. Blood banks are essentially production systems, but they have special requirements for time control (blood expiration dates are a matter of "life and death") and security. Blood banks may not only register donors, but they may also register those not eligible to donate (e.g., those positive for human immunodeficiency virus (HIV) or syphilis or those with hepatitis).

Tissue banks and organ exchanges closely resemble blood banks in structure, but the constraints differ. Tissue banks, except those dealing in materials with a long shelf life (freezer life) or designed purely for research (see National Cancer Institute's Breast Cancer Tissue Registry in Panel 22.5), are tied to systems for registering transplant candidates, and the time window for tissue transplants is usually small. Because of this, tissue banks, organ exchanges, and the relevant registries may be linked together into transnational networks. Such networks offer not only a better possibility of matching but also additional functionality (multipriority waiting lists and double registration detection).

22

4 Summary and Trends

Considering the functionality of HIRs, their basic features are as follows:

- extensive reporting, charting (when numerical data or statistics are available), and graphical presentation;
- integral statistics;
- tools for quality assessment and quality assurance;
- surveillance (vigilance and alerting);
- tools for cost control and financial monitoring (primarily in administrative systems);
- adherence to international or field-specific standards (see also Panel 22.5);

- adherence to national or international security and privacy legislation;
- compliance with information requirements;
- handling of missing data (primarily for vigilance and epidemiology); and
- reliable data identification, incorporating methods for finding and eliminating duplicate records.

Many HIRs are policy oriented and are used either for implementing health care policies or for providing basic information needed for policy formulation. Typically, the data are also used to support research into and to refine underlying mathematical models. Simulation techniques may be used to validate data analyses. When a **DW** or GIS has been implemented, the system will have integral tools for user retrieval, searching, analysis, and display of data.

HIRs cover a wide field that is changing rapidly. The social and economic factors that play a role are:

- legislation (regulation, registration, privacy, accountability, and freedom of information);
- larger commercial aggregations (European Union, North American Free Trade Agreement, and Association of Southeast Asian Nations) with internal standards;
- more international agreements, cooperation, and standards;
- demographic changes (changes in the age distribution of the population);
- government and health insurance pressure to contain rising health care costs; and
- changes in social policies and health care financing.

Technical factors also play a role:

- hardware developments and price reductions (more powerful PCs, larger storage capacities, faster communications, and global positioning systems),
- software developments (better graphical operating systems and applications),
- database technology (DWs and GISs),
- network technology (client servers and intranets),
- new tools for analysis (e.g., knowledge discovery in databases, data mining, and GISs) and presentation,

- wide acceptance of ad hoc standards for textual and graphical information
- exchange across systems and electronic publishing (see Panel 22.4),
- the World Wide Web and Internet services, and
- infrastructure changes (high-speed cable and satellite communications).

The need for more efficiency and lower costs has prompted a trend away from specialized, individual systems toward integrated health information networks. Policies directed toward capture at the source of data for statistics and management information remove a degree of redundancy in the data flows.

It is difficult to reduce the volume of data produced by the numerous computer-based registration systems to meaningful information. Use of knowledge distillation techniques makes it possible for data that would otherwise be discarded to yield insights into the health care process and its efficiency, effectiveness, and costs.

The single factor with the most far-reaching effect on the field is the explosive increase in on-line information resources, especially of Internet services. This has changed the expectations of the average user of health care systems and of the average consumer, resulting in a demand for better, more customized, and more timely information. There are also disadvantages. The enormous volume of available information leads to difficulties in locating a desired item. The majority of information is not peer-reviewed (Internet) or is not extensively cross-checked (on-line data entry and capture at source), and this causes difficulties in distinguishing between reliable and unreliable information. The increasing number of users leads to accelerated changes in infrastructure, which in turn affect possibilities and patterns of use, requiring additional infrastructure.

Key References

Fayyad UM, Piatetsky-Shapiro G, Smyth P, Uthurusamy R. *Advances in Knowledge Discovery and Data Mining.* Cambridge MA: AAAI Press/MIT Press, 1996.

See the Web site for further literature references.

22

VII
Methodology for Information Processing

Authors of Part VII

Chapter 23: Logical Operations
   J.H. van Bemmel, J.S. Duisterhout, Erasmus University Rotterdam

Chapter 24: Biostatistical Methods
   J. Michaelis, Johannes Gutenberg University, Mainz

Chapter 25: Biosignal Processing Methods
   J.H. van Bemmel, R.J.A. Schijvenaars, Erasmus University Rotterdam

Chapter 26: Advances in Image Processing
   C.A. Kulikowski, L. Gong, Rutgers University, New Brunswick; with contribution of A.T. McCray, National Library of Medicine, Bethesda

Chapter 27: Pattern Recognition
   E.S. Gelsema, Erasmus University Rotterdam

Chapter 28: Modeling for Decision Support
   M.A. Musen, Stanford University

Chapter 29: Structuring the Computer-based Patient Record
   A.M. van Ginneken, J. van der Lei, J.H. van Bemmel, Erasmus University Rotterdam

Chapter 30: Evaluation of Information Systems
   J.C. Wyatt, Imperial Cancer Research Fund, London

23 Logical Operations

1 Introduction

This chapter provides an introduction to **Boolean logic**. The reasons for incorporating a short introduction to logic in this Handbook is that an increasing number of decisions in health care are supported by computers and that most **decision-support** programs are of a **qualitative** (also called: **heuristic**) nature (see Chapter 15). Heuristic decision-support systems operate with **logical expressions** that may, in turn, be composed of elementary **binary** (two-way) decisions. These elementary decisions are used to test, for example, whether some symptom is present or whether a measurement is larger than some threshold value. Such a test can be represented by a logical expression *E*. Logical expressions operate with two-valued variables: **TRUE** and **FALSE**. The values may be the result of some **logical operation** (as described in Chapter 15) such as **truth tables**, logical **decision trees**, and *logical expressions*,

as they are encountered in reasoning methods. Logic is a branch of mathematics that has a philosophical origin. As used here, it became operational with the advent of the digital computer, after the second world war, because all circuitry in digital computers operates with rules based on binary logic. The foundation for mathematical logic, however, was laid in the 19th century, when Boole published his book *The Mathematical Analysis of Logic* in 1847. Therefore, mathematical logic is also called *Boolean logic*[1]. The following sections focus on the principles of logical operators and expressions, truth tables, and Venn diagrams (Section 2) and Boolean algebra and Karnaugh diagrams (Section 3). In addition, because modern computers are digital computers, operating on the basis of binary numbers and logical circuitry, we also elaborate briefly on binary numbers and logic (Section 4).

2 Logical Operations and Truth Tables

In logic, a variable or an expression can have only one of two values: TRUE or FALSE. In some cases, instead of using TRUE and FALSE, it is easier to use 1 and 0, respectively (see Section 3).

Logic has a finite number of operators, of which the most important are the **binary operators AND** and **OR** (both operating on two logical variables) and the **unary operator NOT** (operating on one logical variable). All other logical operators can be derived from only two of these three, but generally we use all three of them. A logical variable is commonly denoted by a capital letter. The truth table presented in Table 23.1 summarizes the most elementary operations on two logical varia-

---

[1] *Boolean logic has many versions, known under different names, such as combinatorial logic, symbolic logic, or propositional logic. Each of these names for logic has its own historical background, but they are in fact equivalent.*

Table 23.1
Truth Table for the Binary Operators AND and OR.

A	B	A AND B	A OR B
T	T	T	T
T	F	F	T
F	T	F	T
F	F	F	F

Table 23.2
Truth Table for the Negation: NOT

A	'A
T	F
F	T

bles A and B: AND and OR. Table 23.2 gives the truth table for the negation NOT.

2.1 The Venn diagram

A **Venn diagram** is a graphical representation of all possible objects belonging to a certain class of objects (see Fig. 23.1a). The rectangle of a Venn diagram is the **domain** of a certain class of objects. For instance, a class of objects can be animals. This class can be visualized by all objects within the rectangle. If we want to represent the set of *mammals*, for instance, we position all mammals within a circle and all other animals outside the circle.

In logic, we also use Venn diagrams. For instance, a logical variable A may represent the expression: A = "this animal is a mammal." In Fig. 23.1a, the domain within circle A represents all mammals, that is, there A is TRUE. Outside the circle A is FALSE, that is, the domain outside the circle represents A = FALSE. Similarly, we can draw a circle B representing: B = "this animal lives in the ocean." Typically, the two circles for A and B will partly overlap, called the intersection, for the subset of mammals that live in the ocean.

Using Venn diagrams and truth tables we discuss the logical NOT, AND, and OR operators.

2.2 Logical Operators

- The NOT operation.

The expression

$E = NOT\ A$

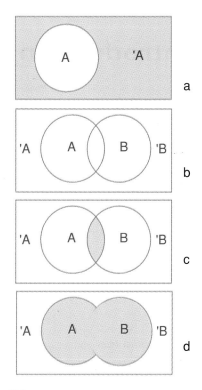

Figure 23.1
Venn diagrams indicating the domains where logical variables are either TRUE or FALSE (see also Table 23.1). (a) The area inside the circle represents the domain of A where A is TRUE; outside the circle A is FALSE. (b) The domains are depicted for both logical variables A and B. (c) The shaded area indicates the domain of the expression E = A AND B. The shaded area in panel d represents the OR operation.

is TRUE if A is FALSE (the area outside the circle of Fig. 23.1b) and FALSE if A is TRUE. In Boolean algebra, the apostrophe is used for NOT:

$E = {'}A.$

- The AND operation

The expression

$$E = A \text{ AND } B$$

is only TRUE if both A and B are TRUE; otherwise, E is FALSE.
This is graphically shown in the Venn diagram of Fig. 23.1c, in which the shaded area (the ***intersection***) indicates the domain of the expression $E = A$ AND B. In Boolean algebra we use the notation:

$$E = A \cdot B,$$

with the dot representing the AND operation or ***logical product***, in a way similar to algebraic multiplication.

- The OR operation

The expression

$$E = A \text{ OR } B$$

is only FALSE if both A and B are FALSE; otherwise, it is TRUE.
The shaded area of Fig. 23.1d (the ***junction*** of A and B) represents the OR operation in a Venn diagram. In Boolean algebra:

$$E = A + B,$$

with the plus sign representing the logical OR or ***logical summation***, which is totally different from the algebraic summation (see Section 3).

2.3 Logical expressions

A logical expression may be:

- a verbal statement that is either TRUE or FALSE,
- a logical variable, or
- statements and logical variables combined by logical operators.

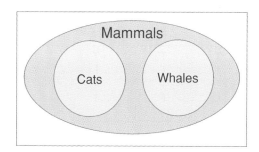

Figure 23.2
Venn diagram of the set of cats, which belongs to the set of mammals, as does the set of whales. Note that the subset of cats has no intersection with the subset of whales,.

A verbal statement is usually placed within double quotation marks.
Examples of some simple verbal logical expressions are the following:

$E_1 =$ "EEG is an acronym for electroencephalogram"
$E_2 =$ "12 is a prime number"
$E_3 =$ "8 + 5 = 13"
$E_4 =$ "a cat is a mammal"
$E_5 =$ "a whale is a mammal"
$E_6 =$ "IF E_4 AND E_5 THEN 'a cat is a whale' "

Every expression E_i is either TRUE of FALSE. In the examples given above, it is immediately apparent that the expressions E_2 and E_6 are FALSE. This seems strange for E_6, because both E_4 and E_5 are TRUE so that the result of the AND operation is also TRUE. Yet, a cat is not a whale. To understand this, we must refer to Venn diagrams (see Fig. 23.2). The set of *cats* belongs to the set of *mammals*, as does the set of *whales*. However, the subset of *cats* has no intersection with the subset of *whales*, so that the expression "A cat is a whale" is FALSE. Therefore, the expression E_6 is a valid logical expression, but with an outcome of FALSE.
Some logical expressions are known from human reasoning, such as the ***implication***, the ***equivalency***, the ***exclusive OR***, and the ***tautology***. We will discuss these four expressions and verify whether they can all be expressed in one of the three basic operations.

23

A	B	A → B	A ↔ B	A + NOT A	Table 23.3
T	T	T	T	T	Truth Table for the Implication, the Equivalency, and the Tautology.
T	F	F	F	T	
F	T	T	F	T	
F	F	T	T	T	

• The implication

In an implication we relate two logical expressions A and B to each other by stating that if A is TRUE, then B is also TRUE. The expression:

$$E = A \rightarrow B$$

is a short notation for "A implies B" or "IF A THEN B." Expressions of the type "if A then B" are seen in **knowledge bases** that are used in **expert systems** (see Section 4.2 of Chapter 15, and Panel 16.2 of Chapter 16). The following is an example of an expression E that is easy to understand:

$E = $ IF "the sun is shining" THEN "the temperature is high".

There are two possible situations, which are the expressions in quotation marks; each of them can either be TRUE or FALSE. The expression E is called

an *implication*, because it says that the shining of the sun implies that the temperature is high. Such a statement is, of course, only TRUE if we measure a high temperature when the sun is indeed shining. However, when the temperature is high and the sun does not shine, the expression E is not violated, because E only tells us of a situation when the sun shines. If the temperature is low while the sun shines, the expression E is no longer TRUE. In fact, we have four possible combinations of the two possible situations:

1. "the sun is shining" = TRUE AND "the temperature is high" = TRUE
2. "the sun is shining" = TRUE AND "the temperature is high" = FALSE
3. "the sun is shining" = FALSE AND "the temperature is high" = TRUE
4. "the sun is shining" = FALSE AND "the temperature is high" = FALSE

The first combination is in agreement with statement E, the implication, so the value E is TRUE. The second condition contradicts the statement of the implication, so the value of the implication is FALSE. The third and the fourth conditions do not contradict the statement of the implication; therefore, the value of the implication is TRUE. We can replace the expression "the sun is shining" by the logical variable A and the expression "the temperature is high" by the logical variable B: results are summarized in Table 23.3.

The implication can also be represented in a Venn diagram (Fig. 23.3a) by shading the three areas for which the expression

$$A \rightarrow B$$

is TRUE. Note from Fig. 23.3a that the expression 'A +

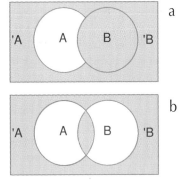

Figure 23.3
Venn diagrams for equivalency (a) and implication (b).

PANEL 23.1

Basic Boolean Operations

$$A \cdot A = A$$
$$A \cdot \text{TRUE} = A$$
$$A \cdot \text{FALSE} = \text{FALSE}$$
$$A \cdot {'A} = \text{FALSE}$$
$$A + A = A$$
$$A + \text{TRUE} = \text{TRUE}$$
$$A + \text{FALSE} = A$$
$$A + {'A} = I$$

Double negation	$''A = A$
Equivalency	$A \leftrightarrow B = A.B + {'A}.{'B}$
Exclusive OR	$A \leftrightarrow {'B} = {'A} \leftrightarrow B = A.{'B} + {'A}.B$
Commutative law	$A.B \leftrightarrow B.A$
Distributive law	$A.(B + C) \leftrightarrow A.B + A.C$
	$A + (B.C) \leftrightarrow (A + B).(A + C)$
Associative law	$A.(B.C) \leftrightarrow (A.B).C$
	$A + (B + C) \leftrightarrow (A + B) + C$
De Morgan's laws	${'(A.B)} \leftrightarrow {'A} + {'B}$
	${'(A + B)} \leftrightarrow {'A}.{'B}$
Implication	$A \leftrightarrow B = {'A} + B$
Tautology	$(A + {'A}) \leftrightarrow \text{TRUE}$, or $(A \leftrightarrow A) \leftrightarrow \text{TRUE}$
Identity	$A \leftrightarrow A$

23

B gives the same logical result for the four possible conditions. This means that :

$$A \rightarrow B = {'A} + B.$$

• The equivalency

The expression A $\leftrightarrow$ B is a short notation for "*A* is equivalent to *B*", which is only TRUE if *A* and *B* have the same value. Table 23.3 and Fig. 23.3b present the equivalency operation.

The expression $E = A \leftrightarrow B$ can also be written by using the basic operators only:

$$E = A \leftrightarrow B = (A.B) + ({'A}.{'B}).$$

(See Panel 23.1 for the use of mathematical symbols and operators used in logic.)

- The exclusive OR

The exclusive OR (in short **XOR**) is a slight modification of the equivalency:

$$E = A \leftrightarrow \, 'B.$$

The expression is TRUE only when one of the operands is TRUE and the other is FALSE. This can also be specified as:

$$E = (A.'B) + ('A.B).$$

- The tautology

The expression $E = A + 'A$ means that E is always TRUE, whatever the value of A (see Table 23.3). The tautology is often denoted by the symbol I (for identity), which is always TRUE. In all composed expressions it is important to inspect whether tautologies are present, because such expressions contain no information (see also Panel 23.1).

3　Boolean Algebra and Karnaugh Diagrams

23

In the previous sections, we followed a formalism for logical expressions that was generally based on **set theory**. Briefly, we also introduced a notation (similar to the commonly known algebra) for logical expressions called **Boolean algebra**. This algebra follows the symbols and formalism of common algebra (such as the plus sign for OR, and the dot for AND, and quotation marks), but there are a few important exceptions. These should be reckoned with when calculating in Boolean algebra. Most of the important logical expressions and laws for Boolean algebra are summarized in Panel 23.1. In this section we give a few examples, based (in part) on what was already described in Section 4.2 of Chapter 15. From that section we borrow Equation (14) in Boolean algebraic notation, which is (if we write for the six variables E_1, E_2, E_3, E_5, E_7, and E_{12}: P, Q, R, S, T, and U, respectively):

$$D = P.Q.'R.'S.'U + P.Q.'R.S.T, \tag{1}$$

which can be written with the distributive law and the **De Morgan**'s law (see Panel 23.1) as:

$$D = '\{'P + 'Q + R + '['(S + U) + '('S + 'T)]\}.$$

This latter equation uses the operators NOT and OR only (see Panel 23.2 for a derivation).
All expressions in logic can be reduced to a combination of only two of the three operators OR, AND, and NOT, but generally, all three are used. It may be easier to derive a logical expression from a truth table not by use of Boolean algebra but by use of a so-called **Karnaugh diagram**, which is a representation of all possible conditions expressed in a truth table. In this case a logical expression is simplified by first generating the Karnaugh diagram and subsequently generating a logical expression.
In a Karnaugh diagram the domain of logical values is divided into two halves (e.g., A and $'A$) or into four squares (e.g., $A.B$, $A.'B$, $'A.B$, and $'A.'B$). These two diagrams are shown below.

Division of the domain in two halves.
At the left side A = TRUE, at the right side A = FALSE.

PANEL· 23.2

Example of De Morgan's Law

Equation (1) in Section 3 was written as follows:

$$D = P.Q.'R.'S.'U + P.Q.'R.S.T \tag{1}$$

With the distributive law we can write:

$$D = P.Q.'R.('S.'U + S.T)$$

Double negation gives:

$$D = '['\{P.Q.'R.('S.'U + S.T)\}],$$

In this formula the three operators AND, OR, and NOT are used. To transform this formula to another formula with only OR and NOT, we need to apply the laws of De Morgan:

$$D = '['P + 'Q + ''R + '('S.'U + S.T)], \text{ or}$$
$$D = '\{'P + 'Q + R + '['(S + U) + '('S + 'T)]\}$$

This latter formula has the operators NOT and OR only.

23

---

results in the Karnaugh diagram:

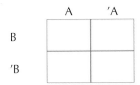

	A	'A
B		
'B		

Division of the domain in four squares.
At the left side A = TRUE, at the upper half B = TRUE.

For example, use of a Karnaugh diagram to simplify the logical expression

$$E = A.B + 'A.B + A.'B \tag{2}$$

	A	'A
B	TRUE	TRUE
'B	TRUE	FALSE

Division of the domain in four squares.
At the left side A = TRUE, at the upper half B = TRUE.

The Karnaugh diagram is always composed of a number of squares equal to the number of possible combinations of logical variables. In an expression involving only two logical variables A and B, each variable is TRUE or FALSE, resulting in 2 x 2 possible combinations of A and B. Therefore, the given Karnaugh diagram will have four squares. For each square we evaluate the logical expression and indicate the resulting value, TRUE (abbreviated T) or FALSE (abbreviated F), in the square. The square in upper left indicates the

---

PANEL 23.3

Example of a Karnaugh Diagram

Given is a logical expression E for four variables A, B, C and D, and we are requested to simplify E by using a Karnaugh diagram:

$$E = A.'B + A.C.D. + 'A.D + 'A.'B.C + 'A.'B.'C.D + 'B.'C.'D$$

The Karnaugh diagram of this expression is:

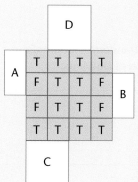

Looking at the area where D is TRUE (T), it is seen that all cells are filled with T's. This means that on that account, E is TRUE for D, and the same applies to $'B$. These two areas cover all values in the diagram where a T is indicated, so for a simplified version of E we can write:

$$E = 'B + D$$

Of course, the same result can be obtained by applying the rules given in Panel 23.1.

It is also interesting to derive the formula by starting from the areas where E is FALSE. We see that this is the case for

$$E = '(B.'D),$$

which is, after applying a law of De Morgan, similar to the earlier solution.

---

condition for A = TRUE and B = TRUE with the result that E = TRUE.

It can also be seen that E is TRUE either for the left column where A = TRUE, or for the upper row where B is TRUE, so that Equation (2) becomes

$$E = A + B.$$

This can also be obtained by applying the rules of Boolean algebra, as given in Panel 23.1. We rewrite Equation (2) as follows:

$$E = A.B + 'A.B + A.B + A.'B,$$

in which the expression A.B has been repeated, which is allowed because $A.B = A.B + A.B$ (see Panel 23.1). By using the distributive law we can write

$$E = (A + 'A).B + A.(B + 'B)$$ or, because $A + 'A$ = TRUE,
$$E = (TRUE).B + A.(TRUE),$$ and
$$E = B + A = A + B$$

PANEL 23.4

Transformations from Decimal to Binary and Vice Versa

Conversion from the decimal to the binary system is comparatively easy; this involves solving the equation

$$237_{10} = a.2^7 + b.2^6 + c.2^5 + d.2^4 + e.2^3 + f.2^2 + g.2^1 + h.2^0,$$

where each factor (a through h) has the value of either 1 or 0. For the conversion the following steps should be taken:

	237		
Step 1	128	1×2^7	$10\ 000\ 000_2$
	-——		
	109		
Step 2	64	1×2^6	$01\ 000\ 000_2$
	-——		
	45		
Step 3	32	1×2^5	$00\ 100\ 000_2$
	-——		
	13		
Step 4	0	0×2^4	$00\ 000\ 000_2$
	-——		
	13		
Step 5	8	1×2^3	$00\ 001\ 000_2$
	-——		
	5		
Step 6	4	1×2^2	$00\ 000\ 100_2$
	-——		
	1		
Step 7	0	0×2^1	$00\ 000\ 000_2$
	-——		
	1		
Step 8	1	1×2^0	$00\ 000\ 001_2$
	-——		
	0		

23

Thus, 237_{10} equals $011\ 101\ 101_2$. The binary number has been written as small groups of three bits, because this enables better pronunciation of this number in octal form:

$$237_{10} = 355_8,$$

because the first group of three bits (011) equals 3_8, the second and third (101) equals 5_8. (Of course, all octal numbers 0_8 to 7_8 are equal to the decimal numbers 0_{10} to 7_{10}, respectively).

For logical expressions in which more than four variables are involved, the use of Karnaugh diagrams often becomes too complex. Panel 23.3 provides an example of the derivation of a logical formula from a truth table via a Karnaugh diagram with four variables.

4 Binary Numbers and Logic

As already mentioned, all present-day digital computers operate with ***binary numbers*** and logical circuitry. Therefore, we also examine the inner operation of computers, with the purpose of demystifying the inner "workings" of the computer (as if it were built with circuits similar to our nervous system). In no way, however, it is possible to compare highly complex human neurons and their interconnections in the brain and electronic circuitry in computers (see also Chapters 3 and 15). Nevertheless, computers do surpass the human brain in processing speed and permanent memory storage.

The tiniest memory cell of a computer can only store a two-valued variable, the binary digit (or ***bit***), that represents either a logical (TRUE or FALSE) or a numerical (1 or 0) piece of information. Electronically, this is realized by, for example, a low and a high voltage or current, a negative and a positive voltage, or a weak and a strong magnetization, respectively. The number of times per second that the computer is able

Panel 23.5

Binary Addition and Subtraction

The rules for adding and subtracting binary numbers are exactly the same as those for adding and subtracting decimal numbers. As an example, the decimal numbers 43_{10} and 78_{10} are added as follows (where 10^1 and 10^0 indicate the base):

base	10^1	10^0	
43	4	3	
78	7	8	
—— +	—— +	—— +	
121_{10}	11	11	
	1 ◄———	┘	← the "carry"
	—— +	—— +	
	12	1	or 121_{10}

The same numbers in binary form are

000 101 011 = 43_{10}
001 001 110 = 78_{10}
———————— +
001 111 001 = 121_{10}

to change, write, or read the voltage, current, or magnetization and the number of parallel operations determines its speed.

The computer stores all decimal numbers, as we use them, in binary form. The user is not concerned with the transformation from decimal to binary or vice versa, or with binary or arithmetic addition, subtraction, multiplication, or division. Yet, it is useful to have a basic idea of the inner operation of the computer, even if it is only to demystify this human artifact. Therefore, this section and Panels 23.4 and 23.5 briefly describe basic binary operations together with their relationship to logic.

The ancient Arabs gave us our decimal number system (base 10), and the Babylonians had a sexagesimal system (base 60), the basis for our clock. All number systems can be transformed to any other number system. The binary system has base 2, the octal system has base 8, and the hexadecimal system has base 16. When counting in the decimal system, we use 10 different symbols from 0 to 9; when counting in the binary system there are only 2 symbols, 0 and 1. Panel 23.4 shows counting by means of three number systems: binary, octal, and decimal. A decimal number is expressed as a series of digits. The position of the digits determines the weight; the weights are powers of 10. For example, the number 237_{10} (the subscript $_{10}$ is used to indicate that it is a number with decimal base ten) can be decomposed as:

$$237_{10} = 200_{10} + 30_{10} + 7_{10} = 2 \times 10^2 + 3 \times 10^1 + 7 \times 10^0.$$

Similarly, the binary number 1011_2 can be decomposed as:

$$1011_2 = 1000_2 + 0000_2 + 0010_2 + 0001_2 = 1 \times 2^3 + 0 \times 2^2 + 1 \times 2^1 + 1 \times 2^0.$$

The example in Panel 23.5 indicates that it is not difficult to transform decimal numbers to binary numbers, and the reverse is also true. The use of octal numbers is helpful in pronouncing large binary numbers. Generally, however, with the increasing *word length* of present-day computers (generally of 32 bits), it is more convenient to replace each group of four binary digits by one *hexadecimal* digit, which implies the use of a numbering system of mode 16; this requires 16 different symbols. Since we have only 10 number symbols (0 to 9) on a computer keyboard we must add 6 additional symbols, to be treated as a hexadecimal digit. Usually, the first letters of the alphabet are used:

A = 10, B = 11, C = 12, D = 13, E = 14, and F = 15.

For instance, the hexadecimal number $B7_{16}$ is: $11 \times 16^1 + 7 \times 16^0 = 176 + 7 = 183_{10}$.

When subtracting two binary numbers, again, the same rules used as for subtracting decimal numbers apply.

23

Key References

See the Web site for literature references.

24 Biostatistical Methods

1 Introduction

Biostatistics is closely related to medical informatics for the following reasons:

1. Many data (e.g., laboratory measurements, documentation of diagnostic and therapeutic measures and their results) that are gathered from routine medical informatics applications can be used for statistical analysis and evaluation.
2. Most medical research is based on the use of computers for data acquisition, data storage, and data analysis.
3. Powerful statistical software packages are easily available for any computer user. Unprofessional use of these systems and misinterpretation of the generated output cause many problems.

Therefore, it is useful to include an introductory chapter on biostatistical methods in this Handbook.

Biostatistical methods are used to describe and analyze the results of biomedical experiments and observations. In addition, they serve for the planning of experimental and observational studies and for describing biological phenomena by mathematical models. The domain of biostatistics (an equivalent term is *biometry*) is too extensive to be covered within the framework of an introduction. Therefore, this chapter presents only a few paradigmatic aspects and some examples illustrating these. For any practical application the reader is referred to specific textbooks (see the References). The reader may also seek biostatistical advice from a professional.

2 Data Description

The first aim of a statistical analysis is to describe *empirical observations* in a condensed, meaningful manner. For this purpose, one must distinguish between different forms of data:

1. *Qualitative data* describe **nominal categorical aspects** (e.g., gender, disease categories, and hair color).
2. *Ordinal data* represent observable quantifications (e.g., disease stages, quality of life, and social status). Corresponding observations may be qualified as *ordered categories*, such as "good", "intermediate," and "poor" or 1 to 5.
3. *Quantitative data* represent countable or measurable observations.
   – *discrete data* correspond to countable observations (e.g., blood cell count, parity, number of medications taken), and
   – *continuous data* represent the results of measured observations (e.g., blood pressures, and serum glucose concentrations).

Disease groups	Frequency		
	Absolute	Relative	
Leukemias	7,435	35.2	
CNS tumors	3,608	17.1	
Lymphomas	2,555	12.1	
Sympathetic nervous system tumors	1,649	7.8	
Soft-tissue sarcomas	1,446	6.8	
Renal tumors	1,397	6.6	
Bone tumors	1,088	5.1	
Germ cell tumors	870	4.1	
Other diseases	1,080	5.2	
Total	21,128	100.0	

Table 24.1
Frequency of Different Childhood Malignancies.

In statistical terms, data are denoted as *observed values* (*observations*) of *variables*.

2.1 Qualitative Data

Qualitative data are efficiently described by means of tables. These tables may comprise absolute or relative *frequencies*, but a combination of both, as shown in Table 24.1, is preferable. Relative frequencies are usually given as percentages to facilitate comparisons of frequencies obtained from different numbers of observations. One should avoid presenting more than the *significant digits*. For instance, it would be misleading to report 14.29% if this result is based on one of seven observations. Computer programs tend to produce many insignificant digits that should not be copied for publication. Graphical representations of observed qualitative data are *bar diagrams*, *block diagrams*, or *pie charts* (see Fig. 24.1). User-friendly graphical presentation programs are available for personal computers.

2.2 Continuous Data

Continuous data are usually reported in form of *classifications* (e.g., age in years or groups of years). The

adequate graphical representation is a *histogram* (see Fig. 24.2). A histogram illustrates the observed distribution of a variable such as age or blood pressure. These distributions may also be characterized by computing their parameters. The two best-known parameters are the *mean value* ($\bar{x}$) and the *empirical variance* (s^2) or the *standard deviation* (s). They are calculated by the following formulas:

$$\bar{x} = \frac{1}{n} \sum_{i=1}^{n} x_i \qquad (1)$$

where n is the number of observations, and x_i is the value of the observation i.

$$s^2 = \frac{\sum (x_i - \bar{x})^2}{n - 1} \qquad (2)$$

The mean value describes the location of the distribution, that is, the average value, whereas the standard deviation indicates the *spread* of the distribution, that is, the variability of the data. The spread of the data may also be characterized by the *range*, which is the distance between the largest and the smallest observations. Many data are "normally" distributed, that is, the distribution can be described by the well-known symmetrical, bell-shaped **Gaussian curve**. If this is the case and if the number of observations is very large, about 95% of all observations fall into the range of $\bar{x} \pm 1.96s$. Many medical data (e.g., laboratory measurements) have a **log-normal distribution** (see Fig. 24.3). If the distribution of the original data is skewed it often becomes Gaussian after a logarithmic transformation (e.g., $y_i = \ln x_i$).

If the data show a **skewed distribution** or contain some **outliers**, that is, observations with extreme values for certain reasons, it may be more adequate to characterize the location of the distribution by calculating the **median value** . The median is obtained by sorting all observations in ascending order and selecting the observation that is right in the middle of the sorted data. If n is an odd number, the median is the value of x_i of the sorted data with $i = (n + 1)/2$.

For even numbers of sorted observations there are two observations in the middle (with $i = n/2$ and $i = n/2 +1$), and the mean value of these two observations is taken as the median.

In contrast to the mean value, the median does not change if the value of extreme observations is changed; hence it is considered to be *robust* against outliers.

The intention of defining the median in this way is that approximately 50% of all observations are $\geq$ and, correspondingly, 50% are $\leq$. The median is also called the 50% **quantile**, or $x_{0.5}$. In analogy, one can define other *quantiles* of a distribution, for example, $x_{0.95}$ or $x_{0.2}$. According to the quantization of the distribution, some of these quantiles have specific names: *percentiles, deciles, quartiles,* and *quintiles*.

To obtain a robust parameter for the spread of a distribution, one may indicate the difference between certain quantiles. For instance, the *central* 50% of the observations fall into the range between $x_{0.25}$ and $x_{0.75}$, the so-called interquartile distance.

A graphical summary of observed distribution parameters is given by the so-called box and whisker plot. This plot is especially well suited for illustrating differences in observed distributions.

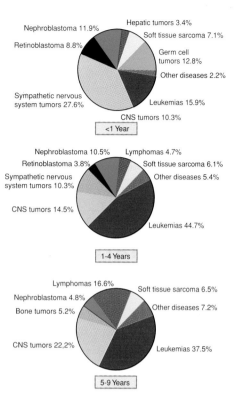

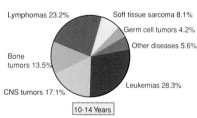

Figure 24.1
Frequency of childhood malignancies in infants and children ages 1 to 14. CNS indicates central nervous system.

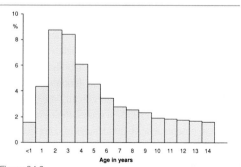

Figure 24.2
Age distribution for boys and girls with childhood leukemia.

24

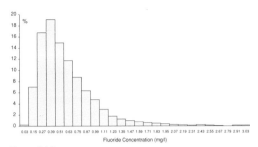
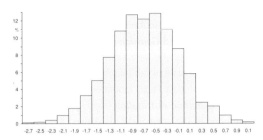

Figure 24.3
Distribution of serum glutamic oxalacetic transaminase (SGOT) measurements before and after logarithmic transformation.

3 Estimation of Parameters and Hypothesis Testing

Almost all observational and experimental medical studies relate to samples from populations. For example, the effects of a prophylactic anticoagulant therapy observed in 100 patients with major surgical operations, such as a hip replacement, will be generalized to all patients who undergo such operations. To perform such generalizations one must use biostatistical *stochastic models*.

A possible outcome of such a study could be that 15 postoperative thromboembolic complications are observed among the 100 treated patients. Suppose that for the above-mentioned operations the frequency of complications in patients not treated with anticoagulants is known to be 30%. What can we tell from the present observation? If an untreated sample of 100 patients was studied, one would not expect to observe exactly 30 complications but – due to chance variation – one would observe a figure relatively close to 30. The amount of expected chance variability can be calculated by using the model of the **binomial distribution** that cannot be described in detail here. The calculation reveals that in 95% of such samples we would expect to observe relative frequencies of complications within the range of from 21 to 40%. In other words, the chance of observing a relative frequency outside this range is small (5%). Of course, more extreme observations – those due only to chance – are possible, but

the probability for more extreme observations becomes smaller and smaller (e.g., 1% for values outside the range from 18 to 43%). Therefore, from the observed frequency of 15% we would conclude that this has not been due to chance but, rather, to the given therapy. This is the first part of the generalization from this study.

The second part relates to the question, "How effective is the therapy?" Again, it may not be assumed that a replication of the study with 100 other treated patients would again show exactly 15 complications, but it may be expected that the result varies within certain limits. It is also possible to calculate such limits by means of the binomial distribution. The result of a corresponding calculation tells us that the unknown frequency of complications in the population of all treated patients, is in a range from 9 to 24%. The underlying procedure guarantees that this statement will be correct for 95% of similar observations. The limits are called the 95% **confidence limits**, and they illustrate how precisely the therapeutic effect may be estimated from such a study. From such considerations we can conclude that in this example we can only be relatively sure that the effect is at least equal to the difference between the population parameter (30%) and the observed upper confidence limit (24%), which amounts to 6%.

Test Result	Real Situation		Table 24.2
	H_0 true	H_0 false	Possible Decisions Based on Statistical Significance Tests
H_0 maintained	correct decision	Type two error probability ß	
H_0 rejected	Type one error probability α	correct decision[a]	

[a] probability 1 - ß = power

The procedures described by this example are called **hypothesis testing** and **parameter estimation**, respectively, in formal statistical terms. The procedures shall now be described in formal terms to facilitate the understanding of more complex approaches.

3.1 Hypothesis Testing

The number of outcomes (x patients with complications in a study of sample size n) can be modeled by a *binomial distribution* with parameters p and n, where p denotes the known chance (probability) for untreated patients to experience the complication. The binomial distribution of x is denoted by the expression:

$$x \sim B(p, n).$$

In this context, x is also denoted as the *test statistic*. If p_1 denotes the unknown probability for complications in treated patients, one can define the **null hypothesis**,

$$H_0: p_1 = p$$

and the alternative hypothesis,

$$H_1: p_1 \neq p.$$

This means that under the *null hypothesis* one assumes that the therapy has no effect (the probability of complications is equal to that known for untreated patients), and under the alternative hypothesis one assumes that both probabilities are different. This type of alternative hypothesis is called *two sided*, because it makes no

assumption on a possible positive or negative effect of the treatment. If one does not really have any definite reason to assume superiority of the treatment under study (which will be true in most practical applications) one should use a *two-sided hypothesis*. This was also done in the above intuitive description of the example. If one has convincing reasons to do so one could also state a *one-sided* alternative hypothesis, for example,

$$H_1: p_1 < p,$$

which is only looking for superiority of the treatment. In this case, the calculated figures for the two-sided hypothesis presented above would have to be adjusted.

The logical procedure of the statistical test is that we reject H_0 (and thereby accept H_1) if the probability that the test statistic (in this example the observed number of patients with complications takes a value as extreme or more extreme than the one actually observed) is smaller than a certain threshold (e.g., 5%) otherwise the null hypothesis is maintained. If one falsely rejects H_0, this is called a **type one error**. The **type two error** denotes the error that H_0 is maintained, although H_1 is true (see Table 24.2). The corresponding error probabilities are denoted by α and β, whereas the probability of the type one error is also called **level of significance**. The corresponding threshold values of the test statistic are called **critical values**.

The definition of hypotheses and the choice of the significance level must be made before the statistical analysis, usually during the planning phase of a study. The choice of the significance level is somewhat arbitrary; conventional levels are 5 and 1%. The selection

24

should be adequately related to the conclusions that will be based on the analysis. For example, it may be more acceptable to decide incorrectly that a new human immunodeficiency virus (**HIV**) therapy is effective than to decide that a new beta-blocker is effective. Such considerations also reflect the probability of the type two error, which usually increases if the probability of the type one error is decreased.

The value 1 minus β is called the **power of a statistical test**. Generally, it is advisable not to perform studies that have a statistical power of less than 80%. Under certain circumstances, for instance, if one wants to detect very subtle treatment effects (as would be the case with HIV), it may be necessary to obtain a power of 90% or more in order not to overlook possible relevant findings. It is one of the tasks of statistical experimental design to calculate the sample sizes in order to maintain adequate levels of α and β.

3.2 Parameter Estimation

The second part of the statistical analysis in the example above was the estimation of an unknown population parameter. Calculating the relative frequency from the sample of 100 patients is the best that we can do to estimate the "true" probability for all patients treated under similar conditions. The confidence limits give an impression of how precise this estimate is. The confidence limits become smaller, that is, our estimate becomes more accurate with increasing sample sizes. The problem of estimating the parameter of a binomial distribution is comparable to estimating parameters of the normal (Gaussian) distribution, which was mentioned in Section 2. The **normal distribution** is defined by the parameters μ and σ^2. These parameters are estimated by calculating $\bar{x}$ and s^2. Calculations of confidence intervals for these parameters are based on the t and χ^2 *distributions*, respectively.

On the basis of the principles described above, a large number of statistical tests have been developed, and these tests suit most of the commonly used experimental designs. It is beyond the scope of this chapter to describe statistical tests in detail, but a few remarks can be made. The comparison between a known parameter

from a population and an observation from a sample is a relatively rare situation. More common is the need to compare the results from tests of two or more samples. To compare relative frequencies from two samples, a procedure called **Fisher's exact test** is in most instances adequate. In most **clinical trials** (see Section 4) one compares observations from two random samples. If the observation of measurement data is of specific interest, the comparison of results from two samples is performed by means of the well known **t-test**. The t-test is based on the assumption that the data are normally (Gaussian) distributed and have equal standard deviations. In this case the null hypothesis is stated as follows:

$$H_0: \mu_1 = \mu_2,$$

where μ_1 denotes the (unknown) parameter for population 1 (e.g., the mean blood pressure of patients treated with an old medication A) and μ_2 is the parameter of a second population (e.g., patients treated with a new antihypertension drug). The two-sided alternative hypothesis is stated as:

$$H_1: \mu_1 \neq \mu_2.$$

If the data are not normally distributed, they can also be examined by another statistical test, and if they cannot easily be transformed into a normal distribution, for instance, by calculating the logarithm of the observed data, one may use the **Wilcoxon-Mann-Whitney test** to test the hypothesis of equal distributions. This test procedure is based on assigning **rank scores** to the observed original data. Therefore, this test is also adequate when the original observations are ordinal data.

In case one does not compare observations from two samples but, rather, compares two observations for the same individuals within one sample (e.g., measurements before and after a therapy), it is possible to use the **paired t-test** (for normally distributed data) or the **Wilcoxon signed rank test** (for other types of quantitative data or for ordinal data). In this case the null hypothesis for the paired t-test is stated as:

$$H_0: \delta = 0,$$

where δ denotes the parameter of the (unknown) distribution of intraindividual differences between the first and second observations. A one-sided, alternative hypothesis could be

$$H_1: \delta > 0.$$

This assumes that the observed differences tend to be positive (e.g., the blood pressure measurements are decreasing after therapy).

For comparison of more than two samples or more than two observations within one sample, more complex methods are available. In the case of normally distributed data it is possible to apply the *analysis of variance* (*ANOVA*). If one must compare k groups, the global null hypothesis is stated as:

$$H_0: \mu_1 = \mu_2 = \ldots = \mu_k.$$

The alternative hypothesis states that a least one inequality is present between the different parameters. If the observations are not normally distributed, the **Kruskal-Wallis test** can be applied, which is also based on assigning rank scores to the individual observations. For com-

parison of multiple observations within one sample, it is possible to apply an adequate ANOVA model for normally distributed data. The **Friedman test** is an analogy for not normally distributed data. If one wants to compare several specific groups of observations individually, in addition to the null hypothesis stated above, several null hypotheses should be formulated. This situation leads to the problem of *multiple comparisons,* and it requires an adequate specification of type one error probabilities. A large number of techniques is available for performing this task. One should at least be familiar with the fact that, for instance, performing a series of t-tests with an α-error probability of 5% would reveal misleading results with a grossly "inflated" type-one error. A well-known approach to overcome this procedure is the *Bonferroni correction:* to maintain the specific level of α one must perform k tests at the level of α/k. This procedure has the disadvantage that it produces "conservative" results. This means that the level of α is correctly maintained; however, the level of β will be largely increased. Therefore, elaborate procedures have been developed to cover specific situations more efficiently. These procedures are beyond the scope of this Handbook.

24

4 Multivariate Analysis

So far, we have only dealt with the analysis of univariate data. This means that we were only focused on the observation of one individual item, such as blood pressure measurements or responses to a therapy. In many situations, however, it is relevant to observe and analyze more than one item simultaneously. For instance, this may become necessary when we want to study the interaction of individual factors or the effect of a therapy on multiple outcome measures.

The best-known *multivariate* approach is to look at two items simultaneously, for example, height and body weight or age and serum cholesterol level. In these examples it may be of interest how weight increases with increasing body height or whether serum cholesterol levels increase with age. In both examples it is assumed that one observation is dependent on the other. One simple way to model such a dependence is

linear regression analysis. If one has obtained n pairs of observations $x_i, y_i (i = 1, \ldots, n)$, where x_i denotes the independent data and y_i the dependent data, it is possible to illustrate these observations by means of a *scattergram* (see Fig. 24.4). The aim of linear regression analysis is to find a straight line that best fits the observed data. One useful way to define the best fit is the *least-squares* principle, which aims to minimize the sum of squares of distances d_i between the individual observation points and the line (as shown in Fig. 24.5). This approach leads to the following equation to determine the line:

$$y = a + bx,$$

where b and a are calculated as follows:

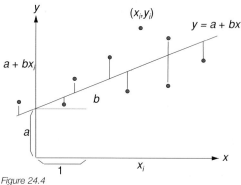

Figure 24.4
Correlation diagram and regression line.

$b = \dfrac{s_{xy}}{s_x^2}$ *and* $a = \bar{y} - b\bar{x}$ *with*

$$s_{xy} = \frac{1}{n-1} \sum_{i=1}^{n} (x_i - \bar{x})(y_i - \bar{y}) \qquad (1)$$

s_x^2 = variance of the observed values x_i, and

$\bar{x}$ and $\bar{y}$ = means of the observed values x_i and y_i.

As illustrated in Fig. 24.4, the slope of the line ascends when b is positive. This means that values y_i are increasing with increasing values x_i. This is denoted as *positive correlation* of x and y. The **correlation coefficient** ρ describes how close this correlation is.

The correlation coefficient ρ is calculated by:

$$\rho = \frac{s_{xy}}{s_x \cdot s_y}$$

By this definition ρ can vary between -1 and +1. Positive values of ρ correspond to an ascending regression line, negative values of *r* indicate that values y_i are decreasing with increasing values x_i. If ρ^2 has the (maximum) value of 1, all observations lie on the fitted line; ρ^2 describes the amount of the variance of y that is explained by x. If ρ^2 has the value of 0, there is no linear correlation between the two variables. By using a specific version of the *t*-test it is possible to analyze whether two normally distributed variables are statistically linearly dependent. The corresponding hypotheses are:

$H_0\colon \rho = 0$ and $H_1\colon \rho \neq 0$

with ρ being the unknown correlation parameter for the population from which these observed samples stem. For not normally distributed data, **Spearman's rank correlation coefficient** may be computed and analyzed by a corresponding test.
If the correlation of two sets of discrete observations is to be analyzed (e.g., disease stage and obtainable degree of clinical remission in cancer patients) the observed results should be presented by means of **contingency**

Survival after 5 years	Tumor Stage							
	I + II		III		IV		Total	
	N	%	N	%	N	%	N	%
Yes	121	89.6	149	63.9	80	15.3	350	39.3
No	14	10.4	84	36.1	442	84.7	540	60.7
Total	135	100.0	233	100.0	522	100.0	890	100.0

Table 24.3
Contingency Table: Tumor Stage and Relapse Frequency.

tables, as shown in Table 24.3. A statistical test for independence of the two variables is based on the χ^2 distribution.

The (bivariate) linear regression analysis can easily be extended to k independent variables and is then called *multiple regression* analysis. The corresponding equation is

$$y = a + b_1x_1 + b_2x_2 \ldots . + b_kx_k.$$

This approach also allows specification of the square of a multiple correlation coefficient that describes the amount of variance of y explained by the variables X_1 to X_k. A further generalization of this approach allows for the analysis of several dependent variables as well. The corresponding analysis is called *canonical regression* analysis.

All above-mentioned types of regression analyses describe linear dependencies within observed continuous data, but other techniques enable the description of non-linear dependencies and they may include discrete data. One popular method that is frequently used in observational studies of risk factors is the *logistic regression*. The corresponding equation is specified as follows:

$$\ln\left(\frac{p}{1-p}\right) = a + b_1x_1 + b_2x_2 \ldots b_kx_k$$

In this formula p denotes the probability of developing a certain disease (e.g., myocardial infarction) and x_i denotes observations of risk factors (e.g., age, serum cholesterol level, and hypertension). Another fre-quently used type of multivariate statistical regression analysis is named after the author of the first publication: *Cox's regression*. It relates to the analysis of observed survival times, and it is described by the following equation:

$$\ln\left[h(t)\right] = \ln\left[h_0(t)\right] + b_1x_1 + b_kx_k,$$

where $h(t)$ denotes the "hazard" that an individual will experience a certain event (e.g., die from a certain disease or suffer from a relapse) as a function of time t after a defined starting point (e.g., the start of treatment). $h_0(t)$ is a *baseline hazard* (without any influence factors being effective), and X_1 to X_k are possible influence factors, for example, type of medication, initial disease stage, and age.

With all of these regression techniques, it is common to perform statistical significance tests on the effectiveness of the observed variables X_i. All these tests examine the null hypotheses:

$$H_0: \beta_i = 0,$$

with β_i denoting the population parameters estimated by b_i. The size of the estimates b_i corresponds to the amount of effectiveness of the analyzed variables x_i. It is also possible to calculate confidence intervals for the true values of β_i and to translate these into a range of possible effects. It is important to recall that a significant result only indicates that the corresponding effect is present; the confidence interval allows for the relevance of such an effect to be judged.

24

5 Biostatistical Aspects Design of Experiments and Observational Studies

An important domain of biostatistics is the design of experimental and observational studies. Statistical study design aims to obtain optimum scientific information from the available data and to minimize the number of observations that are needed to draw firm, scientific conclusions. Application of an adequate methodology for the planning may lead to the exposure of a minimal number of patients to potential risks of an experiment or to a reduction of the resources needed for research. Biostatistical planning also relates to the selection of an adequate statistical model that best describes the underlying medical problem.

5.1 Controlled Clinical Trials

In Section 3 it has been implicitly described that statistical analyses are based on probabilistic approaches. Therefore, when designing studies it is important to provide a correct basis for applying statistical methods. For the estimation of population parameters it is necessary to make sure that samples of the corresponding population are randomly selected. If one wants to compare two treatments given to different groups of patients, one must perform a *randomization* of the therapy by which each observed individual will have the same chance of receiving one of two treatments (an *m:n* randomization is also possible). It is the element of randomization – nowadays, mostly performed by computer programs that generate pseudo-random numbers – which is the essence of so-called *controlled clinical trials*. Such trials are carried out to show the efficacy, superiority, or equivalence of some therapy.

Efficacy is studied by controlled clinical trials, in which one group is given a *placebo* treatment and one or more groups are given substances that are to be tested for their efficacies. The placebo is a nonactive drug that looks and tastes like the drugs to be tested. It is used to indicate the spontaneous course of a certain disease, possibly modified by the suggestive effect (the so-called *placebo effect*) of obtaining an effective drug medication. Only if the effects of active treatment are superior to those of placebo therapy is efficacy regarded as proven. Instead of comparison with a placebo, one frequently compares the efficacies of two drugs, for example, to show the superiority of a new treatment over an old one, or to show that two types of therapy are equally effective ("equivalent").

A study is called *blinded* if the patient is not informed about the kind of therapy he or she is receiving. In most instances it is also necessary that the treating physician not be informed about the therapy to ensure the unbiased observation of the relevant outcome criteria. This type of study is called a *double-blind study*.

If one knows the relevant factors that may influence the efficacy of a treatment (e.g., age or stage of disease) these factors can be built into the design of the study by forming "blocks" (i.e., corresponding groups of patients). Randomization is then performed *within* these blocks.

5.2 Non-randomized Approaches

If it is difficult to recruit the required sample size for a specific study, it may become necessary to perform *multicenter trials*. In this situation it is generally advisable to take the different treatment centers as blocks and to analyze by specific methods whether there are effects due to possible differences between centers.

Randomized studies constitute experiments that form a sound basis for drawing scientific conclusions. For certain research questions it is, however, not possible to perform experiments, for example, if one wants to study the effect of potential *risk factors*, such as cigarette smoking or occupational exposure to mineral

24

fibers. In such instances one cannot perform a randomization of the potential risk factors; rather, one must design observational studies. The two most commonly used designs are the *cohort* and *case-control* studies.

In a cohort study one observes (mostly prospectively) two or more groups in a population that are or are not exposed to the risk factor under investigation. During an adequate time interval, which may be 10 to 20 years in cancer research, one observes how many events of interest occur in the study groups. The observed relative frequency of events is called the *incidence*, and the ratio of incidences is called *relative risk*. If, for example, the observed incidence of myocardial infarctions in a group of 1,000 heavy smokers over a time interval of 10 years is 100/1,000 and in an equally large group of nonsmokers it is 10/1,000, the relative risk is 10. The difference in incidences, in this case 90/1,000, is called the *attributable risk*. The relative risk is approximated by the *odds ratio*, which is defined as the ratio of the numbers of events/numbers of nonevents in the two groups. For rare events and large observational groups, the odds ratio is close to the relative risk (in our example, it is 11).

In a case-control study one defines the study groups not by observing the risk factor but by observing the event to be studied. For the question of cigarette smoking and myocardial infarction, this would be a group of patients with myocardial infarction who would be compared with a group of comparable people who did not have this disease. In that case one would ask the study participants in both groups whether they smoked regularly before. A possible result could be that 90 of 100 patients were smokers and that there were 35 smokers among 100 control subjects. In this situation it is impossible to calculate a relative risk because there is no information on disease incidence. However, it is also possible to calculate the odds ratio (which would be 16.7 with the given figures), which

may be considered an indicator of the relative risk. A relative risk or odds ratio of 1 indicates that the potential risk factor is not effective. For a statistical significance test one formulates, for example,

$$H_0: OR = 1$$
$$H_1: OR \neq 1$$

where the odds ratio (OR) denotes the population parameter that is estimated from the observational study. One also computes confidence limits for the true ratio, to obtain a range of values that reflects the accuracy of the observations. As mentioned in section 4, it is also possible to obtain odds ratio estimates from multivariate logistic regression analysis.

Both types of studies have specific strengths and shortcomings, but these will not be described here. However, it should be mentioned that, whenever possible, it is useful to perform both types of studies to explore a specific question. It should also be stated that epidemiological studies – as nonexperimental studies – are not suitable for proving causal relationships; they can only provide a certain *strength of evidence*. However, epidemiological studies may well be and have been very useful for generating and supporting new scientific hypotheses that may be proven by additional experiments or that may be considered proven, for example, by a summary of evidence obtained from other observations or analogies or from biological plausibility.

Key References

Altman DG. *Practical Statistics for Medical Research*. London: Chapman and Hall, 1991.

See the Web site for further literature references.

24

25 Biosignal Processing Methods

This chapter describes methods that are frequently used in *biosignal processing* systems. We have attempted to limit mathematical formalisms, but their use was at times unavoidable.

For a more superficial discussion of biosignal analysis the reader is referred to Chapter 8, and for a more in-depth discussion of biosignal processing and signal processing methods in general, the reader is referred to the literature in this area.

Some references are listed at the end of this Handbook.

1 Signal-Amplitude Properties

Properties of signals can be expressed in a variety of ways. As an introduction to signal processing, we first discuss some properties of signal amplitudes.

For *deterministic signals*, we have seen in Chapter 8 that the signal waveshape is defined in principle; only the moment of occurrence of the waveshape must be detected (see Section 4 of this chapter). The amplitude properties of deterministic signals, therefore, are fully defined by their waveshapes. Some amplitude properties are of direct diagnostic interest, such as the maximum slope in a *spirogram* during forced expiration or the *ST-T* part of the *ECG* directly after the *QRS* complex. More details on such diagnostic signal properties are discussed in Section 3 of Chapter 13.

In *stochastic signals* we deal with the statistical properties of the signals. Therefore, the parameters that we derive have an inherently statistical character. In the following sections we review some simple statistical parameters related to the amplitude properties of these signals.

1.1 First-Order Amplitude-Density Distributions

In Chapter 8 we described the signal by means of a variable as a function of time. Other representations of signals may also be useful and may reveal signal properties that are not immediately visible in the time domain. One of these representations is the density distribution function (*ddf*), of which the amplitude ddf is an example. To obtain this distribution from sampled signals, we count how often during the observation period T the sampled signal has an amplitude between x and $x + \Delta x$, Δx being a small amplitude increment. This results in a number for each amplitude interval Δx, and all such numbers can be expressed in a *histogram* (see Fig. 25.1). For a relatively short observation period T (or, to phrase it better, for a low number of samples), this histogram will be a rough estimate of the true amplitude ddf, but for a large enough number of samples the histogram will approach the ddf. Then it becomes possible to express this amplitude ddf as a

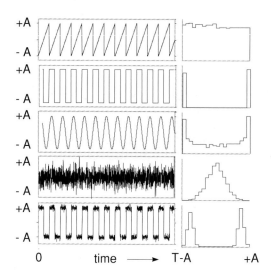

Figure 25.1

Amplitude distribution functions of a sawtooth (where the ddf is uniformly distributed), a block-shaped signal (where the ddf consists of two pikes), a sine wave, normally distributed noise, for instance, an EEG (where the ddf has a Gaussian distribution), and a block wave plus Gaussian noise (from top to bottom, respectively). The effect of a low number of samples is seen in the histograms.

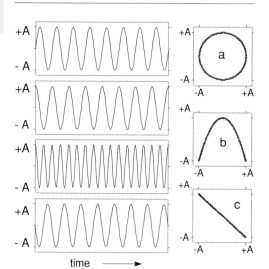

Figure 25.2

Examples of 2-D amplitude distributions: Lissajous figures. A sine and a cosine of the same frequency and no phase difference (a), a sine and a cosine of twice the sine-wave frequency (b), and a sine wave, with amplitudes taken half a period apart (c).

probability function, for example, $f(x)$. In some cases, for instance, in the case of certain types of randomly fluctuating signals, the amplitude ddf will assume the shape of a normal or **Gaussian distribution**.

It is possible to determine for such histograms the values of different statistical parameters, such as the **mean**, **median**, **dispersion**, **skewness**, or **kurtosis** (see Chapter 24 for the meaning of these terms; see Panel 25.1 for some illustrations). The more independent samples there are, the better the estimation of the statistical parameters is. Obviously, the observation time T must be longer when the **sampling rate** is lower, that is, when the signal has a lower frequency content. Figure 25.1 provides some amplitude ddfs of well-known signals with a deterministic character, as well as of random **noise**. It also depicts ddfs of signals plus noise.

Thus far we have discussed so-called one-dimensional or first-order ddfs, which are distribution functions of one parameter only, in our case, the amplitude. In the next section we discuss higher-order distributions, in which more amplitudes of one signal or amplitudes of more signals are involved.

1.2 Second-Order Amplitude-Density Distributions

Above and in Fig. 25.1 we gave some examples of first-order or one-dimensional amplitude distributions. In many instances, however, it is also of interest to examine the relationship between amplitude variations of two different signals or between amplitude variations of the same signal, but at two different time instants, say, τ seconds apart. A so-called **Lissajous figure** (known from physics) is an example of a two-dimensional or second-order distribution function (2-D ddf).

1.2.1 Deterministic Signals: Sines and Cosines

Figure 25.2a shows the relationship (a Lissajous figure or 2-D ddf) between amplitude variations of two deterministic signals, a sine wave and a cosine wave, both with the same frequency, f_s. Figure 25.2b shows the

PANEL 25.1

One-Dimensional Distributions, Means and Variances

In many instances we want to follow how signal properties change as a function of time in order to detect trends in the underlying biological processes. In that case we compute parameters for short observation periods T, in which the periods T may show some overlap. During such an observation period we consider the signal to be stationary, and determine for each period T parameter values that describe the signal. In this Panel we derive parameter values from amplitude ddfs, which may or may not have a stable means, which may be narrow or wide, and which may or may not be symmetric. If the signal can be described as:

$x(t)$, for $t = t_0$ to $t = t_0 + T$, where T is the observation period,

then the sampled signal can be expressed as:

x_i, with $i = 1, 2, \ldots N$, the sample number.

The interval $\Delta T = T/N$ is called the *sampling interval*, and $f_s = 1/\Delta T$ is the *sampling frequency*. The amplitude ddf of x_i can be expressed as $f(x)$, in which no time information or sample number information is kept. The mean of a statistical variable x, for which the ddf $f(x)$ is given, may be written as the *expectation* of x, or:

$$E\{x\} = \int_{-\infty}^{\infty} xf(x)\mathrm{d}x$$

which is also called the *first-order moment* of the ddf $f(x)$. Another way of writing the mean value of the variable x is:

$$\bar{x} = \frac{1}{N} \sum_{1}^{N} x_i,$$

which is a good approximation of $E\{x\}$ for large N. Thus, for the observation period T, $E\{x\}$ is equal to $\bar{x}$. For stationary signals, this equation holds for all observation periods T; for nonstationary signals $\bar{x}$ may vary. In a similar way it is possible to write for the *variance* of the signal (the second-order moment of the ddf):

$$E\{[x-E\{x\}]^2\} = \int_{-\infty}^{\infty} \{[x-E\{x\}]^2\}f(x)\mathrm{d}x. \qquad (1)$$

For a signal with a mean value of zero ($E\{x\} = 0$) this variance becomes:

$$E\{x^2\} = \int_{-\infty}^{\infty} x^2\, f(x)\, \mathrm{d}x. \qquad (2)$$

The *dispersion* σ_x is the square root of the variance. The signal-to-noise ratio (SNR) of a signal that is the sum of a signal plus noise, $x(t) = s(t) + n(t)$ (assuming that $E\{s\}$ and $E\{n\}$ are equal to zero) is defined as the ratio of the variances of signal and noise, S and N, respectively:

$$SNR = S/N = \sigma_s^2 / \sigma_n^2 = E\{s^2\} / E\{n^2\}$$

25

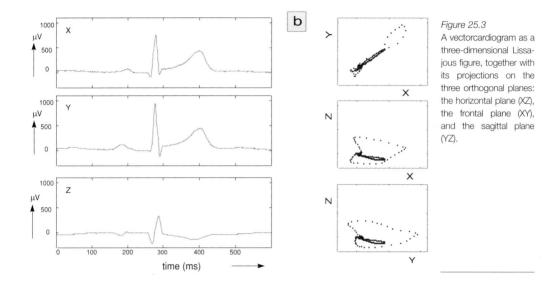

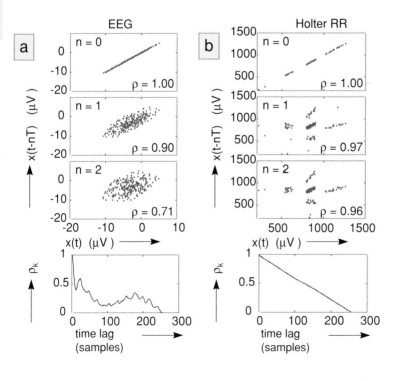

Figure 25.3
A vectorcardiogram as a three-dimensional Lissajous figure, together with its projections on the three orthogonal planes: the horizontal plane (XZ), the frontal plane (XY), and the sagittal plane (YZ).

relationship for a sine wave, and a cosine of twice the frequency of the sine wave shown in Fig. 25.2a (i.e., at $2f_s$). Figure 25.2c shows the relationship between a sine wave and a sine wave at half a period apart.

1.2.2 Deterministic Signals: ECGs

The *vectorcardiogram* (*VCG*) offers a practical example of the composition of biosignal amplitude values in

Figure 25.4
Two-dimensional amplitude ddfs for EEG amplitudes (panels under a) and RR intervals (panels under b) recorded during Holter monitoring. Horizontally, sample n has been plotted; vertically, sample $n + k$. In the upper panels, samples have been plotted for k equals zero (i.e., the samples have been plotted against themselves). In the second and third panels from the top, samples have been plotted for k is equal to 1 and k is equal to 2, respectively. For each panel, with a specific value of k, the correlation ρ_k can be computed. The two lower panels show the correlation coefficients as a function of k, which is also called the *time lag*. These latter functions are called correlograms or correlation functions.

PANEL 25.2

Two-Dimensional Distributions and Correlation

Equations 1 and 2 of Panel 25.1 are, in fact, examples of a special second-order moment of the function $f(x)$. As we have seen from Fig. 25.4, it is possible to plot two-dimensional amplitude density distribution functions (2-D ddfs) of signal samples either from two different signals or from the same signal, taken τ seconds apart. As we can see from Section 1.3 and Fig. 25.4, we can compute correlation coefficients from such 2-D ddfs and plot them as a correlation function $\rho(\tau)$.

If we define the 2-D ddf of two samples taken from two signals x and y as $f(x,y)$, then we may write in general terms the second order-moment as:

$$E\{xy\} = \int_{-\infty}^{\infty} \int_{-\infty}^{\infty} xy\, f(x,y)\, dxdy. \tag{3}$$

This value is called the *covariance*. If we take samples of the signal y at a *time lag* of τ seconds after the samples of the signal x, we can compute the 2-D ddf for x and y_τ in the way mentioned in Section 1.2. For each value of τ the correlation coefficient $\rho(\tau)$ can be computed, which is after normalization:

$$\rho_{xy}(\tau) = E\{xy_\tau\}/[E\{x^2\}E\{y_\tau^2\}]^{1/2}.$$

This value is called the *cross-correlation*. Similarly,

$$\rho_{xx}(\tau) = E\{xx_\tau\}/[E\{x^2\}E\{x_\tau^2\}]^{1/2} = E\{xx_\tau\}/E\{x^2\}.$$

is called the *autocorrelation*, which is equal to one for $\tau = 0$.

25

a Lissajous figure. In vectorcardiography, the heart is considered to be an electric *dipole*, located within a three-dimensional (3-D) volume conductor, the torso. From the body surface three physically *orthogonal* ECGs are derived (along the axes X, Y, and Z), which may be shaped into three 2-D Lissajous figures (in the XY, the XZ, and the YZ planes), the VCG (see Fig. 25.3). When the dipole model would be justified, and when we do not account for the fact that the volume conductor is finite and has an inhomogeneous conductivity, the VCG can be considered to represent the so-called heart vector h. This heart vector is then directly related to the direction and strength of the dipolar field generated by the cardiac muscle. From the shape of the 2-D or 3-D VCG we can make

diagnostic deductions regarding cardiac diseases. (A more extensive discussion of ECG or VCG interpretation by computers is provided in Sections 3.1 and 3.2 of Chapter 13.)

1.2.3 Stochastic Signals and Point Processes

It is possible to present 2-D ddfs for stochastic signals, for instance, for two correlated electroencephalograms (*EEGs*), similar to those discussed for deterministic signals (e.g., for adjacent *RR* intervals computed from an ECG). Such ddfs can also be presented as quasi-3-D ddfs, where the vertical axis represents the density of the distribution functions.

It is interesting to investigate the effect of an increasing time difference τ on the shape of the 2-D ddfs. We have illustrated this effect for the two signals above, an EEG (Fig. 25.4a) and RR intervals computed from an ECG (Fig. 25.4b). As we can see from the series of 2-D ddfs, the shape of the 2-D ddfs gradually changes from a line under 45° to a circular cloud. This reflects a decreasing relationship (i.e., a lower *correlation*) between two different amplitude values, because they are taken at larger time intervals τ. The next section provides a brief introduction to correlations between biosignals.

1.3 Correlation

The relationship between two statistical parameters can be visualized in a 2-D ddf and can be expressed mathematically by a number, called the *correlation coefficient* ρ (for its definition, see Panel 25.2). A maximum correlation between the statistical parameters gives a value of $\rho = 1$; the ddf then has the shape of a straight line. When the 2-D ddf is an ellipsoidal cloud, this correlates with a low statistical correlation that may minimally result in ρ equal to zero for a circular cloud. In a biosignal, it is possible to compute ρ for amplitudes at a distance of τ seconds (i.e., the interval between two samples, also called the *time lag*); ρ can be represented visually by a 2-D ddf (the values of ρ are given under each 2-D ddf in Figs 25.4a and 25.4b). It is obvious that for τ equal to zero ρ will be 1 and that for a circular 2-D ddf, which is to be expected for a sufficiently large value of τ, ρ will approach zero. The different values of ρ can be plotted as a function of increasing τ, which is called the *correlation function*, usually expressed as $\rho(\tau)$. At the bottoms of Figs. 25.4a and 25.4b, the respective correlation functions have been plotted for the EEG and the RR intervals, respectively. (Panel 25.2 describes in more detail the mathematical background of 2-D ddfs and correlation functions.) When we deal with a correlation function, computed from amplitude values of the same signal, we call this the *autocorrelation function*; in case of amplitude values from two different signals, the result is called the *cross-correlation function*.

Computing the correlation between various amplitude values offers several practical advantages. We summarize some of them:

- We can detect the presence of weak periodic or *quasiperiodic signal* components amidst a mixture of disturbing signals, such as small EEG components that are related to stimuli given to patients (so-called *evoked potentials*) or *atrial flutter* in ECGs.
- We can trace the time lag between two different signals, such as the time difference between an electric stimulus to a nerve cell and the response of a muscle cell, recorded by the *electromyogram*.
- More generally, by auto- and cross-correlation functions, it is possible to obtain more insight into the characteristics of biological processes (e.g., the so-called *transfer function*).
- The frequency *power spectrum* of a signal can also be computed from its autocorrelation function (see following Section).

2 Frequency Spectra and Filtering

In the preceding paragraphs we have used the term *frequency* when discussing the process of sampling. Already we see a superficial difference in frequency content between different biological signals such as a *phonocardiogram*, an ECG, or a spirogram (see Fig. 25.5, which shows different biological signals). A *frequency spectrum* represents the number and density of frequency components present in a signal.

2.1 Fourier Transform

The basic concept of a frequency spectrum is that a signal is thought to be composed of a sum of sines and cosines. This is illustrated in Fig. 25.6a and b for a block-shaped signal and a sawtooth-shaped signal, respectively. It can be proven that a signal can be fully represented by its frequency spectrum (i.e., its amplitude and phase components), that is, without loss of information (i.e., without increasing the information *entropy*).

A frequency spectrum may be computed by means of a method called Fourier analysis, after the French mathematician Fourier (1768-1830). His method, called the **Fourier transform** (FT), determines which frequency components are present in a signal $x(t)$. The result of the Fourier transform is the frequency spectrum $X(f)$. For a sampled signal containing $N = 2^n$ samples, a special version of the computation of the Fourier transform was developed by Tukey: the fast Fourier transform (**FFT**). The result of the FFT is a sampled frequency spectrum. Similar to a sampled signal of finite duration, the sampled FFT also contains a finite number of samples. If the signal has a duration of T seconds and has a frequency bandwidth of W Hz, then it must be sampled with at least $f_s = 2W$ Hz so that the sampling results in $2WT$ samples. (Here, we tacitly assume that the signal of duration T is repetitive with period T.) If we apply the FFT to this signal, it also results in $2WT$ frequency components (i.e., WT amplitude components, and WT phase components). We can transform a signal $x(t)$ by the FT to its frequency spectrum $X(f)$, and can transform $X(f)$ by the inverse FT (often written as FT^{-1}) to obtain $x(t)$.

Sometimes, *semantic* signal components (*features*) can be better derived from the frequency spectrum than from the temporal signal or the amplitude ddf. This especially applies to stochastic signals. Figure 25.5 shows an example of a frequency spectrum for an EEG that contains α-**waves** (quasiperiodic EEG components around 10 Hz). Also, Fig. 12.8 in Chapter 12, where we discuss patient monitoring, gives an example of the use of frequency spectra for the detection of changes in nonstationary signals.

The Fourier transform has many advantages, but also severe limitations for nonperiodic signals of rather short duration. Therefore, other types of signal transformations have been developed, of which the so-called **wavelet transform** is one of the most recent and interesting ones (see Panel 25.3).

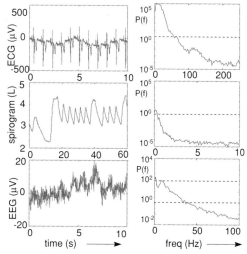

Figure 25.5
Examples of three biological signals (ECG, top; spirogram, middle; and EEG, bottom) with their frequency spectra given at the right. Of the frequency spectra, only the signal power per frequency component is shown. The frequency spectrum of the EEG shows a peak around 10 Hz caused by the so-called α-waves.

25

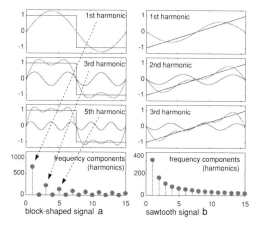

Figure 25.6
Frequency components that compose a block-shaped signal (a) and a sawtooth-shaped signal (b). The different harmonics that contribute to the signals are shown. In the bottommost pair of panels, the different frequency components are shown. Note that for the block-shaped signal, only uneven frequencies contribute to the block-shaped signal.

PANEL 25.3

Wavelet Analysis

In Fourier analysis, a signal is thought to be composed of sines and cosines. By using the *Fourier transform*, a signal can be decomposed in these basic functions. The samples of the transformed signal (Fourier coefficients) represent the contribution of sine and cosine functions at different frequencies. A disadvantage of Fourier analysis is that it is difficult to compose a signal that is *limited in time*, by using functions that, by definition, stretch out into infinite time. It is therefore difficult for a Fourier function to approximate sharp changes in a signal. For example, a very simple and time-limited signal, a spike, is decomposed by Fourier transformation into an infinite number of sines and cosines (see also Fig 25.6a for the decomposition of a block signal).

A way to tackle this problem is through *wavelet analysis*. It uses the same principle as Fourier analysis, namely, that signals are composed of basic functions, called *wavelets*. The most important difference between these wavelets and the sines and cosines used in Fourier analysis is that wavelets are limited in time. The procedure for wavelet analysis is to choose a suitable wavelet prototype function (also called mother wavelet or analyzing wavelet) that meets certain constraints. All composing functions are derived by stretching or scaling the mother wavelet both in time and in amplitude. Using a wavelet transform, the signal is decomposed into these scaled versions of the mother wavelet. In fact, the composing cosines used in Fourier analysis can also be seen as stretched, scaled, and shifted versions of a *mother-cosine*. In Fourier analysis, the composing functions are infinite in the time domain because they represent exactly one frequency. In wavelet analysis, the composing wavelets have a limited extent both in the time domain and in the frequency domain, where contributions from frequencies outside a certain area are negligible.

The most important result of the wavelet transform is the location of the composing wavelets in time. Sharp, time-limited signal parts will be represented by wavelets that are scaled down in duration. As in Fourier analysis, the contribution of the composing wavelets to the signal provides information about the temporal properties of the signal on different time scales. Additionally, the locations of the composing wavelets provide information about the position of a specific signal property. Figure 25.7 shows two examples of a mother wavelet, both from the well-known Coiflet wavelet family.

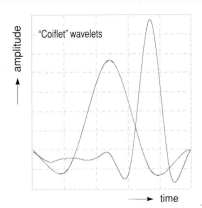

Figure 25.7
Two examples of a mother wavelet, both from the Coiflet wavelet family.

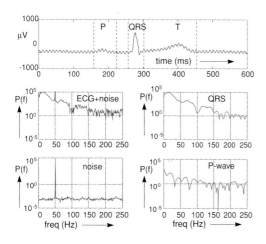

Figure 25.8
Frequency spectra of an ECG plus disturbance and of the QRS complex, the P-wave, and the disturbance separately.

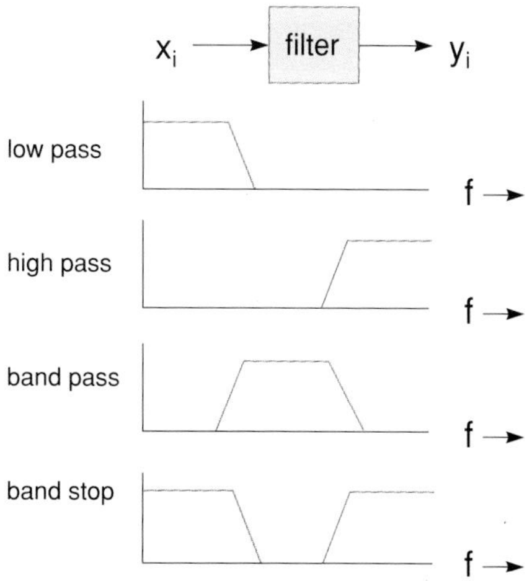

Figure 25.9
Schematic representation of a low-pass, a high-pass, a band-pass, and a band-stop filter.

2.2 Filtering

In this section we briefly discuss digital *filtering*. The intention of this introduction is to convey terminology and some concepts. Filtering of a signal is essentially intended to remove unwanted frequency components. This may, in principle, be accomplished by applying the FT to a signal $x(t)$, resulting in $X(f)$, thereafter removing the undesired frequency components, and, finally, by applying the inverse transform FT^{-1} (see illustration in Fig. 25.8 for an ECG plus disturbance).

Often, instead of using the FT, we apply filters to the temporal signal $x(t)$ itself to remove unwanted frequency components. We discern three different types of (linear) filters, *low-pass*, *high-pass* and *band-pass* filters, with the third one being a combination of the first two filters. Figure 25.9 depicts the three different filters, also showing a band-stop filter.

An example of the use of a band-pass filter is one that removes noise generated by muscle activity and baseline fluctuations on an ECG. According to the American Heart Association the ECG bandwidth that is of routine diagnostic significance ranges from 0.15 to 150 Hz. Baseline fluctuations are, however, lower than, for example, 1 Hz, and muscle noise contains frequencies far above 150 Hz, say, up to

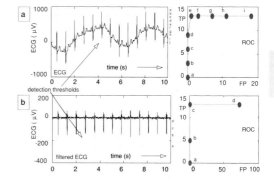

Figure 25.10
Electrocardiogram (left upper panel) and its band-pass filtered version (left lower panel), in a bandwidth to optimize the signal-to-noise ratio (SNR) for the QRS complex. Thresholds have been applied in both signals to detect the presence of QRS complexes. The higher the detection threshold, the fewer FP detections, but also the fewer TP detections; the opposite is also true. The relationship between TP and FP is depicted for various threshold levels in the ROCs at the right-hand side for the unfiltered and the filtered signals, respectively.

1,000 Hz. The latter would require sampling with at least 2,000 Hz. Therefore, we usually apply a band-pass filter between 0.15 and 150 Hz. In principle, a

---

PANEL 25.4

Coherent Averaging

In coherent averaging we compute the sum of, say, K waveforms s_0, which are extracted after detection from a noisy signal $x_0(t) = s_0(t) + n_0(t)$. The original signal variance is $S_0 = \sigma_{s0}^2$ and the noise variance is $N_0 = \sigma_{n0}^2$, so that the SNR is:

$$SNR_0 = S_0/N_0.$$

The sum of the K signal waveforms s_0 will result in a waveform s_1 which is K times as large as the original waveform, that is, $s_1 = Ks_0$. The resulting signal dispersion is also K times as large: $\sigma_{s1} = K\sigma_{s0}$. The variance of s_1 is then $S_1 = \sigma_{s1}^2 = K^2\sigma_{s0}^2$.

We assume that the noise has a *normal distribution*. The K noisy waveforms n_0 are also summed to a new noisy signal, n_1. It can be proven that the variance of n_1 is K (and not K^2) times as large as the variance of n_0 so that $N_1 = \sigma_{n1}^2 = K\,\sigma_{n0}^2$. The SNR after summation is then:

$$SNR_1 = S_1/N_1 = K^2\sigma_{s0}^2/K\sigma_{n0}^2 = K\sigma_{s0}^2/\sigma_{n0}^2 = KS_0/N_0 = K\,SNR_0.$$

This implies that the SNR has improved linearly with the number of summed waveforms.

25

300-Hz sampling rate would then be sufficient. (In practice, 500 Hz is often applied.) Figure 25.10 illustrates the effect of band-pass filtering on an ECG, in this case meant for the detection of the QRS complexes.

---

3 Signal-to-Noise Ratio

In Chapter 2 we mentioned that the transmission of all signals is accompanied by disturbances, or noise. This applies especially for signals of biological origin. Noise hampers the determination of signal features that are of interest for the interpretation. For instance, when recording ECGs during physical exercise, signals are often disturbed by low-frequency baseline disturbances (because of changing electrode impedances and offset potentials) and higher-frequency electromyographic signals, caused by active muscles. In that case, it is not possible to measure depressions of the ST-T segment accurately. Another example are repetitive weak EEG components, triggered by stroboscopic light flashes, that may be masked by other EEG signals and are not visible without the removal of the disturbing components.

From these examples it is obvious that we must take countermeasures to improve the so-called **signal-to-noise ratio** (**SNR**), that is, to decrease the relative contribution of noise to the mixture of signal and noise. The SNR is defined as the ratio between the variance of the signal and the variance of the noise (see Panel 25.4 for a definition of SNR).

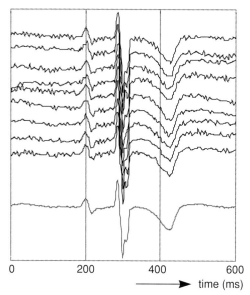

0   200   400   600

→ time (ms)

Figure 25.11
Coherent averaging of complexes in an ECG recording. The averaged complex has a higher signal-to-noise ratio than the original complexes.

3.1 Coherent Averaging

The SNR may be improved by different methods. For instance, in a quasiperiodic disturbed signal, such as an ECG, we may make use of the fact that the waveform is deterministic, whereas the noise has a statistical character. In that case we try to detect the moments of occurrence of the waveforms and apply *coherent averaging*. (Coherent averaging is discussed in more detail in Panel 25.4.) It can be proven that the SNR improves linearly with the number of summed waveforms, when the noise has a normal (Gaussian) distribution. An example of such coherent averaging is seen in Fig. 25.11.

4. Signal Detection

In Figure 8.2 of Chapter 8 we discussed the different types of signals and discerned the point processes within the group of deterministic signals, indicating the occurrence of "events" in a signal. This section provides a short introduction into detection, which is the method used to derive a *point process* from a biosignal. Figure 8.3 of Chapter 8 provides an illustration of the derivation of a point process from a continuously varying signal: the localization of the R-waves in the depolarization waveform generated by the ventricles, the QRS complex. In straightforward circumstances of detection we are generally confronted with four different situations:

1. an R-wave is correctly detected (*true positive*; TP),
2. an R-wave is present but not detected (*false negative*; FN),
3. an R-wave is not present, but some other event (e.g., a noise spike, or a T-wave) is considered by the detector to be an R-wave (*false positive*; FP), and

4. an R-wave is not detected if not present (*true negative*; TN).

These four detection situations show many parallels with decision making, for example, in a *differential diagnosis*, in which a disease may or may not be present and in which we also discern TP (called *sensitivity*) and TN (*specificity*) results (see Chapter 15). In patient monitoring situations, detection of an FP result is often called a *false alarm*. We have generalized these four situations in Table 25.1, in which the situation that an event is present is indicated by S ($'S$ is used if the event is not present), and the decision that an event is detected is indicated by D ($'D$ is used if the event is not detected).

Signal detection and waveform estimation often go together, and in an ideal situation, we have an *estimator* and a *detector* operating in parallel with *feedback* loops to each other (see Fig. 25.12). This feedback means that the estimated waveforms are used to opti-

Situation[a]	Description	S	D
TP	The event is present AND is correctly detected	1	1
FP	The event is not present AND is incorrectly detected	0	1
TN	The event is not present AND is correctly not detected	0	0
FN	The event is present AND is incorrectly not detected	1	0

Table 25.1

Four Different Detection Situations for the Decision D that an event S is Present.

[a] TP, true positive; TN, true negative; FP, false positive; FN, false negative.

mize the detector, whereas the detected events are used as prior information for the estimator.

Instead of giving a rather theoretical description of detection, we will give two examples of detection. The first one is an example of the detection of QRS complexes in an ECG, which could be encountered in practice. The other one is artificial: we have added increasing amounts of disturbing signals to an amplitude-modulated series of impulses so that we are confronted with an increasing amount of FP detections.

4.1 Detection of QRS Complexes in an ECG

Figure 25.10 presents an ECG signal and below it the same signal is shown after band-pass filtering. The

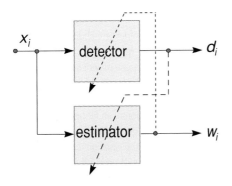

Figure 25.12
Detection and estimation may reinforce each other. Knowledge about the signal waveshape is used to design or optimize the detector, and knowledge about the locations of the events as detected by the detector, leads to a better waveshape estimation.

task is to detect the proper location of QRS complexes in the ECG. In both signals, we have applied detection *thresholds*. We assume that when the signal is above the threshold, there is a QRS complex, and vice versa. It can be seen in the unfiltered ECG that the higher the detection threshold, the fewer FP detections and the more FN detections. Alternatively, the lower the threshold, the more FP detections and the fewer FN detections.

We filter out the baseline fluctuations and much of the high-frequency noise by band-pass filtering in a *bandwidth* that contains most of the frequency spectrum of the QRS complexes (from about 6 to 25 Hz). The *SNR* (see Panel 25.4 for a definition) of the QRS complex has then improved considerably. If we apply detection thresholds now, the effect is a much better performance of the detector: less FP and FN detections.

Apparently, FP and FN detections cannot be changed independently of each other, given a certain signal and a specific detection method. We can see in Fig. 25.10 for both signals that if FP decreases, FN increases, and the reverse is true as well. It is possible to depict this relationship in a so-called relative operating characteristic (*ROC*). (In detection theory an ROC was originally called a receiver operating characteristic.) Often, the expression *ROC curve* is used.

In an ROC, the percentage of TP (or its complement, the percentage of FN) is plotted against the percentage of FP (or its complement, the percentage of TN). Figure 25.10 depicts the different percentages for TP and FP at the right-hand side for both signals. One ROC point is obtained for each signal and every detection threshold. If we had varied the detection thresholds from very low to very high, a continuous ROC curve would have been obtained, indicating the performance of the specific detector (i.e., the combination of some pre-

25

processor such as a band-pass filter, and a detection threshold). The more the ROC approaches the ideal point of 100% TP and 0% FP, the better its performance.

ROC curves are used in all other situations of decision making, such as in making differential diagnoses (see Section 4.1.2 of Chapter 15) The area between the two main axes and the ROC curve is often used as a measure of the performance of the detection (or diagnostic) method. From Fig. 25.10 we can see that an ROC curve for the detector based on the bandpass-filtered ECG is far better than one based on the unfiltered signal.

4.2 Impulse Series plus Disturbance

To show the effect of increasing disturbance we have generated an artificial signal of amplitude-modulated impulses $x(t)$, to which an increasing amount of noise impulses $An(t)$ are added, with A being an amplification factor (see Fig. 25.13 for three different situations: high, medium, and low SNRs). The amplitude ddfs of the peaks of both $x(t)$ and $n(t)$ have Gaussian distributions. By varying the amplification factor A it is possible to change the relative amplitude of the noise. Because we have given the noise impulses the same frequency spectrum as the signal impulses, band-pass filtering offers no further help, so that we apply detection thresholds to the original signal right away. In the middle column of Fig. 25.13 we have plotted the amplitude ddfs for the peaks of $x(t)$ and $n(t)$ for the three different SNRs. The ROCs for these three SNRs are seen at the right-hand side of Fig. 25.13, confirming that there is a given relationship between TP and FP detections and that the detection performance is better for a higher SNR.

4.3 Conclusions Regarding Detection

From these two examples we can draw a few important conclusions regarding detection, which are in full agreement with what we observed in Chapter 2:

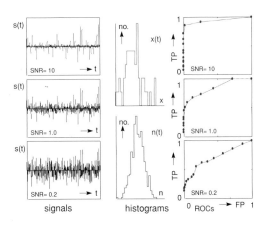

Figure 25.13
An artificial signal of amplitude-modulated impulses $x(t)$ to which an increasing amount of disturbing impulses $An(t)$ are added (A is an amplification factor) for three different situations: high, medium, and low SNR, in the upper, middle and bottom panels, respectively. The amplitude ddfs of the peaks of both $x(t)$ and $n(t)$ have Gaussian distributions, shown in the middle. The ROCs for these three situations are seen at the right-hand side for the various values of the SNR. It may be observed that the detection performance is better for a higher SNR.

25

1. Signals should ideally be recorded close to the signal source (in patients this is not always possible; see also Chapter 2) with an SNR that is as high as possible.
2. Preprocessing (e.g., filtering) should be applied in such a way that the SNR of the signal component that will be detected is optimized.
3. A detection method with a minimal amount of FP and FN detections should be selected (i.e., the proper point on the ROC should be carefully selected).

It should be noted that the selection of the detection threshold in itself does not result in a better or worse ROC. The location of the ROC is determined by the SNR and the preprocessing. The choice of a certain threshold (i.e., the selection of a point on the ROC, e.g., for a low percentage of FP, results in a high percentage of FN) is dependent on the context in which detection takes place. For instance, detection of all possible events in an intensive care unit may result in too many false alarms, but use of a detector that is too insensitive may result in many missed events.

Key References

Oppenheim AV, Schafer RW. *Discrete-Time Signal Processing.* Englewood Cliffs, NJ: Prentice Hall, 1989.

Rabiner LR, Gold B. *Theory and Application of Digital Signal Processing.* Englewood Cliffs, NJ: Prentice Hall, 1975.

Swets JA, Picket RM. *Evaluation of Diagnostic Systems: Methods from Signal Detection Theory.* New York NY: Academic Press, 1992.

Van Bemmel JH. Biological signal processing. In: Ingram D, Bloch RF, eds. *Mathematical Methods in Medicine.* New York: Wiley and Sons, 1984: 225-72.

See the Web site for further literature references.

26 Advances in Image Processing

1. Introduction

Among the many scientific and technological advances related to high performance computing, medical *imaging* stands out because of its powerful visual appeal in showing the inner structures of the human body. It is also a harbinger of automation in health care practice, biomedical research, and education. Medical imaging offers great opportunities for improving health care through technology by increasing the ways with which we can noninvasively visualize, analyze, and interpret the processes of health and disease.

• Three-dimensional imaging

Advances in imaging instrumentation and the design of new modalities depend on high-performance computing for rapid reconstruction and display of large sets of images (see Chapter 9). New techniques of digital image processing, particularly in three dimensions (3-D), are the keys to visualization, manipulation, and analysis, seeking to extract the medical information content of the images (see Chapter 10).

• Diagnostic support

Although the large amount of precisely localizable and measurable information in medical images is already used for individual patient diagnosis and therapy, the accumulated information contained in biomedical image databases waits to be mined for scientific and educational purposes. However, because medical images are concrete and patient specific, they lack the abstract expressive power of language-based descriptions. As a result, their information content is much less easily defined, shared and communicated than are the traditional symbolic descriptions of patient conditions found in the patient record (i.e., the computer-based patient record (*CPR*), see Chapter 7) .

• Integration

The integration of imaging information with data in the CPR in ways that will facilitate standardized communication and interpretation can be considered the central informatics problem of medical imaging. In addition, with the development of *multimedia* and *virtual reality* systems that can capture voice, touch, and other sensory information as well, we may even foresee the emergence of a more general "multimedia medical informatics" to study the problems of coherently representing and integrating such disparate sources of information.

• Image transmission

As high-speed, high-bandwidth networking comes closer to reality, the transmission of multimodality medical images between imaging systems and health care centers will become routine. This will profoundly affect the practice of health care. The ability of *teleradiology* to interactively monitor a measurement as it is being taken and make it available remotely, as well as to efficiently retrieve medical images from image databases for comparison with other related images, not only promises to increase the productivity of radiological procedures (see Section 1 of Chapter 13) but also enables large-scale quantitative studies of the visualizable anatomical changes that occur in disease.

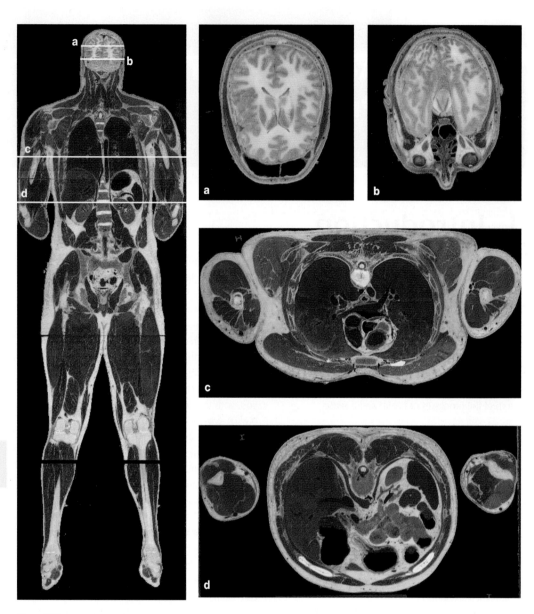

Figure 26.1
Reconstruction of a sagittal cross section and a few horizontal cross sections through one of the visible humans (printed with permission of the National Library of Medicine. See www.nlm.nih.gov/research/vivible/visible_human.html).

• Real-time imaging

Until recently, the 3-D nature of human anatomy was difficult and prohibitively expensive to model on the computer. Advances in hardware, graphics, and imagery software and in modeling methods are finally making it possible to plan for real-time 3-D anatomical modeling and matching to patient data. Sophisticated interactive 3-D display and visualization methods are

PANEL 26.1

The Visible Humans Project

The goal of the *Visible Humans project*, sponsored by the U.S. National Library of Medicine, is to provide image data sets of the human body for use in the study of anatomy, for use in conducting imaging research, and for use in a wide range of educational, diagnostic and treatment planning and simulation applications. The first phase of the project has resulted in *CT*, *MRI*, and *cryosection* image sets for a human male and a human female. The complete male data set consisting of scans taken at 1 mm resolution is 15 gigabytes in size. The complete female data set consists of scans taken at 0.33 mm intervals and is 40 gigabytes in size. Both datasets may be downloaded over the *Internet* by interested individuals for research and experimentation.

Some applications that are already underway by researchers around the world who have begun working with the datasets include prototype systems for non-invasive colon cancer screening, prostate cancer surgical rehearsal, plastic surgery rehearsal, and educational systems for anatomical dissection. Fig 26.1 offers examples of a few cross sections through one of the visible humans.

being widely distributed and are already proving their worth in advanced radiology research and demonstration projects (see Chapter 9 and also Panel 26.1 and Fig. 26.1).

• Imaging software

Despite much progress in picture archiving systems (*PACS*), relatively few centers at present have fully integrated digital processing capabilities for all routinely performed imaging studies. However, their numbers are increasing, and software environments designed specifically for medical image processing and analysis are also becoming more sophisticated and more widely available. The range of software tools for image analysis is also growing: many more sophisticated processing and analysis techniques and methods for image registration are being developed, as are methods for lossless (as well as lossy) *image compression* (see the discussion on *DICOM* in Chapter 13) and *decompression*, facilitating the effective transmission of the large quantity of image data now being generated.

• Image coding

From an informatics perspective, it is also crucial

that parallel efforts are ongoing in the development of CPR systems and the informational infrastructure for them: vocabularies and languages for describing medical knowledge and practice. The Unified Medical Language System (*UMLS*, see Panel 6.3 of Chapter 6) and standards for medical and radiological nomenclature can help in describing the contents of medical images more uniformly and according to shared conventions.

From a practical point of view, current research in modeling radiological concepts is based on analysis of linguistic constructs within reports describing radiographic images.

This chapter highlights present developments and research in medical image processing. Despite slower-than-expected progress in the central problem of automated image *segmentation*, developments in interactive visualization and analysis software have more than compensated for this by providing effective tools for radiology practice and research. The present convergence of technological, scientific, and societal factors makes it very likely that imaging will grow increasingly important to medical informatics in coming years.

26

2 Two-Dimensional Medical Image Processing: Preprocessing

Medical imaging systems almost never provide the radiologist with "raw" image data. Instead, various computational preprocessing methods are used to reconstruct an image that will give the greatest amount of diagnostic information to the practitioner (see Chapter 10). Reconstruction methods are specific to the particular form of imaging (*CT*, *MRI*, *PET*, etc., see Chapter 9). Other preprocessing typically involves general low-level vision-based methods for *filtering* and transforming the image data so that they are better visualized and easier to analyze.

2.1 Computer Vision Versus Human Vision

Since the early days of computing, researchers have been beguiled by the promise of using computers for automating the recognition of visual patterns. Analogies between human vision and machine vision motivated Rosenblatt's *perceptron*, the ancestor of today's artificial *neural networks*. Numerous other *pattern recognition* methods followed, with many being applied to visual problems such as handwriting recognition (see also Chapter 27). In medical imaging, Lodwick used *Bayes' Theorem* (Chapters 15 and 27) for the computer-aided diagnosis of bone tumors with great success after painstakingly and manually extracting the *features* characterizing these tumors in radiographic images from 2,000 cases stored in the Bone Sarcoma Registry of the American College of Surgeons. It is natural to characterize visual objects by sets of features extracted from the natural scene (the X-ray image) in which they are found. Objects are most easily classified by comparing the patterns of features. When the features are noisy and uncertain, this classification approach to pattern recognition is closely related to statistical decision making (see Chapter 15).

2.2 Feature Extraction

When computers became powerful enough, features began to be extracted from image data automatically. In *grey-level* images, typical features could include measures of the intensity level of an object and descriptions of its boundary, shape, *texture*, size, and so forth (Chapter 10). It was recognized early on that segmentation of an object from its background (everything else in the scene) could be accomplished by either identifying a region in the image corresponding to the object or by first identifying the boundary of the object and then extracting the enclosed region.

2.3 Boundary Detection

Region-based segmentation approaches became popular because they could be easily implemented by simple methods (see also Chapter 10):

1. *thresholding* individual pixel intensity values,
2. *region growing*, or
3. *region splitting*.

Thresholding works when object regions have uniformly high contrast in relation to their background (a high *signal-to-noise ratio*, see Chapter 25) and well-defined edges. Thresholding uses some measure of discontinuity in the intensity values of the image, such as the gradient. In images of natural scenes, edges are frequently complex and noisy, so simple step or ramp models of discontinuities prove to be unrealistic. Edges typically present in different sizes or scales in different parts of a scene, requiring application of multiple resolutions of edge-extracting operators for preprocessing of the entire image.

Boundary-based segmentation is usually more complex, since it requires defining an object boundary in terms of the edges detected in the image. An alternative is to detect the most rapidly changing part of an edge through zero crossings of a second-derivative function of the image. To reduce susceptibility to noise it can be combined with a *low-pass filtering* function (see Chapter 25). Tissues in medical images may exhibit differences in texture, color, or other more complex features that can be used for discrimination, also preferably by multiresolution methods. Regardless of the definition of edges and other features, however, medical images with multiple complex objects and various sources of noise are rarely directly segmentable in their entirety by any single method.

2.4 Image Filtering

For simple segmentation methods to have a chance of succeeding, images must be filtered first to smooth out noisy (high-frequency) edges by low-pass filtering and to enhance true edges by high- or band-pass filtering. The problem, of course, is that it is hard to know a priori how to distinguish true from spurious edges. Despite the availability of many sophisticated statistical models for edges, their applicability to and superiority over other models for particular problems can be ascertained only by carefully controlled empirical testing – which may be feasible with phantoms but which is frequently costly and not practical in clinical situations.

2.5 Image Processing Strategies

Given the complex dependencies between image formation processes and environments, it is hardly surprising that attempts to solve the general automatic segmentation problem have not been very successful. A survey of methods for object recognition in 2-D images of natural scenes from aerial photometry, industrial inspection, and medicine illustrated the difficulties of choosing computational strategies for solving problems of this type. Four different classes of computational strategies can be distinguished:

1. Feature vector classification methods
    These methods apply only to the simplest problems with low data and model complexity (no noise and

simple object labeling). They can work directly with the raw data (*pixel* classification) or with abstracted features or regions derived from the raw data.

2. Fitting models to noisy image data
    Here, spatial constraints describe the expected structure of objects to be recognized and can be either fixed or flexible. In fixed models (like the *Hough transform*), mathematical operators with predetermined global characteristics must be parameterized for recognition. Flexible models are specified by generic constraints and delineate the contours or surfaces of an object. In medical imaging various elastic deformation methods are used to model surface contours.

3. Fitting models to symbolic structures
    Scenes containing multiple and different types of objects are best modeled by using descriptions of subparts that are, on the one hand, easily detected from the data and, on the other, easily assembled into the whole scene (i.e., the problem is decomposable, or reasonably so). Recognition can then be carried out by finding efficient search strategies for the best assembly of subparts (or intermediate symbolic structures) that may have generated the image. In medical imaging such situations are rare.

4. Combined strategies
    With the high degrees of complexity of both noisy data and models, combinations of data-driven and model-driven strategies are suggested, with optimization of some subproblems (such as *feature extraction*) being feasible within a generic scheme for recognition. Such approaches characterize the solution of more abstract medical imaging problems: the composition of image processing processes; the planning, experimental design, and learning of such compositions; and the indexing and retrieval of images according to the arrangements of their subparts.

On the basis of the categorization presented above, most 2-D medical image recognition work falls into categories 1 and 2, since applications of recognition

26

techniques have traditionally been demonstrated on very specific (and often highly delimited and idealized) imaging problems. Although the use of combinations of strategies has become more frequent in recent years, the computational complexity of most medical image interpretation problems has tended to make their application very specific and generalizations about broader applicability less than obvious.

2.6 Vision-Based Methods

A very different perspective to recognition methods was taken by Marr in his computational theory of vision. Using an information-processing approach, he differentiated the issues of vision research according to whether they are at the level of (1) computational theory, (2) representation and algorithm, or (3) hardware. This approach has had a strong influence on the active or purposive vision-based methods that have been applied, particularly in *robotics*, in which a reconstructive, top-down, model-based approach is frequently taken when designing experiments in *machine vision*.

Such approaches will have increasing relevance to medical imaging when it is embedded within surgical, robotic, and other controlled environments. General mathematical models of vision illustrate clearly how most 2-D image recognition problems are ill-posed inverse problems for which we cannot expect to find solutions without severely limiting their generality by problem-, method-, and domain-specific constraints.

2.7 Image Compression

The increasing demand for rapid transmission of medical visual information for purposes of *teleradiology*, *telepathology*, and biomedical

research and education poses difficult challenges in image compression. While the use of standard *compression* techniques has greatly improved transmission efficiency, users are still frustrated by long transmission waiting times for even medium-sized pictures (e.g., 512 x 512 pixels). Furthermore, medical applications require very high fidelity for diagnostic and treatment purposes, which has still existing problems in recognizing and differentially compressing the clinically important versus unimportant parts of the image data to further improve image transfer efficiency beyond the limits of standard compression methods.

2.8 Interpretation of Compressed Images

The performance of most standard compression techniques is largely dictated by the nature of the data and their usage. For instance, in some radiological images, lossy compression may sometimes suffice for initial screening (filtering out irrelevant slices). A *region of interest* at full resolution, however, is absolutely necessary for performing diagnostic readings, although the remaining part of the image may be compressed with a lossy compression scheme.

For many specific task environments, a significant portion of the requested image data (e.g., the background of an MRI scan or a *mammogram*) can be safely treated as being irrelevant to the analysis and so does not need to be transmitted. This kind of context- and content-based data compression and reduction will dramatically improve image transfer efficiency. Therefore, it is necessary to study the compression ratios that are tolerable in specific applications such as diagnosis and surgery design for different classes of images by conducting psychophysical experiments.

3 Three-Dimensional Medical Image Processing

In contrast to general natural scene recognition, medical imaging does provide fairly strong constraints, particularly if we use a 3-D model that corresponds to the true underlying patient environment. *Tomographic* measurements in particular yield highly accurate volume-averaged estimates of the values of actual physical properties of the tissue being imaged within each volume element or *voxel* of the body (see Chapter 9). Unlike general-purpose imaging like photography, medical imaging modalities have usually been specifically refined to discriminate between target tissue types. Although still subject to various sources of noise, instrument-induced error, field-of-view *artifacts*, slicing approximations, inadequacies in resolution, and scene complexity and scaling problems for certain tasks, the interpretation of sets of 2-D slice data from most 3-D medical image acquisitions presents few problems for the experienced human observer. Automatic 3-D object recognition, although still unfeasible except for very simple objects in standard settings, may finally be on the horizon due to the recent dramatic advances in imaging and computing hardware, graphics, modeling, and visualization software.

3.1 Three-Dimensional Reconstruction

For 3-D visualization and analysis, 2-D data slices must be combined by *interpolation*, and the corresponding images of different modalities, views, or times of acquisition must be registered. Various sophisticated methods for viewing the inherently 3-D data on 2-D screens have been developed, but they generally fall into one of two categories: surface and volume renderings. A new shell-rendering method, however, combines elements of surface and volume rendering. Fusion of data from multiple modalities is also frequently required for display and analysis purposes. Figure 26.2 provides an example of 3-D pre-

sentation of the chest after boundary detection, labeling, shadowing and coloring of organs (image made available by the University of Hamburg, Germany).

3.2 Image Transformations

Udupa lists how various imaging transformations are specified according to their applicability to the acquired data (scene space); the data extracted for viewing (object space), their rotations, scalings, and transformations (image space); and their 2-D representation on a screen (view space). Transformations for each of these spaces (of scene, structure, geometry, and image, respectively) and mappings between them are described. Mappings are mostly bidirectional, reflecting the emphasis of this work on practical interactive tech-

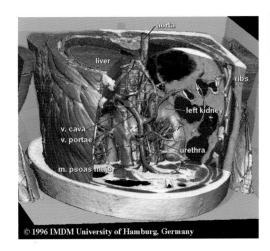

© 1996 IMDM University of Hamburg, Germany

Figure 26.2
Example of 3-D presentation of the chest after boundary detection, labeling, shadowing and coloring of organs (made available by Dr. K.H. Höhne, University Hospital Eppendorf, Hamburg, Germany. See www.uke.uni-hamburg.de/institutes/IMDM/IDV/images).

26

niques for user-controlled selection of different operators by which images can be transformed for more effective analysis (in a parameter space of chosen models). These operators may be mathematical (such as filtering or feature selection) or graphical (selection of views, subscenes, or **rendering methods**). The choice of analysis method (segmentation, image transformation) is left largely to the user.

Although the above description represents a retreat from the goal of fully automatic segmentation, it can be seen as a healthy reaction to what is an overambitious and impractical undertaking for most imaging problems. Instead, the user is encouraged to apply different segmentation methods to various subproblems in intermediate stages of processing. Because alternative geometric models (surface versus volume, projection vs. slice) can be used to fuse multimodal, multislice, and multiview data spatially at different stages of visualization and analysis, the operations of applying filtering, segmentation, feature extraction, and surface or volume estimation and rendering can be applied in different sequences to obtain different results for a given problem. Each sequence represents a different analysis strategy, and the expert image analyst must then choose which of the alternatives to trust the most or try to fuse them into a single coherent interpretation. This is currently left to the human expert.

3.3 Validation of Image Processing

Overall performance results for some combinations of techniques and studies of observer **variability** have been reported, but the methodology is still too young and evaluation methods are still inadequate for systematic and controlled experimentation to compare different strategies for a given problem. Just defining what constitutes a class of problems is difficult, as witnessed by the variability encountered in the literature. Although evaluation methods from signal analysis in the form of **ROC** curves (see Chapter 15) can be applied to individual segmentation and recognition subproblems, more sophisticated strategies will be needed to assess complex system usage.

3.4 General versus Special Solutions

Currently, each imaging modality (and combination of modalities) is analyzed with various filtering and transformation techniques for particular types of problems. Some applications are more general than others. For instance, an image filtering method is reported to be the optimal linear filter for correcting partial volume effects in the fusion of **MRI** modalities, while at the same time segmenting for a specified feature. Scale-space techniques have been successfully used for interactive segmentation, and multiresolution methods like **wavelets** are gaining in applicability. **Neural networks** have been applied with increasing frequency to MRI segmentation. **Morphological**, geometric, and knowledge-directed geometric modeling and knowledge-based frameworks have been tested, with generally successful results for prototype systems.

3.5 Incorporating Domain Knowledge

Combining medical domain knowledge such as anatomical models and image data characteristics with generic image-processing techniques has been demonstrated to be an effective approach to the design of practical image analysis systems in medicine.

The way in which imaging expertise and knowledge are incorporated into a system varies widely from one system to another, with relatively little systematic generalization being reported. Is it usually very difficult to apply a specific knowledge-based system directly to a new class of problems, and it is also inefficient and expensive to modify the existing system for the new problems. A class of more general knowledge-based approaches has been developed to remedy the problem. Most of these approaches view image interpretation as a design or planning process that composes or assembles applicable image processing and recognition procedures for applications to the problem at hand.

The goal is to develop a relatively general design or

planning framework within which problem-specific image processing and recognition processes for different problems can be generated more efficiently and effectively. In this way, we could gain generality at the designing and planning stage, even though it might elude us at the final analysis stage where the interpretation processes are executed. This type of approach can be characterized as an intensive knowledge-based approach to representing both imaging and domain expertise for the solution of a problem, and has been demonstrated to work well, particularly for image domains for which there exist not only a relatively rich class of problems but also well-defined models of objects and image modalities.

4 Medical Image Processing and Informatics Implications

All the techniques of medical image processing are directed to achieving goals in medical practice, research, and education. The most dramatic application of the new visualization and analysis capabilities are those involving computer-assisted surgery and teleradiology. This work builds on a decade of experience with surgical planning and simulation guided by 3-D imaging. With faster imaging modalities and high-performance computing and networking becoming more reliable, cost-effective, and ubiquitous, plans are now under way for image-guided surgery through the superimposition of images from prior acquisitions, as well as images acquired during the course of the surgical procedure. Another related area of high visibility and promise is the evaluation and design of *prostheses*, to which is now added the possibility of automatic milling of prostheses by *robots*.

4.1 Image Databases

From an informatics perspective, the explosion of imaging data from practical and research applications poses interesting opportunities and challenges. As cost-effective storage media capacity increases, so will the temptation to store all records digitally. Meaningful, intelligent retrieval can present problems with current techniques of data representation and storage. While *ACR-NEMA DICOM* conventions have helped standardize communication of images between devices, they do not standardize anything about the content of an image. A review of database issues in medical imaging is given in Chapter 9. Indexing and retrieval of structures within images is difficult by most present techniques, which lack representations of visual objects. New methods of representing, indexing, and retrieving pictorial objects are beginning to appear, and much research is needed on this topic. *Object-oriented* techniques for representing and manipulating dynamic sequences of visual objects are being developed for multimedia applications and may well prove to be essential for handling the processes of visualization, manipulation, and analysis of images within an interactively controlled *feedback* loop of surgical intervention.

26

4.2 Visible Humans Project

The construction of digital atlases and other sets of visual reference data from the large amounts of imagery being recorded in the *Visible Humans Project* and from other anatomical collections, both human and animal, requires research into the registration, structuring, segmentation, visualization, and validation of visual data. Tools for *navigating* through the great volume of visual data are needed, since such collections can range from the level of gross anatomy down to the cellular level. The possibilities for substantive *morphometric* analyses increase as large databases of digital images are built. The greatest challenge is to develop techniques for injecting meaning into large image collections through flexible annotations and logs of our journeys through them, correlating different functional and structural observations with higher level conceptual summaries and interpretations. Developing knowledge-based methods for capturing the *semantics* of imaging sequences in their many facets and relating them to corresponding information from other sensory channels promise to open a whole new chapter in informatics: that of imaging.

Key References

Baxes GA. *Digital Image Processing; Principles and Applications.* New York NY: Wiley & Sons, 1994.

Gonzalez RC, Woods RE. *Digital Image Processing.* Reading MA: Addison Wesley, 1992.

Jain AK. *Fundamentals of Digital Image Processing.* Englewood Cliffs NJ: Prentice Hall, 1989.

Castleman, KR. *Digital Image Processing.* Englewood Cliffs NJ: Prentice Hall, 1979.

Udupa JK, Herman GT, eds. *3D Imaging in Medicine.* Boca Raton FL: CRC Press, 1991.

Höhne KH, Fuchs H, Pizer SM, eds. *3D Imaging in Medicine: Algorithms, Systems, Applications.* Berlin: Springer-Verlag, 1990.

See the Web site for further literature references.

26

27 Pattern Recognition

1 Introduction

Pattern recognition is the application of (statistical) techniques with the objective of classifying a set of objects into a number of distinct classes. Pattern recognition is applied in virtually all branches of science. In an article on interactive pattern recognition, Kanal wrote:

Since recognizing patterns is, in one form or another, intrinsic to intelligent activity and since search for regularities is the principal concern of scientific inquiry, . . . , the field of pattern recognition impinges upon all scientific inquiry and intelligent behavior.

Pattern recognition methods exploit the similarities of objects belonging to the same class and the dissimilarities of objects belonging to different classes. Before we describe various techniques in detail, Table 27.1 provides a number of examples of applications of pattern recognition in medicine; as can be seen, the objects to be classified may be diverse. Adding applications from other fields would further increase the diversity. Yet, all applications approach patterns with exactly the same techniques, which makes pattern recognition an extremely versatile discipline.

Because the field of pattern recognition consists of many diverse techniques, it is useful to subdivide them into groups, in other words, to apply some pattern recognition to pattern recognition methodology. The first general subdivision concerns the distinction between *syntactic* methods and *statistical* methods. Of these, statistical methods are applied much more frequently, but an overview of pattern recognition would be incomplete without at least mentioning the syntactic approach.

27

Field	Objects	Objective
Cytology	Cells	Detection of carcinomas
Genetics	Chromosomes	Karyotyping
Cardiology	ECGs	Detection of coronary diseases
Neurology	EEGs	Detection of neurological conditions
Pharmacology	Drugs	Monitoring of medication
Diagnostics	Disease patterns	Computer-assisted decisions

Table 27.1
Examples of the Application of Pattern Recognition Techniques in Various Fields in Medicine.

2 Syntactic Pattern Recognition

In *syntactic* or *linguistic* pattern recognition, objects are described by a set of primitives. A *primitive* is an elementary component of an object. The object is then recognized by the sequence in which the primitives appear in the object description. A simple example of a set of primitives is the *Morse alphabet*. The objects are the individual characters and the spaces between words. The set of primitives is:

{short sound, long sound, short pause, long pause}.

A grammar describes the sequence in which these primitives constitute the various characters.

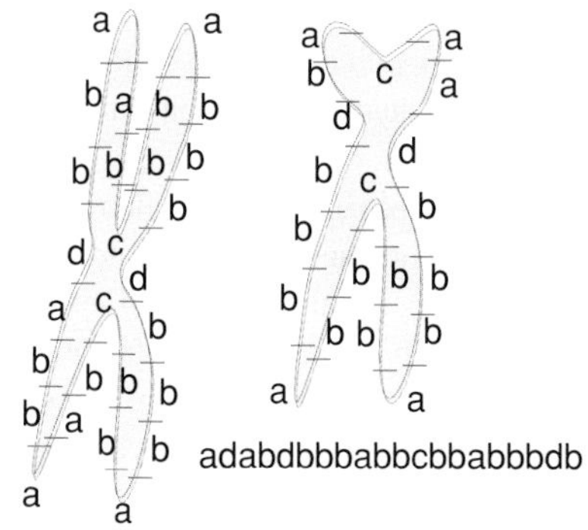

adabdbbbabbcbbabbbdb

abbcbbabbbdbbbabbcbbabbbdbba

Figure 27.1.
Syntactic description of a submedian and a median chromosome in terms of primitives.

Another possible example of a universe of objects is the set of human chromosomes. Suppose that the chromosomes have been isolated as a result of the application of image-processing techniques to a chromosome spread (see Fig. 27.1, showing two isolated chromosomes). They may then be described by their contours. If the aim of the application is to construct a *karyogram* of the chromosome spread, the objective of pattern recognition is to group the chromosomes in pairs, corresponding to the homologes. In this case, the set of primitives describing a contour may be the set (see Fig. 27.1):

{convexity (a), straight part (b), deep concavity (c), shallow concavity (d)}.

Different chromosomes are now described by different grammars. Figure 27.1 gives the syntactic description of a submedian chromosome (the centromere is shifted from the center) and of a median chromosome (with the centromere in the middle). Syntactic pattern recognition therefore consists of two parts:

1. identification of the primitives, followed by
2. identification of the *object class* by recognition of the grammatical description.

Syntactic pattern recognition was very popular in the early days of computer-based pattern recognition, but it has now been replaced to a large extent by methods based on statistical considerations.

3 Statistical Pattern Recognition

In *statistical pattern recognition* objects are described by numerical features (observations). Statistical pattern recognition techniques are commonly subdivided into two categories: *supervised* and *unsupervised* tech-

niques (see also Chapter 15). In supervised techniques the number of distinct classes is known and a set of example objects is available. These objects are labeled with their class membership. The problem is to assign a new, unclassified object to one of the classes. In unsupervised techniques, a collection of observations is given and the problem is to establish whether these observations naturally divide into two or more different classes.

Unsupervised classification techniques are also referred to as *clustering* methods. The art of statistical pattern recognition therefore consists of the determination of suitable *features*. A good feature is one for which the statistical distributions in the various classes are different and, ideally, non-overlapping.

3.1 Supervised Pattern Recognition

In supervised pattern recognition, class recognition is based on the differences of the statistical distributions of the features between the various classes. In real-life problems, especially in medicine, ideal (nonoverlapping) feature distributions do not exist. In such cases, multiple nonideal features are used. Each of these features contributes to some degree to the total classification power. The single feature is then replaced by a *feature vector*, and class recognition is based on the means and standard deviations of the vector components within the classes and on the *correlations* between these components.

The development of supervised classification rules normally proceeds in two steps:

1. In the first step, the *learning* phase, the classification rule is designed, on the basis of class properties as derived from a collection of class-labeled objects, the *design set*. Such classification rules will then have to be validated.
2. Validation is done in the second step, the *test* phase, in which another collection of class labeled objects, the *test set* is used. By subjecting the test set to the rules designed in the first step, for each of the test objects, the class label obtained by the rule is compared to the a priori known class label. Thus, the proportion of correct classifications obtained by the rule can be established. It should be emphasized that for a correct validation, *the objects in the learning set must be different from those in the test set*.

• Bayes' Rule

In most cases, pattern recognition is ultimately based on *Bayes'* theorem (see also Chapter 15):

$$p(c_i|x) = \frac{p(c_i)\, p(x|c_i)}{\sum_k p(c_k) p(x|c_k)} \qquad (1)$$

In this expression, the **a priori probability** of occurrence $p(c_i)$ of class c_i ($i = 1, \ldots, n$) is converted into the **a posteriori probability** $p(c_i|x)$ of class c_i, in the light of the value of the observation x. The function $p(x|c_i)$ is the probability density function for class c_i. It gives the probability that the value of the observation is x, given that the object belongs to class c_i. An object for which a feature vector x has been observed is then assigned to the class c_i for which $p(c_i|x)$ attains the largest value. For example, consider that under the microscope we observe a leukocyte in a blood smear of a mature human. A priori, the probability that it is a neutrophil is about 0.60 and the probability that it is a lymphocyte is about 0.30. These probabilities do not add up to 1.00, because there are a few more possibilities. Therefore, not having made any quantitative observation, our best guess is that the cell is a neutrophil and

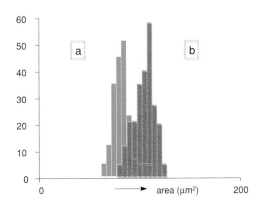

Figure 27.2.
Illustration of Bayes' Rule. The distributions of the cell area for a collection of lymphocytes (a) and for a collection of neutrophils (b) are shown. The prior probability that an unclassified cell is a neutrophil (60%) is higher than its prior probability of belonging to the class of lymphocytes (30%). When an area of 75 μm² is measured, the posterior probability that the cell is a lymphocyte is higher.

27

we would therefore classify it as such. Suppose further that the cellular area for the class of lymphocytes is distributed as illustrated in Fig. 27.2a and for neutrophils as in Fig. 27.2b. For an unknown cell we observe a value of 75 μm^2. Since for the class of neutrophils this value is very improbable, whereas it is a normal observation for the class of lymphocytes, the product in the nominator of Equation 1 is larger for the lymphocytes, and the unknown cell is classified accordingly.

From this example it becomes clear that classification is a trivial application of Bayes' Rule if the probability densities $p(x/c_i)$ for all classes c_i are known. If this is not the case, these class-conditional probability distributions must be estimated. This may be done by using the collections of labeled objects and constructing histograms like the ones in Fig. 27.2. In situations in which classification is based on more than one feature, a separate histogram must be constructed for each of them. In that case straightforward application of Equation 1 for each feature sequentially does not take correlations between features into account. More elaborate methods are available to handle such situations properly.

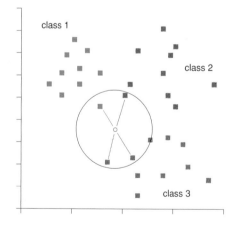

Figure 27.3

Illustration of nearest-neighbor classification. The learning set consists of objects belonging to three different classes: class 1 (blue), class 2 (red) and class 3 (black). Using one neighbor only, the 1-NN rule assigns the unknown object (yellow) to class 1. The 5-NN rule assigns the object to class 3, whereas the (5,4)-NN rule leaves the object unassigned.

- 1-Nearest-neighbor rule

The family of **nearest neighbor** rules (NN rules) constitute an approach to classification that does not make use of Bayes' Rule. Rather than estimating the class-conditional probability densities, the a posteriori class probabilities are directly obtained. In its simplest form this is done by using the single nearest-neighbor rule, which is conceptually easy to understand. This rule does not have a real learning phase. All objects from the learning set are stored, together with their class membership. To classify an unknown object, the nearest object from the learning set is identified. The unknown object is then assigned to the class to which its nearest neighbor belongs.

- *q*-Nearest-neighbors rule

There are a few variations on the simple theme of the 1-nearest-neighbors (**1-NN**) rule. Rather than deciding on class membership on the basis of a single nearest neighbor, a quorum of q nearest neighbors is inspected. The class membership of the unknown object is then established on the basis of the majority of the class memberships of these q nearest neighbors. In a slightly more complicated form (q,m-NN), a minimum majority m may be required to confirm the classification of the unknown object. Thus, in a ($q = 5$, $m = 4$) nearest-neighbor rule, the class membership of five nearest neighbors is inspected. When a majority of at least four of these neighbors belong to the same class, the unknown object is assigned to that class. Otherwise, the object is not classified. Therefore, this form of nearest-neighbor classification is one with a reject option. Figure 27.3 gives an example of classification according to various nearest-neighbor rules.

The nearest-neighbor rules have been demonstrated to possess elegant theoretical properties. It is possible to show that the 1-NN rule has an error rate that does not exceed twice the error rate obtained by using Bayes' Rule, which in turn may be shown to be the minimal attainable error. The error rate decreases with increasing quorum q. Unfortunately, the theoretical properties only hold in the limit of an infinitely large **learning set**.

Classification with a nearest-neighbor algorithm is not without problems. First, as mentioned above, it is possible to prove analytical properties of the rules only in the limit of infinitely large data sets. Use of the rule is

27

justifiable with large learning sets only, and this entails long computation times. In principle, to classify one unknown object, the entire learning set must be searched for the nearest neighbor(s). Fortunately, intelligent algorithms have been designed to reduce computation time.

Another problem is that the classification rule is not scaling invariant. In a multidimensional case, feature vector components with large absolute values dominate those with small absolute values. Therefore, a judicious scaling operation is required to obtain reliable results.

3.2 Unsupervised Methods

Another class of methods is related to a somewhat different problem. As before, objects are available in the form of multidimensional observations. However, the observations do not have any class assignment associated to them, nor is it known how many different classes of objects there are. The problem is to detect clusters, that is, groups of objects, grouped in such a way that in some sense objects within one group are more similar to each other than objects from different groups. Such problems are referred to as *clustering problems* and they are solved by clustering methods, also called methods of *unsupervised pattern recognition*. There is a large variety of such methods. Here we give two examples of clustering algorithms. One is based on measures of distance between a point and a cluster, the other is based on distances between clusters. In the following examples we will assume that distances are Euclidean distances, although other distance definitions exist and are sometimes used in clustering algorithms.

- Object-cluster distances

The best-known representative of this group of clustering algorithms is the **K-means algorithm**. Again, the principle is extremely straightforward. First, the number of clusters to be detected in the collection of objects must be given. For each cluster to be detected, a point in feature space (**seed point**) is chosen, in principle at random. These points act as the initial cluster centers. Then, an iterative procedure is started. For

each object, the distance to each of the cluster centers is calculated. The object is then assigned to the cluster with the nearest center. When all objects have thus been assigned to a cluster, for each cluster a new cluster center is calculated as the mean of the objects assigned to it. Then, a next iteration is started with the updated cluster centers. Iteration continues until no changes in cluster membership occur. Usually, a maximum number of iterations is prescribed to avoid oscillating situations.

In Fig. 27.4, this process is illustrated in a two-dimensional configuration. In this example, the initial cluster centers (indicated as ∗) have intentionally been chosen in unfavorable positions. Even so, the process converg-

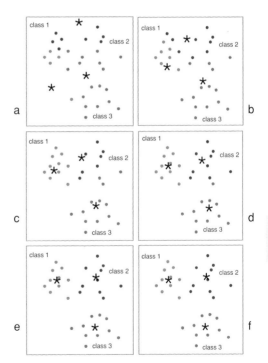

Figure 27.4

Illustration of the K-means clustering algorithm. The object configuration of Fig. 27.3 is used. Initially (configuration a), three seed points (indicated with ∗) are (arbitrarily) chosen. For each object, class membership is assigned according to the nearest seed point and new cluster centers are calculated (configurations b to f). The final configuration (configuration f) displays the clusters according to the true class labels (see Fig. 27.3).

27

es to an acceptable solution. In this example, the final clustering solution is obtained in six iterations.

A problem with this clustering technique is that when different initial cluster centers are selected, the process may converge to a different final solution. Therefore, the entire process is often repeated with different seed points and then the final results are compared. The confidence in a final solution increases if it has been obtained from different initial seed point configurations. In general, however, a criterion for the clustering quality is required. Such a criterion may be based on the compactness of the clusters. This can be expressed in mathematical terms to compare clustering solutions with the same number of clusters. The formulation of criteria to compare clustering solutions with different numbers of clusters is more problematic.

• Cluster-cluster distances

Algorithms based on cluster-cluster distances are of the hierarchical type. Within that family, we can distinguish the *agglomerative* and the *divisive* variants. In a situation with N objects, the agglomerative type of algorithm departs from an initial configuration of N

clusters: each object is its own cluster. At each iteration step, the two clusters that are the closest are merged together. Thus, after N -1 steps, a configuration of one cluster is reached: all observations belong to the same cluster. The most difficult part of the technique is the determination of the best solution of c clusters ($1 < c < N$) between these two trivial extremes. A divisive clustering algorithm operates the other way around: the initial situation is described by a configuration of one cluster, and at each step one cluster is split into two.

It is clear that the performance of these clustering algorithms depends on the definition of a distance between clusters. There are several possible choices for such a distance, and we list four of them:

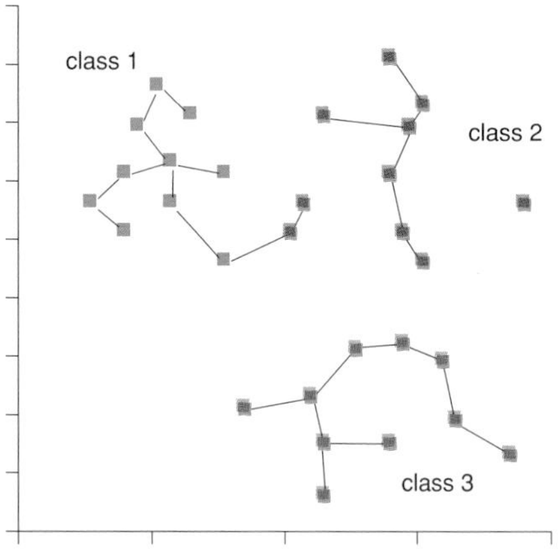

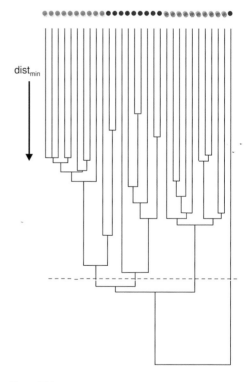

Figure 27.5
Clusters found for the object configuration of Fig. 27.3 by an agglomerative clustering method that was discontinued when four clusters were formed. The distance measure d_{min} was used. The Figure also shows the part of the minimal spanning tree constructed up to that point. The clustering solution is not completely correct according to the true class labels (see Fig. 27.3).

Figure 27.6
Dendrogram corresponding to the clustering procedure illustrated in Fig. 27.5. The procedure was discontinued at four clusters. This corresponds to the dashed line. It is seen that the cluster of class 1 (blue) has integrated two members of class 2 (red) and that one member of class 2 is not assigned to any cluster.

27

1. The distance between two clusters is the distance between the cluster means (d_{mean}).
2. The distance between two clusters is the average of the distances between all possible pairs of objects, in which the two objects of a pair belong to different clusters (d_{avg}).
3. The distance between two clusters is the minimum of the distances between all possible pairs of objects, in which the two objects of a pair belong to different clusters (d_{min}).
4. The distance between two clusters is the maximum of the distances between all possible pairs of objects, in which the two objects of a pair belong to different clusters (d_{max}).

Generally, application of these different distance measures results in different clustering configurations. For a given number of clusters, the best algorithm may be selected on the basis of their compactness. Again, it can be stated that the comparison of clustering results is more problematic with different numbers of clusters. Application of the agglomerative procedure to the object configuration of Fig. 27.3 is illustrated in Fig. 27.5. The clusters found by application of the measure d_{min}, terminated at a number of clusters c equal to 4 is shown. Clustering by using the distance measure d_{min} is a method of building the *minimal spanning tree* (MST). The MST is the graph of the minimum total length of the connections between all the object points. It preserves much of the information about the spatial configuration. It is also customary to illustrate the clustering process with a so-called *dendrogram*. In a dendrogram, all objects are depicted on a horizontal line. The merging process is illustrated by U-shaped structures, the depth of which is given by the distance d_{min} at which the merger takes place. Fig. 27.6 illustrates the dendrogram resulting from the clustering process illustrated in Fig. 27.5.

4 Design of a Pattern Recognition Application

For a given application, for example, the classification of human leukocytes, it is generally unknown a priori which features to measure and which classification rule to apply. The best solutions to these problems are usually found by trial and error: the designer measures all features that may possibly contribute to the classification process. Subsequently, it becomes possible to apply algorithms to detect the best feature or feature combinations and to test various classification strategies. This is best accomplished by using a highly flexible interactive system. One such system, developed in the Department of Medical Informatics of Erasmus University Rotterdam, The Netherlands, is *ISPAHAN*. This system is a collection of various algorithms for feature evaluation, supervised classification, and clustering (and more). These algorithms interact with each other through a data manager. Use of the system relieves users from the administrative burden of data management and enables them to concentrate on the problem at hand.

27

5 Modern Developments

The methods described above constitute the core of what may be called *classical pattern recognition*. It has become clear that for any given application there is not one best technique. Sometimes, a combination of various classification techniques results in substantially better performance. This has given rise to the development of so-called hybrid systems and to a proliferation of comparative studies, in which large, standardized data collections are used.

Also, most of the classical techniques cannot be applied in situations of incomplete information, that is, in situations in which the values of some of the features are unknown for some of the objects. This is one of the reasons why some new developments in pattern recognition exploit other techniques. In particular, *neural networks* are worth mentioning here.

The operating principle of neural networks is not new. Neural networks were invented and implemented in the 1960s, but they were found to be impractical because of the limited hardware capabilities. In the 1980s, when hardware became much more powerful, they were reinvented in various forms. A neural network is a system of interconnected artificial neurons (nodes). Such nodes may be implemented in hardware but almost always are simulated in software. The development of neural networks was inspired by an analogy to the human brain system. When used in various classification problems, their performance is claimed to be superior to that of classical techniques. Their behaviors, capabilities, and limitations are still the subject of many comparative studies. Although statistical properties of neural networks are difficult to prove, neural networks do have the theoretical advantage of improved learning of appropriate classifications when there are nonlinear relationships among input data and concluded output variables.

Key References

Fu KS. *Digital Pattern Recognition.* Berlin: Springer Verlag, 1976.

Duda R, Hart P. *Pattern Classification and Scene Analysis.* New York: Wiley 1973.

See the Web site for further literature references.

27

28 Modeling for Decision Support

1 Introduction

Decision-support systems come in a variety of forms. Many, such as *QMR* (see Chapter 16), are stand-alone applications that users access via personal workstations or via the *Internet*. Others are *software modules* embedded within much larger computer programs – such as within portions of clinical information systems – that operate without users specifically seeking decision-making advice. Developers build some decision-support systems from scratch using generic programming languages. They create other decision aids using expert system-building *shells* that allow them to use *production rules*, *Bayesian probabilistic networks*, or other formalisms to implement the necessary decision-making behavior. The great variety of approaches to constructing, validating, and deploying decision-support systems discussed in Chapter 15 may give the impression that methods for building decision-support systems are necessarily eclectic and ad hoc. Whereas there is indeed considerable variability in the way that developers create decision-support systems, there are many underlying principles that remain constant, despite the details of any particular implementation. These principles concern the ways in which the developers model medical knowledge conceptually and the ways in which the decision-support system itself acquires information about the case at hand and generates its advice for the user.

The principles that underlie decision-support systems have been debated vigorously, and the resulting consensus has been widely disseminated within the computer science community for more than a decade. Unfortunately, these principles have not always been articulated widely within the medical informatics community. Many workers in medical informatics often have been more concerned with the exigencies of installing complex systems within the clinical environment than with the generalizable axioms that transcend particular implementations. We take the position here, however, that the science of medical informatics demands that system builders understand the construction of decision-support systems from a theoretical perspective and that they be able to relate the development of clinical decision-support systems to the development of decision-support systems in general.

Because decision-support systems must represent and reason about knowledge of some domain (the application area), our discussion here emphasizes how knowledge is modeled within computer systems. As a result, our discussion here is somewhat more abstract than other presentations in this Handbook. Moreover, because the practice of building clinical decision-support systems has been changing rapidly as a consequence of recent research, we find it helpful to take a historical perspective on techniques for building decision aids that relates current methodological trends to well-established approaches.

28

2 A Broad View of Decision Support

The term *decision-support system* (*DSS*) is used widely in the literature, yet its meaning is vague. Some authors view a health care DSS to be a stand-alone program that interviews a user about a clinical situation and then generates advice regarding that situation. Thus, the user may enter information about a patient's signs and symptoms to receive a set of diagnostic possibilities or therapeutic recommendations. Other authors have a more encompassing point of view, and consider a DSS to be any software module that demonstrates intelligent behavior regarding a clinical situation and that communicates its findings to a human who can take action. Thus, programs that generate alerts automatically on the basis of data from clinical information systems can be viewed as decision-support systems. Programs that enforce clinical practice guidelines also fall into this category. Here, we define a DSS to be:

any piece of software that takes as input information about a clinical situation and that produces as output inferences that can assist practitioners in their decision making and that would be judged as "intelligent" by the program's users.

We do not restrict ourselves to programs that make their inferences about the current clinical situation by any particular technique. Although the majority of clinical DSSs are implemented with IF-THEN production rules (see Chapter 15), DSSs need not be rule-based systems. Systems can provide decision support using:

- *neural networks,*
- *Bayesian networks,*
- *pattern recognition* techniques, or even
- plain program code.

The underlying principles are completely independent of the details of how inference mechanisms are programmed in the computer. As we shall see, how clinical knowledge might be modeled and how the knowledge might be used to generate inferences are much more important than the mechanics of computer programming. Much of our theory of DSSs has arisen as a result of the experience of the knowledge-based systems community over the past three decades: first, in building *rule-based* expert systems and then in developing second-generation *expert system* architectures. As a consequence of our experience with artificial intelligence techniques, it is convenient to use the terms decision-support system and *knowledge-based system* (KBS) interchangeably. We do so recognizing that KBSs do not need to be rule-based systems and that all computer programs that provide clinical decision support, regardless of how they are implemented, somehow must represent medical knowledge in a machine-processable form and must use that knowledge to generate advice for their users. Many authors use the older term *expert system* as a synonym for KBS, although it is inappropriate to suggest that KBSs solve problems by using the same strategies that human experts use.

3 Rule-Based Systems

The use of IF-THEN *production rules,* coupled with the use of *inference engines* that perform *forward* or *backward chaining* on the rules to derive conclusions for decision support, originated in the 1960s. The Dendral system, which determined molecular structures from *magnetic resonance imaging* data, provided one of the first well-known demonstrations of the use of production systems to perform knowledge-based applications. In the 1970s, the *MYCIN* system, which workers at Stanford University in the United States developed to assist physicians both in determining possible causes of bacteremia and meningitis and in selecting appropriate therapy, is perhaps the best known of the early rule-based systems. The extraction of the MYCIN backward-chaining inference engine as a separate program that could operate on new rule bases in new domains (the *EMYCIN* system) was a significant achievement. Suddenly, developers could encode knowledge for new clinical problems using the same rule-based syntax that had been so successful in the case of MYCIN, and thus could use EMYCIN to generate clinical consultations in the new domain. Writing a set of rules about blood coagulation disorders allowed one group of workers to create a new EMYCIN-based system called *CLOT* that could diagnose the cause of abnormal bleeding, writing a set of rules about interpretation of pulmonary function tests led to another DSS called *PUFF*, and so on.

The availability of EMYCIN thus led developers to create a wide variety of small DSSs by constructing new EMYCIN-compatible rule bases. Two other rule-based shells – *EXPERT* and *OPS5* – became available from academic groups in the United States at Rutgers University and Carnegie-Mellon University, respectively. Numerous developers were able to create working DSSs; several of these systems were demonstrated empirically to perform at the level of human experts. By the end of the 1970s, businesses, such as Digital Equipment Corporation, began to make substantial investments in KBS technology; rule-based systems, such as the XCON program to configure the layout of components on minicomputer backplanes, reportedly led to significant cost savings throughout the industrial sector.

By the early 1980s, a host of start-up companies began to market not only commercial versions of EMYCIN and OPS5 but also more sophisticated shells for building KBSs; such shells formed the substrate of a burgeoning artificial intelligence industry. Nearly all the commercial shells had a rule-based component; many provided mechanisms for developers to encode knowledge using frames and other representation formalisms. By the middle of the decade, excitement about KBSs technology was at its peak. Most of the enthusiasm came from outside the health care arena: many industries saw rule-based systems as a panacea for streamlining their operations and for providing timely advice to workers who might not have immediate access to human experts. At the end of the 1980s, however, much of the excitement had waned, and many of the initially successful start-up companies had gone bankrupt. Many researchers in the academic community were left confused as to why it had been so difficult to transfer their technology to the private sector.

The reasons for the near collapse of the artificial intelligence industry in the 1980s are manifold and complex. It is essential, however, to understand the problems in adopting KBS technology commercially if we are to avoid similar pitfalls when building contemporary DSSs. A primary cause for the "artificial intelligence winter" was that rule-based technology simply did not scale up to the requirements of industrial applications, in contrast to what many of the vendors had promised. It was extremely difficult to develop – and even more difficult to maintain – the large rule bases needed to represent the knowledge required to solve many real-world problems. Despite the expressive power of the available representation languages and the deductive power of the associated inference engines, the lack of principled *software engineering* methodologies for using the shells in the first place made it arduous for many programmers to construct scalable knowledge bases (see Section 4).

Rule-based systems certainly have not disappeared, and there still are many excellent development tools for building KBSs. Rule-based systems continue to be the primary basis for myriad industrial applications, with increasing visibility in the health care setting. For example, the *Arden syntax* (see Chapter 16, Panel 16.2) for encoding *medical logic modules* within clinical information systems is a rule-based formalism. The unbridled enthusiasm for rule-based systems that was existent in the 1980s finally has been replaced by a more rational recognition of the strengths and weaknesses of the technology. For workers in medical informatics, it is particularly instructive to study the software engineering problems that led the computer science community to acquire these more realistic expectations concerning rule-based approaches.

28

4 Abstraction Beyond the Rules

The idea of using production rules to represent knowledge within computer systems can be traced to Alan Newell and Herbert Simon's hypothesis that the application of production rules is a necessary and sufficient property of human intelligence. Early workers in artificial intelligence thought that it was only natural to program KBSs using a production-rule approach. Many of these authors claimed that there was a one-to-one correspondence between the production rules that developers encoded for expert system knowledge bases and the cognitive constructs that human experts actually used to solve problems. Experts, after all, often seemed to articulate rules of thumb (*heuristics*) when describing how they solved problems, and there was little reason to doubt that experts invoked such heuristics during their cognition. (Subsequent research has demonstrated that there often is astonishing disparity between the way that people verbalize their problem-solving strategies when asked to do so and the way that they solve problems in practice.)

Initially, rule-based systems were viewed as computational models of human problem-solving behavior. Few developers of current KBSs, however, would presume that their systems represent models of true cognitive processes, although the precise role of cognitive modeling in the construction of DSSs remains an open question.

Possibly because the early developers of KBSs believed that their production rules represented correlates of true cognitive primitives, these developers did not view their work as software engineering. Indeed, they invented the term *knowledge engineering* to distinguish their work from that of traditional computer programmers. The fundamental problem, however, was that these knowledge engineers needed to use production rules as programming constructs to coerce certain behaviors in the resulting DSS.

The developers of the MYCIN system, for example, were well aware that by changing the order of the clauses in the premise of a rule, they could radically affect the process by which the system arrived at its conclusions. The MYCIN inference engine processed production rules by evaluating the clauses in the premise of each rule strictly in the order in which those clauses appeared. To determine the truth value of each clause in a given rule, the backward-chaining algorithm would invoke different sets of rules of possibly different complexities. Thus, the specific order of the clauses in the rules determined the efficiency of the problem-solving process. Knowledge engineers had to think critically about the order of the clauses in each rule's premise, to minimize the resulting computation, and to streamline the system's dialogue with the user. They would often spend hours tinkering with the order of rule clauses or with the attached certainty factors to coerce the system to behave in a particular way.

Although rules were viewed as "modular" units of knowledge, introducing new rules into a knowledge base would, in fact, have side effects that might be impossible to predict. For example, it might be difficult for knowledge engineers to remember how several preexisting rules depend on parameters concluded by a new rule. At the same time, a new rule might reference existing symbols in the knowledge base, but assume *semantics* slightly different from those shared by several of the previously entered rules. William Clancey called the latter phenomenon concept broadening, and pointed out the problem in the original MYCIN knowledge base. One rule in the knowledge base stated that "IF an organism is cultured from a site that ordinarily is sterile, THEN that organism is significant." Later, a rule that stated the following was added: "IF an organism is cultured at a time when the patient has signs of serious illness, THEN the organism is significant." The concept "significant organism" thus was broadened to mean not only: "an organism from an ordinarily sterile site," but also: "an organism cultured in the setting of serious illness."

It may be appropriate to expand the meaning of the term "significant" in this manner, but the rules in the knowledge base that were written before the new rule was added made assumptions about the nature of a significant culture that did not reflect the subsequently broadened concept. The old rules that were written in keeping with the more narrow meaning of significant might now be invoked inappropriately if the new rule

28

concludes that an organism is significant whenever a patient is seriously ill. Viewing the knowledge base only as a collection of seemingly independent production rules made it impossible for developers to perceive how the rules interacted to generate the system's composite behavior. The inability to predict precisely how a rule-based system's behavior might change as new rules were added or as existing rules were deleted or modified made it essential for system builders to devise new ways of understanding the knowledge base at a higher level of abstraction.

In 1985, Clancey described how the MYCIN system and a large number of other KBSs used a stereotypical pattern of inferences to perform classification problem solving. Clancey did not view MYCIN's use of data about a particular patient to identify potential infectious organisms merely as the result of the almost random interaction of a collection of independent production rules; rather, he identified a reproducible pattern of reasoning that appeared as an emergent inference strategy. This pattern of inferences was evident not only in MYCIN but also in several other KBSs that Clancey studied. This pattern is called **heuristic classification** (Fig. 28.1) and involves three discrete kinds of inferences:

1. The features of the input case are abstracted into higher-level generalizations (e.g., patient data, such as the white blood cell (**WBC**) count, are used to infer abstract characterizations, such as that the patient is in an immunocompromised state).
2. The generalizations are associated heuristically with elements of the set of potential solutions that can classify the case (e.g., the immunocompromised state is associated with possible infection by gram-negative bacteria).
3. Additional information is used to refine abstract solutions into more specific ones (e.g., that the situation suggests that the most likely gram-negative bacterium causing the infection *is Escherichia coli* or *Pseudomonas aeruginosa).*

Instead of being asked to view MYCIN's behavior as the result of arbitrary interactions among more than 400 production rules, workers in medical informatics suddenly could use the heuristic classification model

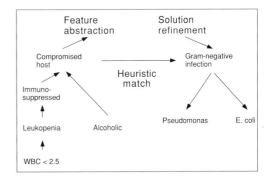

Figure 28.1.
Heuristic classification. The pattern of inferences is one in which (1) case data are abstracted into higher-level generalizations (e.g., the patient is a "compromised host"), (2) these abstractions are associated with potential classes of solutions (e.g., "gram-negative infection"), and (3) the ultimate solutions are selected from a preenumerated set.

to understand MYCIN in terms of three clearly defined inference procedures:

- feature abstraction,
- heuristic match, and
- solution refinement.

The elegant result of Clancey's analysis was that the pattern of inferences in heuristic classification explained not only the behavior of MYCIN when that system was identifying likely causes of infection but also the behavior of the other KBSs that Clancey examined. For example, the CLOT system for diagnosis of coagulation disorders:

1. makes abstractions regarding a patients' illness on the basis of specific input data (e.g., bleeding time),
2. heuristically matches those patient-oriented abstractions to possible defects in the patient's coagulation system (e.g., a pattern of test results suggests a disorder of the extrinsic pathway), and
3. refines the characterization of the possible defects into disorders of specific clotting factors (e.g., Factor VIII deficiency).

28

Similarly, the PUFF system:

1. makes abstractions regarding a patients' illness on the basis of pulmonary function test measurements (e.g., vital capacity),
2. heuristically matches those abstractions to different classes of lung disease (e.g., the low forced expiratory volume suggests obstructive airway disease), and
3. refines the class of the patient's lung disease into more specific diagnoses (e.g., significant, nonreversible obstruction).

Although many DSSs that perform diagnoses use heuristic classification as their underlying problem-solving strategy, many others use alternative patterns of inference. For example, the *QMR* program (see Chapters 16 and 17) uses a pattern-matching algorithm that does not involve any abstraction of patient findings; QMR also presents to the user all diseases that may be consistent with the specified pattern rather than attempting to perform solution refinement. When a diagnostic program does perform its inference-using heuristic classification, construing the system's behavior in terms of feature abstraction, heuristic match, and solution refinement makes it much easier for developers to understand both the program's reasoning and the particular ways in which the program uses medical knowledge during problem solving. Thus, when a developer of a KBS can define the required problem-solving behavior in terms of the inference patterns in heuristic classification, each rule that is entered into the knowledge base can be seen to contribute to the particular inferences in heuristic classification in a specific way. No longer is each new rule added to a soup of seemingly unrelated rules; instead, each new rule can be seen to contribute to the problem-solving process in a well-understood manner.

Heuristic classification is not an appropriate pattern of inferences for many decision-support problems. For example, there are many problems for which the solution set cannot be preenumerated and for which simple solution refinement is inadequate. When the assumptions of heuristic classification do hold, however, the developer suddenly has a structure that can clarify the purpose of each rule in the knowledge base and that makes it clear where new knowledge might need to be added to an evolving system and what rules are likely to interact with a rule that needs to be changed.

Although heuristic classification commonly is considered to be an inference pattern used by rule-based systems, many other kinds of decision-support programs perform heuristic classification. For example, programs written in ordinary programming languages, such as *C* can perform heuristic classification. In fact, the description of heuristic classification as a recurring pattern of inferences that could transcend particular implementation platforms such as EMYCIN helped to clarify the fact that construction of DSSs required developers to think about the overall behavior of the systems, in addition to the particular programming constructs (e.g., production rules) that they would use to implement their work.

5 The Knowledge-Level Hypothesis

In 1980, when Alan Newell gave his presidential address at the first meeting of the American Association for Artificial Intelligence, he articulated a hypothesis about KBSs that was, at the time, remarkable. Newell suggested that developers of KBSs (indeed, everyone concerned with the study of artificial intelligence) were placing undue emphasis on how systems were implemented. True, there were important trade-offs to consider regarding whether developers should implement DSSs using production rules, *frames* or *procedural program* code. Newell argued, however, that such implementation-specific concerns were tangential to the problem of identifying what basic knowledge a given computer program should have in the first place to achieve its problem-solving goals. Just as there were different levels of abstraction at which we could understand computer architectures (basic circuits, logical components, virtual machines, and so on), there was a distinction to be made between how knowledge might be encoded in a computer system (e.g., using frames or rules, at what Newell referred to as the *symbol level*) and, more abstractly, how knowledge might be used by the computer to bring about problem-solving competence (at which Newell referred to as the *knowledge level*). Thus, distinct from any particular computer program was the abstract body of knowledge on which that program operated to generate intelligent behavior.

This distinction between implementation and knowledge is precisely what Clancey was attempting to capture in his description of the heuristic classification model. We can understand MYCIN at the symbol level as an **artifact** that encodes knowledge using production rules and that has a backward-chaining inference engine that processes rules to generate its output. We also can understand MYCIN at the knowledge level as a problem solver that uses heuristic classification to characterize the current clinical situation and to identify potential causes of infection. The advantage of the knowledge-level perspective is that we can describe what MYCIN knows about infectious diseases and how it uses that knowledge for decision support without having to be concerned with how the system's developers ultimately programmed that knowledge into the computer. In the construction of any DSS, once developers understand the required behavior of the system at the knowledge level, the knowledge-level characterization can then serve as a design specification for implementation of the system at the symbol level. The knowledge-level specification also serves as an important reference during maintenance of the completed knowledge base. During the 1980s, when many people were attempting to develop KBSs and were getting extremely uneven results, there was little appreciation for the importance of knowledge-level modeling as a prerequisite to implementation. Current methodologies for building DSSs uniformly emphasize knowledge-level modeling as the initial step.

Heuristic classification provides a valuable framework for understanding systems such as MYCIN in an implementation-independent manner. For many DSSs that perform classification problem solving (i.e., that select an explanatory element from a preenumerated solution set), the heuristic classification model provides an extremely useful set of terms and relationships for describing the system's behavior.

Not all problem solvers, however, can operate via heuristic classification. For example, our previous description of MYCIN was oversimplified. Although the portion of MYCIN that performs the task of identifying potential causes of infection can be understood in terms of heuristic classification, there is another part of the system that so far we have ignored: the component that recommends treatment for the presumptive infection. MYCIN's treatment-planning algorithm does not use classification problem solving. (Although it may be easy to preenumerate all potential causes of bacteremia or meningitis, it is not straightforward to list all possible combinations of all antibiotic prescriptions!) The treatment-planning component must construct a solution (i.e., a set of antibiotics to which all putative pathogens are likely to be sensitive); it cannot simply choose a predetermined recommendation. Development of the means to describe complex behaviors such as that of MYCIN's treatment-planning algorithm at the knowledge level remains a principal challenge for researchers in medical informatics.

For hundreds of years, defining and typifying human knowledge has been a principal business of philosophers. We do not suggest that the creation of knowledge-level descriptions of medical expertise for the purposes of constructing DSSs is in any way simple or that it involves easily reproducible techniques. There are, in practice, relatively few frameworks such as heuristic classification that can be applied readily by system builders who wish to capture the requirements of their applications at the knowledge level, although substantial progress is being made in this area (see Section 6 of Chapter 16). It remains a fundamental element of research in medical informatics to elucidate knowledge-level frameworks for describing clinical expertise. Basic research in medical informatics requires both characterization of generic problem-solving behaviors that are important in the health care setting and description in implementation-independent terms of the knowledge on which clinical practice is based.

28

6 KADS

In the mid-1980s, a consortium of investigators supported by the Commission of the European Community proposed a new methodology for expressing models of expertise at the knowledge level. These researchers, centered at the University of Amsterdam, The Netherlands, recognized that DSSs, no matter how intricate the knowledge on which such systems were based, still were pieces of software and that principles of good software engineering certainly must apply to the development of systems for decision support. By combining the goals of modeling expertise and of applying standard principles of effective software engineering to the creation of KBSs, the consortium proposed a methodology known as knowledge acquisition and design structuring (*KADS*).[1] By the end of the 1980s, KADS had spread throughout Europe to become the de facto standard approach for building DSSs of all kinds. Programmers continue to construct most large commercially available KBSs in Europe using either KADS or a methodology inspired by KADS, and there is an increasing appreciation for KADS worldwide.

An important contribution of the KADS methodology is the separation of the *conceptual modeling* of expertise (i.e., creation of knowledge-level descriptions) from the implementation of working systems (Fig. 28.2). When using KADS, developers start with the data that inform their understanding of the knowledge in an application area; they then construct a conceptual model of expertise, which represents the body of knowledge that drives decision support, in an implementation-independent manner. The conceptual model is distinct from the design model that serves as a programming specification for implementation of the DSS as a running program. By distinguishing between conceptualization of knowledge and construction of a working system, the KADS approach allows developers to perform a structured analysis of the required knowledge before they commit to a particular framework for implementing the system. The developers' analysis of the expertise required for decision support consequently is not biased by programming concerns. Indeed, alternative design models may be derived from a single conceptual model. KADS defines a general outline for conceptual models that allows developers to write down the knowledge required to solve a particular application task in an explicit fashion. There are three general elements in the KADS framework:

1. KADS first asks system builders to indicate the basic concepts in the application area (e.g., that there are patients, organisms, and antibiotics).
2. KADS then furnishes the means for the developers to define primitive inferences that are relevant in the domain (e.g., that treatment of a patient who is infected with a particular organism requires use of an antibiotic to which that organism is sensitive), and then
3. KADS asks to specify the way in which those inferences might be sequenced to solve particular tasks (e.g., that treatment of presumptive infection first requires determination of the potential pathogens

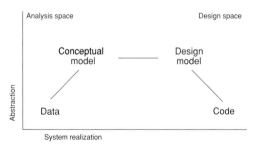

Figure 28.2

Conceptual design in KADS. System developers elicit data about the application domain from a variety of sources and abstract these data into a conceptual model of the expertise required to solve application tasks. In a separate set of steps, the conceptual model informs the creation of a design model, which guides the programming of the final DSS.

---

[1] *Schreiber, G, Wielinga, B, and Breuker, J, eds. KADS: A Principled Approach to Knowledge-Based System Development. London: Academic Press; 1993.*

and second requires determination of an appropriate antibiotic regimen).

A KADS model of expertise thus embodies (1) the set of basic domain concepts (2) the primitive inferences that define relationships between the domain concepts and (3) a task structure that sequences the primitive inferences.[2] This layered framework for modeling the knowledge needed to drive DSSs has proved useful both in medicine and in other application areas. When defining a model of expertise, system builders analyze the relevant knowledge and then enumerate what they perceive to be the various domain-layer, inference-layer, and task-layer constructs.

The KADS approach emphasizes that creation of a model of expertise is a highly subjective activity and that there is never a single correct way to capture the knowledge needed to solve a particular task. The emphasis is on defining the knowledge required to solve the task in as explicit a manner as possible and in a standard, implementation-independent formalism. Because KADS also recognizes that DSSs are, ultimately, large pieces of software, the KADS methodology incorporates general software engineering principles. In addition to creating the model of expertise, developers using KADS ideally model the organization that will use the final DSS, the kind of communication that users will have with the system, the software framework in which the DSS will be embedded, and other aspects of the overall computational system. These models reflect the kinds of considerations required for managing any large

software-development project (see Chapter 35, Section 5). Although it has been a long-term goal of the KADS consortium to offer automated tools that can assist developers in this process, robust tools that support KADS have become available only recently.

In the 1990s, the KADS consortium refined its methodology and released a revised framework known as *commonKADS.* The commonKADS approach clarifies certain aspects of the models that system builders create using KADS and adds facilities for designing KBSs from libraries of reusable components. These components include reusable domain *ontologies* (abstract descriptions of the concepts in an application area) and problem-solving methods (abstract descriptions of the procedures by which families of application tasks might be solved). The investigation of methodologies that allow developers to reuse both domain ontologies and problem-solving methods in the construction of new KBSs has become a major focus of work in the study of decision-support technology. Although reuse of preexisting components in general is often difficult, such reuse has the potential to ease both the design and the long-term maintenance of complex DSSs.

[2] The initial description of KADS included a fourth, strategic layer that allowed for the consideration of alternative problem-solving approaches at the task layer. In practice, the strategic layer was almost never used.

7 Reusable Problem-Solving Methods

At the time that Clancey proposed heuristic classification as a recurring inference pattern that could be identified in KBSs such as MYCIN and PUFF, it was becoming clear that various well-defined problem-solving strategies were reappearing in a variety of KBSs. Chandrasekaran's group at Ohio State University in the United States, for example, identified several such strategies, which they called generic tasks. These generic tasks corresponded to stereotypic control strategies that

could be abstracted from the KBSs that the Ohio State University group was building. John McDermott's group at Carnegie-Mellon University similarly noted a set of problem-solving methods that provided the control structure for a number of other KBSs. All these investigators were demonstrating that many decision aids had highly regular mechanisms for sequencing certain classes of inferences. These domain-independent problem-solving strategies provided standard ways of addressing certain kinds of tasks. Even though the original developers of these KBSs might never have thought about these regularities explicitly, there nevertheless were a number of well-defined, generic strategies that were emerging from analysis of how diverse automated problem solvers addressed their associated application tasks. These generic strategies are now referred to as *problem-solving methods* by nearly all workers in the KBSs community. Problem-solving methods define domain-independent strategies for arriving at solutions to generic problems by sequencing certain classes of inferences, such as the three classes of inferences in the heuristic-classification model.

Several dozen problem-solving methods have been described in the literature. Of these, *heuristic classification* is the best understood.[3] Other problem-solving methods perform procedures such as constraint satisfaction, planning, fault diagnosis, *probabilistic reasoning*, abstraction of primary data into corresponding summaries, and *case-based reasoning*. The enumeration of additional problem-solving methods and the refinement of existing methods continue to be active areas of investigation by a growing community of researchers.

It is easy to confuse the idea of a problem-solving method with that of an inference mechanism such as *backward chaining*. Backward chaining is not a problem-solving method because it is a procedure that operates on production rule representations (i.e., new rules are invoked because they conclude values for parameters that happen to match for those parameters that are referenced in the premise of the rule currently under consideration). Inference mechanisms such as rule chaining or *frame-based inheritance* can be understood only in the context of particular knowledge representation formalisms (i.e., rules or frames). A problem-solving method, on the other hand, is a knowledge-level construct that can be described independently of the particular data structures on which the method

might operate. The heuristic classification model, for instance, is completely neutral to how a system that performs heuristic classification might be built; a programmer can implement heuristic classification by using production rules and backward chaining or by writing software in the programming language C.

Problem-solving methods provide a convenient means of developing knowledge-level models. When a designer can come to understand the domain knowledge needed to solve an application task in terms of a predefined problem-solving method, it becomes clear how each element of the domain knowledge might ultimately contribute to the problem-solving behavior of the system. When designing a heuristic classifier, for example, the developer can readily identify whether a primitive inference is used to perform feature abstraction, heuristic match, or solution refinement (see Fig. 28.1). The heuristic classification model thus becomes a unifying framework by which to relate all the elements of domain knowledge that the developer might acquire. Using the problem-solving method as the basis for conceptual modeling limits the roles that domain knowledge can play in problem solving to those particular knowledge roles (e.g., feature abstraction and heuristic match) that are defined by the method. The role-limiting nature of problem-solving methods makes it clear what domain knowledge is needed to solve a task that can be automated by a given method (all the method's roles need to be filled for the method to work) and clarifies the purpose of each piece of elicited knowledge (each primitive inference must satisfy some role in the underlying problem-solving method, or else the inference is irrelevant to the task at hand). A problem-solving method thus can provide an extremely useful framework for organizing the domain knowledge needed to automate an application task; the knowledge roles defined by the method merely need to be filled with appropriate domain knowledge. Of course, the designer needs to select an appropriate problem-solving method in the first place; it is not always obvious a priori whether a given problem-solving method will be sufficient for a particular task, unfortunately.

When associated with a piece of program code that implements it, the problem-solving method becomes much more than an abstraction useful for conceptual

---

[3] *Clancey, in his original description of heuristic classification, did not make any commitment to the order in which the individual inferences might be carried out. He therefore presented heuristic classification only as a pattern of inferences rather than as a problem-solving method.*

28

modeling; the method becomes a building block in the design model that a programmer can use to implement a working system. System builders can use the method conceptually to help them to model the domain knowledge that they need to acquire to build the DSS and can then use the operational form of the problem-solving method to implement the decision aid. In this manner, the problem-solving method functions like an element from a mathematical **subroutine library**: it provides a reusable piece of software that facilitates implementation of the required computer program.

In the 1980s, several research groups began to experiment with the idea of creating tools for building DSSs that were based on particular problem-solving methods. Such tools would use the knowledge roles of a given problem-solving method to structure their interactions with developers, who would fill the knowledge roles, providing the domain knowledge needed to perform problem solving at run time. For example, one well-known knowledge acquisition system, **MOLE**, was developed by Larry Eshelman and others working in John McDermott's group at Carnegie-Mellon University. MOLE embodied a diagnostic problem-solving method known as *cover-and-differentiate*. The general strategy for cover-and-differentiate is as follows:

1. Ask the user what symptoms need to be explained.
2. Conclude what diagnostic hypotheses will explain or cover these symptoms (using covering knowledge).
3. Conclude what additional information about the current situation might allow differentiation between the hypotheses that cover each symptom (using differentiating knowledge).
4. Ask the user for that information.
5. If there still are symptoms that are not covered, return to Step 2.
6. Conclude the best combination of diagnostic hypotheses that will explain all the symptoms (using combined knowledge).
7. If there is additional information about the current situation that might affect the likelihood of any combination of hypotheses, then (a) ask the user for that information and then (b) return to Step 2.
8. Report the best combination of hypotheses.

The MOLE knowledge acquisition tool uses the cover-and-differentiate method to drive its dialogue with the system developer. The tool asks the knowledge base builder for covering knowledge (associations between symptoms and diagnostic hypotheses) and differentiating knowledge (additional associations that alter the degree of belief that a symptom can be explained by a given hypothesis).[4] The tool also asks for combining knowledge, which allows the problem solver to propose an appropriate and parsimonious combination of diagnostic hypotheses that can explain all the symptoms. Thus, the knowledge acquisition dialogue is structured by the three major knowledge roles associated with the cover-and-differentiate method. To provide decision support, an implementation of the cover-and-differentiate method (written in a rule-based language) operates on the domain knowledge that fills the method's knowledge roles to generate appropriate diagnostic problem-solving behavior.

If a developer were to use MOLE to create a medical diagnostic system, it would be necessary to enter the covering knowledge (e.g., that sore throat may be a symptom of either streptococcal pharyngitis or infectious mononucleosis), the differentiating knowledge (e.g., that infectious mononucleosis is associated with generalized lymphadenopathy, whereas streptococcal pharyngitis is not), and the combining knowledge (e.g., that serologic evidence for mononucleosis should cause the system to suggest that diagnosis, even if the differentiating knowledge weights the likelihood of streptococcal pharyngitis to be higher).[5] Thus, to create a DSS with a knowledge acquisition tool such as MOLE, the developer must cast all the domain knowledge in terms of the three kinds of knowledge roles

28

---

[4] *Covering knowledge is analogous to the heuristic-matching knowledge used by the heuristic classification problem-solving method; differentiating knowledge is analogous to solution refinement knowledge. The cover-and-differentiate problem solving method does not incorporate the notion of feature abstraction.*

[5] *MOLE was never used to build an actual medical knowledge base. Most experience with MOLE was gained by people constructing DSSs to perform fault diagnosis for electromechanical systems.*

assumed by the cover-and-differentiate method. The developer's dialogue with the knowledge acquisition tool is completely independent of the ultimate implementation language for the DSS. More important, the tool can use its knowledge of the problem-solving method to suggest to the user where knowledge may be missing, contradictory, or incomplete. For example, MOLE can analyze the emerging knowledge base and will inform the developer whenever a symptom lacks the covering knowledge needed to suggest a corresponding diagnostic hypothesis or whenever there is inadequate differentiating knowledge to distinguish between two potentially competing hypotheses.

Knowledge acquisition tools such as MOLE ask the system developer to create a knowledge base by filling the roles of an assumed problem-solving method. The ability to view the domain knowledge in terms of how a well-defined problem-solving method will operate on that knowledge offers considerable advantages over viewing a knowledge base in terms of symbol-level production rules and other data structures. At the same time, the tight coupling between the knowledge roles of the method and the representation of the knowledge in the knowledge base results in a significant disadvantage: There is no way to view the domain knowledge independently of how that knowledge is processed by the problem-solving method. For example, we can see from

the few facts that we associated with the cover-and-differentiate problem-solving method in the preceding example that it is not easy to ask questions such as: What can the knowledge base tell us about the system's understanding of infectious mononucleosis? Knowledge about the typical symptoms of mononucleosis is stored as part of the covering knowledge required by the cover-and-differentiate method; knowledge about other symptoms of mononucleosis that may help to verify the diagnosis is stored as part of the differentiating knowledge; other knowledge about mononucleosis is stored as part of the combining knowledge. There is no direct way to obtain a coherent view of all the knowledge pertaining to any of the diagnostic hypotheses in the MOLE system, because each hypothesis is the subject of a variety of inferences, each of which is associated with different knowledge roles. Although this situation is an improvement over that associated with rule-based approaches – where it is impossible to obtain any coherent view of either the system's behavior or the domain knowledge by examining the rule base – workers in the knowledge acquisition community began to recognize in the 1990s that the use of problem-solving methods alone as the basis for structuring DSSs had certain limitations. To overcome many of these problems, they turned to a knowledge modeling approach that had been adopted within the initial KADS system.

8 Reusable Ontologies

The KADS methodology (see Section 6) mandates that developers create conceptual models of expertise that include distinct layers for

1. domain concepts and relationships,
2. primitive inferences, and
3. task-oriented sequencing of inferences.

When they model expertise in the domain layer, developers who use KADS define the various concepts that are important within the application area, the attributes of those concepts, and the relationships between concepts. The domain layer element of a KADS model

of expertise provides an explicit description of domain concepts independently of how those concepts will be applied at either the inference layer or the task layer.

Both in the recent commonKADS framework and in other modern approaches to building DSSs, there is particular emphasis on modeling the classes of domain concepts that are important for problem solving and on defining the attributes of and relationships between those classes. Ultimately, the developer will have to define how a given problem-solving method will operate on the domain knowledge; initially, however, focus is on describing the classes of domain concepts in a coherent fashion. When creating the description of relevant classes of concepts (e.g., diseases and patients' symptoms), the developer is not initially concerned with enumeration of the instances of those classes (e.g., infectious mononucleosis and sore throat), but considers merely the categories of **concepts** that need to be considered by the DSS.

This notion of a description of the classes of concepts relevant in an application area has become increasingly important to developers of intelligent systems. Just as modern **database** systems are driven by **conceptual schemas** that define the classes of entities about which the database stores specific data, modern DSSs incorporate as a central component of their knowledge bases a model of the classes of entities about which problem solving takes place. Workers in computer science often refer to such a model as an **ontology**, borrowing the term from the branch of metaphysics concerned with the characterization of what exists in the universe.

As we use the term ontology in this chapter, it is a kind of model of an application area. An ontology characterizes the concepts relevant in an application domain, typically ignoring the instances of those concepts. The ontology defines the attributes that concepts may have, but generally is silent regarding the specific values of the attributes that are assumed by particular **instances** of the concepts. For example, an ontology may indicate that there is a concept called *disease* that has an attribute called *common name*; we would not expect the ontology to indicate that there is an instance of a disease called *streptococcal pharyngitis* that has the common name *strep throat*. Of course, an ontology is not constructed without considerable forethought regarding what instances ultimately will need to be represented. Consideration of potential instances informs the developer's conceptualization of the classes that need to be included in an ontology; once the ontology has been defined, the instances are then represented in terms of the applicable classes and relationships.

A more detailed example might help to elucidate what we mean by an ontology. Figure 28.3 demonstrates a concept hierarchy for the ontology that underlies an experimental reconstruction of the **INTERNIST-I** system (see Chapter 16) created at Stanford University. Although the original developers of INTERNIST-I

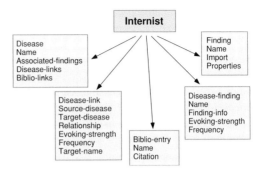

Figure 28.3

An ontology of the experimental INTERNIST-I domain. Each box represents a different class in the ontology. Attributes of classes appear in italics.

designed the knowledge base more than two decades ago and certainly would not have thought to define an explicit ontology for the system's domain, Fig. 28.3 shows what an ontology for the knowledge in INTERNIST-I might look like. (The ontology in Figure 28.3 also incorporates additional distinctions made by the more recent QMR program.) The ontology is relatively simple, with classes that specify the notions of diseases, findings, and so forth. Note that one class represents "findings" as isolated entities, whereas another class ("disease-finding") defines the relations between instances of findings and instances of diseases (defining the corresponding frequencies and evoking strengths). The disease-finding class thus provides a specification for the kind of knowledge contained in INTERNIST-I disease profiles. Because ontologies generally provide information about only abstract classes of concepts, the representation in Fig. 28.3 does not describe any individual diseases. The ontology also defines the additional concepts of disease-disease links and of bibliographic citations that justify particular disease-finding relationships, although these were not features of the original INTERNIST-I knowledge base.

Because ontologies are models, there is not a single correct way to define ontologies; there are essentially infinite distinctions that we can make about a particular application domain. An ontology merely represents a convenient way of characterizing a set of concepts

28

and relationships in an application area, and thus of creating the domain of discourse for talking about those concepts and relationships.

The tree of classes and attributes in Fig. 28.3 certainly appears to be a hierarchy of frames and slots, as we would expect in traditional **frame-based** or **object-oriented** data representations. Indeed, developers typically use frame languages to model ontologies, because these kinds of hierarchies are often perfect for documenting classes of concepts and relationships among the classes. Not all ontologies, however, can be modeled simply as frame hierarchies. For example, some ontologies explicitly include additional constraints on allowed relationships between concepts that are not expressible declaratively in traditional frame languages or object systems. Conversely, nearly all frame systems and object-oriented languages allow program code to be associated with individual frames, a procedural specification that has no place in an ontology, which simply defines a domain of discourse. Despite the convenience of using frame systems to model ontologies, we must remember that ontologies are knowledge-level constructs, distinct from the symbols that we may choose to represent them.

The notion of an ontology is powerful because explicit ontologies provide KBSs with something that databases have had for some time: a machine-processable representation of how domain-specific content is organized. The ontology provides a computable reference of the concepts about which the system "knows something," and defines a framework for organizing concepts in a knowledge base. More important, when two different DSSs can reference the same ontology, the two systems have the potential to share knowledge about the application domain and even to work in concert to solve complex problems.

Current work on the design of cooperative problem solvers that can run on different computers depends on the availability of common ontologies that offer a unified view of the knowledge in the relevant application area. A major role for reusable domain ontologies in modern computer architectures is to govern the interchange of data and knowledge between software modules that may be implemented in substantially different ways and that may require communication among distributed processors connected via networks. For example, one could imagine two different software agents that would share the INTERNIST-I ontology depicted in Fig. 28.3. One agent would perform automated diagnosis, whereas the other would perform bibliographic searching for the literature references associated with particular diseases. The common ontology would ensure that the two agents shared the same vocabulary for talking about the world (they both would operate on "diseases" and "findings", rather than on "ailments" and "manifestations"). Because the two agents would have a shared domain of discourse, they could be guaranteed to exchange data in a consistent manner.

Just as problem-solving methods capture at the knowledge level reusable, stereotypic behaviors for DSSs, ontologies provide a knowledge level means of describing the classes of domain concepts on which problem-solving methods operate. It is impossible to describe a DSS at the knowledge level without considering both the program's problem-solving method and that program's ontology of the application area.

9 Modern Architectures for Decision Support

Modern architectures for building DSSs allow developers to select (1) reusable problem-solving methods and (2) domain ontologies from libraries and to incorporate these components explicitly into the systems that they construct. Although such architectures are still largely experimental, it is important to understand the principles that these development environments embody, because the principles are still relevant when we are using conventional software development techniques. Fortunately, computer **workbenches** that sup-

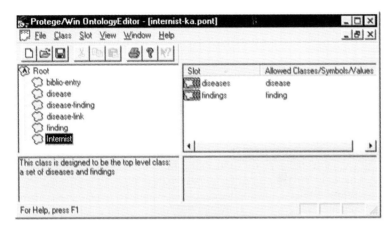

Figure 28.4.
The INTERNIST-I ontology as viewed from the Protégé Ontology Editor. Developers describe classes on concepts using the panel on the left. They define the attributes of these classes using the panel on the right. The small icons that appear before each attribute description provide a graphical shorthand for summarizing the data type of the corresponding attribute. In this case, the top-level INTERNIST class includes two slots, which contain multiple instances of diseases and findings, respectively.

port structured development of DSSs are becoming common. Recent research projects, such as those leading to the development of **PROTÉGÉ** (at Stanford University) and of **GAMES** (created by a collaboration involving, among other institutions, the University of Pavia, Italy, and the University of Amsterdam, The Netherlands), have made available to the medical informatics community both tools and methodologies that embody these ideas.

Several modern methodologies for building KBSs advocate the development of domain ontologies and the mapping of those ontologies to the data requirements of reusable problem-solving methods. In commonKADS (see Section 6), for example, the principles for constructing ontologies and for assembling problem-solving methods are particularly well worked out. Although commonKADS provides an extremely useful software engineering approach for building DSSs, the methodology has not yet led to widely disseminated computer-based development tools that can ease the construction of large-scale systems. Whereas commonKADS provides descriptions for a large library of reusable problem-solving methods, there are no standard software implementations of these methods that developers can put to use in their own applications. Both the original KADS system and commonKADS provide a set of extremely valuable guidelines for building KBSs, but it is largely up to individual developers to operationalize these guidelines.

The Protégé approach represents an alternative philosophy regarding the development of DSSs. The creators of PROTÉGÉ have put particular emphasis on the availability of computer-based tools to assist in the construction of intelligent systems, at times omitting several of the finer distinctions noted in approaches such as commonKADS. A hallmark of the PROTÉGÉ methodology concerns the division of labor between those developers who are concerned with conceptual modeling and those whose job it is to fill in the details of the knowledge base in a manner consistent with the conceptual model created by other project members. The contention is that construction of a conceptual model is a highly creative, labor-intensive task that requires considerable interaction between skilled analysts and professionals in the application domain; filling in the details of the knowledge base, on the other hand, is a task that can be performed by an application specialist, often working independently. In PROTÉGÉ, developers first use one tool to construct an ontology of the application area. They then map that ontology to an appropriate problem-solving method. The PROTÉGÉ system automatically generates a domain-specific tool that application specialists can use to enter the detailed content knowledge for the DSS.

Workers at Stanford University have used Protégé to reconstruct an experimental version of the INTERNIST-I system. Understanding of this reconstruction provides insight not only into the Protégé approach per se but also into principled approaches for development of KBSs in general.

Protégé comprises a collection of automated tools. One of these tools is the Ontology Editor. Figure 28.4

28

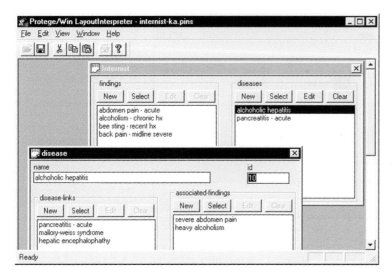

Figure 28.5.
A knowledge acquisition tool for INTERNIST-I generated by Protégé. The forms in this tool were created automatically from the domain ontology shown in Fig. 28.3. Here, the user is entering information concerning the disease *alcoholic hepatitis*. (Hx indicates history.)

shows the experimental INTERNIST-I ontology entered into the Ontology Editor. The editor provides basic functionality for declaring and describing classes of concepts, relationships between classes, attributes of classes, and data types for class attributes. When another module in the PROTÉGÉ system takes as input a domain ontology, it generates programmatically as output a knowledge acquisition tool that is custom-tailored for the corresponding domain. In the case of the INTERNIST-I ontology, Protégé creates a tool that allows developers to specify a list of diseases and patient findings, the relationships between those diseases and findings, and references to the clinical literature (Fig. 28.5). In using the tool, the developer creates the knowledge base that defines the content knowledge for the emerging DSS, where that knowledge base conforms to the structure of the domain ontology shown in Fig. 28.3. With the aid of the knowledge acquisition tool, the developer can build a knowledge base that contains much of the static information present in systems such as INTERNIST-I and QMR. Naturally, when Protégé generates knowledge acquisition tools from other domain ontologies, they look markedly different from the tool shown in Fig. 28.5; they incorporate forms and blanks that reflect the concepts in the corresponding domains.

A static knowledge base alone is insufficient for problem solving. PROTÉGÉ therefore has a library of reusable problem-solving methods that can operate on the static knowledge. PROTÉGÉ also allows developers to create new problem-solving methods when the need arises. In the case of the INTERNIST-I example, a programmer had to devise a new problem-solving method that could automate the kind of diagnostic reasoning performed by the original INTERNIST-I system. A set of explicit mappings between the data requirements of the problem-solving method and the domain ontology (as in Fig. 28.3) provides the glue that allows the ultimate DSS to solve diagnostic cases in a manner similar to that of the original INTERNIST-I program. For example, one mapping indicates that a disease in the domain ontology corresponds to the method's more general notion of a hypothesis; another mapping defines how the method's input known as *finding with respect to hypothesis* maps to the domain-specific concepts of the evoking strength and frequency of a finding within a disease, as declared by the INTERNIST-I ontology.

If there is a need to create a DSS with a somewhat different reasoning behavior, the developer could map the same INTERNIST-I ontology to an alternative problem-solving method. For example, one might relate the INTERNIST-I ontology to the data requirements of the cover-and-differentiate problem-solving method used by the MOLE system (see Section 7). Because the cover-and-differentiate method does not generate quantitative scores of how well a given hypothesis is covered by the findings requiring an explanation, a decision aid that comprised the INTERNIST-I ontology (and corresponding knowledge base) and the cover-and-differentiate method would not be able to rank order the likelihood of potential diseases; the system simply would ignore the frequency and *evoking strength* information in the knowledge base. Because different problem-solving methods have different competencies, system builders often may need to experiment with alternative methods, possibly refining such methods as they come to understand the nuances of particular tasks that they wish to automate.

In modern architectures for building DSSs, emphasis is placed on translation of knowledge-level conceptual models into working, implemented programs. In such approaches, developers can craft domain ontologies that describe the structure of the concepts in an application and can map those ontologies to reusable problem-solving methods that provide stereotypic behaviors for arriving at solutions to application tasks. Unlike both rule-based systems such as MYCIN (see Section 5) and method-based systems such as MOLE (see Section 7), decision aids built with both explicit domain ontologies and problem-solving methods clarify the manner in which domain knowledge is organized and document the role that each element of domain knowledge plays in problem solving. The conviction is that as the knowledge required for decision support becomes increasingly complex, systems implemented in this more transparent fashion will scale up to the requirements of these new tasks, facilitating the ability of developers to maintain these systems over time.

10   Summary

There have been rapid changes in the practice of general software engineering during the past two decades. The adoption of principled methodologies for building decision-support software, however, has been slower in coming. Given the relative complexities of most useful KBSs, it is particularly unfortunate that structured approaches for the construction of decision-support software are only now beginning to receive widespread attention. In medical informatics, where workers must process knowledge and data that are notoriously complex in terms of composition, time dependency, and uncertainty, there is an urgent need to adopt more principled approaches to knowledge modeling.

Performing conceptual modeling of a DSS requires understanding the required problem-solving behavior at the knowledge level independently of how the system ultimately may be implemented. Although early KBSs were viewed as inference engines that operated on particular data representations (e.g., production rules and frames), it now is more helpful to construe such systems as containing well-defined problem-solving methods (such as the heuristic classification and cover-and-differentiate methods) that operate on knowledge bases that reflect some explicit ontology of the application area. Problem-solving methods and domain ontologies are knowledge-level constructs that are useful for conceptual modeling. They also can be reflected in reusable software components that can facilitate implementation of knowledge based systems in an almost plug-and-play manner. The use of well-documented ontologies and problem-solving methods in component-based architectures may also lead to enhanced system maintenance: The purpose of each module in the system can remain clear, and software engineers can adapt individual components or can replace them with new ones as problem-solving requirements change.

Key References

David J-M, Krivine J-P, Simmons R, eds. *Second Generation Expert Systems.* Berlin: Springer-Verlag; 1993.

Marcus, S, ed. *Automating Knowledge Acquisition for Expert Systems.* Boston: Kluwer Academic; 1988.

28

Musen MA. Dimensions of knowledge sharing and reuse. *Computers and Biomedical Research.* 1992;25:435-67.

Musen MA, Gennari JH, Wong WW. A rational reconstruction of INTERNIST-I using PROTÉGÉ-II. In: *Proceedings of the Nineteenth Annual Symposium on Computer Applications in Medical Care.* New Orleans, 1995:289-93.

See the Web site for further literature references.

28

29 Structuring the Computer-Based Patient Record

1 Introduction

Clinicians are increasingly aware of the benefits of computer-based patient records (*CPRs*). The data in CPRs are primarily used for:

1. direct patient care,
2. quality assessment of care,
3. management and planning support, and
4. research and education.

The intent is for the patient data collected in a CPR to be usable for all four goals. This can only be accomplished if patient data are properly coded (see Chapter 6) and all clinical events and interventions are properly documented. Ideally, a CPR contains all data on the patient's history, physical examinations, diagnostic tests, and therapeutic interventions done to support patient care (see Chapter 8). The realization of a CPR is one of the most difficult and challenging endeavors in medical informatics research. This is all the more difficult and challenging if the data in such records are to serve the other three goals as well: assessment of the *quality* of care, management and planning support, and research and education. The diverse requirements for these data may actually conflict and may threaten the proper use of the patient record.

2 Four Levels

Information systems in health care are generally used on four levels:

1. on the personal level, that is, the physician, the nurse, and the patient;
2. the clinical department, the outpatient clinic, or the primary care practice level;
3. the health care institution level (the hospital or an organization of health care providers); and
4. the regional level (country, state, or province).

Patient data are exchanged between providers on the same level (e.g., between different general practitioners [GPs]), and between the different levels (e.g., data flowing from the GP to the national authorities). Both the nature of the patient data and the required perspective may differ, either on the same level (e.g., the data required by an orthopedic surgeon may differ from those required by a pediatrician), or between levels (e.g., a clinician requires a patient-oriented approach, but a policy maker requires a more global perspective). The exchange of data – be it on the same level or between levels – should be subjected to well-defined rules and regulations, and inappropriate or indiscriminate transfer of data should be prohibited; this requires proper regulation. The need to monitor

29

the use of data will pose additional requirements for data acquisition, coding, storage, and processing.

On all four levels, users may benefit from CPR data. Patient care centers on the use of individual patient data. On the level of departments or hospitals one is interested in information on a broader scale. Statistical reports and bills can automatically be generated on the basis of data contained in the patient record. On a higher level the benefit of CPR-coded data enables the generation of cost-efficiency reports, and the data can serve as input for management and planning. Examples of reports are the number of admissions and outpatients per department or specialty, disease profiles of in- and outpatients, the average cost per diagnostic category (e.g., per *diagnosis-related group*, see Chapter 6) or per type of intervention, or overviews generated as a func-

tion of resources and utilization of tests. Researchers, too, may benefit from the CPR by electronically retrieving information about patients according to specified criteria. The information retrieved can then be processed by statistical programs. The same holds for applications that are directed toward the assessment of the quality of care.

Network technology and communication (also called *telematics*) are now prominent developments in information technology and have a large impact on health care (see Chapter 5). By using standard communications networks and standard software, there is a more efficient data interchange between the four levels. A fully operational exchange of patient data between systems, with proper authorization, is one of the present challenges in health care.

3 Generic Structure of CPRs

In this chapter we discuss the structure of the CPR. A structured approach toward the CPR is required if the data contained in the CPR must be used at all four levels and for all four purposes mentioned above. Such a CPR should bear a *generic* character.

A long experience with developing CPR systems in many institutions has led to an increased insight into how future CPR systems might be constructed. In this section we describe some central elements of a CPR. In the following sections we sketch the requirements that a CPR should fulfill if it were to be used for the entire health care spectrum:

- First, the *structuring* of CPR data is described.
- Next, the issue of *time* in CPR data will be discussed.
- This is followed by the description of a *model* for CPRs.
- Finally, the way that patient data can be *entered* into a CPR is described.

Some countries, especially in Europe, have extensive experience with the introduction of CPRs in primary

care. The main lesson learned from that experience is the following: if CPR systems are not based on an explicit model and if CPR data are not well structured, then it will not be possible to use CPR data for different goals, nor can such data be exchanged between health care providers to support *shared care*. Data in CPRs are also used for *electronic data exchange*, research, and shared care. The use of CPRs for different purposes exposes the limitations of these CPRs. As experience is being accumulated, important lessons are being learned: particularly the need to develop structured patient records based on a clear conceptual model. This is the main reason for elaborating on structuring the CPR.

3.1 Structuring CPR Data

In this part we briefly allude to health care events in the patient history as documented in a CPR, relationships between patient data and clinicians' actions, different views on CPR data, and reliability of CPR data if they are to be used for different purposes.

29

3.1.1 Events

A patient record describes *events* as a function of time (Fig. 29.1). Examples of an event are a patient visit or a hospital admission. A surgical operation or the arrival of an X-ray report are also events. Each event contains different *data components* (e.g., patient history data, laboratory results, an *ECG*, an X-ray picture, a prescription, or a surgical report). All separate data components require some activity from the physicians, nursing staff, laboratory technicians, or systems. Therefore, the data components, which are the result of such activities, are called *actions*. In short, the events contain one or more actions, and actions may contain different data components. The different data are collected as a function of time during the diagnostic-therapeutic process, which gives a further ordering of the data in a patient record.

Events and their data components, the actions, repre-sent what the clinician *observed, thought,* and *did.* Therefore, events may contain data components pertaining to the three stages of the so-called *diagnostic-therapeutic cycle* (see Fig. 1.2 in Chapter 1): (1) observations, (2) decisions, and (3) interventions (therapies). Observations include complaints, findings, and test results and are descriptions (as objective as possible) of what the clinician has heard or seen. Examples of decisions are diagnoses or diagnostic hypotheses that require further examinations. Interventions encompass test orders, drug prescriptions, referrals, and other components of workup and treatment plans.

3.1.2 Relationships

Data on these three types often co-occur in patient records. Cardiac complaints may go together with ischemic *ST depressions* in the ECG, the prescription of an *ACE inhibitor* may be followed by side effects.

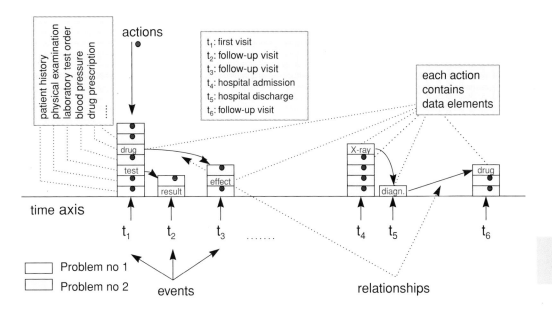

Figure 29.1

A computer-based patient record describes events as a function of time (e.g., a patient visit at time t_1 or a hospital admission at time t_4). Each event contains different actions (e.g., patient history taking, ordering a laboratory test, prescription of a drug). The actions result in data components (a blood pressure, diagnostic code, ECG, or an X-ray). The CPR should support the definition of links between the different components (indicated by arrows). Actions may be related to one or more problems by defining multiple links. The CPR should also support problem-oriented recording of patient data (not indicated in the graph).

When using patient data for, for example, medical auditing, it is important to have insight into how the data in the record are interrelated. These relationships are not self-evident; the temporal order will only tell part of the story. When treating their own patients, clinicians are often able to infer relevant relationships based on their personal acquaintance with the patient and on their medical knowledge and experience. Therefore, even when patient data are not complete, the treating clinician is often able to draw correct conclusions from the available patient data. This is, regretfully, not so when dealing with other patients, for example, after referral, or in situations of shared care, or when using the patient data in a large *database*. Studies have shown that ambiguous descriptions and missing data may hinder proper interpretation. Explicit recordings of indications for treatment and diagnostic tests are, for instance, essential for assessment of the quality of care.

Relationships between the data components are not necessarily defined by the mere fact that they may have the same time stamp. For instance, the result of an incoming laboratory test may be related to a request that was made during an earlier patient visit, and a prescription may pertain to a patient problem that was defined previously (Fig. 29.1). In addition, a patient may have different concurrent problems. Therefore, a CPR should support the definition of links between the components in the record. The issue of time is discussed separately in Section 3.2.

The user should be able to define different problems and to denote reasons why an intervention is done. Actions may then be related to one or more problems by defining multiple links. Actions can also be interlinked to each other, for example, by stating that "an *exercise ECG* was made because the patient showed signs of angina pectoris." The links between actions and patient problems reflect the clinician's *insight*. To make the process of care more transparent and to be able to use the data for multiple purposes, the context of patient data and possible relationships between the data must be made explicit in the CPR. Weed's *problem-oriented medical record* is an early example in which *semantics* are added to the patient record (see Chapters 6 and 7). By relating *SOAP* labels to a single problem, it becomes clear that subjective or objective observations (S and O), assessments or decisions (A),

and plans or interventions (P) are related to each other in the context of a problem.

3.1.3 Views

Certain data generally occur in every patient record: demographic data, signs and symptoms, current medications, test results, diagnostic assessments, and treatment plans. The partitioning of data into categories gives structure to a patient record, which can be called the *macro level*. At the *micro level* we discern the contents of the categories, such as actual complaints and findings. Categories are characterized by the procedure by which the patient data were acquired (laboratory, X-ray, ECG, etc.) and are, in fact, *source-oriented* views on the patient and the data contained in the patient record.

The *source-oriented* view is in contrast to and, in a way, *orthogonal* to the *problem-oriented* view. Both views are important to the clinician, but the fundamental difference between the two is that a source-oriented view is content-independent, whereas a problem-oriented view is not; problem-oriented views depend on semantic relationships between the data in the record, as indicated above. For example, in a source-oriented view, the result of a serum potassium analysis will always be located in the category "laboratory results," irrespective of its actual value. In the problem-oriented view, it might be related to a prescription for a diuretic (the serum potassium level is required to monitor a possible side effect of the diuretic), and its result (a low potassium level) might be an indication to change the drug regimen. Therefore, a problem-oriented view varies for each patient record, whereas the source-oriented view reflects the more general structure of a patient record. In other words, it lends itself to structuring the CPR. Data categories that are source oriented are hierarchically structured: "additional tests" may be subdivided into laboratory tests and X-rays. Progress notes may be subdivided in the patient history and physical examination categories. Differences in the

[1] Rector AL, Nowlan WA, Kay S et al. Foundations for an electronic medical record. *Meth Inform Med* 1991;30:179-86.

granularity of categories correspond to different levels in the same hierarchy.

The data views explained above are based in part on the work of Rector and colleagues[1], who distinguish two levels in the patient record:

- Level 1 encompasses facts from the clinician's observations, thoughts, and actions.
- Level 2 provides the links between the components at the first level to make explicit how they fit into the decision-making process and the clinical dialogue.

The explicit recording of indications for tests and treatments corresponds to the second level. The latter level provides the links to elucidate decision making. The items to be recorded should serve to provide a dynamic explanation. When interpretations are made explicit in relation to their underlying observations, this purpose is served with more clarity than by recording the interpretation alone. In the section on temporal aspects of CPR data (Section 2.2) we elaborate on this growing and possibly changing insight as a function of time.

3.1.4   Reliability

If computer-stored patient data are to be used for many purposes and by different health care professionals, then the **reliability** of patient data is of utmost importance. CPR systems should improve data reliability with **validity checks** and stimulate completeness *during* data entry (see Section 3.4, Data Entry). In clinical practice, clinicians do not record everything that occurred, but only record those data that they consider *relevant* at the time of recording. Relevance is subjective, but, regretfully, insight only comes after a series of events have taken place, not beforehand. Fortunately, experienced clinicians are able early on to identify events that might be relevant for future patient care. However, if people other than the clinician who entered the data will use the patient data at a later stage (e.g., in situations of shared care; see Section 3.3), then at data entry the clinician should be encouraged to enter complete data, and the system may assist with checking the consistency and the reliability of the data.

3.2   Temporal Aspects of CPRs

The patient record not only consists of different categories of data but is also a *chronological* account of observations, interpretations, and interventions. Time is present in medical knowledge and facts, it is absolute or relative, and it may vary greatly in precision. Time may be expressed in *absolute* terms ("July 4th 1996, 6:04 p.m."), as a *relative* expression ("1 month after"), or as a *duration* ("lasted 10 seconds"). Relative time is used in the context of medical knowledge, such as a disease description or a clinical protocol. Facts may also involve relative time, especially when a patient or a physician describes the progress of disease: "the pain lasted for two hours," or "I started to feel nauseous one hour after eating an omelet." Absolute time is usually found in the context of events, such as an operation or a myocardial infarction. The degree of granularity of time varies. A patient may have undergone cardiac surgery in 1995, a chest X-ray in May 1996, or the recording of an ECG after an impending infarction at 11:15 a.m., on June 6th, 1996. Which granularity is appropriate depends on the medical context. In a coronary care unit, minutes or seconds may be important, whereas for the assessment of the effect of antihypertensive drugs, months are appropriate.

For automated interpretation of temporal relationships between data in the patient record, time stamps need to be recorded in a standardized format. Time stamps in patient records are often inaccurate or incomplete. Temporal inaccuracy means that the true moment of an event lies within an *interval*. A time stamp, such as March 5th, 1996, denotes the entire 24-hour period of the 5th of March. The required precision of temporal data will vary according to the use of these data.

Although the insight of the physician may grow or evolve over time, patient data, once collected, may not be changed at some later date, nor is it permitted to overwrite decisions documented in the past. This would have severe legal implications if this were done. In medical auditing, for instance, it is important to know when the physician was informed about an event and could be expected to have included it in his or her medical considerations.

29

The CPR should, however, allow clinicians to document their new insight in the patient record when they later change their opinions on the basis of new evidence or better insight. Therefore, a CPR should permit the labeling of the CPR with three time stamps on data related to an event:

1. the moment when the data are entered,
2. the moment when the insight is gained, and
3. the moment when the insight became applicable.

For instance, a patient visits the GP on April 1st because of thirstiness. Because of the raised blood sugar level the GP suspects diabetes mellitus. On April 10th, another blood sample is taken at a specialized laboratory for further assessment of the patient's hormone levels. The GP receives the result by mail on April 20th. The GP now diagnoses with certainty that the patient has suffered from Cushing's disease since the 10th of April (when the blood sample was taken). Because it is probable that the patient suffered from Cushing's disease at the time of the first visit, the GP may enter in the CPR that it is considered that the patient had the disease from April 1st onward, but certainly on April 10th. This sequence of events is shown graphically in Fig. 29.2. In case the patient was treated for diabetes after the first visit, this cannot be blamed on the GP, because at that time the GP had no evidence of Cushing's disease. Different time stamps are

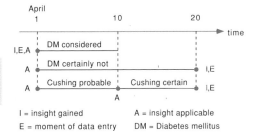

| April |
| 1   10   20 |

I = insight gained   A = insight applicable
E = moment of data entry   DM = Diabetes mellitus

Figure 29.2
Example of how clinicians may change their insight regarding a diagnosis. The assignment of an expression of certainty should be expressed with each diagnosis, together with the specification of the time period when the insight applies.

therefore of importance for building a record for *evidence-based medicine.*

3.3 Models for CPR Data Representation

Patient data in CPRs must be structured so that they are usable for purposes other than only patient care by the treating clinician. The requirements, in short, are as follows:

1. Data should reflect *events* during the different stages of the diagnostic-therapeutic loop: observations, decisions, and interventions.
2. Each event contains different *actions* that reflect some activity by all people (or systems) involved in patient care. The actions contain different data elements.
3. Actions may belong to one or more *patient problems.* The *semantic relationships* between the different data elements should be documented.
4. All data should have a *time stamp,* because the documentation of actions at one particular moment may not give sufficient information for evidence-based medicine.
5. Data should be collected with *multiple purposes* in mind: patient care, shared care, and assessment by others. Different *views* on the data should be possible.
6. At the stage of data entry, *completeness* should be promoted and the *reliability* of the data should be checked.

These different purposes require a general approach to the documentation of patient data in a CPR, involving a knowledge model that defines which data and which expressions are allowed and operational instantiations of that knowledge that represent the actual patient data.

The structure of a CPR along the lines explained above is totally hidden from the clinician who uses the system. However, as soon as she or he requires some functionality from the system other than for direct patient care, the advantages and limitations of a system will become apparent. One of the most important aspects of such a system is the way that the user interacts with the system, and structured data entry is a crucial part of this interaction. For that reason data entry is discussed in the following section.

3.4 Data Entry

For a CPR to have benefits, the data in that record need to be, at least to a certain degree, structured and coded. Obtaining structured and coded data, however, has proven to be a significant hurdle. Clinicians are accustomed to paper-based records. How clinicians use these records has been the subject of a number of European projects. From such investigations it became apparent that clinicians are far more lenient in using computers for consultation of data in patient records than for patient data entry. This is not surprising: Data entry requires more effort from the clinician than browsing through the record. Some researchers have argued that direct input by clinicians must wait for radical improvements to the human-machine interface, such as speech input.

Views on CPR data, for patient care, decision support, scientific data analysis, or assessment of the quality of care require patient data to be highly structured and unambiguous. It is extremely difficult to fulfill these requirements with narrative (textual) data. Ideally, therefore, patient data should be acquired directly from the clinician in a structured format and should preferably also be entered by the clinician herself or himself. To accomplish this, two different approaches to *data entry* will be addressed: *natural language processing* and *structured data entry*. The last two methods are the focus of several research projects, also in Europe. We complete the following overview of data entry by summarizing experience with *patient-driven data entry*.

3.4.1 Natural Language Processing

Natural language processing (NLP) is intended to automatically extract coded medical data from free text. European research in this area has mainly been done by Baud and colleagues and by Sager and Friedman in the United States. The basic advantage of NLP is that clinicians do not have to alter the way in which they express their findings or document their decisions. In principle, they may continue to use audiotapes or manually written text, although both are prone to transcription errors. Ideally, computerized **speech recognition** may also be applied. NLP makes use of knowledge about textual **syntax**, frequently used terms, and **semantics** in the medical domain. Only when its application domain is strictly confined can NLP offer advantages. A fundamental disadvantage of NLP is that the data-capturing process itself cannot be influenced and improved. Data that the clinician has not written or spoken remain unknown. Freedom of expression is inherent to free text. Therefore, it is difficult to impose structure on data that are used as input for NLP.

3.4.2 Structured Data Entry

Another mode of data entry is context sensitive and is adaptable to different clinical domains. It is called structured data entry (SDE) and consists of forms of which the content is knowledge driven. In an SDE-oriented European project, the forms are structured, but their contents can continuously be adapted to accommodate the user's requirements and personal preferences. Besides a knowledge model, the system contains a predefined vocabulary (see Section 2.3 above) and specifications on how the terms of the vocabulary may be combined into meaningful expressions. During data entry, the system "intelligently" follows the user input, and, on the basis of the knowledge contained in the model, it generates the most appropriate questions to be asked. The level of detail of the forms is fully determined by the user. This method can be characterized as **knowledge-driven structured data entry** (see Moorman et al).

SDE is also an efficient tool for enhancing data completeness and testing for data reliability. Yet, all structured methods including SDE, however "intelligent" they may be, are hampered by intrinsic limitations. For this reason, all data entry methods should also contain escape routes to allow for the expression of observations, events, or actions in free text. Narrative data may have low scientific relevance but may be useful for patient care. Graphics and voice input may also serve

29

to enhance the capabilities of SDE.

Data entry based on descriptive medical knowledge has several advantages: Its level of flexibility is high and the maintenance effort is relatively low. It must be realized that data entry and data *retrieval* are fundamentally different tasks. During data entry, flexibility is what counts; during data retrieval, data must be accessible in a consistent way, although different kinds of views should be permitted. Research in knowledge-based SDE methods may result in interfaces that fulfill both of these requirements.

3.4.3 Patient-Driven Data Entry

We complete this overview of activities in the field of data entry by outlining research that has been done on *patient-driven data* entry. This is not illogical now that increasing numbers of patients are acquainted with computers and growing numbers are connected to the **Internet** at home. The crucial question is whether a patient-driven patient interview may partly replace a clinician interview or precede it.

Ever since computers first made their appearance in health care, attempts have been made to use them to support patient history taking. Before interactive equipment became available, many techniques were used to acquire primary patient data with or without the assistance of a physician or a nurse, such as coding sheets, **mark-sense** forms, **punched cards**, sortable pictures or cards, audio- and videotapes, and so on. Later on, some interaction between computer and patient became

possible, first by the use of typewriter terminals, next by *visual display units*, and now by *PCs*.

Few studies have been done to investigate the impact of the computer-based patient history on diagnosis and therapy. It was investigated whether paper-based patient interviews completed by clinicians and computer-based interviews (constructed as a set of forms with multiple-choice questions) completed by patients themselves contained identical patient data and complaints. It was also investigated whether the diagnostic hypotheses generated on the basis of either the computer-based interviews or the clinicians' interviews were comparable (see Quaak et al).

It appeared that patient histories entered by patients themselves are much more complete than written histories based on oral interviews. However, although the patient history completed by the patient contained more *data*, it contained less *information* than the clinician interview. Diagnostic hypotheses formulated on the basis of a computer-based patient history were considered by clinicians to have a higher degree of certainty (38%) than hypotheses generated from paper-based records (26%). It seems that **computer-based history taking** by patients themselves can be recommended for certain patients (first referral, chronic diseases, and follow-up), but should precede and not replace the oral interview. This is an interesting finding, because in the future, home care will be encouraged in all countries, and electronic communication will penetrate the homes of all citizens.

4 Realization of CPR Systems

4.1 CPR Systems in Primary Care

In some countries, especially in The Netherlands and the United Kingdom, there is a rapid increase in the use of information systems by GPs in primary care. CPRs are incorporated in these information systems and are quickly replacing existing paper-based

records. The use of CPRs, especially by GPs, is rapidly gaining ground. In 1996 it was estimated that more than 90% of all GPs in The Netherlands and in the United Kingdom used information systems in their practices, with a large percentage using CPRs. This is directly related to the fact that in both countries GPs are the "*gatekeepers*" in health care. Most GPs run a practice by themselves or with a small number of colleagues. In contrast, specialists work in large institutions in a more complex setting, involving a much larger number of departments and personnel. Furthermore, GPs keep less extensive records so that data entry is less time consuming and less detailed.

The actual situation in primary care offers a good example of both the success and the potential of the use CPRs. This can be attributed to the four factors described below.

1. Role of GPs

Professional organizations of GPs have played an active role in setting guidelines for information systems in general practice and in assessing the systems available on the market. Furthermore, they announced to industry that they would recommend to their members only those systems that would meet their requirements. In this way a de facto standard was established. Since then, systems requirements are regularly refined and extended, and vendors must submit their systems for reevaluation by professional organizations. This iterative way of refinement of guidelines and assessment of systems gives potential buyers of systems a basis on which to judge the available information systems and gives vendors clear-cut guidelines that their products must meet. Definition of guidelines started with requirements for patient administration and evolved into guidelines for diagnostic coding (in all systems the **ICPC** has been implemented, see Chapter 6), guidelines for drug prescriptions (all systems use the same national **thesaurus** for drugs), guidelines for the type of data to be contained in a basic CPR, and requirements for electronically interchanging patient data between different systems in primary care, that is, from one GP's system to that of another GP (see Chapter 5).

2. Training

The success of information systems is largely determined by the clinicians' expectations. Education at universities nowadays prepares clinicians in the use of computer-based information systems and CPRs. Also, the professional organizations have ensured that postgraduate training of GPs conveys a realistic set of expectations (if expectations are too high, they lead to disillusionment; if they are too low, they may impede the introduction of new systems). The training emphasizes that proper use of systems and CPRs reduces administrative workload; increases the accuracy of billing (no accountable patient data are lost), and enables the production of referral letters, the use of **electronic data interchange**, and the tracking of certain categories of patients. Potential users should realize that, certainly at the beginning, investments must be made. These investments can be expressed not only in financial terms but also in time and personal efforts. For instance, for a typical practice with about 2,500 patients, it takes about 2 years before all patient data have been entered into the system's CPR. This data transcription from paper to computer is generally done when patients come for a consultation, since the majority of patients pay a visit to their GP once in 2 years. A GP who is just starting to use a CPR system needs an extra 2 to 3 minutes during a consultation. The GP's assistant prepares all administrative operations, such as patient admission, patient scheduling, and so forth, but GPs themselves enter the patient care-related data into the CPR.

3. Structure of Health Care

The two factors described above are, perhaps, easily transferable to most countries; the third factor, however, is strongly related to the structure of health care in the United Kingdom and The Netherlands, and, for example, Canada and the Scandinavian countries. Patients in The Netherlands and the United Kingdom have a single GP who coordinates their health care, acting as a gatekeeper to other specialists; the latter report back to the GP. Several projects are now under way to use electronic data interchange for this GP-specialist communication (see Chapter 5). Thus, the GP coordinates the health care-related data of a single patient, in principle over his or her lifetime, and is requested by other specialists to share the patient's information. The GP's role as coordinator eases the introduction of CPR systems because the demands of care are easier to meet when the data are available in electronic form.

4. Population-Based Care

A fourth reason for the success of accepting CPRs is when primary care is also population based, in contrast to institution or clinician based. Such population-based orientations create demands that are easier to

29

meet when CPRs are introduced. For instance, the use of a *gender-age register* to report on statistics in primary care or active case finding, for example, for periodic cervical smears or cardiovascular risk, are much facilitated by having CPRs with properly coded data. The same applies to studies on the use and effects of drugs in the population (*postmarketing surveillance of drugs*).

4.2 CPR Systems in Hospitals

Information technology has been introduced in many hospitals. This is no longer restricted to special areas of care only, such as radiology or the laboratory (Chapter 13). In principle, we now have technology that allows central and *monolithic* hospital information systems to be transformed into hospital-wide *networks* with "intelligent" *workstations* or PCs all over the hospital, up to the consultation room and close to the bedside. At present, graphical workstations and network technology are leading developments in the computer industry. *Client-server* protocols ease the integration of systems and the distribution of processing tasks. Workstations offer, in principle, an environment that make all applications, running either locally or through a network, act as a single integrated system from the user's perspective. In several institutions promising developments in health care workstations, enabling integration of patient data that are scattered over different systems, are under way. In principle, such systems offer the clinician on one computer screen patient data, images, and biosignals, on whatever computer they are stored and on whatever system they are processed.

While the technical issues involved in the integration of various systems are being solved, the absence of a *conceptual model* for a CPR may become a major stumbling block. Technical integration alone, although a necessity for a CPR, does not facilitate the *navigation* through that information. As the amount of available data increases, the need to provide a conceptual data model increases accordingly. Thus, there emerges the trend in which a technical infrastructure (the platform for the CPR) takes care of the communication with

the numerous systems available in the hospital. At the core of this integration platform, CPRs are developed. This distinction is not trivial. When developing the platforms, questions such as how to embed an already existing system are addressed on a technical level. On the level of CPR development, questions are, for example: "How do we present the data to the user in a consistent manner," or "What additional data must the clinician record?" We address two important issues: the *platform* for the CPR and the hierarchical structure of a clinical CPR.

4.2.1 Platforms for CPRs

Clinical workstations that offer an environment for systems integration do exist. Communication between applications is automatically arranged for by the workstation and follows *ISO* standards. Instead of having one large central database of patient data, all existing databases and applications are left unchanged and patient data are combined on demand. This has advantages compared with building one large integrated database:

1. data can be distributed and remain stored at places that are most convenient (i.e., close to where the data are collected and used), and
2. commercially available applications can be used for data processing without modifying them.

Such platforms for systems integration generally operate in a *UNIX* or a *Windows* environment. In the last few years, the Internet – in particular the *WWW* – is receiving attention for interface development. The advantage of Web applications is their platform independence: only a widespread Web *browser* is required to use them.

4.2.2 Structure of Clinical CPRs

A CPR for group practices or health care organizations should be based on two main principles:

1. There must be one *central clinical CPR* for the entire clinical department or, preferably, the entire organization. This central clinical CPR is extended

with subrecords, each fulfilling the requirements of a specific domain of care.

2. The CPR structure must support *flexible consultation*, efficient data entry, data analysis, and decision support. Flexibility is important in many respects; even though every specialist has his or her own domain, he or she will probably be confronted with findings outside one's direct field of expertise.

Whereas the subrecords may be designed to meet the needs within a specific domain of care, the central record is intended to provide a place to record all findings for which no explicit subrecord has been created. The availability of a generic model for the different CPRs (central or specialized) is essential for the structured representation of patient data, as well as for a reliable interpretation and analysis of patient data. The clinical CPRs should follow the demands (as outlined in Section 2) described above for the requirements of a generic CPR.

5 Use of CPR Data

To illustrate the use of patient data in CPRs for goals other than direct patient care, we give two examples of applications in which CPR data are used: for decision support, and for the assessment of the quality of care. Finally, some remarks are made on the clinician's responsibility in using CPR data instead of data from paper-based patient records.

5.1 Decision Support

Some projects have investigated whether CPRs contain sufficient information to support decision making by generating critiques with **critiquing systems**. This was done, for instance, by critiquing the treatment of hypertension and chronic obstructive respiratory diseases. Both systems rely on CPRs to obtain patient data.

The critiquing systems generate comments in a two-stage process. First, CPR data are automatically interpreted to review the actions of the GP at a given visit (e.g., starting a new drug, continuing treatment with a drug, or replacing one drug with another drug). Second, each action is assessed. The system searches the CPR for conditions that contraindicate that action (e.g., **contraindications** to specific drugs), determines whether preparations required for the action have been performed, determines whether the GP has performed the routine monitoring required by the action, and searches for any undesirable condition that might have resulted from the action. Reviewing the CPR requires detailed knowledge about drugs, such as on customary dosages, contraindications, side effects, interactions, workup requirements, and criteria for judging the efficacy of the treatment. In the limited area of mild hypertension, computer-based critiquing of care was compared with critiquing by peer review. The comparisons revealed the following:

1. Automated assessment of CPR data by the critiquing system could compete successfully with peer review.
2. The system was not able to reproduce some comments of experts. This was caused either by insufficient CPR data, by the absence of sufficient medical consensus, or by omissions in the knowledge base of the critiquing system.

On the basis of the outcomes of this and other studies reported in the literature, the following can be concluded:

1. Systems for the assessment of patient care should be able to acquire patient data automatically from the CPR.
2. Ideally, the care assessment system should be functionally integrated with the CPR system.

5.2 Quality Assessment

It is to be expected that CPRs will also be increasingly used for the assessment of the quality of care in practices, departments, and institutions and, for instance, for the support of postmarketing surveillance (PMS) studies. Pressure from law-enforcing bodies, third-party payers, peer-review organizations, hospitals, clinicians, and patients themselves may lead to this use of automated review of CPRs. An example of the use of data in CPRs is *PMS* of drugs.

PMS is the research into the beneficial and adverse side effects of drugs on human health, starting from the moment that these drugs are marketed. PMS consists of two stages: a hypothesis generation stage in which a side effect is suspected and a hypothesis verification stage in which the hypothesis is tested. Hypothesis generation is typically based on spontaneous reporting of potential side effects by clinicians. Studies, however, have shown that this spontaneous reporting leaves much to be desired. For instance, in some studies it was shown that computerized monitoring of adverse drug events in hospitals, using computer-stored patient data, offers many advantages over voluntary reporting of such events.

5.3 Clinicians' Responsibilities

Now that CPR data are becoming available for the different goals mentioned in the Introduction to this chapter, it is of great importance to protect the data, to guard the *privacy* of patients, and to protect the professional interests of health care professionals. In the different European countries, privacy laws exist to control health care data (see Chapter 34). Yet, it will be difficult to totally prevent the improper use of data stored in CPRs.

When patient data are stored in CPRs it is important to discern between *permanent* and *variable* patient data. Many parties (employers, insurance companies, etc.) are interested in patient data and so the data should be extremely well protected in CPR systems. In Europe there may be more sensitivity toward improper use of patient data than elsewhere; it could even impede the introduction of CPRs in some countries and for some purposes or hamper the use of CPR data for goals other than patient care alone.

Medical data can be categorized into *permanent* data

(e.g., one's genetic profile) and *variable* data (e.g., a blood pressure). The protection of the data in the first category is perhaps the most privacy-prone. Generally, the use of these two types of data is also different: variable medical data (including **alphanumeric** data, biological signals and pictures) are primarily used for the diagnosis and treatment of transient diseases, whereas permanent data are often strongly related to an individual's life and may possibly predict his or her future health. The latter category is also of interest for one's next of kin: parents, siblings, and children. Genetic data, for instance, do not change or age; they are valid for an entire lifetime.

Both the patient and the clinician must be protected against improper, let alone illegal, use of computer-stored medical data. Privacy implies several issues. For instance, it means the "right to be left alone," but it also signifies that everyone is entitled to decide for himself or herself how, when, and to what degree others may dispose of one's data, including one's medical data. In many countries, this right has been incorporated into law. In Europe it has been anchored in the *Treaty for the Protection of Human Rights and Fundamental Freedom.*

Essentially, the privacy of the patient is guarded by the clinician's professional obligation to keep his or her patient's medical data secret. This secrecy is also a right of a patient; a patient should be able to transfer all medical information to his or her clinician without fearing that the clinician will pass these data to third parties without the patient's approval. This professional secrecy is regulated by the laws of most countries.

If clinicians want to fulfill their responsibilities to guard the patient data, they should ensure that the data are well protected. This entails the use of measures against loss, theft, or damage; against unintended abuse and false interpretations; and also against intended abuse and misuse. The latter also includes the fact that medical data should not be unjustly used for purposes other than for which they were collected without the consent of the provider of the data. To accomplish this, measures are required to address the legal and scientific (e.g., prevent data from being improperly used and interpreted), technical (e.g., safeguarding the data against damage or fire), software (such as the use of **passwords**, **auditing trails**, confined functionality, and *encryption*), and hardware (e.g., use of *backups* and double installation of essential parts such as disks) aspects.

Because modern health care provision often requires *shared care* instead of care by a single clinician only, the individual clinician is no longer capable of personally guaranteeing the patient's privacy. For that reason, after the regulation of professional secrecy, modern societies must lay down the right to privacy. This means that in the different countries, for all automated registrations of personal data, including patient data, written regulations must be required, and these

regulations should be supervised by a privacy committee. These regulations should contain descriptions of the purpose of the registration, the disposal of data to third parties, and the right of all people concerned to inspect, alter and destroy their data. In principle, these regulations do not concern *anonymous data*.

It is of utmost importance that in all future CPR systems proper measures be taken to protect the privacy of patients and to protect the data. This issue is also the subject of discussions at the European level, for example, in the standardization committees that were established for health care informatics and telematics (see Chapter 34).

6 Final Remarks

From what has been discussed in this chapter, consider the following.

- Benefits

CPR data may benefit health care either directly or indirectly. Directly, they serve patient care itself; indirectly, they can be used for the assessment of care, biomedical research, education, and health care management. Patient care benefits from the fact that computer-stored patient data can be rapidly accessed, wherever they are stored, and can be shared among care providers; by the generation of referral letters and discharge summaries; by the generation of critiques, reminders, or warnings; and by advising clinicians via integrated protocols and decision support. Although in some countries GPs have been eager to introduce CPRs in their practices, clinicians have generally been slow to accept CPRs in their practices. With new generations of clinicians who are familiar with information technology from childhood onward, this attitude will rapidly change.

- Integration

A CPR can be introduced as a separate software package, but it should preferably be implemented within a context of all kinds of other practice-support subsystems, such as for patient administration and scheduling, correspondence and electronic data interchange, drug prescription and laboratory reports, statistical

overviews, access to images, *biosignals* and diagnostic function reports. It should also generate reminders and warnings, allow for case retrieval, and give access to the literature. A CPR should ideally replace the paper-based record; only then can it become fully accepted.

- Structuring

In all CPRs, structured data entry is most essential. If data are not structured the CPR is decreased to, at best, an "intelligent" *word processor*. It should be realized that until data entry has become truly "intelligent," that is, when the system "understands" what the clinician-user intends to say, there remains a certain tension between standardization and structure versus the time that it takes to enter the data.

- Barriers

The introduction of a CPR in clinical practice is inhibited not by the present technology but by the great variety of specialized care, the existing differences in culture between different clinics and (particularly in Europe) between different countries. Only flexible and user-adaptable generic models for the generation of a CPR may help to overcome these problems. Specialized health care institutes, where there is a continuous introduction of new insights and methods, render the maintenance of a CPR very complex. A last issue is

29

how in a clinical setting an old, paper-based situation can be transformed into a new, computer-based environment. This transformation deals not only with technological problems and the entering of written patient data into computer databases, but also with the logistics of the transformation process and psychological and social barriers. Training of users is essential to making this transformation successful. Finally, there is the financial aspect. It should be investigated whether there is a favorable balance between investments and benefits. The question is whether the person or the health care institute that makes the investment also receives most of the benefits.

Key References

Dick RS, Steen EB, eds. *The Computer-based Patient Record. An Essential Technology for Health Care.* Washington DC: National Academy Press, 1991 (first ed.) and 1997 (second ed.).

Baud RH, Rassinoux AM, Scherrer JR. Natural language processing and semantical representation of medical texts. Meth Inform Med 1992;31:117-25.

Sager N, Lynman M, Tick LJ, Ngo TN, Bucknall CE. Natural language processing of asthma discharge summaries for the monitoring of patient care. In: Safran C, ed. *Proceedings of the 17th Symposium in Computer Applications in Medical Care.* New York: McGraw-Hill, 1993:269-73.

Rector AL, Nowlan WA, Kay S, Goble CA, Howkins TJ. A framework for modelling the electronic medical record. Meth Inform Med 1993;32:109-19.

Quaak MJ, Westerman RF, van Bemmel J.H. Comparisons between written and computerized patient histories, patient complaints and diagnostic hypotheses. BMJ 1987;295:184-90.

Moorman PW, van Ginneken AM, van der Lei J, van Bemmel JH. A model for structured data entry based on explicit descrip-tional knowledge. Meth Inform Med 1994;33:454-63.

See the Web site for further literature references.

29

30 Evaluation of Clinical Information Systems

1 Introduction

This chapter introduces the reader to a very broad topic: the evaluation of clinical information systems and their impact on clinical attitudes, decisions, and actions. For the purpose of this chapter, we define *evaluation* as "measuring or describing something, usually with a question in mind."

1.1 Why Evaluate?

Although engineers in some disciplines, such as civil engineering, can rather confidently predict the performance of an *artifact*, such as a bridge, this is not always so with information systems, especially if they are complex. Thus, empirical evaluation is required to understand system performance. This is even more true when we recall that the purpose of clinical information systems is to improve clinical performance and patient outcomes. We cannot predict how an information system will influence complex human and organizational behaviors, so we must measure them empirically. This means that evaluation is important for both the certification of clinical information systems by bodies such as the *Food and Drug Administration* in the United States, and for medicolegal reasons: Clinicians would be unwise to use any system unless it has been shown to be safe and effective. A final reason for evaluating clinical information systems is that it is our only method for advancing the science of medical informatics. Unless we perform evaluations, we cannot hope to improve our theories about what works and why.

1.2 Subjectivist and Objectivist Approaches to Evaluation

As suggested in the definition of evaluation given above, there are two complementary approaches to evaluation, and these approaches reflect different attitudes to the world as we see it.

One approach, the subjectivist or qualitative approach, aims to describe the world and the information systems in it as they appear to individual people. The emphases in such studies are careful, unbiased observation, the identification of themes or questions as they emerge from study subjects, and attempts to confirm and refine these by further observation. Such studies use ethnographic techniques such as analysis of documents, structured and unstructured interviews, participant observation, and video analysis. Data are painstakingly collected and analyzed by well-documented techniques, and a report is drafted in collaboration with the people under observation. Such methods are often used at the two extremes of system development: to help define user requirements and to assess the impact of an installed system on the experience of individual users and the organization in which they work.

The alternative, the objectivist approach, assumes that there are truths in the world that, given satisfactory measurement methods, can be recorded and that all rational people or judges will agree to these truths. To formalize this approach, objectivists believe that there are *objects* in the world (e.g., information systems or clinicians) that have real but unobservable **attributes** (e.g., diagnostic accuracy) which *judges* can infer by observing one or more *items* of information (e.g., the system's advice for each of 100 test cases). Much work by psychometricians and others has led to "classical measurement theory", which describes how to select and improve the items of information (e.g., questions on a questionnaire) and how many cases or judges need to be used to achieve a given reliability.

1.3 The Range of Evaluation Techniques

Given the fundamental importance of evaluation to medical informatics, it is hardly surprising that many techniques are available and many disciplines are involved. These range from needs assessment exercises carried out by medical informaticians and ethnographers to calculation of the **cost effectiveness** of installed information systems by health economists. Table 30.1 lists some of the common techniques that are used.

1.4 General Framework for an Objectivistic Evaluation Study

To perform a satisfactory objectivistic study, investigators must complete the following stages:

- define and prioritize study questions,
- define the "system" to be studied,
- select or develop reliable, valid measurement methods,
- design the demonstration study:
  - design a descriptive, correlational, or comparative study,
  - eliminate potential **bias**, and
  - ensure that study findings can be generalized;
- carry out the study, and
- analyze and report the results.

These stages are discussed in the section that follows.

2 Planning and Executing an Objectivistic Evaluation Study

2.1 Defining and Prioritizing Study Questions

As discussed above, there are many stages in system development, each with corresponding evaluation methods and relevant study questions. Without a list of prioritized questions, it is hard to evaluate a system. The questions and the resources available for answer-

ing them depend on who is asking and who is funding the evaluation study. For example, **software engineers** are unlikely to be concerned with measuring cost effectiveness, whereas health service managers are. Evaluators must be sensitive to the differing concerns of various stakeholders in a project and help each group of stakeholders to define the questions of most interest to them. It is up to the stakeholders to merge their lists and give the evaluator a finalized set of questions in priority order.

Table 30.1
Range of Evaluation Techniques Available.

Technique	What it measures	Who carries it out
Needs Assessment	Describes information problems amenable to support	Ethnographer, medical informatician, software designer
Informal Assessment	Function, potential value	Development team
Verification	Static aspects of system against its specification	Software engineer
Validation	Dynamic aspects of system against user requirements	Systems analyst, software designer
Laboratory Tests of Performance	System performance on new test cases *in vitro*	Medical informatician, external experts / judges
Laboratory Tests of Usability and Impact	Usability, impact on users' decisions in the laboratory	Medical informatician, psychologist, users
Field Tests of Usability, Performance, and Impact	System usability, performance *in vivo*; impact on users' actions, patient outcomes	Medical informatician, clinical epidemiologist, statistician, users, patients
Organizational Impact Study	Effects of system on organization, hierarchies, and relationships	Ethnographer, occupational psychologist, users, patients
Cost Effectiveness Analysis	Cost of system per procedure assisted	Health economist

2.2 Defining the "System" to be Studied

It may seem that an information system is well-defined, but often this is not so. A classic example is the **Leeds Abdominal Pain System** (see also Chapter 16), a **Bayes**ian decision-support system (**DSS**, see Chapter 15) used for emergency room patients suspected of having appendicitis. Patient data were captured by clinicians on a one-page paper questionnaire and then entered by a research assistant. During an evaluation of its impact on diagnostic accuracy it was found that using the paper questionnaire alone improved diagnostic accuracy by 10%; in addition, when clinicians were given monthly feedback about their performance by using these data, their performance improved by a further 10%. The computer-generated advice contributed an average of only 4% more to diagnostic accuracy, so it would have been misleading to claim that the 24% overall improvement in accuracy was due to the computer's advice.

A similar question arises when evaluating **telemedicine**. It makes little sense to compare telemedical consultations with conventional consultations, because a closer analogy would be to mail a Polaroid photograph or video of the patient to the specialist and conduct a two-way discussion by telephone. Thus, to assess the contribution due solely to interactive **videoconferencing**, this should be compared to a scheduled phone discussion of a mailed video or Polaroid pictures.

30

2.3 Selecting or Developing Reliable, Valid Measurement Methods

In the study of the Leeds Abdominal Pain System described above, the crucial question was whether the system improved the admitting clinicians' diagnostic accuracy. Since it was relatively simple to record the admitting clinician's diagnosis for each patient, diagnostic accuracy was taken as the number of patients for whom the clinician made a certain diagnosis divided by the number of cases in whom this was the true diagnosis. However, the true diagnosis was not always clear. It was obviously impossible to carry out a postmortem examination for every patient because only a small proportion died, so the investigators came up with an alternative method of measuring the correct diagnosis, or a *"gold standard."* They chose to use the patient's discharge diagnosis, which was usually informed by several days of observation, the opinion of a consulting surgeon, and the results of laboratory tests and X-rays.

Although this seems reasonable, we still need to know whether this discharge diagnosis was reliable and valid. The words "reliable" and "valid" are crucial. *Reliable* means that the measurement method produces similar results, irrespective of who measures it or when – assuming that the quantity being measured is static. This means that the within- and between-observer *variability* should be low. The within-observer variability could have been measured by asking the original surgeon to review the same notes and record the discharge diagnosis a few weeks later, without seeing the original diagnosis. Between-observer variability would mean asking another surgeon to review the notes and record the diagnosis, without seeing the first surgeon's diagnosis. *Validity* assesses how much the measurement result reflects what it is intended to measure, for example, diagnostic accuracy. To be sure that a measurement is valid, it must be compared to a gold standard, which for diagnostic accuracy might be the results of a postmortem examination. Although we cannot carry out this gold standard test for every patient, the investiga-

tors could have compared the discharge diagnosis with the diagnosis made at the postmortem examination for the small proportion of patients who did die, to assess the validity of the discharge diagnosis.

This illustrates a general evaluation problem: Making reliable, valid measurements is hard. Sometimes, a validated method can be used, unchanged, to make measurements in an evaluation study. This might be a questionnaire or some other measurement "instrument" that has previously been shown to have satisfactory reliability and validity. However, in medical informatics we are usually measuring properties of information systems or their impacts on clinicians and cannot rely on finding a published instrument. This means that we must often develop our own instrument. Once we have developed it, we need to conduct "measurement studies" to show that our new technique is indeed reliable and valid. To allow others to benefit from this work, we should strive to publish a description of the technique and the results of our measurement study as a service to the field. Only when we are satisfied with our measurement technique can we go on to use it to answer the evaluation questions in appropriately designed demonstration studies.

2.4 Designing the Demonstration Study

The aim of a demonstration study is to answer the questions about the information system posed by the stakeholders. These questions are answered by analyzing variables of two types. The main variable of interest is the dependent variable, for example, the clinicians' diagnostic accuracy in the example given above. The independent variables are the other variables that may be relevant to the question, for example, the kind of decision support that was available to the clinician.

2.4.1 Descriptive, Correlational, and Comparative Studies

To answer evaluation questions, three kinds of demonstration study can be performed:

30

Table 30.2
Common Bias in Demonstration Studies.

Name of biases	Mechanism	How to eliminate / measure it
Volunteer Effect	Volunteers perform better than others	Recruit a random sample of users, patients
Assessment Bias	Knowledge of gold standard or system output may influence judges' decisions	Blind judges to gold standard, system's output, whether the system was used in this case
Placebo Effect	Patients' symptoms improve if "high tech" computers are present	Measure objective outcomes; provide computers to control patients / clinicians
Checklist Effect	Performance improves if clinicians use a checklist	Provide checklist to control group
Hawthorne Effect	Performance improves if clinicians know they are being studied	Conduct low-profile baseline study; use balanced incomplete block design
Carryover Effect (contamination)	Clinicians learn from the system, so performance improves on control cases	Randomize clinicians or clinical teams, not patients
Allocation and Recruitment Bias	Clinicians may fail to recruit a patient if they know that they will be a control case	Ensure patients are recruited before it is known if they are a control or computer case
Data Completeness Bias	More data are collected in computer versus control cases, so assessment is more accurate	Ensure same data are collected in control and computer cases
Secular Trends	Known or unknown changes over time may influence dependent variable	Randomize patients or clinicians to use of the information system; avoid before-after studies

- Descriptive study, describing the attributes of an object or a class of objects (e.g., counting the number of questions asked by a DSS, or the accuracy of a DSS). Here there are no independent variables.
- Correlational study, comparing two or more measured quantities and attempting to correlate them without attributing cause and effect (e.g., exploring how clinicians' perceptions of the perceived usability of a DSS varies with the number of questions that it asks). Technically, we are attempting to correlate changes in the dependent variable with changes in the independent variables.
- Comparative study, comparing the properties of two objects (e.g., the accuracy of two DSSs) or one object in two states (e.g., a clinician unaided versus a clinician aided by a DSS), often to attribute cause and effect. The main independent variable here is the state of the object.

Understanding these different kinds of studies and distinguishing dependent from independent variables helps the evaluator to formulate appropriate questions and guides the evaluator in selecting an appropriate experimental design.

30

2.4.2 Eliminating Potential Bias

Bias or *confounding* means that one cannot rely on the study's results because there is some unknown systematic effect that may account for the findings. There are many kinds of bias, ranging from measurement bias to bias in attributing cause and effect in demonstration studies. Some are listed in Table 30.2, together with their mechanisms and a brief note on how to eliminate them. Evaluators need to be aware of these before they design measurement or demonstration studies so that they can take steps to eliminate them or to measure how much they may be affecting their study.

2.4.3 Ensuring that Study Findings can be Generalized

Some studies are conducted in one specific setting with one group of users to answer a specific question about a unique information system with no intention of applying the results elsewhere. However, in most evaluation studies it is hoped that the results obtained from the specific subjects, patients, clinical setting, information system, and measurements can be generalized to other subjects in similar settings with similar systems. To achieve this generality, investigators must ensure that they do not select, deliberately or accidentally, patients, clinicians, settings, information systems, or measures that are unusual or even unique.

Study clinicians should be representative of those to whom one wants to generalize the study results. This means avoiding those who have helped to develop the information system and volunteers, who are typically early adopters of technology, better informed, and psychologically atypical. The best subjects are a random sample of all those meeting predefined eligibility criteria, such as clinicians working in an emergency room for more than 3 but less than 12 months with no previous exposure to a computerized DSS.

Patients must also be representative. However, patients with the same problem in two similar settings, such as asthma patients attending a chest clinic and a general medical clinic, can differ markedly in disease severity and age profile. Thus, the patients and clinical setting should be chosen with care, because some collaborators in medical informatics projects are at tertiary referral or even national specialist centers. If the study aims to demonstrate benefit to general hospitals, it should be carried out in general hospitals. This is because the resources and the patient case mix are typically very different in different health care settings.

We have already discussed the importance of defining the information system, to ensure that any claims made reflect the system component being evaluated. However, in an evaluation study it is natural to try to get the best from the clinical information system. Thus, developers and evaluators typically provide extra support, training, tailoring of the system to its users, and even progress reports to enhance user participation. Unless all of these will be provided as part of the system package wherever it is installed, it is impossible to generalize from the findings of such a study. This is why evaluation is usually best carried out by an independent team who could not provide extra support or training even if they wanted to.

Finally, we have discussed how to ensure that the measurement methods used in the study are reliable and valid. To ensure that they are also generalizable, evaluators need to check that the validation procedures use generally acceptable definitions of the gold standard, not some local variant.

2.5 Carrying out the Study

Once the study is designed, it needs to be documented in a study *protocol*, which explains the selection and numbers of subjects, how to make measurements, and the mechanics of carrying out the study in detail. If the study requires use of confidential patient data or will lead to changes in patient care, approval from an ethics committee needs to be sought before starting the study.

2.6 Analyzing and Reporting Study Results

Analyzing the results of a demonstration study often requires **contingency table** and **analysis of variance** techniques, which are partly discussed in Chapter 24, and other statistical techniques covered by other authors. When analyzing and reporting study results, it is important to keep in mind the original question. Thus, if the major question concerns the effect of a diagnostic DSS on diagnostic accuracy, it is important to compare the accuracy of clinicians who were and were not provided with the DSS rather than those who used it with those who did not. This is called "analysis by intention to provide information" and allows evaluators to estimate realistically the benefit of providing the DSS, allowing for the fact that a certain percentage of clinicians will refuse to use it or will ignore its advice.

3 Conclusions

Evaluation is important for many reasons and can be performed at each stage in the development of a clinical information system. Careful evaluation provides valuable information to system developers, users, potential purchasers, and medical informaticians and should be considered an integral part of any system development project. There is no shortage of methods for carrying out evaluations, but the choice of technique is usually obvious once the questions are clearly framed. System developers should usually budget 15 to 25% of their resources for evaluation and should budget more for demonstration projects, but when studying the impact of information systems on clinicians or patients, the budget may need to be several times the development cost, as is the case with drug trials. Many such studies of the impact of decision support and other clinical information systems have in fact been carried out, although few were very rigorous.

Key References

Altman D. *Practical Statistics for Medical Research*. London: Chapman and Hall, 1991.

Friedman C, Wyatt J. *Evaluation Methods in Medical Informatics*. New York: Springer-Verlag, 1996.

Mays N, Pope C, eds. *Qualitative Research in Health Care*. London: British Medical Journal Publishing, 1996.

Wyatt JC. Clinical data systems, Part III: Developing and evaluating clinical data systems. Lancet 1994;344:1682-88.

See the Web site for further literature references.

30

VIII

Methodology for Information Systems

Authors of Part VIII

Chapter 31: Human-Computer Interaction in Health Care
V.L. Patel, A.W. Kushniruk, McGill University, Montreal

Chapter 32: Costs and Benefits of Information Systems
A.R. Bakker, University of Leiden; C.J.W.A. Enning, Hiscom, Leiden

Chapter 33: Security in Medical Information Systems
A.R. Bakker, University of Leiden

Chapter 34: Standards in Health-care Informatics and Telematics in Europe
G.J.E. de Moor, University of Gent

Chapter 35: Project Management
H. Lodder, A.R. Bakker, University of Leiden

31 Human-Computer Interaction in Health Care

1 Introduction

Health care is becoming increasingly dependent on computer technology. The quality of the interaction between health care workers and computers is at the heart of the effective use of technology in medicine. The study of **human-computer interaction** (**HCI**) in health care is concerned with the design, implementation, and evaluation of interactive computing systems for health care that are both *usable* and *effective*. Important aspects of HCI include the understanding of:

- human *cognition*, and the motivations and actions that constrain the use of computing systems, and
- technological issues and advances in the use of computer systems and the development of user interfaces for health care.

Advances in HCI promise to have important effects on medical informatics. From the human side, progress is being made in understanding the psychological and cognitive aspects of the interaction between health care professionals and computers. From the technological side, innovations range from new forms of input devices, including **pen-based** and **speech-based input**, to advances in the development of innovative methods for the presentation of information.
In this chapter we address both the cognitive and the technological aspects of human-computer interfacing in health care. The focus will be on understanding the interplay between the cognitive aspects of the human-computer interface and the emergence of technological innovation.

The lack of good human-computer interfaces has been identified as being a major impediment to the acceptance and routine use of many types of computing systems in health care. Strenuous demands are placed on the *interface* by health care professionals and their work environments. As a result, a variety of issues and challenges have arisen in human-computer interfacing in health care. Some of these deal with a need for commonality in the design of interfaces. The maintenance of a consistent user interface style allows users to quickly learn and adapt to new parts and features of the overall system. On the other hand, for computing systems to be acceptable to a wide range of health care professionals they must be flexible enough to meet the specific information needs of those professionals. A better understanding of the issues related to cognitive processes involved in HCI is essential to designing interfaces that can be used intuitively by and that are acceptable to health care professionals. New techniques for characterizing the information needs and cognitive processing of health care professionals are beginning to appear. Such work will be required to ensure that there is a match between the designer's conceptualization – or model – of the system and the end user's (i.e., the physician's or the nurse's) understanding of the system. A better understanding of the health care worker's cognitive capabilities and limitations will be central to the development of a wide range of medical systems.
In considering the problem of a lack of acceptance of computerization by many medical staff, it appears that

31

this resistance can be reduced when systems are designed to take into account the needs of health care staff and their existing work practices. Often, the dominant perspective of HCI focuses on understanding the interaction within a very narrow context. However, there is a growing awareness of the importance of considering the cognitive activities of groups of people working together on joint problems (see also the discussion on shared care in Chapter 11). In health care this perspective extends the traditional human information-processing model of HCI to include the effects of computer systems on the social and organizational context. A number of other practical and technological issues are currently being addressed regarding human-computer interfacing in health care.

- Technical aspects of HCI, such as data entry, have in the past been major obstacles to the acceptance of many medical information systems.
- The development of physical input-output devices that are appropriate to the users' requirements and work context is essential.
- The inclusion of facilities for customizing and personalizing the user interface is becoming another requirement.
- Advances related to professional-computer interaction include the development of *graphical user interfaces*, the use of effective interface metaphors, and the integration of various media within the human-computer interface.
- Professional-computer interaction styles need to be examined to arrive at context-sensitive interactions.
- Issues dealing with the presentation of information, such as information density and *navigation*, must be addressed.
- It has also been recognized that the evaluation of human-computer interfaces must be given high priority, because it is only through careful consideration of the problems encountered by users that roadblocks to effective development can be eliminated.

The objective of this chapter is to provide a guide to important and emerging areas of human-computer-interaction in health care. Section 2 focuses on the cognitive aspects of the health care professional's interaction with computer systems and provides a framework from which to view HCI. Section 3 deals with the technological aspects of HCI in health care. This is followed by a discussion of emerging technologies in health care user-computer interfaces in Section 4. Section 5 considers design methodologies and interface evaluation. Finally, Section 6 presents basic principles for the design of health care interfaces.

2 Cognitive Aspects of Human-Computer Interfacing

The purpose of this section is to provide a background for understanding the human or cognitive aspects of human-computer interfacing in health care. The topics discussed include the role of *cognitive psychology* in understanding and building more effective interfaces, as well as aspects of human perception, learning, and expertise.

2.1 Why Consider Psychology?

The *user interface* is the part of a computer system that communicates with the user. The objective of users of health information systems is to carry out tasks in which information is accessed, manipulated, or created. From this perspective, HCI is largely cognitive, that is, it involves the processing of information by the user, in conjunction with a computer system. The application of principles,

31

ideas, and findings from cognitive psychology in the design of interfaces is important in that it can facilitate the design of systems that allow information processing to take place as effectively as possible, given the limitations of the processing capabilities of the human mind. Specifically, cognitive psychology can help improve the design of interactive health care systems by:

- providing knowledge about what users can and cannot be expected to do,
- identifying and explaining the nature and causes of user problems,
- characterizing the problem solving and decision-making processes of health care workers,
- determining the cognitive needs of users (e.g., what kind of information should a computer display in order to support physician decision making processes?),
- supplying input into the design of improved systems through the iterative evaluation of user interactions, and
- providing models and frameworks for conducting HCI research and applications.

2.2 Cognitive Frameworks for HCI

The study of HCI is about designing computer systems that support people so that they can carry out their activities productively and safely. The design of the human-computer interface is one aspect of HCI that deals with those aspects of the system with which the user comes into contact. Over the past several decades, research from cognitive psychology has begun to be applied to a variety of problems in HCI. An emphasis of much of this work has been on developing and testing theories concerning the ways in which users behave in the course of interacting with a computer. Some of the theories deal with areas such as perception, language comprehension and production, memory, problem solving, intention, and the control of actions. In addition to developing theoretical perspec-

tives for HCI, researchers in applied cognitive psychology are developing and refining techniques that can be used to characterize the needs, information processing limitations, capabilities and level of expertise of users. The information processing model has been very influential in shaping the development of cognitive models of the user in HCI. The underlying theoretical framework has provided a means of conceptualizing user behavior that enables predictions to be made about user performance. One such model, called "model human processor," consists of three interacting systems: the perceptual system, the motor system, and the cognitive system. The model provides a means of characterizing the various cognitive processes that are assumed to underlie the performance of a task. One family of such models, the GOMS (goals, operators, methods, and selection rules) models, attempt to model the computer users' goals and action (e.g., keystrokes) in describing user performance. HCI is an interdisciplinary area of applied research and design practice. Its key concern is to understand and facilitate the creation of the user interface. It draws on many disciplines, including psychology, computer science, anthropology, management science, and industrial science, with psychology and computer science being possible candidates for qualifying as foundation sciences. The applied psychology of HCI addresses the understanding of how human motivation, action, and experience place constraints on the usability of computer equipment and to support the development of new computer technology that exploits these constraints. Psychology has borrowed computer science concepts to construct models of the human information processing. Now computer developers seek out psychological knowledge as a guide to the design of systems. The need to design displays and keyboards for interactive computer systems led to the increasing interest of perceptual and cognitive psychologists. The study of human information processing is often categorized into studies of sensation, perception, cognition, and motor control, all of which are relevant to system design. However, most direct influences from cognitive science come from its parent disciplines of artificial intelligence, psychology, linguistics, and philosophy.

31

2.3 Resources in Human Information Processing

A basic concept from psychology, namely, resources, has its analog in the computer domain (e.g., memory processing cycles and *bandwidths*). Two kinds of resources have similar properties in humans:

- *Critical resources* are those required to perform a particular task or to execute a particular process.
- *Limited resources* are the ones that may be in short supply relative to their needs.

In cognition, as in operating systems, problems arise when critical resources are limited and supply cannot meet the demand. Various tasks and cognitive activities can be discussed in terms of the type and quantity of resources that they consume. Processes are limited by:

- available processing resources, such as memory, and
- the quality of the data being processed.

Since there is usually a trade-off between resources and data quality, a primary design objective should be to minimize resource consumption by improving data quality. This is because cognitive resources are in short supply and there is a high demand. A good measure of the complexity or difficulty of a task is its demand on resources. This measure is called *cognitive load*, and this correlates with factors such as learning time, fatigue, stress, proneness to error, and inability to "time share". Cognitive load is an important consideration for design, but its calculation is not simple. This distribution of load may differ from isolated tasks to large systems.

Sometimes, a critical resource is limited and cannot be allocated to a task. This may occur when performing a task requiring a high cognitive load or when two tasks make simultaneous demands on the same resource. Degradation in the performance of one task because of competition with another task for a critical resource is known as *interference*. Many tasks performed with a computer require a high cognitive load and, thus, are susceptible to such inference. One design goal would be to reduce the likelihood of interference by:

- reducing the load associated with task performance,
- improving the quality of data available to users, and
- minimizing the likelihood of competition.

2.4 Expertise, Skilled Performance, and Learning

Empirical studies of expertise and skilled behavior of expert practitioners and novice learners have contributed to our understanding of how to reduce cognitive load in task performance. Studies of expert performance inform us that experts perform tasks in their own domain of expertise effortlessly. They are skilled in that particular activity, and many aspects of this skilled task performance are automatic, consuming negligible cognitive resources. This means that skilled performance is less susceptible to interference. The resources thus released can be available for other tasks performed simultaneously.

Achieving a skilled level of proficiency in most tasks is difficult. As one moves from simple to complex tasks, repetition, although necessary, is not a sufficient condition for the development of skill acquisition. Thus, training in skill acquisition is a part of human-computer interfacing that is becoming important. This demand for learning and training increases with a growing number of features in applications, the number of applications available, and expansion of network availability, and as more people become computer users.

However, it should be noted that although skilled performance has the desirable property of minimizing the cognitive load during task execution, acquiring skill takes time and effort. Training is not a good investment if a skill is rarely exercised. It is desirable to characterize expert behavior and its relationship to trainees such that we can develop a stepwise model of skill acquisition from novice to expert. Since most novice trainees come to a domain with some prerequisite skills, we may get a head start in training by using existing skills as a basis for performing new tasks. This is known as "skill transfer." There are four guidelines for successfully designing an interface to maximize this transfer:

- build upon the users' existing set of skills,
- keep the skills required by the system to a minimum,
- use the same skill wherever possible in similar circumstances, and
- use *feedback* to identify similar contexts and distinguish ones that are dissimilar.

The underlying cognitive principle is that if interfaces require the same skills in similar contexts, the exploitation of existing skills is minimized. As computer use becomes more widespread, the problematic side of transfer of training is increasingly important to developers.

2.5 Perception and Attention

Perception is a fundamental aspect of human interaction with computers. Users need to be able to visually perceive information presented on a computer in meaningful way. Other perceptual modalities, such as sound and touch, are also beginning to appear and are becoming important in the human-computer interface (e.g., in *multimedia* and *virtual reality*). The psychological study of perception, in the context of HCI, is important, particularly in medicine, where large amounts of complex visual information often must be presented to health care workers in that they can be perceived and understood unambiguously.

Closely related to issues of perception is attention, which refers to our ability to filter out and make sense of the mass of information that our senses are constantly bombarded with. However, due to our selective attention, the ability of humans to perform many tasks and to attend to large amounts of information at the same time is limited. This has important implications for the design of effective user interfaces. Effective user interfaces need to help users focus attention on

information that needs to be dealt with (e.g., the display of patient alerts in medical information systems). This is facilitated by presentation of information by the computer system in ways that facilitate:

- presentation of information in a logical and meaningful way,
- use of attention-getting cues (such as alert messages or highlighting), and
- the organization of the display into partitions or *windows* (discussed in Section 3)
- that can help users focus attention on particular operations or information contained in the windows.

2.6 Recent Approaches to Cognition and HCI

With the development of computing, the actions of the brain have sometimes been characterized as a series of programmed steps, using the computer as a metaphor. Concepts such as buffers, memory stores, and storage systems, and the types of process that act upon them provided psychologists with a means of developing more advanced models of information processing that could be tested. A move away from the information-processing framework in cognitive psychology occurred in parallel with the reduced importance of the model human processor in HCI and the emergence of other theoretical approaches. These are the computational and connectionist approaches. More recently, other alternative approaches have been developed. These approaches have situated cognitive activities in the context in which they occur. This perspective focuses on how our interactions in the world affect individual, social, and cultural development.

The principal advantage of these emerging approaches is that they view people, such as computer users, not as static information processors but as individuals who are continually shaped by their ongoing patterns of activity. This type of perspective alerts people to issues that are pushed into the background by other approaches, including individual differences, cross-cultural differences, and differences based on experience or occupation. There is a growing concern that if computer systems are to be designed to match users' needs, then it is necessa-

31

ry to consider the context in which they are to be used. An emerging theoretical framework, namely, distributed cognition, attempts to conceptualize cognitive activities as embodied and situated with the work context in which they occur. Principally, this involves describing cognition as it is distributed across individuals and the settings in which it takes place (i.e., cognition is viewed as being distributed among any number of information processing systems, including both humans and computers). This conceptualization of "cognition in the wild" can inform system design by examining the coordination and breakdown of interdependent activities and their implications for future technological developments.

2.7 Usability

Designing systems that are easy to learn and use is an important objective of HCI work. *Usability* can be defined as the measure of the ease with which a com-

puter system can be learned and used, its effectiveness and efficiency, and the attitudes of users toward it (i.e., its enjoyability). To develop systems with good usability, a number of practical areas need to be considered:

- understanding how computers and people can operate together most effectively (this requires understanding of psychological, ergonomic, and social factors),
- creating tools that can aid in the development of systems with a high degree of usability,
- developing and refining methodologies for guiding the process of interface design,
- determining the degree of match between the designer's model, or conception, of the system and that of the end user (mismatches between the designer's and the user's mental models are potential causes of interface problems), and
- developing effective methods for accurately assessing the usability of both completed systems and systems in development.

3 Technological Aspects of Human-Computer Interfacing

A wide range of technological developments and advances are rapidly changing the nature of HCI in health care. This section discusses some of the more prominent developments. When considering the application of these technological developments, it is important to keep in mind human issues such as how the technology affects the current work patterns and the implications of the technology for medical staff with various levels of expertise, experience, age, and educational background. Over the past several years, remarkable advances have been made in the development of computer *hardware*, including dramatically increased processor speeds and storage capacities. These advances are beginning to be matched by improvements in technologies for HCI, such as pen-based and speech-based input (see also Chapter 7), which are likely to have a major impact on the nature of the human-computer interface in health care. It has

been suggested that in the past issues such as data entry have been major obstacles to the acceptance of many medical systems by health care professionals. The design of physical input/output devices that are appropriate to the users' requirements and work context is essential. The inclusion of facilities for customizing and personalizing the user interface is also becoming another requirement of systems for clinical use.

With a perspective to understanding the HCI derived from considerations presented in the previous section of this chapter, major technological issues in the professional-computer interaction will be described. Specifically this section focuses on the following aspects of the professional-computer interaction:

- Interaction style

The use of graphical, *windows*-based interfaces has become prevalent and a wide variety of media, including *alphanumeric* texts, graphics, and images are beginning to be integrated into health care user-computer interfaces.

- Data entry

The development of effective input devices is an essential area in the development of human-computer interfaces in health care. Use of devices for inputting data must be intuitive, and the devices must match the particular needs of health care professionals.

- Standardization

The issue of the development of user interface standards is an area that is becoming more prominent. Although there is a need for development of open user interface standards, de facto proprietary or industry standards, such as Microsoft **Windows**, have emerged and continue to influence the design of human-computer interfaces.

- Customization

The capability to customize medical user interfaces is also required to allow for the diverse needs of users, including their particular information requirements and work contexts.

- Emerging interface technologies

A number of emerging technologies, including *multimedia*, *hypermedia*, and *virtual reality* and developments in computer supported cooperative work environments are beginning to have important impacts on computer use in health care.

3.1 Interaction Style

Information systems in health care can greatly improve access to and retrieval of medical information. However, the large volume of data that can be retrieved by computer-based systems must be carefully presented in order not to overwhelm the user's ability to obtain the most relevant and significant information. Indeed, early attempts at providing health care professionals with comprehensive computer-based information often led to cognitive overload. Issues related to human cognition, including the comprehension of information and the limits of the human perception and memory, must be taken into account. The presentation of information to health care workers should reflect the meaning of the data and should also be sensitive to the context of the

patient, provider, and task. This will greatly facilitate comprehension of the information presented to the user and increase the acceptability of the system. Developments in HCI, such as the emergence of graphical user interfaces and the incorporation of multimedia technologies, have provided interface designers with tools that can greatly facilitate the presentation and comprehension of medical information.

The exchange of information and instructions that goes on between a computer user and a computer system can be looked at as a form of communication dialogue. For example, the computer may present the user with **prompts** for which the user replies with *responses*. User responses involve the input of data or instructions of some form into the computer system. A number of different styles of communication have been designed for human interaction with computers. This section describes the two most common styles:

- the use of **command languages**, and
- the use of graphical interaction.

3.1.1 Command Languages and Character-Based Interfaces

For many years the predominant style of HCI involved *keyboard* input by users of commands for effecting com-

```
C>copy file1 file2

File not found - FILE1
    0 files copied

C>dir

 Directory of C>

 COMMAND COM 47845 04-09-95 5:00a
 OLDNOTES DOC    184  11-11-94 6:40a
 AUTOEXEC BAT    56 03-08-94 4:20p


```

Figure 31.1
Human-computer interaction with a character-based interface. The characters that were typed in by the user have been underlined.

31

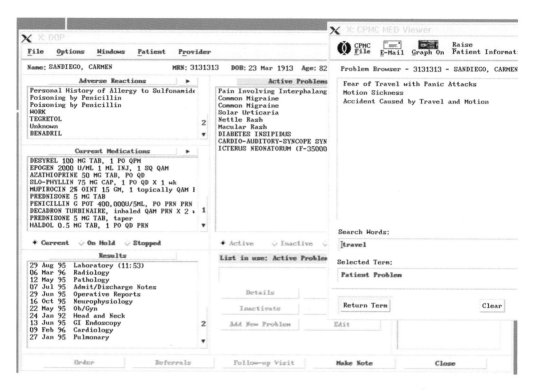

Figure 31.2
Windows-based interface for a patient record system (see text).

puter operations. Interfaces based on command languages constrained the user to typing in exact commands at the keyboard. For example, Fig. 31.1 shows a dialogue between the user and a character-based computer system (the **DOS** interface on IBM compatible computers).

In the example dialogue in Fig. 31.1, the user has typed in the command to copy a file to another file as a response to the prompt. The computer has responded with a message indicating that the file to be copied was not found (i.e., it is not in the directory that the computer is searching). The user then proceeds to use the "dir" command to check what files do exist in the current directory, with the system responding with the name of three files. The problems that computer users often have with such command languages in **character-based interfaces** have been well documented. These include the limitations of humans for remembering complex command names to enter into the computer, or difficulty in interpreting complex error messa-

ges returned by the computer. This type of user interaction was the predominant form of user interaction in the 1970s and still represents the mode of interaction for many health care computer applications. Keyboard interaction also remains an important means for mass data entry in medical interfaces. However, there is a clear trend toward the development of medical user interfaces with graphical capabilities.

3.1.2 Graphical Manipulation

During the 1980s user interface design began to be dominated by the style of user interaction offered by **graphical user interfaces**. Graphical user interfaces allow for more flexible HCI styles and for computer use by nonspecialists. These interfaces typically use a direct manipulation style of interaction, which means that the user can point and click on objects displayed by the computer (e.g., using a **mouse** or **tracking ball** to select from menus or activate parts of a computer display). This style of interaction, compared to command-driven systems, allows the users to recognize, rather than recall, the computer operations that they wish to effect. In many health care applications, being able to quickly recognize information and easily perform operations with a computer, without having to memorize complex command sequences, can lead to considerable improvements in the efficiency of the HCI. In addition, easy-to-use interfaces can greatly improve user's satisfaction with computer technology. User interfaces that include windows, buttons, boxes and icons are commonly known as *graphical user interfaces* (or *GUIs*) or *windows*-based user interfaces. Windows refer to bordered areas on the computer screen, with each window having a title bar across the top (see Chapter 3). For example, the windows-based interface shown in Fig. 31.2 contains two windows, with the window on the right hand side overlapping the window beneath it. Windows may contain text, images, *menus*, or *buttons*. Buttons refer to areas on the screen (usually, labeled boxes or circles) that can be selected (i.e., clicked on) by the user. Clicking on a button results in some particular activity (e.g., the display of another window).

The example in Fig. 31.2 is from the interface for a patient record system currently being used at the Columbia-Presbyterian Medical Center in New York (see Chapter 20). The system (the Decision-Supported Outpatient Practice System) allows clinicians to record patient problems, allergies, and medications through a windows-based interface. Figure 31.2 shows a sample screen with two windows displayed. The larger window is the system's main window, which displays various components of the medical record, including adverse reactions, current medications, and medical terms. In this example, the user had selected (i.e., clicked on), "Problem List" on the main screen and then the button "Add New Problem." When the look-up screen appeared, the user then entered the word "travel" and the system responded by displaying three terms that could be selected from in order to describe the patient's problem: "Fear of Travel with Panic Attacks," "Motion Sickness," and "Accident Caused by Travel and Motion." This type of interaction is typical of windows-based interfaces.

3.2 Principles for the Display of Information

How successful a human-computer interface is depends to a large extent on the organization and content of information displayed to users. Well-organized information that is presented in a logical and meaningful way leads to a higher degree of usability. On the other hand, display of information in a cluttered, illogical, or confusing manner leads to decreases in user performance and user satisfaction. There are a number of guidelines for organizing computer-based information displays in ways that can greatly facilitate usability:

• Grouping of information
The organization of information by grouping related information items together is important in allowing users to focus their attention. For example, the use of different windows for containing different types of information facilitates good information organization.

• Minimizing amount of information overload
Due to human limitations in information processing, a good design heuristic is to minimize the amount of information presented by techniques such as using concise wording, and familiar data formats and presenting only what the user really needs.

• Standard information display
Consistency in user interface layout and properties is one of the most important attributes of a user-friendly system. A consistent format for information displayed (e.g., patient data always appearing in a certain part of a window) facilitates user comprehension.

• Information highlighting
The highlighting of important information (using any of a number of techniques including underlining, boldface, coloring information so that it stands out, and *reverse video*) greatly facilitates the communication of essential information to users.

• Use of graphics
Graphs and tables can be extremely useful for concisely summarizing and presenting information. This is especially true in health care applications, where large amounts of patient data often must be presented to

31

Table 31.1
Input Devices.[a]

Device	Description
Keyboard	Most commonly used, especially for data entry
Mouse	Very useful device to point to the display screen but with limitations for use in health care
Trackball	Is a rotating ball and similar to the mouse to point to the display screen
Graphics tablet	Is a touch-sensitive surface which lies apart from the display screen. Can be operated by using finger, pencil, or stylus. Is sometimes used for data entry in computer-based patient records
Touch screen	Does not require any other device but rather the user touching the display screen with his or her finger
Pen	A lightpen allows the user to point at spots on the display screen. More advanced versions of computer pens allow users to handwrite on the screen
Speech	Voice input to the computer, allowing to use natural language. In the future this holds much promise for health care.

[a] For a further description, see also Chapter 4.

Table 31.2
Data Entry Communication Styles

Input Style	Description
Form filling	When the same type of data have to be entered repeatedly, the use of forms (having the appearance of a paper form) can facilitate data entry
Question and answer dialogues	Here the system prompts with a question to which users respond (e.g., by selecting from preset choices). This is a style for data entry which is useful for novices but often frustrating for expert users.
Menus	Menus provide users with a limited set of options from which to choose. Types of menus include: • fixed menus (which stay in place), • pull down menus (which are dragged from a title or menu bar), and • pop-up menus (which appear when a user clicks a particular part of the screen)
Natural language	This is to allow users to enter data in unrestricted natural language. This has proven to be a difficult problem to solve because of the complexity of natural language. A solution is to limit the domain to a subset of language.
Direct manipulation	Instead of making users remember commands, direct manipulation allows the users to select objects and actions by using a pointing device

31

health care workers. Appropriate graphics can greatly facilitate comprehension of complex data. A variety of graphics can be applied, including line graphs, *pie charts*, *bar graphs*, *simulated meters*, and *scattergrams*.

• Optimal text presentation

The spacing, font, color and size of the text displayed are important attributes in determining the readability of displayed text.

• Use of icons

Different aspects of a computer system, including things such as files, programs, and applications can be neatly represented by using small graphic images or icons. *Icons* pictorially represent (on the computer screen) objects such as file folders or trash cans. They can thus serve as metaphors that can facilitate ease of use and understanding of a system. It is important, however, that such representations be easily understood by users and be representative of the task domain in which they are used.

3.3 Data Entry

A wide variety of input devices are now available and can be used in human-computer interfacing in health care. The selection of which device is suitable for a particular user and application should be based on an assessment of the specific needs of the prospective users. For example, an operating surgeon might need voice input since his or her hands are occupied, whereas a radiotherapist might require a *digitizing tablet* when planning treatment. As with other aspects of the design of health care systems, flexibility and the allowance for diversity is important. Table 31.1 provides a list of input devices that are candidates for health care applications.

It may be that for the short term, development of improved pen-based input may be most promising for a range of medical applications, whereas for the long term, research is needed to improve speech-based input. In addition to considering the type of input device that can be used in medical systems, the overall of type of user-system interaction can be characterized according to the data entry style, which ranges from very system-directed input involving the filling in of forms and answering of computer-posed questions to more user-controlled forms of input, including use of direct manipulation interaction or even entry of *natural language* (see also Table 31.2).

In the context of health care systems, the form in which information should be entered into a system by users is an issue of current debate. In general, medical data can be organized according to three basic structures, described below:

• Free form

The clinical information entered into the system is in whatever form the user desires. This assumes the ability to encode some of the content of the text to facilitate organization, retrieval, and presentation. Research is being conducted into the design of computer systems for analyzing medical *free-form text* and translating the text into computer-based representations that can be later retrieved on the basis of content and meaning. Input in free form could be done by using any number of input devices, including a keyboard, pen, or speech.

• Semistructured approach

An intermediate position, between allowing free-form input and imposing a high degree of structure on input, is a semistructured approach, which is used in some applications such as *computer-based patient records*.

• Structured, codified approach

Selection of *coded* entries provides a way of entering textual information by allowing the user to select appropriate words or phrases from menus or lists.

31

4 Emerging Technologies in Medical User-Computer Interfaces

Technologies from a number of emerging areas promise to have important implications for the design of medical computer interfaces. The rapid development and application of multimedia and hypermedia technology, with the improved integration of text, graphics, and images, has led to advances in user interface design in a number of areas in health care. This section will examine some developments that have implications for the design of human-computer interfaces in health care.

4.1 Visualization of Medical Data

Data and scientific information can be visualized in the form of graph displays, chart displays, histograms, and, more recently, elaborate screen images. Rapid progress has been made in the development of visualization techniques, with three-dimensional (3-D) *imaging* appearing in diagnostic medicine as well as in medical education (see Chapter 26). However, the effective graphical display of information still presents a number of challenges. Work is being conducted in developing methods for determining important relationships in the large quantity of medical data that could be displayed to end users and for restricting the display of complex data to those parameters that are most relevant to the patient context.

Bedside critical care *monitors* that are typically available often provide limited types of display: for example, all monitored signals over some time period (e.g., the last 30 to 60 seconds) or a summary view through the last few hours or day. Research is being conducted in transforming such numerical data into novel and concise visual metaphors.

Medical *imaging* techniques have developed to an advanced stage, and complex medical images have begun to be incorporated into a variety of medical user interfaces. Medical workstation interfaces capable of integrating complex radiographic images with text and graphics are becoming more common, and *multimedia* capabilities are emerging in computer-based patient record systems. Advanced medical workstations support real-time, 3-D graphics, with HCI methods emerging from work in *computer-aided design* and *computer-aided manufacturing* industries being applied to medicine. Experimental visualization software that uses 3-D graphics to reconstruct views of the body and aid in surgery are already being developed. Furthermore, the simplification of graphics programming by the availability of *open* graphics libraries should speed the development of such advanced visualization technologies.

4.2 Multimedia

Over the last several years, multimedia has become one of the most popular topics in information technology and has already begun to change the user-computer interaction in significant ways in a number of areas, including the development of educational and clinical systems. The rapid increase in multimedia applications is an example of a technology-driven phenomenon, made possible by advances in *optical disk* technology, high-quality graphics and imaging, *network* developments and the decreasing costs of computer processing and storage. Multimedia systems allow for the presentation of a variety of forms of information, including text, sound, and images. An important element of multimedia systems is related to their interactivity, that is, to interrupt and be interrupted by the user. This feeling of close involvement of the user implied by such interactivity is a characteristic of multimedia.

A variety of multimedia technologies and applications have appeared, such as:

- Educational *videodisk* programs, which have evolved to include digital systems such as laserdisk col-

31

lections on topics such as brain anatomy and inter-active videodisk and laserdisk educational systems that allow for a high degree of user interaction.

- CD-ROM and *World Wide Web* technology : CD-ROM disks and Websites can provide digital text, graphics, audio and video images and have been used for a wide range of educational programs and scientific databases in medicine. Currently available medical applications include a multimedia version of *Scientific American's* textbook *Medicine*, as well as a number of medical journals and reference sources.

A number of large-scale projects with implications for medical education have also appeared, including the Anatomy Project, a multiformat, multi*platform* application of multimedia technology combining anatomical and clinical content, and the *Visible Humans Project* of the National Library of Medicine in the United States (see also Panel 26.1 in Chapter 26), consisting of a digital library of images of volumetric data representing a complete normal adult human female and male.

Multimedia is also having an impact on the development of interfaces to medical record systems and clinical workstations, allowing clinical staff to obtain patient information that integrates text, graphics, and radiographic images at windows-oriented terminals or workstations. A variety of computerized patient record systems now incorporate multimedia capabilities, with charts of laboratory test results and graphic information and images all displayed in a coherent manner at the user interface (see also Chapters 7 and 29).

4.3 Hypertext and Hypermedia

A closely related advance in HCI has been the development of hypertext and hypermedia systems. The fundamental principles underlying *hypertext* and *hypermedia* are the following:

- Units of screen-based information are reactive (i.e., users can click on highlighted text or graphics, which can result in the display of a new screen of information).

- The linking together of information units is an essential aspect of hypermedia applications, that is, users can click on a highlighted part of one screen, go to another screen, and again click on text or graphics to go to yet further levels of linked information (hypertext systems are restricted to linked nodes consisting of text, whereas hypermedia systems contain displays of various media).

- Such systems allow users to *navigate*, or *browse* through information at their own pace (e.g., by clicking on highlighted text or images), enabling them to explore connections between concepts in educational applications, and allowing users access to information in large databases.

Multimedia applications in medicine often include various degrees of hypertext or hypermedia capability. Multimedia and hypermedia technologies are already exerting an important effect, particularly in computer-based medical education. The application of hypermedia concepts to the design of instructional systems has the potential of improving the usability and adaptability of systems from the perspective of the user. From a psychological perspective, the presentation of information through the integration of a number of media more fully engages human sense perception, and the linking together of semantically related units of information in hypermedia systems can be considered as being analogous to the organization of human memory. However, a number of fundamental issues remain that deal with aspects of hypermedia design and user interaction remain to be resolved. Although the flexibility that such environments provide users can greatly facilitate information retrieval, this flexibility can also lead to common problems:

- *User disorientation.* A common criticism of hypermedia systems is that users may encounter a feeling of being lost in a sequence of information displays, especially when the number of linked information units is very large.

- *Cognitive overload.* Hypermedia techniques should simplify access to large bodies of information; however, if that information is not well organized (i.e., linked), users may have difficulty in accessing the desired information.

31

Related work is being conducted in developing better navigational tools and the integration of hypermedia systems with knowledge base components that can apply intelligent means to alleviate information overload.

4.4 Advances in Pen-Based Input

The human-computer interface has been a major challenge and technological barrier to the widespread implementation of medical computing systems, in particular computer-based patient record systems (see Chapters 7 and 29). Problems with input devices have been singled out as being a major component in the problem of acceptance of such systems. In response to health care professional-stated preferences regarding input, there have appeared computer systems that allow health care professionals to use an electronic stylus to point, draw, and handwrite on a computer "pad," thus allowing for some of the input flexibility that they are accustomed to in using paper-based records. The "pen and paper" metaphor that these systems support is flexible, and the use of this form of input in conjunction with portable, *laptop* computer hardware have made this direction in HCI very attractive. As a result, a number of commercially available products incorporating *pen-based* input have recently appeared. However, a number of areas warrant further work and will likely improve greatly over the next few years. These include the need for:

- portable pen-based systems with thinner, lighter pads,
- extended battery life, and
- improved handwriting recognition capabilities.

Other possible developments include wireless connections with host systems and, ideally, any stylus. These developments will allow for pen-based input devices that can be flexibly used in clinics or medical offices and other health care settings.

4.5 Advances in Speech Recognition

It has been argued that *speech input* will provide the ultimate form of input for many types of health care applications. However, a number of environmental considerations and technical problems are associated with this technology (see also Chapter 7). For example, speech input may not be feasible in noisy clinical environments. Furthermore, more research needs to be conducted in the areas of developing methods for computer recognition of continuous, speaker-independent speech. Limitations of some conventional speech recognition systems include:

- the requirement to "train" the system to recognize a particular speaker,
- the inability to interpret continuous speech of a significant duration, and
- limited use of systems in noisy environments, like clinics and emergency rooms.

Some of the issues and problems related to speech input stem from problems and challenges regarding the input of free text in general, regardless of the input device. Specifically, the interpretation of natural language input remains a major challenge for medical informatics researchers. However, the promise of speech input is considerable for use in health care, and some clinical information systems that use speech have already begun to appear commercially. Recent experimental work in the integration of speech recognition systems with medical information and decision-support systems indicates that limited grammar speech recognition systems are feasible and already allow for some degree of continuous speech recognition, given current technology.

4.6 User Interfaces to the Internet

One of the most interesting developments in the area of user interfaces is the development of multimedia user interfaces to global computer networks. Advances in wide area networking technologies have led to the development of the *Internet*, which supports millions of users worldwide. The World Wide Web, is the most advanced information system deployed on the Internet and has already begun to be used by the medical community. Multimedia user interfaces, such as the widely used *Netscape browser*, allow for access to the ever increasing amount of information available on wide area networks. Netscape allows users to navigate the information available on the Internet by supporting access to a wide range of information sources and allowing users to browse through audio, graphic images, and video using hypertext links.

A variety of medical applications, ranging from those targeted at medical education to multimedia applications providing information resources for oncology have appeared on the Internet. Document languages have also appeared. These languages, for example, the hypertext markup language (*HTML*), allow authors to structure a document for use on Internet. HTML allows the author of the document to include hypertext links to images, sound or movies, and has been used to create a variety of medical applications deployed on the Internet. The Website of this Handbook, too, uses HTML. The use of such standardized methods for implementing health care applications has been a critical factor in the increasingly widespread use of the Internet for health care applications. Such methods allow for the creation of platform-independent applications. The integration of a variety of medical applications on the Internet, in conjunction with standardized methods for their deployment and access, has greatly facilitated this trend.

4.7 Cooperative Work Environments

New perspectives from which to view HCI in complex domains have emerged. It has been argued that the social context in which humans interact with computer systems is an integral part of that activity. It has also been argued that a clearer understanding of HCI must take into account the real-world context in which that interaction takes place and should be based on a characterization of the cognitive activities of groups of people working together. From this perspective cognition is seen as being distributed among individuals. This view of distributed cognition has important implications for the development of health care systems. In

line with the distributed perspective, a number of technologies for computer-based group support are beginning to appear in health care, including group decision-support systems and computer support of collaborative work (CSCW). The cognitive assessment of work practices in health care can provide an important basis for the development of such systems. In general, computer support of collaborative work can be characterized along two dimensions:

- mode of interaction between users (i.e., occurring synchronously or occurring at different times) and
- geographical location (users are situated in the same environment or in different locations).

Several CSCW applications have appeared in health care. To provide medical care and education services between remote hospitals, a variety of distributed medical communications systems have been developed. For example, a variety of *telemedicine* systems that allow remotely located physicians to cooperate and aid each other in making medical diagnoses have been designed. These systems may use graphical multimedia interfaces, available at all locations. The results of medical actions and the retrieval and storage of data are communicated to other users via manipulation of *objects* (e.g., file *folders*) in the user interface. Other recent applications involving computer-supported cooperative work include the use of interactive large-screen computers to serve as "electronic whiteboards" in medical education. Such computer powered wall screens allow for user input with wireless pens, allowing for collaborative work "at the board."

4.8 Customizable and Adaptive User Interfaces

A key issue that has been identified by a number of authors as being of importance in the delivery of systems that will be accepted by end users is that of flexibility. A number of studies examining user acceptance of medical computing systems have indicated that an important criticism voiced by many users of

31

many conventional systems deals with their perceived inflexibility. Displays should be flexible enough that they may automatically modify their presentation mode on the basis of the importance of the information to be displayed for the particular context in which it will be viewed. Such highlighting may take place at the level of the institution, provider (i.e., clinician), or patient. In addition to customizable presentation, interaction styles (e.g., menu and direct selections) and interaction modes (for users with different levels of user experience, e.g., experts and novices) could also be customized. The method of implementation of such customizability could vary from vendor-provided facilities to allowing users to specify their interface preferences. Users could be able to customize the presentation view (e.g., problem-oriented, review of systems-oriented, chronological, graphical, or tabular views), the interaction style (e.g., a menu-driven or a command-driven style), and the interaction mode (e.g., expert system user, novice system user, domain expert, or domain intermediate mode). However, most users would like the system default configuration to be very good from the beginning, requiring only fine-tuning by the user.

5 Methods for the Design and Evaluation of User Interfaces

This section of the chapter deals with the process of user interface design in health care. A number of methodologies for guiding the design and development of user interfaces have emerged. Recent work in HCI has indicated that many aspects of traditional approaches to designing computer systems, which proceed in sequence from requirements specification through software development and maintenance (see Chapter 19, Section 3.2), may not be appropriate in the development of user interfaces. Indeed, several general principles seem to have emerged from work in the development of user interfaces:

1. Development should include early and continuous empirical testing involving real users (e.g., physicians or nurses) performing representative tasks (e.g., entry of patient data).
2. As development proceeds, it should incorporate iterative refinement procedures (to determine the most appropriate changes to make to the design of the user interface).
3. Expertise from different disciplines related to HCI (including cognitive psychology) should be brought to bear on the design of interfaces.

A variety of techniques have been applied in the complex problem of creating effective user interfaces in health care. These range from the use of cognitive task analysis, to techniques based on an ethnographic study of physician work practices. In this section, individual types of analyses will be considered in the context of the entire process of interface development. Hix and Hartson have argued for a model of interface development in which activities such as analysis, requirements specification, design, and implementation are all subject to continued evaluation by users and experts.

5.1 Stages in the Development of User Interfaces

A description of the steps taken in developing user interfaces for medical systems is provided below. Although a rigid adherence to a fixed ordering of stages is not prescribed in this chapter, the following steps highlight key activities that should be considered in the development of human-computer interfaces in health care.

Table 31.3
Design Methodologies for User Interfaces

Methodology	Description
Rapid prototyping and iterative design	Involves building models or mock-ups of the user interface that can be rapidly developed, presented to end users, and modified before the actual system is implemented. This allows designers to find out right away how a change in the design of the interface will affect its usability. It can be used as a method to support the iterative design of user interfaces
User-centered design	Involves the continuous input of the users throughout the process of interface design. The users interact as consultants in the design process and are involved in all aspects, including how the implementation may affect their jobs
Socio-technical design	An approach that focuses on developing a coherent human-computer system, based on an understanding of both the social system and the technical system. In general, an emphasis during design on the users and on how they will interact with the system is recommended
Scenario-based design	Involves development of scenarios that involve actors (e.g., physicians, nurses) and events to help the designer explore design decisions in particular situations. This approach has been applied in the process of designing health care workstations

1. Product description and description of context of use

The capabilities and features of the system and its interface are defined, and the requirements of the end user are determined. A variety of techniques can be applied at this stage to gain information about the users and their work context, including ethnographic study of the work environment and interviews (both structured and unstructured) with end users. The system's users, purpose, and environment (physical, technical and organizational) are defined.

2. Task analysis

Several different types of analysis can be conducted in delineating the tasks that users will be able to perform. These include (1) a hierarchical task analysis involving the identification of user tasks to be performed with the computer system and their decomposition into simpler tasks (at the lowest level, tasks are described as physical operations performed with the computer) and (2) cognitive task analysis, which characterizes the cognitive characteristics of user tasks, including the skills and knowledge required of the users.

3. User interface specification

An appropriate user interface metaphor should be selected, to simplify the cognitive complexity of the interface. Metaphors vary from the well-known *desktop metaphor* (in which the screen contains *icons* of objects such as file *folders* and trash cans) to the 3-D rooms metaphor (in which the interface could organize information for the user pictorially in terms of rooms, e.g., an operating room or a waiting room). Specification of the human-computer dialogue is also required, including specification of user actions, type of feedback, and the general dialogue style.

4. User interface design

A number of methodologies have been proposed and applied in the design of user interfaces. This includes design decisions regarding:

– functionality of the interface (e.g., what the interface will allow users to do);
– the layout and sequence of computer screens and displays;
– determination of the interaction mode, including

31

allowable user inputs and system responses;

– issues related to selection of an appropriate programming tool(s) for developing the interface (described below);

– consideration of access to other software systems by the user interface (e.g., input from medical devices or access to underlying medical databases and vocabularies); and

– plans and schedules for interface development and usability evaluation throughout the development process.

There are a number of promising approaches to designing user interfaces. These are described in Table 31.3.

5. User interface implementation

A number of programming languages and tools that support and speed the implementation of user interfaces have been developed. Special software libraries have been developed for graphics workstations (e.g., the *X11* window system library), and a variety of commercial software libraries are available to interface developers on systems with windowing capabilities (e.g., Microsoft Windows and the Macintosh *toolkit*). Such libraries can greatly speed implementation of user interfaces by providing programming code for developing windows-based user interfaces (e.g., for creating buttons, menus, and windows). Such toolkits can be flexible in that they provide ready-made screen items. However, in the past they have been inflexible in not allowing the interface developer to easily change the look or behavior of the item supplied (e.g., the *menu*). However, with the advent of current interface toolkits, the customization and extension of built-in graphics capabilities is often supported. For developing interfaces on the Internet, HTML and the *Java* programming language are beginning to be widely used.

6. User interface evaluation

Evaluation is critical in the development of successful user interfaces and according to a number of researchers, evaluation should take place throughout the process of designing and developing the user interface to feed back valuable information into the design and development process. The evaluation of human-computer interfaces is also of key importance in judging system success and in determining problem areas that may be holding up acceptance of medical computing systems.

Traditionally, interface designers have had only simple performance measures and subjective evaluations to rely on in the evaluation of interfaces. Some of these measures included error rates, task completion times, and subjective questionnaire ratings of user preferences. Another approach has involved the development of metrics for evaluating interfaces for specific characteristics. A number of basic software metrics have been developed, including metrics for measuring the maintainability, accessibility, robustness, understandability, and *portability* of user interfaces and software systems. Both task-independent metrics (e.g., measures of the complexity of screen displays) and task-sensitive metrics (e.g., measures of appropriateness of screen layout), which can be used to evaluate the efficiency of the organization of the objects in an existing or proposed interface, hold promise for assisting interface designers.

5.2 Advances in User Interface Evaluation

It may be that noncognitive methods for analyzing the usability of computer systems are inadequate. Traditional methods should be complemented by methods that support more explicitly the analysis of cognitive processes and how knowledge is developed and used. These considerations certainly apply to the issue of evaluating health care interfaces, especially because cognitive issues have been identified as being barriers in their development and acceptance. Work is being conducted on developing user interface evaluation techniques that are based on methods of cognitive analysis and that have relevance for the evaluation of health care interfaces. Although evaluation is central to continuous improvement, the evaluation of user interfaces has too often been conducted late in the design process (when reworking the interface is usually prohibitively expensive). It is recommended that a variety of complementary techniques (e.g., cognitive studies as well as ethnographic techniques) be considered early in the design of interfaces. It is also important to emphasize the need to conduct evaluations in realistic health care settings.

A general framework for considering methods used in the evaluation of human-computer interfaces is contain-

Table 31.4
Comparison of Usability Assessment Techniques.

Usability Assessment Method	Advantages	Disadvantages
Observation (ethnography)	• Rich qualitative data • Provides valuable initial information	• Cannot apply experimental rigor • Analysis of data difficult
Questionnaires; surveys	• Easy to administer • Can be used for large numbers of users	• Possible bias in interviews • Questionnaires cannot always tell what users are *actually* doing
Usability inspection; cognitive walkthrough	• Few resources needed • High potential return • Can complement usability testing	• Broad assumptions of users' cognitive operations • Does not examine actual user behavior • Needs an inspector
Usability testing; video analysis	• Can identify severe problems • Reveals users' cognitive processing • Scientific rigor and control • Reliability and validity	• Higher resource demands • Cannot always generalize

ed in Table 31.4. Observational or field study approaches allow us to study computer systems in real work environments (e.g., clinical settings). This typically involves observation (which could include videorecording of HCI) while trying to disturb the environment as little as possible. A commonly used approach to evaluating the usability of user interfaces involves presenting users with questionnaires or interviewing them after they have used a computer system. Such questionnaires typically ask users to rate a computer system or interface in terms of such attributes as how easy the program was to learn, how clear the graphics were, and so forth. Although collecting such data is easy to do, there are problems related to people's recollection of their interaction with the system when they are given questionnaires or interviewed after the fact. Alternative methods, also described in Table 31.4, include the usability inspection methods, in which usability "inspectors" (i.e., human factors experts) methodically step through a user interface in an attempt to identify possible user actions, goals, and

problems. This type of technique can be cost-effective since end users are not required for the analysis, but they do require skill in conducting the evaluation.

A variety of new techniques have appeared for assessing usability, the most recent being usability testing involving the use of video analysis. Video recordings of health care professionals as they interact with human-computer interfaces in performing specific tasks (e.g., entry of patient data) can provide data on system usability and key aspects of HCI. This type of system evaluation can provide a wealth of information about user preferences and problems when designing and implementing health care systems. A useful technique used in such studies involves asking subjects (e.g., physicians, nurses, and other health care workers) to think aloud as they interact with a particular user interface. In conjunction with audio and video recording of this type of interaction, session logs of the computer screens can also be collected. In this way, particular points in the user-computer interaction can be played back and analyzed in terms of what the user was doing at that point in the interaction (e.g.,

31

users may be experiencing difficulty in entering patient data or comprehending a graph displayed by the system). The output from such an evaluation can be presented to the system designers and can provide a rich source of data for improving user interfaces for health care systems, particularly during the iterative development of user interfaces. This type of evaluation has been used in the design of a number of health care systems, including computer-based patient record systems.

6 Principles for the Design of Health Care User Interfaces

All user interfaces have a number of requirements independent of the domain. In addition, the area of health care imposes a number of specific requirements for effective human-computer interfaces. The following attributes are considered critical to the successful development of human-computer interfaces in health care:

• Ease of use
The system should be perceived by end users as being easy to use and as leading to few user problems. User satisfaction should lead to continued and enhanced use of the system.

• Effectiveness
The system should do what is functionally required by a specified population of target users within a specified range of environments.

• Ease of learning
Users should be able to learn the operation of the system within some specified time from the start of user training, based on some specified amount of training and user support.

• Ease of understanding
Users should be able to develop a coherent model of the system that will allow them to use the system accurately and effectively.

• Predictability
The system should provide users with consistency in input operations, option selection, and presentation of output.

• User control
The user should be able to control the interaction rather than being forced to follow a rigid computer-controlled dialogue. In certain situations, however, it may be more appropriate for the dialogue to be controlled by the system (e.g., when the user conducts an unfamiliar procedure).

• Robustness
Due to time pressures and the occurrence of life-threatening emergencies in many health care settings, the system may require a high degree of robustness.

• Adaptation to different user levels and styles
The system should have flexibility in allowing for adaptation to some specified percentage of variation in users, tasks, and environments.

• Input flexibility
Intuitive and flexible forms of input should be available, and these should be suited to the type of users and their particular work environment.

• Appropriate amount of output
The system should not overwhelm the user with large amounts of data that lead to *cognitive overload.*

• Adequate user help and error recovery
Although it is better if the system can be used without documentation, any on-line help that is necessary should be easy to search for, be focused on the user's task, and list the concrete steps to be carried out. Error messages should precisely indicate problems and con-

structively suggest solutions.

• Adequate response times
Response times of less than 1 second are needed for

many patient-related tasks, whereas for ad hoc queries and tasks requiring retrieval of computer images longer response times may be acceptable.

7 Conclusions

Usability is at the very core of the interactive computer technology that is profoundly changing health care. The ongoing revolution in health care information technology has two important directions. The first direction, which is already well under way, is the development and widespread dissemination of affordable computer hardware. Indeed, the trend over the last several years has indicated a consistent doubling of computer processing capability and a halving of cost approximately every 2 years. The implications of such rapid improvement in computer hardware has made possible new technologies such as multimedia and computer imaging over *local area networks*. The second frontier that must be addressed is the challenge of creating *usable* interactive health care systems. This has often proven to be the more challenging of the two directions in the development of computer systems in health care. Indeed, this frontier is at the very core of future work in successfully integrating computing systems in health care and is the frontier on which progress will ultimately depend. As illustrated in this chapter, the area of cognitive psychology can provide a needed foundation for considering the human-related

aspects of computer systems and their interaction with health care professionals that constrain usability. Along these lines, a broad perspective to considering HCI is argued for. To facilitate this effort, it is clear that contributions are needed from a variety of disciplines.

Key References

Preece J, Sharp H, Benyon D, Holland S, Carey T. *Human-Computer Interaction.* New York: Addison-Wesley Publ Comp, 1994.

Shneiderman B. *Designing the User Interface* (2nd ed). New York NY: Addison Wesley, 1992.

Hix D, Hartson HR. *Developing User Interfaces: Ensuring Usability through Product and Process.* New York NY: John Wiley and Sons, 1993.

See the Web site for further literature references.

31

32 Costs and Benefits of Information Systems

1 Introduction

The introduction of information systems in an organization requires a meticulous assessment of the costs and the potential benefits of such a system. From an economic point of view, *costs and benefits* should at least keep each other in balance. Although analysts are generally quite good at measuring the costs of new technology, it often is problematic to calculate actual benefits. Benefits are often intangible and difficult to quantify. Even when the benefits can be measured on a numerical scale, it may be difficult to compare the scaled value to the monetary units used to measure costs. For this reason, economists often are content to compare the cost of an intervention with its *effecti-*

veness, measured in a unit of currency that allows direct comparison with the technology's cost.

This chapter provides an overview of the various costs, the possible benefits, and measurable effectiveness of information systems. Following that a brief consideration is provided of the questions of how costs and benefits of information systems may be determined and how they may be related to each other in such a way that it is possible to make well-founded economic decisions on whether to introduce a specific information system. The chapter concludes with an example to which these considerations are applied.

2 Costs of Information Systems

Before discussing the costs of information systems, the costs of all components must be identified. Many factors affect the costs of applications of large information systems. Hardware and software may not only be purchased but can also be rented, leased, or developed in-house. Operation of the complete information system, including management and support, may even be contracted out to a third party. This is called *outsourcing*. Despite this complexity, it is possible and useful to start a cost analysis by distinguishing the costs of various components:

1. hardware,
2. consumables,
3. software,
4. personnel,
5. housing, and
6. overhead.

These components are described in detail in the following section.

2.1 Hardware Costs

Hardware comprises the equipment necessary for input, communication, archiving, and processing of data. It includes:

1. central hardware, such as computers, *disk* and *tape* units, and control units and peripherally installed *terminals*, *workstations*, and printers;
2. communications equipment, including network and data communication equipment and public-access telecommunications capabilities;
3. additional equipment for *backup* purposes; and
4. air-conditioning equipment in the computer room.

Equipment costs are not restricted to the initial purchase costs (or depreciation costs). It is also necessary to perform technical maintenance, and interest costs must be paid on nondepreciated capital. Depreciation is usually divided into five equal one-year terms of 20%. The reasons for this relatively short period are, among others, the rapid developments in information technology – resulting in more value for less money – but also the changing requirements and notions with respect to applications. Considering the improved price-performance ratio over time, a nonlinear, degressive depreciation might be better than five equal terms, but such a scheme is rarely applied in practice.

2.2 Costs of Consumables

The costs of *consumables* such as magnetic disks, magnetic tapes, paper, and ink ribbons or cartridges should also be taken into account. The rule of thumb that the yearly cost of a printer for depreciation, maintenance, and consumables is equal to its purchase cost illustrates that this cost component is not negligible.

2.3 Software Costs

Purchased, rented, or leased *software* can be distinguished into:

1. system software, such as software for *operating systems*, *database management systems*, *data communication* software, and *compilers*, and
2. application software used by the end user.

Software costs also include depreciation, interest costs, and maintenance costs. Cost calculations for privately developed software are more complex, since the costs of this software must be determined on the basis of development costs. These are, in turn, determined by all cost components that have already been mentioned. The cost of maintenance, which should certainly not be neglected, is determined in the same way. It is wise to count on yearly costs of about one-third of the initial development effort.

2.4 Personnel Costs

A sensible cost analysis should also include the cost for the personnel charged with the management, maintenance, and development of the information system and for personnel charged with providing support and instruction on use of the system. Large information systems need personnel for routine operations (operators and job planners) and for management (database and network management). It should be kept in mind that some maintenance tasks are executed by the end user, for instance, setting up the workstation and the accompanying software. A nonnegligible part of personnel costs consists of costs for support and instruction.

Although the information systems are developed with the aim of allowing the user to be able to use the system autonomously, the user will require support and instruction, especially during the period of introduction of the system. When users are confronted with problems afterward, a *help desk* should be available to set them on the right track or to solve the possible technical defect. Support will also be necessary when new versions of the software are introduced. Note that support and instruction costs consist of two parts: time spent by the instructor and time spent by the instructed users. Personnel costs consist of salaries and social security premiums.

2.5 Costs for Housing

Housing costs relate to the purchase, maintenance, and management of real estate. Depreciation and maintenance are to be considered, but the costs of heating and electricity, security, cleaning, and taxes must also be considered. Calculations are generally based on the amount of floor space. There is, however, a difference between a square meter of archive space and space for computer rooms.

2.6 Overhead Costs

Finally, it should be mentioned that some organizational costs, such as the costs of management, financial and personnel administration, catering, telephone, and mail should be included in cost analyses. These overhead costs are generally accounted for as a proportion of the number of employees.

As mentioned before, determining the costs of information systems is more complex than just listing the components mentioned above. However, using this list as a starting point, some parts may be left out or some may be expressed in more detail in specific situations. The result will be a complete overview of the costs of applying the information system. Some components are often overlooked, for instance, the hidden costs of management or the costs of instructing the end user.

32

3 Benefits of Information Systems

Information systems are usually introduced in health care with the expectation that the effectiveness of care will improve, that the efficiency of care will increase, or that the efficiencies of processes will increase. These aspects are indeed potential benefits of an information system. Unfortunately, history teaches us that it is not easy to make benefits in health care visible. In general, three types of benefits may be distinguished:

1. nonquantifiable benefits,
2. quantifiable benefits that can be expressed quantitatively, although not in monetary terms, and
3. quantifiable benefits than can be expressed in monetary terms.

It will be clear that the last category is the easiest to handle. The decision maker is able to perform an investment analysis in which monetary costs and benefits can be balanced. The first and second categories are less suitable for such an analysis, and they can only lead to qualitative considerations. They are, however, not less important. Nowadays, techniques that are applied in technology assessment allow for a conversion of formerly nonquantifiable benefits into the second

category. There are also methods of weighing the effects of category 2 on a monetary balance. Below we provide examples of the three categories mentioned above. All are taken from health care practice.

3.1 Nonquantifiable Benefits

The following are some examples of nonquantifiable benefits:

1. An information system often leads to a more complete and more accurate recording of data at the workplace.
   Uniformity of registration and reporting will increase.
2. Improved on-line accessibility of data makes it possible to bring together the data available for a particular patient.
   Moreover, a reduction of copying by hand also reduces the probability of errors, which is a quantifiable benefit.
3. Information stored in a database is, in principle,

accessible for management purposes and for scientific research. This adds a new dimension to information technology, since statistical analysis of data that are only recorded on paper is usually impractical.

4. With the help of an information system, patient cases that might be relevant for medical education can quickly be selected.

3.2 Quantifiable, Nonmonetary Benefits

The following are some examples of quantifiable, non-monetary benefits:

1. The time needed to report the results of laboratory tests may be reduced, which will reduce the percentage of *stat reports*.
2. An automated appointment system may reduce the waiting time for patients in the outpatient clinic and may allow patients to combine several appointments in the hospital on the same day. This will save the patients time and it will reduce the crowds in waiting rooms.
3. An automated nursing information system that allows nurses to record data at the point of care may reduce the time needed for the registration of these data.
4. Application of digital *imaging* in radiology departments (where images are no longer stored on film, but available by means of image workstations) can reduce the time between ordering an action and the reporting of its results.

It is possible to make some items quantifiable in a certain sense by the application of techniques from social sciences. Examples are the work satisfaction of the user and the quality of care. It should be remarked, however, that such a mapping of nonquantifiable benefits onto quantifiable benefits should be applied with the utmost care and should be supported by good arguments.

3.3 Quantifiable, Monetary Benefits

Monetary benefits are probably the easiest category to consider, since they concern tangible results. A few general examples also apply to hospital information systems:

- The introduction of a material management system may lead to a reduction of stocks and a reduction of losses of perishable goods.
- Financial systems may lead to faster invoicing and a reduction of the accounts receivable total.

Less direct, but certainly important effects are those on staff. The introduction of an information system in an organization generally means a shift of tasks from employees to the information system, and sometimes a different way of working as well. These changes may influence the use of resources. Personnel costs may decrease, because the information system takes over part of the work. Sometimes this means that the same amount of work can be done by fewer people. The extent to which an increase in productivity can effectively be converted into a higher level of production depends on the existing situation. In general, this does not happen automatically. The time saved may be used for other, new tasks or for a regular extension of existing duties, or the time may become superfluous, so that it becomes impossible to reduce the number of employees, either by natural personnel turnover or by other means, such as layoff. Moreover, small reductions in time spent by large groups of personnel can rarely be turned into savings equal to the sum of these time reductions.

This type of benefit is sometimes motivated as follows: in the future, smaller personnel increases will be sufficient to achieve increases in activity equal to those that would have been achieved before implementation of the information system. This last benefit is then introduced without a solid investigation.

It should also be remarked that tasks are sometimes not taken over by the information system but are merely replaced, so that the responsibility ends up with other employees. If the organization is not adapted, an increase in personnel costs may even occur. Application of information systems may lead to savings on the costs of materials and equipment. Introduction of digital imaging, for instance, may make film and film development materials superfluous, as well as the accompanying equipment for development.

4 Evaluation of Information Systems

A cost-benefit analysis is generally performed before an information system is developed or selected. It is also important to *evaluate* the actual costs and benefits after the information system has been operational on a pilot scale for some period of time, but before the system is introduced on a large scale. This evaluation may be performed by measuring the system's effects on the basis of an experimental setup. For the effects to be measured, the situation before introduction of the system is compared to the situation after its introduction. The problem with such a comparison is that other aspects may also have changed during the trial period of the information system, and these changes also have effects.

Examples of changes are reduction of working hours, changes in the general social climate or the economic situation, organizational changes, the introduction of new diagnostic and therapeutic methods, and so forth. This dilemma may be solved by using a control group, which in this case means an environment that sufficiently resembles the experimental environment but in which the information system is not introduced. This approach is derived from classical randomized trials.

By this approach, the choice of trial and control groups is determined at random, and the involved groups are not told whether the system to be evaluated will be introduced. It is clear that this approach is not feasible when applying it to the introduction of an information system. It is not possible to choose a group at random, since often only one group is involved, and a *double-blind* investigation is fundamentally impossible because of the nature of the system to be introduced. Therefore, in the literature this approach is characterized by the term *quasi-experimental* setup. For obvious reasons, such a quasi-experimental setup should be applied with care: the fact that the decision has been made to introduce an information system could indicate that this group is not an average group. For instance, it may be the case that there is an enthusiastic management team or that the users are interested in applying information technology in their work.

In balancing costs and benefits it should be noted that the costs of automation, especially the equipment part of it, have a tendency to decrease over time because of improved price-performance ratios. Although this effect is not as large as is sometimes suggested, it should not be neglected. It may be significant when measured over a number of years, and it may tip the balance in favor of the information system. Therefore, an information system that is not interesting now might show a positive cost-benefit ratio within a few years. This effect is increased by the fact that the costs of manual processing tend to increase, especially personnel costs.

In conclusion it may be stated that to arrive at a correct cost-benefit analysis, the following questions should be answered:

1. Which alternatives are considered in the analysis?
2. What are the cost components in the analysis, and how should they be specified?
3. What are the potential benefits, and what is their nature? If they are nonquantifiable or not monetarily quantifiable, on the basis of what criteria should the investment decision be made?
4. What is the influence of time on costs and benefits? This dynamic aspect may provide insight into a possible breakeven point in the future.
5. How are costs and benefits checked against reality in an experimental setup?

The answers to these questions will lead to the construction of a model of the cost-benefit analysis for the system that is being considered. This model may sub-

32

sequently be improved on the basis of discussions with experts and with the people involved. This increases the subjective reliability. Next, the objective reliability of relevant parts of the model may be established by validation. The model constructed in this way may be used for the cost-benefit analysis. In the ideal situation, it is possible to generalize the model so that it is valid for arbitrary applications of the information system being evaluated. Such a generalization should be made carefully. Sometimes the postulated effects are only applicable to a specific user's environment, and then a reformulation of the model is necessary. An experimental setup can also provide insight into this situation.

5   Example

This section provides a specific example to illustrate the topics discussed earlier in the chapter.

A hospital considers purchasing an information system for electronic presentation, processing, and storage of nuclear medicine images. In this hospital, such images are now acquired digitally, printed on a film printer, and stored on **optical disks**. Reporting by the nuclear medicine physician takes place on the basis of the printed images, and the resulting reports are made available (after typing) to the requesting physicians by means of the hospital information system that is already present. The film is stored in a dedicated archive, where one can also find earlier images of the patient. The department of nuclear medicine expects to improve the process by introducing an automated system and performs a cost-benefit analysis, in which the present situation is compared to the working methods foreseen with the information system in place. Only those costs that change because of the introduction of this system are considered:

- Hardware
- a central computer for management, distribution, and storage of images;
- a special workstation for diagnosing and reporting; and
- a number of workstations for image retrieval by the requesting departments.

- Consumables

After introduction no consumables are required. Storage on digital media already occurs in the present situation and does not change.

- Software must be acquired for:
- the **operating system**,
- the network management, and
- the processing, presentation, and storage of images.

- Personnel

Extra staff is needed for the management and support of the information system. Overhead for these personnel will be included. Furthermore, it is expected that reporting by the nuclear medicine physician will require more time because of the additional possibilities available with the information system.

- Housing

No extra housing is needed for the use of the information system.

In the next step, the potential benefits are summed. The expected consequences of the introduction of the system are:

1. Improved patient care because of improvements to the diagnostics and the understanding of the requesting clinician, who can simply retrieve the images through a workstation.
2. No more problems with missing films.
3. Better access to images relevant for education.
4. A reduction in turnaround time from the time of a request for a nuclear medicine examination to the time of presentation of the report to the requesting clinician.

32

5. Fewer technicians and administrative personnel will be needed in the department of nuclear medicine.
6. Space for the film archive is no longer required.
7. There is no longer a need for film or for film development chemicals or equipment.

The hospital then considers this inventory and concludes that benefits 1, 2, and 3 may occur, but they will not be measurable in practice. Thus, they are classified as potential benefits that will not be considered in the investment decision. The hospital considers benefit 4, that is, a decrease in the turnaround time, to be an important prerequisite before proceeding with an extensive implementation of the system. Related to a possible reduction of personnel, it is assumed that the reduction of administrative personnel will not be realized, because there is already a shortage of staff in that area. The free technician time arising from the fact that they do not have to process film will be used to manage the information system. The monetary benefits of the reduction of archive space, film development equipment, film, and chemicals will have to be quantified. The time needed for instruction and support will also be included. Considering all aspects, the hospital decides to perform a cost-benefit analysis, as follows. Costs and monetary benefits will be listed and compared. The dynamic aspect, for instance, when computer equipment will become cheaper, will also be considered. If the result of this analysis is positive, the system will be implemented experimentally in the department of nuclear medicine, so that in this trial setup it will be possible to determine whether or not the turnaround time is indeed reduced. In this way the hospital will also gain insight into the extra time spent on reporting. Such a trial setup does not realize the most important monetary benefits, that is, the elimination of costs for film, chemicals, and so forth. Once the result of the study is known, this cost-benefit analysis will be the basis for the final decision with respect to a broad implementation of the system.

The outline of the analysis described above is well balanced and provides an objective view of the postulated effects of the system. A disadvantage of this approach is that in case of a negative decision, the system will have to be removed from the department. This must be included in the contract with the vendor, and it may lead to problems with the staff of the department of nuclear medicine. In a good cost-benefit analysis, such practical considerations should also be included.

32

33 Security in Medical Information Systems

1 Introduction

The amount of data stored in *databases* as well as the accessibility of these data will increase as a result of the introduction of *computer networks* both within health care institutions and within regions. The positive aspects of this trend have already been discussed elsewhere in this Handbook, but negative aspects are also connected to these developments. These negative aspects are discussed here.

First, improved accessibility may be a threat to the *privacy* of those whose personal data are registered. This is especially the case for information systems used in health care, where privacy-sensitive data are stored. Measures should be taken to prevent the unauthorized use of data.

A second important aspect is the *quality* of data and software. Information systems in health care are important at both the operational and the management levels. The risk of errors in data and *software* must be kept within acceptable limits. Protection against the loss or corruption of data is part of this aspect.

A third aspect is the availability of data and the functions of the information system. More and more organizations in health care become directly dependent on the reliable functioning of their information systems. Therefore, actions are needed to reduce the probability of service disruption, along with the pre-

vention of unauthorized use. The purpose of data protection measures is the protection of:

- privacy,
- quality of medical data and software, and
- availability of data and functions.

Measures may concern equipment, software, and *procedures*. They should be adjusted to each other, and they should be balanced. It must be mentioned at the outset that it is impossible to realize 100% protection. However, it is possible to reduce risks or to restrict possible damage because of misuse or abuse. Until recently, terminology in the area of data protection has been far from uniform and has often been incoherent. Now a standard is emerging in which the area of data protection is indicated by *data security*, with the following as subareas:

- confidentiality,
- integrity, and
- availability.

However, various terms are still being used and are found in somewhat older literature. Therefore, it is always advisable to give some thought to the meaning of a particular term.

2 The Scenario for Data Protection

The development of medical science has led to a high degree of specialization. This implies that knowledge and skills essential for patient care are divided between several health care workers. Within health care we even distinguish several "shells" of care: first-line, second-line, and third-line care. Thus, a patient is confronted with various elements of the health care system and with various health care professionals, such as a general practitioner, a specialist, a nurse, a pharmacist, a physiotherapist, or a social worker. For efficient patient care, exchange of patient-related data between the health care professionals is necessary in one way or the other.

Data are recorded in many different places, such as in the medical and the nursing records or billing records, even when computers are not in use. Therefore, it is also important to control access to the data, which does not always happen. The increasing application of computers, however, increases the accessibility of the data, especially when modern techniques, such as a network of terminals directly coupled to computers and local area networks (*LAN*s, see Chapters 4 and 5), are applied. Unauthorized use of the data is not an illusory danger. Therefore, the access to these data must be regulated. The fact that not everybody has access to the data is a logical consequence of the right to privacy.

The right to privacy with respect to data means that the individual can decide which personal data he or she wants to be made available and to what extent these data may be exchanged with other people. This fundamental right to privacy of a patient may be endangered in many ways: by another patient, by somebody working in the institution (e.g., an acquaintance or a family member), or in general, by family, neighbors, an employer, the government, the press, and so forth. The introduction of computers has increased people's fear that their private life will be jeopardized. Therefore, laws to protect privacy have been introduced in many countries. These laws are very different among the various countries of the world. The European Commission, for example, has issued for the European Union the "Directive for the Protection of Individuals with Regard to the Processing of Personal Data and on the Free Movement of Such Data" to reduce these differences in laws in European countries. Member states will have to bring their legislation in line with the directive, which in several ways allows for the inclusion of elements particular to a given country.

The privacy sensitivity of data is strongly context dependent. Data on psychiatric or genetic diseases are often considered to be sensitive. Many diseases, however, are generally not considered to be sensitive, but they may be for people in some professions. If it were known, for example, that a person had a particular disease, it might influence the development of that person's career. Take a top manager requiring an examination for a complaint that is assumed to be possibly caused by stress. The mere fact that the manager has an appointment in a hospital, for instance, with the department of cardiology, could be privacy sensitive for such a person. As another example, some people do not want the outside world to know what medication they are taking. In this context, privacy means that the individual decides to what extent she or he will put data at the disposal of others.

In addition, the individual must be able to check what has been registered about him or her and to whom data are distributed.

3 Policy with Respect to Data Security

Each organization that uses an information system must formulate its policy with respect to data security explicitly, which means that this policy should be laid down in a *regulation*. It should be realized that the regulation of data security to an acceptable level – acceptable, since 100% protection cannot be attained – will not be obtained automatically. It requires an emphatic will and a controlled decision-making process. In this process a number of elements or steps may be distinguished. They are discussed below.

- Raising the awareness of the management of an organization

As a first step, the management of the organization must consider data security to be important. This may be realized by a bottom-up approach, in which, for instance, health care workers or patients draw attention to the necessity of a good privacy regulation. The awareness of the management may be raised by a top-down approach, for example, by legal or governmental measures. Of course, it is also possible that the management of an organization will spontaneously recognize the importance of having a privacy regulation.

- Raising the awareness of the employees in the organization

A second important element is the awareness of the importance of data protection within the organization. Activities are necessary to make the members of an organization aware of the importance of data protection. This process will stimulate the recognition of the existence of risks on the one hand, and it will enhance the acceptance and the effects of measures to be taken on the other. This is a continuing activity in the organization, since new staff will always be joining the organization. There is also the danger that the attention to data security of those who have been in service for a longer time will relax over time.

3.1 Rules for Data Security

Making the purposes of security explicit in rules for data protection is an important step. The organization must define criteria concerning the acceptable number of errors in the data set, the acceptable chance of data loss, and the availability of data. Such explicit descriptions of the objectives of data security rarely exist. Although it is a difficult process, explicit objectives are indispensable if we have to take data protection measures and if we want to do this in a practical way.

The elaboration of the objectives will generally depend on the type of information system for which regulations must be established and on the specific organization to which the regulation applies. Important items are the type of data that are stored, the functions that the system performs, and the size of the system. An example of a norm for the availability of data in a hospital information system is as follows: for an integrated hospital information system (see Chapter 21), system availability at least 99.7% of the time 24 hours a day, 7 days a week is considered a reasonable norm.

3.2 Confidentiality

The access rights of users must be defined to protect data confidentiality. These access rights will depend on current legislation, public opinion, policies within the organization, the attitude of professional organizations, and so forth. Rules for data access depend, among other things, on the professional status of the user within the organization, the patients concerned, the type of data, the relation between the user and the patient, the supplier of the data, and the age of the data. Finally, access will also depend on the user's intended action with the data, for example, read, write, edit, or delete.

3.3 Privacy Regulation

The policy of the authority responsible for protecting registered data should be established in a regulation, usually called *privacy regulation*. There is the danger that the privacy regulations used in various organizations will be so different that patients will lose track of all of the different regulations. It is advisable to set up model regulations that prevent confusing differences among the regulations of various organizations.

4 Threats

Security measures are intended to reduce the threats concerning data confidentiality, integrity, and availability. These threats are elaborated in this section.

4.1 Threats to Confidentiality

Confidentiality is violated when data pass into the wrong hands, either on purpose or accidentally, within or outside an organization. This could happen directly, for example, by burglary, or by intentionally or unintentionally abusing the information system. This can happen indirectly as well, for instance, by the use of careless procedures when distributing printed reports. The most common way to break into a system is to use the *password* (i.e., the code giving a user access to the system) of an authorized user, obtained in an illegal way (by copying the password or by trying different passwords until the correct one is found). It is also possible that a user who formally has only restricted access rights, may illegally try to extend his or her access rights. Tapping of data communications lines by connecting terminals or computers to other computers is possible as well. Illegal distribution may also occur via operating errors and by careless management of access authorizations.

The increase in the use of automated information systems has increased the danger of uncontrolled distribution of data. Moreover, the technical possibility of collecting data relating to the same person in various files (the so-called coupling of files or *record linkage*) is a real danger to a person's privacy. Such a coupling is only allowed under strict conditions.

4.2 Threats to Data Integrity and Availability

Concerning data integrity, there is a danger that data sets are inconsistent or that their contents are corrupted. This may or may not be done on purpose. The inconsistency may have various causes, such as an error in the software, a malfunction in the equipment, or operating errors.

The availability of functions of the information system may be endangered by failures of equipment or network facilities, and the availability of functions of the software may be endangered by errors in operating the system and by insufficient environmental facilities.

Software development on a computer system that is also used as an operational information system along with its corresponding data files, is very risky. If these files are supposed to be confidential, software development on that computer system should not be allowed; this can be achieved by not supplying *editors* or *compilers* for program development on the operational system.

5 Measures

Measures may improve data protection in two ways; some measures may reduce the probability of something going wrong (e.g., fire prevention, access regulations for the space where the computer is located, or the use of passwords). Other measures are aimed at reducing the level of damage in case something goes wrong, Examples of the latter include copying data files, the availability of spare equipment, and setting up and rehearsing crisis procedures. This section mentions a few of the measures that are frequently taken. For further details refer to the literature. Panel 33.1 lists some possible measures that can be taken to protect information systems.

PANEL 33.1

Protection of Information Systems

Equipment measures

Provisions with respect to the computer system belong to this category. Sometimes all central equipment is duplicated. In case of emergency it is possible to fall back on the extra system. This is also an advantage for data availability and data integrity, since production and program development can be completely separated and tests of the quality of new versions of software can be performed on the extra computer system.

Provisions with respect to communication and the network include the possibility of choosing another communication line between a terminal and a computer when a line fails, so-called rerouting. *Cryptographic* techniques, which make data illegible by means of secret encoding, can be used to send messages in the data communication network. At *terminals magnetic card* or *chip card* readers may be used for user identification.

Very simple measures often reduce the probability of disturbances caused by mistakes. Distinct indications on equipment that show for what purpose the equipment is being used at any moment, as well as the further distinct identification of information carriers (disks and magnetic tapes), may be considered. Environmental provisions also belong to this category. They include:

- a computer center that can be well locked (e.g., with magnetic card readers),
- fire protection, often by an automatic fire-extinguishing installation, because in case of fire, smoke is often one of the biggest threats,
- air-conditioning controlling temperature and humidity, and
- protection against flooding.

Software measures

An important aspect of this category is the systematic design of software. The verifiability of software must be taken into account beforehand. Moreover, tests confirming the validity and consistency of data must be incorporated into the programs. These tests must be of a dynamic nature (i.e., testing per *transaction*) as well as static (e.g., periodically checking the contents of files for their validity and consistency). The use of a well-tested *database management system* (see Chapter 4) may contribute to data security. Measures must be taken within the software to arrange data access. Identification of the user is a condition, often met by using a personal password that must be typed before getting permission to use the computer. Provisions must be made to prevent the use of easy passwords and to enforce people to periodically change their passwords. The risk of passwords becoming publicly known and other people taking over the privileges of the owner of the password is not illusory. It should be possible to *log* transactions, such as entering or changing data in a file, which is comparable to registering transactions in a log book. Moreover, software should be available to reconstruct the database by using these logged data and an old copy of the database that is kept in a safe place. ▶

33

Organizational measures

Regulating the operation of the information system is one of the most important organizational measures. Separation of duties is also an important measure. This prevents too many privileges from being the responsibility of any one person, a situation that increases the risk of abuse. Along with dividing up the regulatory authority, data may be classified into different types, and people may be given access only to certain types of data. User's authorizations can be divided into different categories, so that access checks are made between the function of the user, the data type, and the patient whose data are requested. Further refinements to data access may be related to the age of the data, the supplier of the data, and the time and place where the data are requested.

A *handbook of operations* is also indispensable. Such a handbook should indicate what to do in various situations, including crisis situations when the system does not function or conform to certain specifications. In such situations it is important that authorizations be clearly established. Documentation is also important for good data integrity, since data integrity is also served by proper specifications. Documentation may, on the other hand, threat confidentiality, since it can indicate to nonauthorized people how to access the data. Procedures for copying files (the backup mentioned above) and storing these files (preferably outside the computing center, in a fireproof vault) should be meticulously described as well.

Procedures regarding the implementation of new software and new versions of software should be elaborated carefully. Errors in software may be disastrous for the functioning of the system. Some imaginable errors are so serious that recovery of the database (using old copies and entered mutations) is no longer possible. Such a situation occurs when errors in the application software have caused incorrect mutations in the database.

The *management of authorizations* must be elaborated carefully. In large organizations with thousands of users, such as a university hospital, it may not be expected that one person can manage all authorizations. A decentralized structure should be established in which submanagers are designated for specific authorizations. The issuing of passwords must be done carefully. In connection with the software measures mentioned above, organizational measures should be taken to change these passwords regularly and to make sure that easy-to-guess passwords are not applied. Strict procedures should be available in case a user forgets his or her password. It is difficult to prevent users from forgetting a password, since they are specifically requested not to write it down. When issuing a new password, managers should make sure that they are indeed dealing with that user.

The measures taken may involve the equipment, the software, or system operating procedures (i.e., organizational measures). It is important that the protection measures chosen consist of these three types of measures. After all, excellent technical measures for controlling access to a computer center will loose their value considerably if the procedures have not been carefully set up and maintained.

An example of a software measure is the so-called *logging* and *recovery* software that enables the reconstruction of the database after a disruption by using **backups** made earlier. This is only useful if the procedure for regularly copying the database is actually followed.

6. Choice of Measures to Be Taken

As soon as the objectives for the measures with respect to data integrity, confidentiality, and availability have been established, specific measures must be taken to achieve the desired goals. Some possible measures were mentioned above. In practice dozens of measures are possible. Therefore, it is desirable to have some system for choosing the right measures. The following provides a theoretical nine-step approach to choosing among the required measures. This approach is not a recipe book, but describes the questions that should implicitly or explicitly be answered to select the appropriate security measures.

6.1 Identify the Threats

Before measures can be taken, threats and how and when they may occur should be identified. When considering these threats, questions about the information system could be asked, such as the following:

- What could happen with the data?
- Who is able to cause such a situation?
- When and where can they cause such a situation?
- Under what circumstances and why would such a situation occur?

In this analysis all aspects of the information system, not just those concerning the department of information services, should be considered. This first step results in a list of threats to be used for the next steps.

6.2 Estimating the Chances of an Incident

The chances of the occurrence of an incident identified in Section 6.1 may vary substantially. The probability of an incident enters into the choice of a set of measures. For instance, *cryptographic* techniques almost completely exclude the possibility of tapping telephone lines, but introducing a cryptographic technique is hardly sensible when the chances that lines will be tapped are very small. The chances of an incident may be highly dependent on the local situation. In Western Europe the chances of an earthquake are very small, whereas in some areas of Western Europe a computer center might be flooded. In California, the situation is just the opposite. Estimation of the probabilities is not simple, but it may be facilitated by comparing the chances of the threats on the list and ranking them from those with the smallest to those with the largest probability of occurring. In estimating the chances of occurrence it is recommended that a restricted number of frequencies (e.g., on a logarithmic scale) be chosen, such as once every 400 years, once every 10 days, or 100 times a day.

6.3 Estimating Expected Damage

Probability is not the only important aspect. The expected amount of damage should also be considered. The probability of a fire in the computer center will be relatively small, but the amount of damage expected from a fire is usually large. Estimation of the expected amount of damage implies that the consequences of an incident should be considered. For some incidents, it is possible to quantify the damage immediately, that is, it may be expressed as the cost for lost materials, costs for replacement, costs for repair of equipment or reconstruction of the database, loss of personnel time, and so forth. First, the threats should be considered and the damage should be quantified, and then other, more subjective threats may be considered. Although this is a subjective estimate, making a subjective quantification is better than taking haphazard measures when an incident occurs. The subjectivity can be reduced to a certain extent by having several people perform this step independently and making them try to attain a common view in a later consultation.

33

6.4 Probability of Occurrence and Expected Damage

Multiply for each listed threat its probability with the expected amount of damage. The resulting quantity will be called *risk* (the mean expected risk per unit of time). Threats can now be ranked by risk.

6.5 List the Considered Measures

We should realize that measures may influence risks in two ways: they may reduce the chances of occurrence or they may limit the expected damage. Before we are able to select an appropriate set of measures, it is advisable to make a list of measures that may be considered. This list may be established from the literature or from the experiences of other computer centers. It is recommended that a professional organization provide such lists. Not all measures will be applicable in every system: beware of unthinkingly copying existing lists.

6.6 Estimate the Costs of Each Measure

The costs of measures highly depend on the system and its environment. The following are some important cost components:

1. environmental facilities for equipment; they can be written off over a certain period, for instance, 10 to 30 years for the building and 4 to 10 years for the necessary equipment (for instance, air-conditioning);
2. depreciation and maintenance costs for equipment or lease costs (generally 4 to 7 years);
3. program development and maintenance (these can also be written off over 4 to 7 years);
4. costs for software *licenses* (i.e., the right to use software packages);
5. costs for organizational changes;

6. costs for education and instruction of personnel involved in the use of the system;
7. additional time that the user must spend because of measures for data security; and
8. additional capacity of the computer system for processing and storing the data.

6.7 Group the Measures

The process of choosing a set of measures is complicated by the fact that the choice of a specific measure may influence the effects of other measures. The installation of a **badge reader** for identification at each terminal will, for instance, influence the effect of personal **passwords** considerably. Therefore, it is desirable to group highly related measures.

6.8 Relationships between Threats and Measures

In this step the possible effect of the measures on the various threats are classified either as none, weak, slight, or considerable. By using this classification as well as the costs, the effect of a measure becomes clear. A measure may affect several threats, which complicates the selection process indicated in step 6.9; moreover, the dependence indicated in step 6.7 is possible.

6.9 Select Measures

As a result of the foregoing step, some measures may immediately be rejected, since an alternative with a better effect is available. Some measures are imposed by regulations. They must be selected, of course. For the final selection, performance of a *cost-benefit* analysis is important. It implies that for the suggested set of measures the reduction of the total risk and the total costs are determined. In comparing a few suggested sets of measures, a choice can be made on the basis of these figures.

PANEL 33.2

Seismed Guidelines

Because it was believed to be necessary to develop and test guidelines for dealing with security in medical information systems within the Advanced Informatics in Medicine (AIM) program of the European Union, the *Seismed* project was carried out between 1992 and 1995. Guidelines were produced and published for the following:

- security risk analysis;
- high-level security policy;
- baseline security;
- security in medical database systems;
- network security;
- secure systems procurement, development, and design;
- secure system implementation; and
- cryptographic mechanisms.

The guidelines were produced in three versions, directed toward:

- health care management,
- health care information technology and security personnel, and
- health care system users.

33

---

7 Introduction of the Measures

As soon as a set of measures have been selected, they must be introduced, taking the necessary care. This is easier with a new system, which still must be developed and then introduced, than with an existing system.

For many of the existing systems, the current data security measures are insufficient. In general, many data security elements of existing systems must be changed. User's habits must also be changed, and this is a complex task. Yet, for new systems it may also be expected that requirements for data protection will change over time. These changes may result from changes in legislation or because the system is being developed further and will contain new functions or data. The organization management should continuously pay attention to this topic.

---

8 Responsibility for Data Security

The manager of the database, generally the highest authority within the organization, is formally responsible for data security measures. In large organizations this authority will be the board of directors. In smaller organizations it may be the individual professional. Although in a large organization the highest authority is formally responsible, professionals remain at least partly responsible for the protection of the data that they manage as part of their job.

In larger organizations the highest authority will generally not have the expertise or time to bear this responsibility in person. In practice, a specific person within the organization will be held responsible. Nowadays, this is generally the head of a department of information services. This is undesirable, since that person has other responsibilities that might conflict with the responsibility for data security. Therefore, it is advisable to hire a particular person to be responsible for data security, and this person should report directly to the head of the organization.

Finally, it is desirable that periodic external audits be performed on the chosen data security measures and on the way that they are kept, so-called **EDP auditing**.

9 Legislation and Regulation

Until now legislation and regulations have mainly been concerned with privacy aspects. It may be expected that because of the increasing importance of information systems in health care, legislation for data integrity and availability will be realized in due course.

Key References

Bakker AR. Security in medical information systems. In: van Bemmel JH, McCray AT, eds. *IMIA Yearbook of Medical Informatics.* Stuttgart/New York: Schattauer Verlag, 1993:52-60.

Barber B, Treacher A, Louwerse K. *Towards Security in Medical Telematics.* Amsterdam: IOS Press, 1996.

Watson BL. Liability for failure to acquire or use computers in medicine. New York: IEEE Comput Soc 1981:879-83.

See the Web site for further literature references.

34 Standards in Health Care Informatics and Telematics in Europe

1 Introduction

Health care information infrastructures and *telematics* services are becoming essential parts of health care business strategies and the day-to-day provision of health care. Providing a high-quality service to patients involves having the right information at the right place at the right time.

Cost-benefit analyses have been conducted and seem to justify expenditures in telematics, given the constraints of scarce resources and competing demands in health care. Consequently, health care organizations have already started to communicate electronically at both local and national levels. Areas in which action is still needed are the interconnection of networks and the *interoperability* of services and applications. At present, it is recognized that the timely development of health care informatics and telematics standards is necessary for improving the interoperability of systems within health care information infrastructures.

2 Telematics Requirements in Health Care

Although the health care sector is data and information intensive and most of its actors (hospitals, clinics, service departments, and a growing number of individual physicians' offices) are computerized, it has lagged far behind other sectors in applying communications technology. Even though most hospitals and clinics do have computers, they delegate to them isolated and relatively small segments of the organization's clinical operations. Today, there is a clear need for more integration of and better communication between these health information systems.

The necessity for communication of information in the health care sector becomes evident when studying the variety of interested parties and the multitude of applications and their importance. The potential exchange of information between heterogeneous and independent information systems in hospitals, *ancillary departments* (e.g., clinical laboratory and radiology), private medical offices, public authorities, and the health care industry is large and complex. The nature of health care data is also diverse; for example, health care data are in the forms of text, coded data, voice, signals, or images. The list in Table 34.1 illustrates user requirements with regard to exchanging messages in health care.

The environment of medical electronic data interchange (*EDI*) applications is extremely heterogeneous and complex, and it is changing continuously. This also applies, among other things, to the structure of health care as such, the organizations and number of parties involved in the communication scenarios, the diversity of medical

Clinical messages

Table 34.1
Different Types of Messages Exchanged in Health Care.

- Exchange of service requests to and reports from laboratories, radiology departments, and ancillary services
- Prescriptions from physicians to pharmacies
- Hospital admission data and discharge summaries
- Multimedia patient-centered electronic health care records
- Transplantation data, such as registrations, waiting lists, and organ matching
- Data from pharmaceutical industry, e.g., information on drugs, drug surveillance, and pharmaceutical trials
- Interpersonal mail between practitioners, e.g., between general practitioners and specialists
- Information retrieval from external literature and knowledge bases
- Communication with public authorities in connection with epidemiology, quality assessment schemes, or utilization review

34

Logistics and financial messages

- Communication between hospitals and suppliers; purchasing, invoicing, and logistics
- Exchange with insurance agencies and third-party payers; billing and reimbursement

Medical images, biosignals, and multimedia data

- Multimedia patient record
- Conventional X-ray images from radiology departments
- Digital images from computed tomography scanners, magnetic resonance imagers, and ultrasound equipment
- Images processed for radiotherapy and neurosurgery
- Scanned documents (e.g., for the electronic multimedia patient record)
- Digital voice reports
- Biosignals (electrocardiograms, electromyograms, electroencephalograms, etc.)

events, the high number of standardized message types required, the specificity of the message contents, and the number of message syntaxes currently in use.

The parties involved in medical EDI cover a wide range of organizations, each with different goals and priorities, from individual general practitioners (GPs) to large hospital organizations, from regional specialized user groups to international committees, and from small software suppliers to multinational hardware and software vendors. An objective in Europe and the United States is to realize a network of networks, based on common standards, linking GPs, specialists, hospitals, and institutions. Patients will benefit from a substantial improvement in health care, for example, improvement in diagnosis through on-line access to specialists, on-line scheduling of examinations and hospital services by practitioners, and transplant matching. Taxpayers and governments will benefit from better cost control and cost savings in health care spending and from speeding up reimbursement procedures.

To maximize efficiency, effectiveness, and quality in health care delivery, it is necessary to *standardize* all these electronic messages. Studies have shown that the use of *standards* is a key factor in electronic communication, which, in turn, significantly increases the effectiveness of computers. A breakthrough in systems on the health care market will probably result from the introduction of such telematics applications that stimulate the use of computers (also called the *loop effect*, see Fig. 34.1).

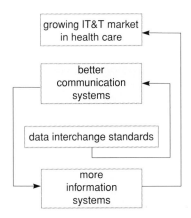

Figure 34.1
The loop effect induced by telematics standards.

3 Definitions

3.1 Standardization

Standardization describes and provides the quality requirements that products, processes, and services must fulfill. It is a systematic activity that creates order, makes selections, and formulates rules. For the purpose of this chapter, the following definitions for standards and standardization from the International Standards Organization (*ISO*) and the International Electrotechnical Committee (*IEC*) apply:

Standardization
Activity of establishing, with regard to actual or potential problems, provisions for common and repeated use, aimed at the achievement of the optimum degree of order in a given context.

Standard
A document, established by consensus and approved by a recognized body that provides, for common and repeated use, rules, guidelines or characteristics for activities, or their results, aimed at the achievement of the optimum degree of order in a given context.

Consensus means general agreement, characterized by the absence of sustained opposition to substantial is-

sues by any important group among the concerned parties and by a process that involves an effort to take into account the views of all parties concerned and to reconcile any conflicting arguments. The standardization process must be open so that all parties can be represented. Consensus requires that all views and opinions be considered and that concerted action be taken toward their resolution. Consensus means much more than decision by a simple majority, but not necessarily unanimity.

In Europe, the recognized standards body for the purposes of health care computing is the Comité Européen de Normalisation, Technical Committee 251 (*CEN/TC251*). It has the scope and responsibility for organizing, coordinating, and monitoring the development of standards in health care informatics, as well as the promulgation of these standards. Publications resulting from the work of *CEN* are called designated European Standards, European Prestandards, or CEN Reports.

A European Standard (EN) is a CEN standard drawn up by consensus of the members and adopted in accordance with a weighted voting procedure. When such a standard is adopted, it must be implemented at the national level by being decreed a national standard and by withdrawal of any conflicting national standards. In other words, once the EN has been adopted, it will rigorously replace the national one. Variations are not allowed. A European Prestandard (ENV) is established as a prospective standard for provisional application in technical fields in which the innovation rate is high (e.g., in information technology). The standard should not be used when the safety of people and goods is endangered. Members must make the ENV available at the national level and announce its existence. Meanwhile, conflicting national standards may be maintained.

A CEN Report (CR) must be approved by simple majority vote of the Technical Board of CEN. CRs are of two types. The first arises when consensus cannot be reached but when the information is so useful that it should be made public. CRs of this type are, in effect, failed standards. The second type is different and does not include failed standards. These are normative documents that are communicated as CEN reports rather than standards. A Harmonization Document (HD) is a standard adopted in the same way as an EN, but national variations are permitted if existing national regulations or particular technical requirements are required for a transitional period. Documents that are still used as CEN working documents are known as prEN, prENV, or draft reports. ENs correspond to ISO standards; ENVs correspond to ISO technical reports.

3.2 Telematics and Electronic Data Interchange

Telematics gives access to any form of data or knowledge anywhere, it speeds up the diffusion of information, it saves time, it increases collaboration between individuals and groups, and it may improve the quality of decisions. However, there is a threat that telematics may also speed up the diffusion of inaccurate or false information.

EDI is defined in many different ways. The following definition is often used: EDI is

the transfer of structured and coded data, by agreed message standards, from computer to computer, by electronic means.

The data are essentially structured. Unstructured information such as *fax* or free-text electronic mail does not strictly fall into the category of EDI, although such information can be included as part of a message. The data are also primarily intended for processing by computer applications rather than for direct interpretation by human users.

Current EDI standards are primarily concerned with the nature of the interchanged data, and they cover three main areas:

1. a common *syntax*, equivalent to the syntax in natural language;
2. definitions of common data elements equivalent to the *semantics* in natural language; and
3. standard messages, which combine data elements and syntax into structured data aggregates, suitable for interchange and processing.

Open EDI is defined as "EDI that uses public standards; that is aimed toward interoperability over time; that covers various business sectors, information technology systems, and data types; and that is capable of multiple and simultaneous transactions."

4 Benefits and Role of CEN

4.1 Benefits

In industry, standards are known for increasing market opportunities and for lowering the cost of equipment and services to users. The same arguments hold for information systems in health care. Common standards reduce the cost of health care information systems and they open up the market.

Thanks to technology (e.g., the *Internet* or the *World Wide Web*), information is no longer limited by location, but is limited only by the availability and quality of the information itself.

34

"Information" implies a proper organization of the data, and this is exactly why standards in health care are of crucial importance: They provide common message descriptions and formats, as well as definitions of medical concepts and codes. The ability to exchange data, both clinical and administrative data, between different information systems is therefore one of the major challenges to health care informatics. Unfortunately, in many cases a situation of heterogeneous and incompatible data exchange protocols exists. However, especially in Europe, where information (e.g., administrative patient data) crosses management boundaries and in many cases regional and national boundaries, agreement on the data structures and the information content of messages is necessary. Standards in health care informatics will contribute to the health of patients by improving the abilities of public administrations, research centers that study the effectiveness of medical care, and health care professionals to share critical patient information.

4.2 CEN

When telematics was introduced in health care, a need arose for standardization and a common use of standards, securing compatibility, connectivity, and interchangeability. Therefore, in 1990, the European standardization committee CEN established a Technical Committee for Medical Informatics (TC251). First, CEN assessed the current situation of standardization in medical informatics (*CEN/TC251*) and described the tasks for its working groups and project teams. The objectives of CEN/TC251 are the organization, coordination, and follow-up of the development of standards in health care informatics, at a European level, comprising 18 countries, as well as a growing number of Eastern European countries.

CEN/TC251 is composed of delegations, officially appointed by the members of CEN. It covers the following activities, for each of which there is a separate working group (WG):

1. health care *information modeling* and *medical records*;

2. health care terminology, *semantics*, and *knowledge bases*;
3. health care communications and messages;
4. medical *imaging* and *multimedia*;
5. communication with medical devices;
6. health care security, privacy, quality, and safety; and
7. intermittently connected devices, including "intelligent" cards.

Each working group supervises a number of project teams, consisting of small groups of trusted people preparing documents.

CEN/TC251 establishes priorities based on health care market priorities, and it identifies both publicly available specifications and outputs that are suitable for transformation into standards (Fig. 34.2).

Since standardization is a worldwide activity, CEN/TC251 works in coordination with the American National Standards Institute (*ANSI*) and its Health Care Informatics Standards Board (HISB). *ANSI-HISB* serves as an umbrella organization for the activities of the American Society for Testing and Materials (*ASTM*), the activities on *MEDIX* (medical data interchange) of the Institute of Electrical and Electronics Engineers, Health Level 7 (*HL-7*), the *DICOM* activities of the American College of Radiology/National Electrical Manufacturers Association (*ACR-NEMA*), the activities concerning data interchange of the National Council of

34

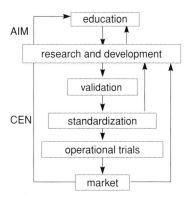

Figure 34.2
Relationships between R&D, standardization, and exploitation.

Prescriptions and Drug Programs (*NCPDP*), and other standardization organizations in the United States. In Europe *ISO*, *IEC*, the Consultative Committee of International Telegraph and Telephone (*CCITT*) and the United Nations Economic Commission for Europe (*UN/ECE*) have agreed to coordinate the future development of EDI standards among their organizations, to avoid divergent approaches to standardization of electronic data exchange.

CEN/TC251 was established simultaneously with the European program for research and development in medical informatics (Advanced Informatics in Medicine, *AIM*). Research and development (*R&D*) and standardization cross-fertilize each other and are of great significance to the future of health care informatics and telematics.

5 Description of Present European Standards

5.1 The Medical Informatics Vocabulary

The Medical Informatics Vocabulary prestandard provides definitions of terms that label key concepts in medical informatics standards, and it describes their interrelationships in a systematic index. This will ensure that those who develop or use information systems have a consistent understanding of the concepts covered by standards in all the working groups of CEN/TC251. The first vocabulary is restricted to the English language. To support a global information infrastructure, agreement on concepts and terms across language boundaries will be essential.

prestandard fits, and it provides pointers to the subjects that will become amenable to standardization as medical informatics matures further. These pointers will offer an essential structure on which future standards makers can build. Because it was necessary to limit the normative scope at this stage, the prestandard may appear sparse and remote from the practical applications that the program of medical informatics standards making as a whole is required to support. However, the intervening standards will be valid only if they are built on the fundamental principles set out in this framework. The prestandard is positioned in relation to extant work on frameworks and architectures, in particular, the seven-layer stack of the open systems interconnection (*OSI*) Reference Model.

5.2 The Health Care Information Framework

The Health Care Information Framework prestandard is a first step to standardizing the architectures that support the delivery of health care information systems.

Associated with the normative clauses, an informative section describes the whole context within which the

5.3 The Electronic Health Care Record Architecture

The prestandard on the *Electronic Health Care Record Architecture* defines the basic architectural components of an electronic health care record and their logical interrelationships. Standardization at this level is necessary if health care records are to support teamwork between clinicians in different

34

disciplines and to enable mobility within and between countries of people who give and receive health care. If these objectives are to be achieved, and this prestandard indicates the types of further work required, further standardization below this basic level will also be required.

The architecture is defined in such a way that it enables clinicians to make their own decisions about what to record and in what format to record it. It supports a common understanding of the necessary variety of the content and format of records. It is not a system specification, nor is it aimed at a standardized patient care record. In building the architecture, the results of a wide range of earlier work have been taken into account, including relevant research projects in the *EU*-funded Fourth Framework Programmes. It has already been used as the foundation for clinical record systems by at least one group of small or medium enterprises. The nature of the source materials is described in a supporting document. The relevance of the architecture to a variety of clinical situations is illustrated in a set of scenarios.

5.4 The Standard Architecture for Health Care Information Systems

The intention of this prestandard is the promotion of *modular* and *open* systems in health care. It also deals with integration with existing systems. It specifies the characteristics of common components regarding the services that they provide and the structure of the data used by each component, without making any assumption about the component's internal structure.

5.5 Classification and Coding

5.5.1 Nomenclature, Classification, and Coding for Clinical Laboratories

This prestandard provides a structure for systematic naming, *nomenclature*, *classification*, and *coding* of properties, including quantitative variables in laboratory medicine. It will facilitate the electronic interchange of messages by using a standard structure for nomenclatures that are used in routine laboratory practice.

5.5.2 Classification and Coding of Surgical Procedures

This prestandard is to be used for all interventional procedures, not only for surgical procedures. It represents a controlled vocabulary related to basic surgical concepts, and it supports the exchange of surgical information between different national terminology classifications within Europe, expressed in *natural language*. The reason is that European countries use different procedure classifications or coding systems, hampering the exchange of health information. The prestandard is complementary to existing classifications, and it will facilitate the international comparison of interventions. This prestandard is to be used by organizations that develop or maintain surgical procedure classifications, but it is not intended for use by individual clinicians or hospital administrators.

5.5.3 Structure of Concept Systems; Vocabulary

Medical informatics deals with many large, overlapping coding systems (e.g., classifications, nomenclatures, dictionaries, and *thesauri*) (see Chapter 6). Each coding system is specialized with respect to either a user group, an environment, a purpose, or a specific information system. Such coding systems may be incompatible in an integrated health care information environment. Computer-based coding systems should be coherent, and it should be possible to map the code

34

between the systems. The standard provides the vocabulary and the guidelines for the structure of a concept system. In the long run, comparison of overlapping concept systems will facilitate convergence of different computer-based coding systems into a comprehensive reference structure, such as covered by the Unified Medical Language System (*UMLS*) (see Chapter 6).

5.5.4 Coding Systems for Drugs

This project will set up a system for the unambiguous identification of medicinal products that are registered in medical informatics applications and about what data are exchanged between different systems. The project does not intend to develop a coding system for these products.

5.5.5 Coding Systems for Medical Devices

Medical devices can be classified into some 6,000 medical device groups comprising an estimated 750,000 or more brands, modes, and sizes. There is no international agreed upon classification system for such devices. The different classification and inventory systems that are used today classify and register the devices in numerous and often incompatible ways, thereby making data exchange concerning medical devices difficult or impossible. This prestandard defines a categorical structure for medical device groups; that is, it outlines a system of descriptors and it provides rules that specify how to combine the descriptors to formulate sensible expressions.

The intention is that each medical device group may be described within the system of concepts and that names may be generated to identify each separate medical device group.

5.6 Standards

5.6.1 Standards for Quantities in Clinical Sciences

Measured data can be expressed in quantities (e.g., a concentration) specified for a component (e.g., creati-

nine) from a substrate (e.g., blood of a known person at a known time). Formal quantitative statements should accept data in any format or font (e.g., roman, italic, subscript, superscript, and different font sizes). Interchange should allow data in local formats to be converted to the International System of Units (*SI units*). Besides SI units, the system should be able to comprehend other units, including those not recognized by the International Bureau of Weights and Measures. The standard might include guidelines on quantitative information, transmitted in graphical form.

5.6.2 Time Standards

The notion of time is omnipresent in medical language and medical information exchange, and there is potentially no limit to the various ways in which time-related information may be expressed (see also Chapter 29). The standard concerned provides a set of basic entities, with precisely defined properties and interrelationships among them, which are sufficient to allow an unambiguous representation of time-related expressions. The prestandard does not confine itself to a particular temporal *ontology* or to an underlying theory on time, because this would be too restrictive with respect to past and ongoing research. The framework proposed for time is general enough to bridge the gap between such preconceived theories or particular systems that deal explicitly with time-related information.

5.7 Data Interchange

5.7.1 Syntaxes for Data Interchange

Health care messages may be expressed in many different interchange formats, so consensus is needed on which ones to use in the future. If it is possible to standardize messages on the basis of a limited number of syntaxes, software will become reusable and better equipped to handle a wide variety of message types. None of the existing interchange formats such as *HL-7*, *ASN.1*, *EDIFACT*, *EUCLIDES*, or *ODA* has been able to support all functionality requirements required so far. Standards such as EDIFACT and ASN.1 are preferable to health care-specific syntaxes that have only limited local implementations (see also Chapter 5). The semantic content of all messages, however, is more important than the syntactical structure.

5.7.2   Registration of Coding Schemes

Coding schemes are frequently used in messages to provide precise and unambiguous representations of the data. Coding schemes that are used in health care communications need proper registration. Throughout the health services in different countries many coding schemes are being used, and therefore, adoption of a single coding scheme for health care data cannot be expected. Therefore, the coding scheme should at least be identified so that the data may be understood by the receiver. This standard specifies a procedure for registering and issuing a unique identifier for each coding scheme that is used in health care. In 1994, the *World Health Organization* in Geneva, Switzerland, became the Registration Authority.

5.7.3   Exchange of Laboratory Information

Clinical laboratories have been computerized for many years (see Section 5 of Chapter 13) and there is an increasing need for EDI of test requests and laboratory reports. This standard covers messages sent between laboratory computer systems and the computer systems used by those who order tests and receive reports, such as GPs' systems, hospital information systems, and clinical information systems. It covers *clinical chemistry*, hematology, and microbiology.

Samples may be collected at the time that the order is issued, or the order may include instructions for the sample to be collected later by the laboratory or other staff. All usual laboratory reports are supported, including partial, supplementary, final, complete, and cumulative results. Test reports may include the normal ranges for that test. They may also include details of the clinical history, previous results, drug treatment, and proposed procedures. Previously issued reports may be modified or canceled. The standard is intended for use by message developers and is of interest to system developers of laboratory computer systems, clinicians, and GPs.

5.7.4   Registration of the Data Sets Used in EDI

This standard provides for the allocation of unique identifiers to the information objects used in health care messages, and it registers information about their functions and characteristics. Communication between computer systems requires the sender and the recipient to have a common understanding of the information objects at issue, and it requires that they have the ability to process them. This implies that with each application it must be able to identify data objects without ambiguity. The standard specifies the content and procedures for maintaining a register and for facilitating the reuse of objects, and it allows for comparisons between similar objects. The information objects to be registered include messages, logical groupings of data elements, and their *attributes*. The standard is supported by a *database*.

5.7.5   Messages for Diagnostic Services

There is a demand for report and request messages to be used between hospital diagnostic services departments and agents requesting services from them. These messages concern services such as X rays, *computed tomography* scans, *magnetic resonance images*, *scintigrams* and *ultrasound* scans, electrocardiograms (*ECGs*), lung function tests, and anatomic pathology reports. The work is based on messages that are used in clinical chemistry, hematology, function laboratories and microbiology laboratories (see Chapter 13). The diagnostic service messages permit explicit references to image, *biosignal*, and other non-character-based information. However, the scope is limited to character-based messages. The messages for diagnostic services departments differ from messages for clinical laboratories in the following respects:

- They include the need to schedule examinations and to transport the patient to the department.
- There is an extensive use of *free text*.
- They consist of structured reports that may contain a mix of logically grouped factual observations and subjective opinions.

34

- They describe studies of the patient, rather than of a sample taken from the patient.

The standard documentation includes:

- Description of the scope of the messages and their functionality.
- A basic information model relevant to these messages.
- Implementation guidelines for different scenarios.
- Documentation of the messages, including definitions using the *EDIFACT* syntax, and an implementation guide.

5.7.6 Messages for Exchange of Health Care Administrative Data

Patient administrative data are needed to support safe, efficient, and effective health care delivery within hospitals and primary care. Patient *identification* data are needed to positively identify the patient. The availability of EDI reduces the number of instances in which *demographic* data need to be transcribed. Patient registration and identification data include:

- the identification of the patient,
- the address of the patient,
- the name of the person who is responsible for this patient or the patient's next of kin, and
- authority for payment.

Additional information will cover, for instance:

- references to contracts or insurance policies and
- addresses of health care providers and health care organizations.

These messages do not cover reimbursement or admission, discharge, or transfer, but they make such processes much easier because of the availability of registration and identification data.

5.7.7 Messages for Patient Referral and Discharge

The term *referral* also covers requests for specialist services, and the term *discharge* covers reports by the specialist service provider, including clinic reports and discharge summaries. The specialist service request message is intended to be used by a health care professional or an insurer who wishes to request a range of specialist services from another health care professional or organization on behalf of a patient. This request concerns both inpatient and outpatient care, home visits, telephone consultation, or notifications of details about the patient's demographics, next of kin, and registered GP and insurer, plus details about the patient's medical problems, current therapy, family, social group, relevant findings, and whatever else is requested. The most frequent occurrence of such a message is the referral of a patient by a GP for advice or treatment from a specialist, but interspecialist referrals and referrals to other disciplines may also be considered. The specialist service report provides a means of transmitting the result of a patient contact, such as a clinical visit or hospital stay, back to the referrer and other parties, giving full details of the care that has been supplied or proposed, together with relevant medical and administrative details. This is normally done when an episode of specialized care has come to an end and patient-related clinical information needs to be transferred to establish continuity of care.

5.7.8 Methodology for the Development of Health Care Messages

The main goal of this CEN/TC251 activity is to develop standardized health care character-based EDI messages. It contains the following main components:

- study of the user requirements in the selected message domain;
- specification of message scenarios in both formal and informal ways; this • includes definition of the communication roles, the services to be supported by each party, and the interrelationships between different EDI message types within a particular domain;
- definition of the information that is shared;
- definition of the messages required to support the information exchange needs, independently of the EDI syntax used; and

- guidelines for implementation, using a standard EDI syntax such as EDIFACT or ASN.1.

5.8 Images

5.8.1 Imaging and Related Data Interchange Formats

This standard refers to the so-called *DICOM* standard, developed by *ACR/NEMA*. By basing this standard on DICOM, CEN has facilitated worldwide harmonization of medical image communications standards with existing industry standards. For some application areas, especially teleservices, such as teleradiology, the MEDICOM standard can be a basis for application development.

5.8.2 Medical Image Management Standard

The DICOM standard was developed by ACR-NEMA to accomplish standardized communication of medical images and related data either by on-line or by off-line means. This prestandard specifies network services to control the safe storage of medical images and related data in a network environment, but it does not cover the issue of data ownership, nor does it provide management with master copies of data. The term *safe storage* implies that it must be possible to retrieve the images at a later time. However, it does not imply that the location where the images have initially been stored will be the only location where they can be retrieved.

5.8.3 HIS, RIS, and PACS

This prestandard specifies information objects and services to be used when transferring information between medical imaging modalities and information systems in a health care environment, such as a hospital information system (*HIS*), a radiology information system (*RIS*), or a picture archiving and communication system (*PACS*). It does not specify particular information systems, because these vary according to local and national practices. It provides:

- a description of the content of the messages that transfer the work list information and
- a communication mechanism to transfer these messages.

This prestandard is applicable to character-based (i.e., *alphanumeric*) information, but it does not apply to information presented as images or graphics.
It does not cover information objects and services to be used when transferring administrative data, requests, reports, and diagnostic service information between departmental information systems (e.g., imaging departments) to or from hospital information systems.

5.8.4 Media Interchange of Medical Images

This prestandard parallels the electronic interchange of medical images and associated information by using removable large-capacity storage media. The development of media-based interchange in addition to networking is required to address the needs for medical image interchange by media in the short term, and it is also required to support the cost-effective exchange of medical images within and between locations where patient care and diagnostics are performed. For instance, the European Society of Cardiology needed standardization of storage of images on *CD-ROM*s for cost reduction in *catheterization* laboratories.

5.9 Biosignals

5.9.1 Computerized ECG Interchange

This standard provides specifications for the interchange format of *ECG*s, but also requirements for data compression and accuracy of signal reproduction. Thus, it supports quality assurance in processing and electronic interchange of ECGs. Electrocardiography is the most frequently used noninvasive technique for the detection and verification of *ischemic heart disease*, *myocardial infarction*, and cardiac rhythm disorders. More than 100 million ECGs are recorded yearly, both in the United States and the European Union, for routine diagnostic and screening purposes. Almost all new

34

electrocardiographs use digital recording, interpretation, and communications techniques. The interchange and documentation of ECGs is regulated in the so-called Standard Communications Protocol (*SCP*-ECG). Characteristic of this communication standard is its high degree of flexibility, which allows for transmission not only of interpretation results but also, when applied in its most extensive form, the transmission of the complete ECG recording, including interpreted waveforms, measurements, diagnoses, and manufacturer-specific diagnostic codes, along with identification data. Furthermore, compression algorithms have been precisely defined, ensuring data integrity within defined error limits.

5.9.2 Vital Signs Information Representation

This work is related to the documentation of *vital signs* of patients as recorded, for instance, in intensive care units. It contains, for example, inventories and proposals on scenarios, a domain information model, service specifications, biosignal interchange formats, and real-time data interchange formats. A proposal for a dictionary of the managed medical objects within intensive care units has been drafted.

5.10 Security

5.10.1 User Identification, Authentication, and Security

This prestandard applies to all information systems within health care that handle or store sensitive health data about people, and it uses *passwords* as the only means of authenticating the entered user identifier (i.e., verifying the claimed identity of a user). Systems included are, for example, computer-based patient record systems, patient administrative systems, and laboratory systems containing personal health data.
The use of passwords that are kept confidential by each user and that are constructed in such a way that others will not be able to compromise this confidential authentication information easily is the most common means of authentication in current computer systems,

and it will remain so for some time to come.
Conventional passwords have several disadvantages. Some of these are as follows:

- They can easily be shared among several users.
- The use of unprotected network technology makes them easy targets for eavesdropping.
- To be secure, they may be hard to remember.

Other technologies that provide more secure means of authentication, such as *chip cards, have been introduced, and they will eventually phase out the use of passwords (see also Chapter 33).*

5.10.2 Security for Health Care Information Systems

The risk of corruption or the loss of health care data is always present, from the point of origin to the point of use. Risk and errors are already associated with data acquisition. Such errors can compound, with subsequent risks in the data-to-information chain, and they may introduce overt risks to the patient or staff member. All staff have a duty to provide the best care for clinical data, but they can only act within the limits of their knowledge. Often they are unaware of what the real risks and threats are. To enhance their understanding and thereby improve the quality of handling of health care data, a coherent scheme that indicates possible consequences of relevant threats is needed.
The objectives are:

1. to develop a library of real risk scenarios in health care information systems, describing the impacts and consequences of possible security breaches;
2. to develop a classification of health care information systems, classified according to their level of security and operational environments; and
3. to develop standardized security profiles for the various classes of health care information systems.

5.10.3 Digital Signature Services

The use of data processing and telecommunications in health care must be accompanied by appropriate security measures to ensure data confidentiality and integrity, in compliance with a legal framework. These measures are aimed at protecting patient privacy as well as professional accountability. An example of such measures is a *digital signature*, which may be described as data appended to a data unit or a cryptographic transformation of a data unit that allows a recipient of the data unit to prove the source and integrity of that unit and to protect it against forgery, for example, by the recipient. Examples are:

- authentication of computer users, organizations, and systems;
- authentication of document originator;
- protection of document integrity and assurance that its contents and the signature are bound together;
- nonrepudiation of origin and receipt of messages;
- time stamping; and
- proof of authorization as a registered professional and other qualifications.

In health care, with an increasing need for open secure communications between all parties involved, it is essential that at least one standard algorithm based on digital signature techniques be able to be used for all services. This prestandard, therefore defines a digital signature algorithm, should such an algorithm be required. The algorithm defined in this standard is the well-known and widely used *RSA algorithm*, named after its inventors, Rivest, Shamir, and Adelman.

5.10.4 Intermittently Connected Devices

This prestandard proposes a framework for data structures used with respect to intermittently connected devices (ICDs). An ICD is a device that stores and transmits person-related data in such a fashion that the originator of the information may not receive confirmation of receipt by the recipient. ICDs include portable computerized medical patient records and, in particular, patient data cards, portable computers, ambulatory monitors, and similar devices to store and transmit identifiable person-related data.

The prestandard describes the data structures in both free text and descriptive ASN.1 notation, and it allocates the appropriate tags to compound data objects that are designed for specific purposes. This includes identification, record linkage, administrative and clinical processes, and images and other nontextual data. The prestandard includes a structure for data interchange, but the document does not prescribe the physical exchange mechanism, thus allowing both ASN.1 and EDIFACT to be used in the exchange between host and ICD units. The design of the data structures is such that a minimum of data is required, thus reducing overhead in terms of implementation. However, implementers may pick and choose from the nonmandatory elements, realizing that they preserve both upward compatibility and the ability to exchange data with other ICD users.

Key References

De Moor G. Standardization in medical informatics in Europe. Med Inform 1994;35:1-12.

See the Web site for further literature references.

34

35 Project Management

1 Introduction

A **project** is a cluster of related activities, and one of its typical features is the presence of a clear beginning and a clear ending in time. Means (money and personnel) are limited. The product that is to be delivered by the project will obtain its final description during the project. These characteristics require special attention for the management of a project.

This chapter discusses all aspects of projects for the development of information systems (electronic data processing (**EDP**) project). Such a project is the total of all human activities directed toward the realization of an information system. It may include the design, development, and introduction of the system. Activities that follow after the system has been accepted – with acceptance being the formal end of the project – such as use and maintenance of the system, are also considered. Not all activities are present in every project.

EDP projects may vary substantially in type and size. Projects may range from the realization of a simple, straightforward registration system or the selection and implementation of already commercially available software to the realization of a complete hospital information system. The complexity of a project should be taken into account when establishing an organization for the management of a project.

The general characteristics of an EDP project will be described below. The intention of the description is the following:

* To give a frame of reference to future users enabling them to answer questions such as:
  - In which order should parts of the information-system be realized? and
  - How is the realization of the information system progressing?
* To outline which problems tend to arise in many projects; this will make it easier to recognize these problems at an early stage.
* To show which solutions are available for some of these problems and what users themselves can do in this context.

2 Information Systems and Projects

Various components can be distinguished within an information system (see also Chapter 4), namely:

1. the equipment (hardware),
2. the computer programs (software),
3. the data,
4. the users of the system, and
5. the procedures to be applied by the users.

When a complete information system is so large and complex that it is impossible to grasp it as a whole, a modular approach is generally applied. Modules are also called *system parts* or *program packages*.

The development of an information system, followed by its **implementation**, is often executed as a project. In all cases a clear ultimate goal must be formulated and organizational measures must be taken to safeguard the progress of the project.

3 Functions in an EDP Project

People connected with an EDP project can roughly be divided into the users (i.e., management and end users) who offer their knowledge of the subject matter and computer scientists who have knowledge of informatics.

Different functions on the on the EDP project side are described below:

1. Management

The management tries to create favorable conditions and to supply capacity. It controls all projects and makes sure that the contents of the projects are in line with the general information policy of the organization.

2. Project leader

The **project leader** has the day-to-day responsibility for the complete project. Making a comparison to the world of the construction industry, we could say that the project leader's role is comparable to the role of an architect. The architect coordinates all activities during the design, programming, introduction, and acceptance of a system and may also be involved in the initial use of the system.

3. Information analysts, systems designers, and systems analysts

The **information analysts**, **systems designers**, and **systems analysts** are the technical draftspeople. These three comparable positions can be distinguished by the level of detail of their work: the information analyst analyzes the current flows of information, the systems analyst analyzes ways to put these flows into a system, and the systems designer designs the system itself. In general, the result of this last step consists of a number of schedules, which will be translated into a computer program by a **programmer**.

4. Programmers

The programmer is comparable to the constructor or the builder. Already, a significant portion of programming activities are taken over by software development tools, which consist of *code generators* closely integrated with design software tools (i.e., the developers' **workbench**).

5. Operators

The task of the **operators** becomes apparent after the information system has been realized. For example, equipment must be operated, external storage media must be mounted, paper must be torn off and distributed, and contact must be kept with maintenance companies. The number of people that operate the computer installation (to be distinguished from the users of computer terminals and workstations) should be kept to a minimum.

In a somewhat larger computer center tasks have been divided among operators, a system manager, a database manager, a job planner, who controls the task division, and a network manager, who takes care of the communication network between the system and the workstations and terminals. These functions can gradually change with respect to form and content, depending on the size of the organization and the project.

In a large university hospital, the EDP staff may consist of about 25 people, about 10 of whom are in charge of the service of the computer center and the network.

4 Cooperation Between EDP Professionals and Users

In small organizations and for small projects, the cooperation between EDP professionals and users can be very simple: the user speaks to the EDP professional (sometimes they may even be the same person). In organizations that are larger in size and complexity, the communication must be formalized more precisely. The structure of the various consultative bodies within a project results from the task areas that can be distinguished within projects. These areas are described below:

1. Policy preparation and policy execution
This includes the supply of information and proposals for the definition of policy regarding the project, as well as the supervision and coordination of the defined policy. This activity is usually prepared by a policy group at the executive level of the organization.

2. Supervision of development projects
The activities within the project are specified, detailed, and surveyed. This is mostly done by experts in the area of health care in which the project is carried out, together with computer scientists. At this stage a steering committee is established for the supervision of the activities.

3. Carrying out development projects
The technical and organizational activities for the realization of the required information applications are performed by one or more project groups.

4. Introduction of applications
This concerns the activities in the users' organization and the EDP department that are needed to be able to use the results of the development. In this context the word **implementation** is often used. Contrary to what is commonly thought, the emphasis on implementation is more on organizational aspects than on technical aspects. A feasible definition of implementation is "the optimal tuning of the possibilities of the application to the required working practice of the users." It may be useful to establish a semipermanent users committee for the introduction and maintenance of the system.

35

5 Development of an Information System

The development of an information system is often a lengthy and complex process. The typical characteristics of a project, mentioned in the introduction, require special measures by management, and EDP professionals to keep the system under control. Essentially, these measures amount to a division of the problem into smaller ones that are more easily manageable, such as in a modular approach, dividing the development into well-defined stages in time. Between two consecutive stages there is a moment to make a decision: a **checkpoint**. It is important to realize that a system development method should be used as a guide for phasing the project and as a checklist for project activities and certainly not as a straitjacket preventing all flexibility. Various "schools" use a slightly different way of dividing projects into stages and sometimes quite different terminologies (see Chapter 19). The basic pattern, however, is more or less the same (for an example, see Fig. 35.1). The following describes the stages in this example and provides a few remarks regarding alternative possibilities.

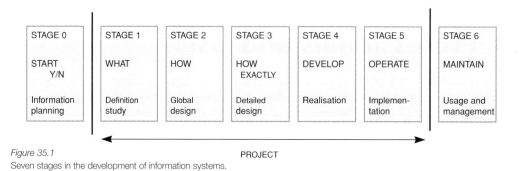

Figure 35.1
Seven stages in the development of information systems.

At a certain point somebody in an organization comes up with the proposal to use a computerized information system for some task. The exploration of the possibilities may give rise to the phased development of an information system, as described below.

Stage 0: Information planning
At this exploratory stage attempts are made to divide the problem of the user into components and to get an impression of the extent of the project and the possibilities for realization. Usually, this is performed by interviewing the user. This stage is primarily intended to furnish the management of the organization with the information needed to decide whether or not to actually start the project. Once the decision has been made to proceed with the project, development starts with a definition study.

Stage 1: Definition study
During the definition study a more specific investigation is performed to discover what users really want to be realized, how their wishes can be fitted into the arrangements of their organizations, and what the connection is with other information systems. In this stage about the same work is done as was done in the preceding stage, but it is done more thoroughly. The quantitative analysis concerning which *transactions* and how many transactions are involved requires much effort. The computer scientist now acts as an information analyst or a system analyst. The division of the future system into modules and possibly into functions (which are parts of modules) is also started. An outline of a *cost-benefit* analysis (see Chapter 32) is part of the results of the definition study. At the end of

this stage the decision is made whether or not to make a global design. At this stage, the intended end user becomes increasingly more involved; this early involvement is an important phenomenon and is known as *participatory design.*

Stage 2: Global design
This stage of the development involves the most user participation. The users determine the outlines and the functionality of the information system, in close cooperation with EDP professionals. They specify which data must be processed for each part, which relations exist between these sets of data, and how the system must control these relations. Finally, they decide how they want the data or the results of the processing to be presented. In this stage the EDP professional acts as a *system analyst* or a *system designer*.

Stage 3: Detailed design
In this stage the global design is elaborated in such a way that the resulting detailed design can be used for realization of the information system. Theoretically, the detailed design succeeds the global design. However, there will usually be an overlap, in the sense that the global design may be changed while the detailed design is worked out. When the user wants a function that can only be realized at high costs, the user might adjust his or her wishes; on the other hand, however, apparently less important user requests can sometimes be realized with little extra effort. As soon as the global design and the detailed design have been approved by the established steering committee, the realization stage will start.

Stage 4: Realization (building and testing)
In this stage the programmer translates the specifications of the detailed design, mostly consisting of schedules and text, into computer programs. The data files are set up by using the detailed data structures. When all software has been thoroughly tested and the EDP professionals are convinced that the system is free of errors, the users will execute an **acceptance test**. The users check whether the system fulfills the requirements by using input data that are as realistic as possible. It is important to check for rarely occurring extreme situations . The preparation of the user's manual, the training of the users, and the setting up of emergency procedures (e.g., what to do when system parts break down or when data in files are not accessible) are also part of this stage.

Stage 5: Implementation
When no errors have been found during the acceptance test, the introduction or implementation of the system can be started. This stage includes the adaptation of the organization that will be confronted with the new system. In many cases measures have already been taken to **convert** data, that is, to transform the existing data that are available in manual form or in another system into a form that can be used in the new system.
The final introduction, when the system is transferred to the users' organization, is usually preceded by a trial implementation. Such a trial implementation allows for a test of the system's functional and technical performance in a real production environment. For safety reasons the old system runs parallel to the new one. This means that for a certain period the information processing is done in the old way, as well as by the new information system. In the event of failure of the new system, processing can continue in the old way. In practice, a gradual implementation plan is followed. In case of a first implementation the plan is completely executed, and in case of a follow-up implementation (a new version or release) it is partially executed.

Stage 6: Usage and management
Once the system is operational, the stage of usage and management is entered. In this stage the system is no longer being developed. However, from time to time the system is maintained. Reasons for maintenance can vary:

1. correction of errors in the software;
2. adaptation and extension of the software because of changes in the technical environment or changes in regulations; this is called *passive maintenance*; and
3. changes in the software resulting from new requirements of the users related to the functions of the system; this is called *active maintenance*.

Maintenance implies changes in the software. Because of these changes the software must be tested again and reaccepted by the users. Not only the software but also the documentation must be modified.
Various deliveries of the software are often classified in numbered versions and releases. A version is associated with substantial functional changes, whereas a release generally concerns corrections of imperfections and errors. This explains the numbering of program packages, for instance, PATIENT 3.2 indicates version 3, release 2, of the package with the name PATIENT.

35

6 Problems During an EDP Project

During an EDP project certain problems are often encountered. The problems can be divided into the following three categories:

1. The system does not perform exactly as the user presumed. In most cases this is caused by problems during the design.

2. The system is ready for use later than expected (a problem concerning the scheduled time from initiation to completion).

3. The system is more expensive than expected (the cost problem).

We discuss each of these categories of problems,

since, sadly enough, most users will be confronted with them sooner or later.

6.1 Problems with the Design

One of the most important problems with EDP projects is that the global design (the result of stage 2) appears to be incorrect. The following are the most important causes:

1. The work that must be done to achieve a global design is very abstract. For EDP professionals this is not a major problem, because they are used to this type of work and they have been trained for it. For users, however, this type of work is mostly new and very difficult. Therefore, they are not able to survey the implications of the specifications on which they have agreed with the EDP professionals.
2. Closely related to the problem of abstraction is the problem of a lack of a description method that is clear to both EDP professionals and users. The existing documentation techniques are not really helpful in the communication between EDP professionals and users.
3. For a complex information system the global and detailed designs are often documented in a voluminous book that can be understood only after serious study. Users usually do not spend enough time studying it, and hence, they overlook the consequences of the design.
4. During the preparation of the design a situation that frequently occurs is that both users and EDP professionals overlook problems and defects in the specifications because they have been involved in the project too closely and for too long.

• Consequences
The consequences of these problems depend on the stage in which they become apparent. It is comparable to the placement of a water pipe system in a concrete foundation. If everything is still on the drawing board, a change can be made simply. When the pipe system has been placed into the steel reinforcement, changes can be made, but it is much more complicated. Once the concrete has set, changes are hardly possible.

The most obvious consequence of errors in the design is that one must go back to an earlier stage of the project. When, for instance, it becomes clear during programming that something has been forgotten, the detailed design and sometimes also the global design must be changed. If these relapses occur too often, one can be certain of a decrease in the motivation of all people involved in the project.

• Possible solutions
In the first place, users should spend enough time and effort in cooperating in the preparation of the global design. A useful means of helping to increase the effective participation of users is to work with **prototypes**. They show the users the main functions of a system in a realistic way. There are even system development methods (e.g., rapid application development) that use prototypes in the first stages to circumvent the problems of abstraction. So-called **fourth-generation programming languages** and powerful software tools make it possible to build representative prototypes with relatively little effort.

To circumvent the problem of designers being blind to problems in their own product, it is advisable to present the specifications of the system to others who are not involved in the project.

Users can help considerably by explicitly requiring the documentation of all preceding stages before a succeeding stage can start.

For the quality of a system, it is important that criteria for acceptance be explicitly formulated beforehand.

6.2 Problems in the Field of Elapsed Time

The following are some of the main causes of delays in EDP projects:

1. The project falls back to a preceding stage, causing a repetition of work that has already been done on the project, making some of the work that has been done useless.
2. Time schedules appear to be unreliable, because the time for certain efforts has been inaccurately estimated in the design stage. This can be caused

by the use of inappropriate techniques or guidelines. Optimistic estimates may also be the result of commercial or policy matters.

3. EDP professionals spend insufficient time on a project because they are confronted with essential maintenance activities on other projects. Again, this is a consequence of in accurate planning.

4. Excess consultations concerning the information system are made. The meetings themselves do not take so much time, but they may cause delays since it is often difficult to get the involved policy makers together at short notice.

• Possible Consequences
1. The team tries to complete the project in time for the scheduled delivery date by employing more people. These people are drawn away from other projects, where scheduling problems will now occur as well. When the number of EDP professionals assigned to a project becomes too large, the law of diminishing returns applies.

2. Quality requirements are attenuated. First, documentation is neglected and then the problem is tackled with quick and dirty solutions. Both approaches show that what first seems to be a good bargain usually works out to be expensive in the end.

3. It is decided that the project will be introduced in stages. First, a few parts of the system will be released, and afterward, the software will be extended. In practice, this implies considerably more effort for the introduction of the system; for instance, more acceptance tests will be necessary. However, splitting a system into smaller parts is not necessarily a bad solution, provided that a good framework exists and that the modules are well chosen. Such a method is called *incremental development*.

• Possible solutions
1. Avoid falling back to the preceding stages. New ideas and requirements during development should be written down and taken into account afterward for a possible revision of the system (i.e., a next version).

2. Employ the proper people in time, both qualitatively (the right person at the right place) and quantitatively (appropriate for the volume of the work).

3. Restrain the maintenance efforts on already operational systems, which can best be obtained by releasing high-quality, well-documented systems.

4. Invest in the development of utility software and standard modules that can be reused for the development of systems.

6.3 Problems in the Field of Costs

The estimated costs of an EDP project are frequently too low.

• Causes
1. Problems during development (see above) may make it necessary that EDP project professionals spend considerably more time than was estimated beforehand, which causes an increase in costs.

2. Benefits are less than expected because of disappointing functionality, and hence, the cost/benefit ratio becomes less favorable.

3. Insufficient attention is paid to the enforcement of planned organizational measures. Manual activities continue, even though in principle they are no longer necessary, and the expected benefits fail to appear.

4. No decisions are made on where to use the personnel (on the user side) that becomes available once the system functions properly. These people then tend to find tasks themselves.

• Possible solutions
The best solution for the problems mentioned above is to survey the project carefully, so that strict control is kept on the realized and the expected costs. This is with regard to the development of the system and the required human capacity. It is of paramount importance to incorporate checkpoints in the project, that is, points in time when the state of affairs can be evaluated. Project management techniques such as network planning and measuring the rate of progress, which can assist in tuning the various parts of the project, either by performing these parts at the same time or in sequence, are important remedies. Various software packages are available to support the planning of an EDP project.

35

7 Final Remarks

From this chapter it becomes clear that the development of a computerized information system of a considerable size requires much time and money. The key responsible persons should thoroughly investigate beforehand whether the goal can be reached with commercially available applications. If such applications are not available and the decision has been made to start the project (stage 1), then the facts that the estimation of costs and scheduled time could turn out to be too optimistic should be taken into account.

35

IX

Medical Informatics as a Profession

Authors of Part IX

Chapter 36: Education and Training in Medical Informatics
    R. Haux, University of Heidelberg; A. Hasman, Maastricht University; F.J. Leven, School of
    Technology, Heilbronn; D.J. Protti, University of Victoria; M.A. Musen, Stanford University,
    Stanford

Chapter 37: International Developments in Medical Informatics
    M.J. Ball, First Consulting Group and Johns Hopkins University, Baltimore; J.V. Douglas, First
    Consulting Group, Baltimore; J.H. van Bemmel, Erasmus University Rotterdam

36 Education and Training in Medical Informatics

1 Introduction

Health care professionals who are well-trained in medical informatics are needed to improve the management of data and knowledge throughout the clinical enterprise. Formal education programs in medical informatics are becoming increasingly widespread and range from special components of curricula for professional development to dedicated programs in medical informatics and continuing education in this field (see Panel 36.1). This chapter provides a brief survey of the training programs in medical informatics and recommendations for medical informatics education.

2 Medical Informatics Courses and Programs

Worldwide, training in medical informatics is fragmented because there is great variety in the types of students who seek training. Many medical informatics programs represent undergraduate- or graduate-level academic units that provide a specific education to students who wish to acquire specific credentials in medical informatics, preparing the students for careers either in academic institutions or in the commercial sector. The same medical informatics programs may offer training to students who are studying to become practitioners in health care-related specialties, whose needs in understanding medical informatics are clearly different from those of students who wish to become medical-informatics professionals. These programs may also offer more limited training opportunities to practicing health care workers, medical librarians, or health care administrators who wish to learn more about the role of information management in their professional work. Some academic groups offer advanced courses for practicing specialists in medical informatics who wish to learn about new theories or emerging technologies.

Given the variability in the goals of the trainees and the differing strengths of medical informatics faculties, it is not surprising that there are substantial differences in the kinds of academic programs in medical informatics that are available worldwide. Because the particular offerings of different training programs change rather frequently, it is inappropriate to list comprehensive curricular details in this Handbook. Nevertheless, it is still helpful to provide an overview of the kinds of training opportunities that are available at a variety of centers. Detailed information about particular academic programs in medical informatics can be found in the annual editions of the *Yearbook of Medical Informatics* published by the International Medical

Informatics Association (*IMIA*). Since 1994, the *IMIA Yearbook* has routinely published synopses of training opportunities available at different sets of academic institutions (see Chapter 37).

In addition, a database of the programs and courses in health and medical informatics is offered by IMIA (see Section 3).

Table 36.1
Courses for Medical and Health Sciences Students at the University of Maastricht, The Netherlands.

Medicine

Year 2
Introduction to epidemiology, statistics, and medical informatics

Years 3-4
Elective courses in medical informatics:
- Databases
- Decision support
- Communication
- Medical records
- Signal analysis

Health Sciences

Year 1
Basic skills in information processing:
- Windows
- Word
- Excel
- Access

Year 2
Computer-assisted instruction in physiology

Year 3
- Simulation of outpatient clinic
- Bayes' rule
Elective courses in medical informatics:
- Design of health care organizations
- Analysis and interpretation of biosignals
- Problem solving and programming

Year 4
- Management information
- Decision support
- Information delivery in hospitals

2.1 Medical Informatics as Part of Educational Programs

2.1.1 Medical Informatics in the Medical and Health Sciences Curricula

In several countries, medical students are being trained in medical informatics as part of the medical curriculum. Usually, medical informatics courses in such curricula provide an introduction to the potential use of computers and information systems in medicine. Education in computer applications ranges from documentation of patient data and *signal* and *image processing* to information systems in health care and decision support in medicine.

Medical informatics is taught either as a separate training or education program, for instance, as a course Introduction to Medical Informatics, or within other education tracks, such as a course Decision Support for Internal Medicine, introducing the use of *knowledge-based systems* in internal medicine. Such courses focus on methods and systems for information processing with respect to clinical problems and primarily from the viewpoint of the clinician. Other courses may be given for students in the health sciences. For example, Table 36.1 presents an outline of the courses for health sciences students at the University of Maastricht in Maastricht, The Netherlands.

2.1.2 Medical Informatics in Computer Science Educational Programs

In various countries, special tracks in medical informatics are offered to computer science (or informatics) students. There, medical informatics is usually offered as a complementary course or as a set of dedicated courses for a bachelor's or a master's degree. For computer science students, the courses usually comprise introductory courses in medicine (medical terminology, anatomy, physiology, biochemistry, and an introduction to the clinical disciplines), courses on information systems in health care (e.g., hospital information systems), and a subset of courses on biosignal processing, medical image processing, coding and docu-

---

PANEL 36.1

Why Teaching Health and Medical Informatics?

Well-trained health care professionals raise the quality of information processing. The quality of information processing influences the quality of health care itself. Therefore, for a systematic processing of information in health care, health care professionals who are well-trained in medical or health informatics are needed.

- Existing medical or health informatics education

Medical or health informatics education has become an integral part of education and training for physicians, nurses, and administrators in different countries all over the world. In addition, medical informatics courses are offered to informatics students, and dedicated programs are organized for specialists in medical informatics.

- Types of programs and courses

Training and education in medical informatics are done at various levels of education and range from educational components in curricula to dedicated programs in medical informatics or continuing education:
- Courses in medical informatics as part of educational programs: (1) medical informatics courses for medical students, (2) medical informatics courses for informatics and computer science students, and (3) medical informatics courses as part of other programs (e.g., epidemiology or nursing).
- Dedicated programs in medical informatics: (1) Ph.D. programs in medical informatics, (2) bachelor's and master's programs in medical informatics, and (3) programs for medical data administrators and medical data technicians.
- Courses for continuing education and fellowship training in medical informatics.

36

---

mentation in health care, knowledge-based systems in medicine, and other subjects. These courses focus on methods, applications, and tools for information processing in health care from an informatics point of view.

2.1.3 Medical Informatics in Other Educational Programs

Medical informatics courses are also offered in educational programs for nurses, medical laboratory assistants, and radiology assistants. Medical informatics and health informatics courses are also offered in programs for public health, biomedical engineering, medical statistics (also called *biometry*), and *epidemiology*. Some bachelor's and master's programs in economics are offering tracks on health economics with respect to health information management.

2.2 Dedicated Programs in Medical Informatics

Dedicated Ph.D. programs in medical informatics exist, among others, in Germany, The Netherlands, and the United States. Such programs may be different because of the different educational systems of the countries. Usually, such programs are offered by medical faculties to people with a master's degree in medical informatics, computer science, or medicine.

For instance, Stanford University offers both M.Sc. and Ph.D. degrees in medical information sciences.

Students spend approximately half their time working on research projects throughout their course of study at Stanford. Students seeking a master's degree prepare a report of their research. Students seeking a doctorate must complete and defend an appropriate doctoral dissertation. Table 36.2 presents an outline of this Ph.D./M.Sc. program. In the United States, where there are still only a handful of degree-granting programs in medical informatics, many students interested in the application of information technology in medicine

Table 36.2.
Courses Offered by the Medical Informatics Section at Stanford University in the Framework of M.Sc. and Ph.D. Degrees in Medical Information Sciences.

1. Medical Informatics

- Computer applications in medical care
- Computer-assisted medical decision making
- Algorithms and representations for molecular biology
- Medical imaging
- Project course

2. Computer Science

- Machine architecture
- Programming languages
- Analysis of algorithms
- Artificial intelligence
- Databases

3. Decision Theory and Statistics

- Probability
- Statistical inference
- Decision analysis
- Experimental design

4. Biomedicine

- Clinical diagnosis
- Introduction to clinical environments
- Human physiology for informaticians

5. Health Policy

- Public health
- Medical ethics
- Medical economics

obtain their diplomas in more traditional fields of study – such as computer science or biomedical engineering. Students in such programs obviously need particular guidance from their dissertation committees to develop research projects that satisfy the requirements of these other departments, while simultaneously pursuing research that makes significant contributions to medical informatics.

A survey of dedicated programs in health and medical informatics leading to a specific master's or bachelor's degree can be found via the **World Wide Web browser** of this book that points to other Web sites listing actual programs. For instance, some programs mentioned are:

- the Graduate Student Program of the University of Utah, Salt Lake City, Utah, United States;
- the Medical Informatics Program of the University of Heidelberg and the School of Technology Heilbronn, Heilbronn, Germany;
- the Graduate Program of Health Informatics of the University of Minnesota at Minneapolis-St. Paul, Minneapolis-St. Paul, United States;
- the Program of Health Information Science at the University of Victoria, Victoria, British Columbia, Canada;
- the Programs of Health Information and Health Services Management of the University of Manchester, Manchester, United Kingdom; and
- the Graduate Program in Health Information Management of the University of Alabama, Birmingham, Alabama, United States.

In Europe, there also exists a program on European Education in Medical Informatics, Statistics, and Epidemiology (EuroMISE). Courses were held at the Charles University, Prague, Czech Republic, in cooperation with several European universities. In Greece, an international master's course in health informatics is organized by the Athens University School of Nursing. Other dedicated programs have been established or are being planned. The intention of such curricula is to impart knowledge and practical skills in medical informatics with a breadth that could hardly be offered in medical or informatics curricula. Table 36.3 presents an outline of the Health Information Science Program

36

Table 36.3
Health Information Science Program at the University of Victoria, Canada.

Health/Management Stream

Introduction to health information science I

Hospital organization

Introduction to the structure and management of health care

Medical methodology

Human communications and relations in health care

Fiscal management in health services

Legal issues in health informatics

Principles of community health

Introductory epidemiology

Health care systems

Issues in community health

Quality assurance and ethics

Epidemiology in health services management

Informatics Stream

Introduction to health information science II

Introduction to health informatics applications

Principles of health database design

Hospital information systems

Nursing informatics

Information management and technology

Patient care support systems

Distributed processing in health care

Principles of health information systems design

Table 36.4
Courses in the Medical Informatics Program[a] at the University of Heidelberg/School of Technology Heilbronn, Germany.

FIRST SECTION (2 years)

• Mathematics
• Basics of informatics
• Basics of medical informatics
• Basics of medicine
• Physics and measuring techniques
• Basic economics

SECOND SECTION (2.5 years)
Mandatory Lectures

• Medical informatics
• Medical biometry and stochastics
• Informatics

Major Subjects in Medical Informatics

• Economics and organization in health care
• Signal and image processing
• Model building
• Information and knowledge processing

Elective Subjects

• Additional courses in medical informatics
• Additional courses in informatics

Final Thesis (Diploma) [b]

[a] Thirty-five students per semester; total duration: 9 semesters of approx. 16 weeks each (4.5 years).
[b] Diploma: "Diplom Informatiker der Medizin" (M.Sc. in Medical Informatics). In total 900 students have received a diploma and 90 have received a Ph.D.

36

at the University of Victoria, Canada, leading to a bachelor's degree. Table 36.4 presents the structure of the medical informatics program at the University of Heidelberg/School of Technology Heilbronn leading to a master's degree.

Several professional schools offer special training for medical data administrators and medical data technicians. These programs concentrate on coding of medical records data, on documentation of clinical care, and on management of health records. Such curricula provide numerous practical exercises for their students.

2.3 Continuing Education and Fellowship Training

2.3.1 Continuing Education

Several countries offer formal programs for professional qualifications of clinicians (see the Web site for more information). In addition, in Germany a certificate in medical informatics is offered to professionals qualified in medical informatics. The certificate attests that the professional has sufficient qualifications in medical informatics related to academic education or continuing education in medical informatics and has completed 5 years of professional activity in medical informatics.

In addition to courses offered at universities, tutorials offered at medical informatics conferences play an important role in the continuing education of informatics professionals. At the same time, courses offered at the professional meetings of physicians and other health care workers provide important opportunities for practicing clinicians to obtain ongoing exposure to topics in medical informatics. For example, in the United States, the American College of Physicians (ACP) takes a particularly active role in educating its membership about issues in medical informatics. ACP views the future role of all medical specialty societies as one of organizing and delivering the specific clinical knowledge of greatest importance to those clinicians whom the societies serve. As purveyors of medical information, health care professional organizations are thus paying increasing attention to issues in medical informatics and are working to educate their members accordingly.

2.3.2 Fellowship Training

In the United States, more than a dozen academic centers offer postdoctoral training in medical informatics. Although most of these training programs are supported by the National Library of Medicine, some are sponsored by agencies such as the U.S. Department of Veterans Affairs. Typically, these centers provide an educational experience lasting 1 to 3 years to health care professionals who wish to pursue careers in clinical applications of computing. Although some institutions combine postdoctoral fellowships with opportunities to obtain formal graduate degrees in medical informatics, the typical postdoctoral fellowship in the United States comprises a more informal curriculum than would be associated with graduate education combined with significant practical experience in building clinical information systems. Some institutions, such as Columbia University, offer both formal graduate training and more applied postdoctoral fellowships, allowing trainees to tailor their educational experience based on their particular academic goals.

3 Working Group on Health and Medical Informatics Education

A Working Group (WG1) of **IMIA** (see Chapter 37) on health and medical informatics education is concerned with the promotion of medical informatics programs at a high professional or scientific level.

In accordance with the aims of IMIA, WG1 seeks to advance the knowledge of:

- how informatics is taught in the education of health care professionals around the world,
- how in particular health and medical informatics is taught to students of computer science and informatics, and
- how informatics is taught within dedicated curricula for health and medical informatics.

Details of medical informatics programs can be found in the proceedings of the IMIA WG1 conferences (see the References). IMIA WG1 has established a Web site to provide up-to-date information about its work (see the Web site of this Handbook). The core of the site is an underlying database providing information on health and medical informatics programs and courses worldwide. In addition, a mailing list was installed to facilitate communication between all people interested in health and medical informatics education.

4 The International Situation in Medical Informatics Education

4.1 Europe

In Europe, the situation with respect to education and training in medical informatics was surveyed in 1993. In the survey, the situation with respect to education and training opportunities for different types of health care staff (physicians, nurses, administrators, managers, technicians, etc.) was examined. The knowledge that professionals possess about information technology (IT) was also reviewed. Although the survey emphasized the situation with respect to health care professionals, attention was also paid to the extent and quality of graduate education in medical informatics in the various European countries. Observations were made for some countries.

- In France, medical informatics is a medical specialty. In 1993, a new medical curriculum was introduced. The association of teachers in medical informatics has recommended 30 hours of medical informatics during the second year of medical school. This suggestion is followed by about two-thirds of all medical schools.
- In Germany, education in medical informatics is well established at professional schools and universities. Most medical schools have a chair in medical informatics, usually combined with biometry. A dedicated medical informatics curriculum is offered by the University of Heidelberg/School of Technology Heilbronn, and related informatics programs are offered, for example, by the University of Lübeck. Medical informatics training is offered to physicians and medical informaticians by universities, private teaching institutes, and a newly founded Medical Informatics Academy.
- In The Netherlands almost all universities have a chair in medical informatics. The number of hours devoted to medical informatics in medical schools, however, is still low. By contrast, more hours are offered to students of health sciences. At the University of Amsterdam a 4-year graduate program in medical informatics is offered. At the Erasmus University in Rotterdam, both an M.Sc. and a Ph.D. program in medical informatics is offered. The program is primarily intended for physicians. Institutes of higher professional education have developed a special curriculum in medical informatics. In The Netherlands courses for managers, nurses, and physicians are offered by universities, institutes of higher professional education, and private teaching institutes.
- In the United Kingdom, the National Health Service Training Directorate is developing appropriate education and training programs to support the implementation of a new *IT* infrastructure concerned with both information management and information technology.
- In Denmark, a few postgraduate courses at the technical universities offer the possibility of specializing in biomedical engineering. Aalborg University, the Danish Hospital Institute, and the Danish Institute for Health and Nursing Research are developing the framework for a study program in health care informatics. The study program is offered as an "open university" course, using computer networks for distance learning.

36

4.2 United States

In the United States, the recommendations of the GPEP report of the Association of American Medical Colleges (see the References at the end of this chapter) have not yet been adopted by the majority of medical schools. Nevertheless, the teaching of medical informatics in U.S. medical schools is becoming increasingly common. In their later years of medical school, some students are able to spend elective time working on medical informatics research projects. Since the late 1970s, the National Institutes of Health (NIH) has offered a special elective course in medical informatics that has been tailored to the needs of U.S. medical students who wish to pursue special training in medical informatics during a several-week period on the NIH campus outside of Washington, D.C.

Medical informatics courses are also offered in educational programs for other health care workers, such as dentists, veterinarians, nurses, laboratory specialists, and radiology technicians. The nursing informatics community has been particularly active in defining curricula that help nursing students learn about the processing of clinical data and the use of those data in decision making.

4.3 General Observations

The following general observations can be made:

- In almost all of the surveyed countries, health care professionals lack adequate knowledge with regard to the possibilities and limitations of computer systems.
- The amount of knowledge about IT varies not only by country but even by regions within countries; it varies for different professional groups and depends on the age of the professional.
- Professionals usually do not have a total view of the system that they are using. Their mental image of the system is confined to the part that they are working with, and even then they sometimes are not familiar with all possible uses of even that part.
- In a number of countries, IT is mainly used for administrative and financial purposes.
- Although courses in IT are usually satisfactory for teaching how to use specific programs, they are often insufficient with respect to offering a broader overview of the potentials of IT.
- In almost all countries, stand-alone personal computers (PCs) are used by health care workers. Generally, the use of PCs is greatest among physicians and administrators. PCs are usually not connected to hospital information systems.
- In most countries, medical schools provide some courses in medical informatics. This does not mean, however, that all schools have a department of medical informatics.
- In nursing schools some courses in nursing informatics are offered, but usually, the number of hours is restricted, equipment for practical work is seldom available, and the number of teachers is low.
- In several countries there are still no chairs in medical informatics. The courses that are offered are frequently devoted to the technical use of computers.
- In general, there is a shortage of medical informatics teachers.

The general conclusion is that the degree to which medical informatics is taught in universities is far from satisfactory. Postgraduate courses are organized by some universities. Sometimes, physicians can obtain an officially recognized specialist qualification in medical informatics (such as in Germany).

5 Recommendations for Medical Informatics Education

Although many medical informatics educators have paid considerable attention to the notion of developing and instituting standard curricular goals, currently no established curricular guidelines for medical informatics are in widespread use. In 1979, for example, the Special Interest Group in Biomedical Computing (SIG-BIO) of the Association of Computing Machinery (ACM) released a model curriculum for Ph.D. programs in the field of health computing. Recommendations on medical informatics education exist, among others, from:

- the Association of American Medical Colleges,
- the Committee for Medicine of the Royal Netherlands Academy of Arts and Sciences, and
- the German Association of Medical Informatics, Biometry, and Epidemiology (GMDS).

A framework for recommendations on health and medical informatics education is presented in Panel 36.2. The reports containing the recommendations of The Netherlands and Germany are briefly summarized here:

- Dutch Recommendations

The Dutch recommendations for education and training in medical informatics were formulated in 1987 by the Subcommittee on Medical Informatics of the Committee for Medicine of the Royal Netherlands Academy of Arts and Sciences. The taxonomy of the skill levels presented in the report *Physicians for the Twenty-First Century* from the Panel on the General Professional Education of the Physician (GPEP report of the Association of American Medical Colleges) were taken as a starting point for describing the contents of an introductory education in medical informatics. It was recommended that an introduction to medical informatics should cover Levels 1 to 3, as described in the GPEP report:

1. the use of basic information-handling tools,

2. independent learning about computers and information management, and
3. the use of computer systems and accessing databases.

The subjects to be taught were divided into three categories:

1. general introduction (taxonomy of applications, systems and hardware, life cycle of software, information and communication, and data management),
2. methods (documentation and registration, signal and image analysis, pattern recognition, decision support, and simulation and models), and
3. applications (information systems, clinical support systems, and systems in health care). It was recommended that hands-on laboratories be organized to enable students to obtain experience with information systems.

- German Recommendations

The GMDS recommendations describe a two-dimensional educational framework, with different educational levels in one dimension and various types of educational needs and orientations in the other one. At the university level, the recommendations comprise both specialized curricula covering the total spectrum of medical informatics and informatics curricula with medical informatics as a subsidiary subject. Besides these informatics-oriented approaches, health care-oriented ways of education in medical informatics are recommended, for instance, postgraduate education in medical informatics for physicians based on foundations in medical informatics as part of their primary education in medicine. At the level of polytechnical schools, curricula in medical documentation and informatics are recommended and at the level of professional training curricula in medical documentation are recommended.

The intention of all these recommendations is to suggest adequate frameworks for medical informatics edu-

36

PANEL 36.2

Recommendations on Health and Medical Informatics Education

Because a variety of educational systems and health care systems exist throughout the world, programs and courses in health and medical informatics may vary among the different countries; the quality of such education may be different as well. Despite these differences, common recommendations on such education can be given.

• Need for education
Systematic processing of information is needed to maintain the quality of health care. Therefore, training and education are needed at various levels, for different types of education, for various health care professionals, and for different specialties. Recognized positions for qualified teachers in medical and health informatics should be available.

• Levels of education
Health and medical informatics courses should be offered within the different educational programs where information processing is of importance and within bachelor's, master's, and doctoral programs. These programs and courses should be offered at universities and professional schools. In addition, continuing education courses should be offered for health care professionals. In those countries where courses have not yet been sufficiently realized, for instance, summer schools for health care professionals should be offered.

• Modes of education
Besides lectures, it is of importance that practical exercises be offered. Besides traditional lectures and exercises within universities, distance learning should be actively pursued.

• Professions involved
Practically all health care professions should be considered with respect to education in medical and health informatics, such as physicians, nurses, health care administrators, coding clerks, medical librarians, and informaticians who follow special programs in medical and health informatics. Computer scientists and engineers who intend to work in health care also need such education.

• Types of specialization
The types of specialization range from courses in curricula to dedicated programs. Many health care professionals need to be aware of the potentials and the risks of information processing in health care. Students should be able to learn the basic principles of medical and health informatics. These principles should include an introduction to the methodology of information processing, its importance for health care, and the use of computers as information-processing tools. In addition, it should be possible to specialize in medical informatics. Such a specialization could, for instance, be offered within programs that lead to a diploma.

cation in relation to the educational systems of the different countries. It is generally recognized that for systematic processing of data, information, and knowledge in health care and medicine, well-trained scientists and qualified personnel must be available. Health care providers and professionals should be in a position to fulfill the existing tasks of information processing in medicine in an expert manner and, apart from the technical possibilities of information processing, also take into account the effects of using methods from medical informatics on patient care and employees in the health care sector.

6 Conclusions

Throughout the world, health care professionals generally lack knowledge of the possibilities and limitations of systematically processing data, information, and knowledge and of information technology. They are often asked to use computer systems of which they have limited appreciation, and could enhance their practices substantially via better use of information resources. It will only be through improved education of health care professionals and through an increase in the number of well-trained workers in medical informatics that this situation can begin to reverse itself.

Current programs and courses in medical informatics are quite diverse in their content and educational goals. There is substantial variation not only from one country to another but also from one institution to another. There are differences both in the scope of what is taught and in the depth to which educators explore the theoretical underpinnings of medical informatics. This variability reflects both the newness of the discipline and the substantial variation in health care

organizations that exists internationally. As medical informatics becomes more established as a profession, and as health care professionals better recognize their information needs and the ways in which methods and tools for the systematic processing of data, information, and knowledge can help them in their work, we can expect professional societies to promulgate comprehensive standards for curricula in medical informatics – standards that should be adopted by the diverse academic groups that now provide training in this area. At the same time, the inherent interdisciplinary nature of medical informatics ensures that there always will be considerable room for training programs to place emphasis on different aspects of their curricula and to take advantage of the particular strengths of their individual faculty.

Key References

Haux R, Leven FJ, Moehr JR, Protti DJ, eds. *Health and Medical Informatics Education.* Special Issue (3/94) of Meth Inform Med 1994; 33: 246-331.

American Association of Medical Colleges. *Physicians for the Twenty-First Century* (The GPEP Report). Association of American Medical Colleges, Washington, D.C., 1984.

Hasman A, Albert A, Wainwright P, Klar R, Sosa M, eds. *Education and Training in Health Informatics in Europe.* Amsterdam: IOS Press, 1995.

See the Web site for further literature references.

For WG1 of IMIA, see: www.ix.urz.uni-heidelberg.de

36

37 International Developments in Medical Informatics

1 Introduction

From the onset, medical informatics has had an international character, which is now growing even stronger because of the proliferation of information systems throughout health care.

This chapter documents some of the most prominent international developments in medical informatics and describes their effects on theory and practice.

2 International Medical Informatics Association

In the world of international health informatics, the International Medical Informatics Association (IMIA) is a recognized leader. The association draws on a long history, tracing its origins back to 1967 when the International Federation of Information Processing (IFIP) formed a committee (Technical Committee 4; TC4) to focus on health-related computing. Over the next decade, TC4 grew in membership. In 1978, *IMIA* was established and today remains an affiliate member of IFIP and is recognized by the *World Health Organization* as a nongovernmental organization.

2.1 IMIA Membership

As an association of societies, IMIA has more than 45 national and corresponding member societies, each with an officially designated representative to IMIA's General Assembly. It also recognizes three regional groups: the European Federation for Medical Informatics (EFMI), the Federation of Health Societies in Latin America and the Caribbean (*IMIA-LAC*), and the Asia Pacific Association for Medical Informatics (*APAMI*). The societies and the regional groups work to strengthen medical informatics across national boundaries and are key to IMIA's strategy. IMIA has also encouraged the formation of a regional group for Africa, helping to organize and fund conferences on that continent.

2.2 IMIA Goals

As a bridge organization, IMIA strives to

- move theory into practice by linking academic and research informaticians with caregivers, consultants, vendors, and vendor-based researchers;
- lead the international medical and health informatics communities into the 21st century;

- promote the cross-fertilization of health informatics across geographical and professional boundaries; and
- serve as the catalyst for ubiquitous worldwide health information infrastructures for patient care and health research.

2.3 IMIA Activities

IMIA pursues its goals through a range of efforts, including its sponsorship of a triennial international congress on medical informatics known as **MEDINFO**. The first congress of this type was started in 1974. The congresses draw attendees from around the globe and their proceedings are published and are widely referenced in the medical informatics literature.

IMIA also sponsors a special interest group (SIG) on nursing informatics and a fairly large number of working groups (WGs) (see Table 37.1). The WGs have also been very active, sponsoring working conferences and publishing proceedings. The range of IMIA activities is designed to help IMIA and its members to further medical informatics by

- monitoring the range of special interest areas and focusing support on new developments,
- capitalizing on the synergies and collective value of IMIA's constituents and components,
- minimizing fragmentation between scientific and operational medical informaticians,
- harmonizing the efforts of competing organizations that emerge to address informatics issues;
- adapting successfully the changes in the medical informatics workplace and discipline,
- raising the profile and awareness of IMIA within and outside the IMIA organization,
- balancing equitably the support to emerging and already existing IMIA members, and
- positioning IMIA as the gatekeeper for medical informatics issues.

WG	Working Group
1	Information Science and Medical Education
4	Data Protection in Health Information Systems
5	Primary Health Care Informatics
6	Coding and Classification of Health Data
7	Biosignal and Pattern Interpretation
9	Health Informatics for Development
10	Hospital Information Systems
11	Dental Informatics
13	Organizational Impact of Medical Informatics
14	Health Professional Workstations
15	Assessment and Quality Development in Health Informatics
16	Standards in Health Care Informatics
17	Computer-Based Patient Records

Table 37.1
IMIA Working Groups.

37

3   Yearbooks of Medical Informatics

The best available comprehensive guide to international informatics activities and interests is the *Yearbook of Medical Informatics*, published annually since 1992 under the auspices of IMIA. The Yearbook reports on IMIA activities, invites review articles, and republishes articles that appear in the refereed literature on key informatics issues. The Yearbook stands as a guide to IMIA as an organization and is widely distributed by the national member societies to their individual members (see Table 37.2).

The information on IMIA makes the Yearbook a valuable resource; each annual volume contains about 550 pages. A total of about 50 pages are devoted to invited review articles on key issues. The remainder of the volume includes articles selected as seminal by a panel of referees and are grouped within topic areas, each of which is accompanied by short synopses writ-

Table 37.2
Topics of Yearbooks of Medical Informatics.

Year	Yearbook Focus
1992	Advances in an Interdisciplinary Science
1993	Sharing Knowledge and Information
1994	Advanced Communications in Health Care
1995	Computer-based Patient Records
1996	Integration of Information for Patient Care
1997	Computing and Collaborative Care
1998	Medical Informatics and the Internet

Table 37.3
Selection of Journals in the field of Medical Informatics (in English).

Journal	Publisher
Artificial Intelligence in Medicine	Amsterdam: Elsevier Science
British Journal of Healthcare Computing	Weybridge, UK: BJHC Ltd.
Bulletin of Medical Library Association	Chicago: Medical Library Association
Computer Methods and Programs in Biomedicine	Elsevier Science Ireland
Computers and Biomedical Research	Orlando: Academic Press
Computers in Biology and Medicine	New York: Pergamon Press
Computers in Nursing	Philadelphia: Lippincott-Raven
IEEE Transactions on Biomedical Engineering	New York: IEEE Press
International Journal of Medical Informatics	Elsevier Science Ireland
Journal of the American Medical Informatics Association	Philadelphia: Hanley and Belfus
Journal of Medical Systems	New York: Plenum Publ Comp
MD Computing	New York: Springer Verlag
Medical Decision Making	Basel: Birkhäuser Verlag
Medical Informatics	London: Taylor and Francis
Medical and Biological Engineering and Computing	Herts, UK: Peter Peregrinus
Methods of Information in Medicine	Stuttgart-New York: Schattauer Verlag
Technology and Health Care	Amsterdam: IOS Press

37

ten by guest editors. These articles come from different journals, such as *Academic Medicine* and the *New England Journal of Medicine*, and also *Artificial Intelligence in Medicine* as well as *IEEE Transactions on Biomedical Engineering*. In addition, articles are selected from journals in medical or health informatics, as listed in Table 37.3.

As indicated in Table 37.2, each volume of the Yearbook addresses an area of special interest to the international informatics community. After an initial focus on inter-disciplinary matters, collaboration, and networking, five consecutive volumes (1994 to 1998) have also empha-sized patient-centered computing and clinical care.

The Yearbook gives added insight into how interests are supported and pursued within the international informatics community.

4 Other International Activities

International activities within IMIA draw on the participation and contributions from a wide range of academic and industrial groups. Collaboration occurs on the intellectual and organizational levels, and many researchers are active in a wide range of associations and endeavors. Two, one based in Europe and the other in the United States, are cited below.

Headquartered in Geneva, Switzerland, the Health on the Net Foundation (*HON*) brings together informa-ticians from Europe and the United States. Its focus is on the appropriate and optimal use of health information on the World Wide Web. The HON server takes many thousands of hits each day. HON addresses the critical issues raised by the proliferation of Web sites with health information and has advanced a code of conduct, developed by its staff and approved by its international advisory board.

37

Table 37.4

Some International and Large National Organizations Organizing Conferences in Medical and Health Informatics in the English Lan-guage.[a]

Congresses in Medical Informatics	Organization
AMIA Fall Congress[b]	American Medical Informatics Organization
AMIA Spring Congress[b]	American Medical Informatics Organization
Artificial Intelligence in Medicine Europe Congress[b]	European Society for Artificial Intelligence in Medicine
Computers in Cardiology[b]	Society for Computers in Cardiology
ISCE Congress[b]	International Society of Computerized Electrocardiology
Medical Informatics Europe Congress[b]	European Federation of Medical Informatics
MEDINFO[c]	International Medical Informatics Organization

[a] For other congresses see, for instance, the IMIA Yearbooks of Medical Informatics.
[b] Annually
[c] Triennial

In 1996, the National Library of Medicine (*NLM*) held the first meeting of its newly established planning panel on international programs. With membership across the United States, the Americas, and the United Kingdom and with input from regional panels from around the globe, the planning panel is addressing the need for NLM to have a number of libraries actively promoting NLM's programs and services and a somewhat more independent International Network of Libraries of Medicine involving three levels of international collaborators: partners, centers, and affiliates. These will build upon a strong international base. Today 50% of *MEDLINE* titles are foreign, 25% of search activity at NLM comes from foreign sites, and many countries have acquired data from the *Visible Humans project* (see Chapter 26).

5 Other Organizations

Many other health care organizations, institutions, and boards are also active in organizing congresses or working conferences or in publishing journals and books. Table 37.4 list some of the international organizations that organize conferences with a strong contribution of medical computing and medical informatics. Some of these conferences have a basic character, and others have a strong applied orientation. Table 37.2 lists the journals in the field of medical or health informatics. The addresses of journals and organizations will be updated on the Web site of this Handbook.

See for Web-sites:
www.mieur.nl/mihandbook
www.mihandbook.stanford.edu
www.ix.urz.uni-heidelberg.de
www.hon.ch

37

Glossary

Authors of Glossary

J.C. Helder, J.H. van Bemmel, Erasmus University Rotterdam, M.A. Musen, Stanford, University

Glossary

This Glossary explains acronyms and specific terms used in the Handbook. It contains cross-references to itself, indicated by *hyperlinks* and it contains backreferences to sections in the Handbook.

Within the Glossary, Syn stand for synonym, Ant for antonym.

α waves	*Quasiperiodic* waves in the *EEG* with a *frequency* of about 10 Hz.
:=	Sign meaning that the variable on the left-hand side becomes (gets the value of) the (value of the) expression on the right-hand side. This sign is used to avoid confusion with the = sign, which means "equals" but which is also used to mean "becomes."
3-D reconstruction	Mathematical reconstruction of a three-dimensional image from a set of two-dimensional images. From this reconstruction images can be displayed by *pseudo-3D* techniques.

A

a posteriori probability	See *posterior probability*.
a priori probability	See *prior probability*.
A-D conversion	Transforming an analog signal or an image into a series of numbers (a digital signal or image, respectively) that can be processed by a computer by taking *samples* with a certain *sampling frequency* or *pixels* of a certain size, respectively (see Chapter 8, Section 4). Syn: discretization, digitizing.
A-mode	Amplitude mode: visualization of *ultrasound* reflections in which the amplitude of the signal is displayed against the time interval between the transmitted pulse and the echo (thus corresponding to twice the distance between the *transducer* and the reflecting tissue). (See Chapter 9, Section 2.1).
acceptance test	A final test of an information system, performed by the users to check whether a system performs as it has been specified.
Access	A relational *database* program, offered by Microsoft.
access control	Protection of data against unauthorized use, a feature of a *DBMS* (see Chapter 4, Section 2.2).
accuracy of data	*Correctness of data* and *conformity of data*.
ACE inhibitor	A drug that inhibits the angiotensin-converting enzyme, used against cardiac diseases.
ACR	American College of Radiology, the professional society for radiologists in the United States.

A

ACR	See *automatic character recognition*
ACR/NEMA	A collaboration of the American College of Radiology (*ACR*) and the National Electrical Manufacturers' Association (NEMA) which developed initial *standards* for storage and transmission of radiological images. See also *DICOM*.
ADC	Analog-digital converter: a piece of equipment that performs *A-D conversion*. Ant: *digital-to-analog* converter.
address	Number denoting the location of data or the location of a program part in the *central memory* or on *disk*, or the location of a computer in a *network*.
Adobe Acrobat	A *desktop publishing* system.
ADT	Admission, Discharge, and Transfer: a module of an *HIS* that collects insurance and demographic data for a patient to enable billing on a per-diem basis.
age-gender registry	Database of personal data that can be ordered according to age and gender.
AI	Artificial intelligence.
AIDSLINE	An on-line abstract journal.
AIM	Advanced Informatics in Medicine: a program of the European Union for research and development in medical informatics.
algorithm	A set of unambiguously defined rules describing how to obtain the solution to a problem.
alias	Record of a patient with a different patient *identification*.
alphanumeric data	Contraction of alphabetic and numeric: the set that consists of the alphabetic characters a to z and the digits 0 to 9. Sometimes a few special characters such as = and - are also considered to belong to this set.
alternative hypothesis	A hypothesis in statistically comparing populations that is tested against the null hypothesis (see Chapter 24, Section 3.1).
ambulatory monitoring	Acquisition of biosignals from a person who is connected to the analysis equipment by wireless transmission. Syn: telemetry.
AMIA	American Medical Informatics Association.
analog signal	Signal that is measured continuously. It is a direct transformation of the original signal, obtained by a *transducer* (see Chapter 8). Ant: *digital signal*.
analog-to-digital conversion	See *A-D conversion*.
analysis of variance	See *ANOVA*.
anamnesis	Patient history.
ancillary department	Hospital department that assists clinicians in diagnosis and therapy (e.g. a laboratory).
AND	*Binary logical operator*, yielding only TRUE when both operands are TRUE.
angiography	Examination of blood vessels by means of *X rays* and *contrast medium*.
anonymous data	Data that do not contain the identifying data of a person or data from which the identity of a person cannot easily be derived, such as an address or a rare disease.
anonymous log-in	Ability to *log-in* on a computer without using a *password*.
ANOVA	Analysis of variance: for comparison of more than two *normally distributed* samples or more than two observations within one sample.
ANSI	American National Standards Institute.
anti-coagulation therapy	Pharmacological therapy to reduce the probability that blood will clot.
APAMI	Asia Pacific Association for Medical Informatics.
API	Application programming interface: documented interface of an application.
application	A program or system part to solve a specific problem or to perform a specific task.
application layer	Functions of a communication program accessible by the user.

A

application program	A program used to solve a specific problem or to perform a specific task.
application server	A computer system that runs the application in a *distributed system*.
ARA	American Rheumatism Association.
ARC/INFO	A powerful *GIS* software package.
architecture	The framework or the concepts from which a *system* is developed, for instance, *information architecture*.
Arden syntax	A standard language for writing situation-action rules that can trigger alerts based on abnormal clinical events detected by a clinical information system.
artifact	1. A product of human art and workmanship. 2. A disturbance that does not belong to a signal or an image.
artificial neural network	A system (in hardware or software) of interconnected nodes (artificial neurons), developed in analogy with the human brain. Used in various *classification* problems.
ASCII	American Standard Code for Information Interchange: an international 7-*bit* code for representing *alphanumeric* characters.
ASN.1	Abstract *Syntax* Notation, a meta-standard to define *standards*, mainly used in the area of telecommunications.
assembly language	*Programming language* with statements very close to a computer's *machine code*. Requires programmers to write code that operates on machine-level elements such as registers and locations in memory.
associative law	An algebraic rule that states that the result of two identical operations is independent of the sequence of these operations, e.g., $a + (b + c) = (a + b) + c = a + b + c$.
ASTM	American Society for Testing and Materials: an organization that issues *standards*.
ATC	Anatomic Therapeutic Chemical code: a systematic and hierarchical classification of drugs (see Chapter 6, Section 5).
ATM	Asynchronous Transfer Mode: enables fast digital transmission over networks.
atrial flutter	Rapid and *quasi-periodic* excitation of the atrium of the heart, visible on the *ECG* as a regular corrugated or sawtooth appearance of the baseline.
attenuation coefficients	Amount of attenuation (of X rays) by body tissue. It is characteristic for the chemical composition and density of tissue.
attributable risk	The relative difference of the *incidence* of a disease in two populations differing in the exposition to a *risk factor*.
attribute	1. A quality ascribed to a person or a thing. 2. A characteristic quality of data in a file. 3. A column of a *table* in a relational database.
audiography	The examination of the hearing function.
audit	An official and methodical examination and verification.
audit trail	Means for documentation of actions on data, such as "enter" or "change."
authentication	Verification of the identity of a computer user, document originator, organization, or system (see Chapter 34).
authorization	In clinical laboratory procedures: the procedure in which the analytical quality criteria of a preliminary laboratory test result are verified and are checked against other test results of the same run or earlier test results for the same patient (*deltacheck*) before the test requester is allowed to see the results (see Chapter 13, Section 5.4).
autoanalyzer	Mechanized and automated analysis equipment in *biochemistry*.
autocorrelation	*Correlation* between values of the same signal (see Panel 25.4). Ant: *crosscorrelation*.
automatic character recognition	Data entry in which the computer reads typewritten or even handwritten text.

A

autonomous DSS	A **DSS** that **monitors** incoming patient data and on the basis of these data takes action without human interference (see Chapter 16, Section 4).
AV node	Small area of slowly conducting cells between the cardiac atria and the ventricular conduction system. In case of conduction disturbances between the atria and the AV node, the AV node itself can issue a pacing pulse.
axis	1. Fixed reference line for measurement of coordinates or for plotting a parameter in a graphical plot. 2. A class of terms in a controlled terminology in which each term refers to a related dimension according to which a **classification** might be made.

B

B-mode	Brightness mode: see **M-mode**.
back propagation	An **algorithm** for training an **artificial neural network** to produce appropriate outputs when presented with a set of previously classified **cases**.
back-projection	Technique to compute the **attenuation coefficients** from intensity profiles covering a total cross section under various angles. It is used in **CT**, **MRI**, and **SPECT** (see Panel 9.2).
backup	Copy of all data on a **mass storage device**, made at certain times (see Chapter 4, Section 2.2).
backward chaining	See **backward reasoning**.
backward reasoning	A recursive **inference mechanism** that starts with a **production rule** in the **knowledge base** and checks whether data are available to confirm the rule; if no data are available to confirm the truth value of the rule, then other rules are evaluated to try to determine the necessary data values (see Chapter 15, Section 4.2.3). Syn: goal-driven reasoning. Ant: **forward reasoning**.
badge reader	Equipment that can read a **magnetic card** or a **smart card**.
band-pass filter	**Filter** that reduces both the high and the low **frequencies** in a signal or in an image.
bandwidth	1. The difference between the highest and the lowest **frequencies** in a data communication channel. 2. The capacity of a channel.
bar code	A code made up of a number of vertical lines of various widths that can be transformed into a binary code by a special reading device.
bar diagram	A graphical presentation in which the values of the dependent variable are represented by vertical or horizontal bars.
batch processing	Computer **transactions** that are withheld and then processed in a batch at certain times. Ant: **transaction processing**.
baud	Unit for the speed of data transmission.
Bayes' Rule	A rule used to calculate the posterior probability of having a disease when some symptoms are observed, based on the conditional probability of showing symptoms when the disease is present and the **prior probability** of having the disease (see Chapter 15, Section 4 and Panel 15.2).
Bayesian belief networks	Graphical structures representing the probabilistic relationships of causes on effects. Given **prior probabilities** of causes, Bayesian belief networks allow for the automatic calculation of **posterior probabilities** of effected outcome states.
Bayesian probabilistic network	A decision-support method for multiple diseases or classes that uses **Bayes' Rule**.
bedside terminal	A terminal at the bedside of the patient (see also **point-of-care system**).

bias	The amount in which the mean of a set of values deviates systematically from a reference value (see Chapter 30, Section 2.4).
binary	1. Mathematical representation of a number with base 2, that is, that representation of a number only consists of zeros and ones. 2. Everything that can be expressed by two values, e.g., 0 or 1, or TRUE or FALSE.
binary number	A number expressed with base 2, the way that a computer usually stores numbers.
binary operator	An operator on two variables, e.g., p AND q.
binomial distribution	Distribution for the probability that an event occurs x times in N independent trials.
biochemistry	Chemistry dealing with the compounds and the processes in organisms. In health care human specimens are investigated in clinical chemistry and hematology laboratories (see Chapter 13, Section 3.5).
biometry	See *biostatistics*.
biopsy	The withdrawal and examination of tissue, cells, or fluid from a living body.
biosignal	Contraction of biological signal: signal delivered by a living organism (see Chapter 2, Section 2, Examples 5 and 8).
biostatistics	Applied statistics in the medical and biological domains used to plan and interpret experiments and observations. Syn: *biometry*.
bit	Contraction of binary digit, the smallest amount of information. The value of a bit can be represented by 0 or 1.
black box	Description of a *process* or *system* by its input and output only, without considering what occurs inside.
block	Unit of data storage on a disk.
block diagram	A graphical presentation in which the values of the dependent variable are represented by vertical or horizontal blocks, drawn at coordinates on the other axis of the corresponding values of the independent discrete variable (see, e.g., Figure 2.4).
BMDW	Bone Marrow Donators Worldwide: a coordination of donor registries for bone marrow transplantation (see Panel 22.5).
body of knowledge	The sum of what is known.
Boolean algebra	A set of rules for *logical variables*, comparable to algebraic rules for numbers. Syn: Boolean logic, symbolic logic, combinatorial logic.
Boolean expression	See *logical expression*.
Boolean logic	See *Boolean algebra*.
Boolean variable	See *logical variable*.
boot	Starting up a computer.
brachytherapy	Application of radiotherapy with radioactive sources placed close to the tumor.
branching-logic program	A decision-support program that uses logical statements.
browse	Following a nonconsecutive way through a multimedia file. Syn: *navigate*.
browser	A program package to perform *browsing*.
budget system	A measure to contain health care costs by only funding an established number of diagnostic and therapeutic actions per health care organization or physician.
bulletin board	A file containing public messages accessible over a network.
business model	A description at a high level of abstraction of the main processes occurring in an organization (see Chapter 19, Section 3.3).
button	An imitation of a physical button on a *VDU* screen that by a point-and-click operation evokes an action.

B

byte	The smallest addressable storage unit of a computer, mostly consisting of 8 *bits*

C

C	A *programming language* originally designed for *UNIX* environments, but now in general use.
C++	*Object-oriented* extension of *C*.
C-scan	Compound scan: *ultrasound* technique in which the crystal can move (see Chapter 9, Section 2.3).
CAI	Computer-assisted instruction.
canonical regression	*Regression analysis* with multiple dependent variables (see Chapter 24, Section 4).
cardiac defibrillation	Conversion of ventricular *fibrillation* into a regular rhythm by applying an electrical shock.
CARE	The language for writing clinical decision rules created for the Regenstrief Medical Information System (*RMIS*) at the University of Indiana School of Medicine. CARE was one of the rule languages that inspired development of the *Arden syntax* for *medical logic modules*.
CAS	Chemical Abstracts Service: a chemical structure and dictionary database containing records on substances (see Panel 22.6).
case	A set of circumstances or conditions (of patients or healthy persons).
case finding	Selection of *cases* of an illness or another condition for research purposes (e.g., to compose *trial groups*) or to obtain cases for educational purposes.
case mix	The composition of *cases* in a group for a *clinical trial* such that no unwanted *bias* occurs.
case-based reasoning	A *DSS* that uses a *database* of similar *cases*.
case-control study	An investigation of two or more groups of a population that differ in the occurrence of an event (e.g., myocardial infarction) over time to explain the influence of *risk factors*.
catheter	A tubular device for insertion into canals, vessels, etc., to permit injection or withdrawal of fluids or transducers.
catheterization	1. Insertion of a *catheter*. 2. More specific: invasive method to determine properties of veins and arteries (e.g., pressures, flows, cross sections).
causal networks	Graphical structures implementing cause-effect relationships. Used to facilitate logical reasoning.
CCD	Charge-coupled device: solid-state sensors configured in arrays of light-sensitive silicon elements to acquire images (see Chapter 10, Section 3.1).
CCITT	Consultative Committee of the International Telegraph and Telephone: an organization that issues many *standards* on the *hardware* and *syntactic* levels of *data communication*.
CCP	Canadian Classification of Diagnostic, Therapeutic, and Surgical Procedures.
CD	Compact disk: high-capacity storage device in which the data (sound, images, and computer data) are stored (mostly only once) by burning small holes and from which data are repeatedly retrieved by means of a laser beam. See also *CD-ROM*.
CD-ROM	Compact Disk Read Only Memory: a *CD* used as a computer memory (see Chapter 3, Section 3.3).
CDC	Centers for Disease Control and prevention (United States).
CEN	Comité Européen de Normalisation: European standardization committee.

CEN/TC251	*CEN*'s technical committee for medical informatics.
central memory	Computer memory directly under control of the *CPU*.
central processing unit	See *CPU*.
channel	A path for electronic transmission between points or between pieces of equipment.
character-based interface	A *user interface* in which only keyboard symbols are used (see Chapter 3, Section 2).
CHD	Coronary heart disease: see *ischemic heart disease*.
chemotherapy	The use of chemical agents in the treatment of diseases, especially in the treatment of cancer.
chip	An integrated circuit consisting of a large number of electronic components.
chip card	See *smart card*.
CISC	Complex Instruction Set Computer: a computer that, in contrast to an *RISC*, has a large number of instructions, including intricate instructions. Ant: *RISC*
classification	Ordering of objects into groups (or classes) on the basis of their relationships (see Chapter 6)
client server	Architecture in which an application is divided over at least two computers: the client issues requests to the server, who provides the requested data or programs (see Chapter 5, Section 5.4); database handling may be performed by another computer. See also *application server* and *database server*.
clinical chemistry	The department responsible for performing chemical and enzymatic analyses of body fluids and tissues.
clinical epidemiology	Principles and methods of *epidemiology* applied to research in clinical medicine.
clinical information system	Patient-oriented information system. Ant: administrative hospital information system (see Chapters 20 and 21).
Clinical Practice Guideline	A predefined policy that allows a health care organization to manage patients with a certain presenting condition in a standardized manner (cf. *protocol*).
clinical trial	An investigation assessing the difference between two (clinical) populations, for instance, with respect to the outcome of a therapy (see Chapter 24, Section 3.5).
clock speed	The rate of the internal clock of a computer that is used to synchronize fetching and execution of instructions.
CLOT	An *EMYCIN*-based *DSS* for the diagnosis of abnormal bleeding.
cluster	A set of objects that belong to each other according to certain criteria.
clustering	Grouping a set of objects into clusters according to their *features*.
CNS	Central nervous system.
code	1. A set of rules that unambiguously describes the form in which data may be represented. 2. A part of a computer program. 3. The representation of a concept by a string of alphanumeric characters.
coding	The process of replacing a concept with a combination of numbers and characters in a defined way.
cognition	The process of knowing, including both awareness and judgment.
cognitive load	A measure of the complexity and difficulty of a task, correlating with factors such as learning time, fatigue, stress, proneness to errors, and possibility of performing parallel tasks.
cognitive psychology	The part of psychology that studies mental processes such as thinking, language, and decision making.
coherent averaging	Averaging the repetitive complexes in a signal or image to reduce the effects of *noise*.
cohort study	An observational investigation using two or more groups of a population that differ in,

C

	for instance, the exposition to a *risk factor* over time, to measure the difference in the *incidence* of an event.
COIN	Clinical Oncology Information Network: cancer registration project of the *NHS* (United Kingdom)
collimator	Device to obtain a beam of parallel radiation or particles or a beam with restricted area.
combinatorial logic	See *Boolean algebra*.
command language	A formal language used to communicate with a computer.
commonKADS	A revision of *KADS* that models explicit, reusable problem-solving methods.
communication	The process by which information is exchanged between individuals or computers through the use of a commonly accepted set of symbols.
communication link layer	Part of a communication program that sends and receives messages to and from the network.
commutative law	An algebraic rule that states that the sequence of an operation can be interchanged, e.g., $a + b = b + a$. Three-dimensional rotations are not commutative.
compact disk	See *CD*
compiler	Program that translates a program written in a high-level language into *object code*. See also *interpreter*.
compression	Reducing data, a signal, or an image to minimize storage and communication requirements. Loss-less techniques make use of the *redundancy* in the original signal; lossy techniques are not completely reconstructable. A standard for image compression is included in *DICOM* (see Chapter 10, Section 3.8). Ant: *decompression.*
computed tomography	See *CT*.
computer	A device capable of acquiring, storing and outputting data and processing these data under the control of programs that are also stored in the computer.
computer language	See *programming language*.
computer memory	Component of a *computer* in which data can be inserted, stored, and extracted. The *central memory* is fast, but it is relatively restricted in capacity; auxiliary memory (e.g., a *hard disk*) is slower but can contain more data.
computer network	A set of interconnected computers and their connections.
computer system	A *system* consisting of computer equipment, computer programs, people and procedures.
computer word	A number of *bytes* (usually 1, 2, 4, or 8 bytes) that can be *addressed* and processed simultaneously.
computer-aided design	Design supported by a *computer system*
computer-aided manufacturing	Manufacturing supported by a *computer system*.
computer-based history taking	See *patient-driven data entry*.
computer-based patient record	(CPR) Administrative and medical patient data electronically stored in a consistent way. A computer-based patient record may contain characters, signals, images, and sounds (see Chapter 7).
concept	General notion or idea defining a class of objects.
conceptual data model	Description of concepts in a domain with their relationships, e.g., by an entity relation diagram (*ERD*) (see Chapter 4, Section 2.1).

C

conceptual graph	A visual representation of logical sentences in which *logical variables* are represented as boxes connected by labeled lines that relate the variables to one another.
conceptual model	A model of a domain consisting of the main concepts and their relationships (see also *model*).
concurrency control	Protection of data against simultaneous updating (see Chapter 4, Section 2.2).
conditional probability	The probability that an event will take place given that some other event also will occur. See also *prevalence*.
confidence interval	The area of a probability distribution where most (usually 95%) of the observations of an event are found. Observations outside this area are more unlikely.
confidentiality	See *privacy*.
conformal radiotherapy	Radiotherapy in which the dimensions of the high dose volume are, as much as possible, equal to the shape of the target volume (the tumor).
conformity of data	Extent to which data conform to the rules of a *coding* system (see Chapter 2, Section 6.2).
confounder	See *bias.*
confusion matrix	A table in which the results of a decision model are compared with an independent reference.
consumables	Articles to be used in a computer environment: *magnetic tapes* and *disks*, paper, ribbon, ink, etc.
context-sensitive help	Help that depends on the phase that a program has reached when help is requested.
contingency table	A table in which the observed results of two or more sets of discrete observations are presented to analyze their correlation (see Chapter 24, Section 4).
continuous data	Data that must be represented by a *real* number, such as the results of measured observations.
contour extraction	Manipulation of an image such that only contours remain.
contraindication	Reason why a treatment or a procedure is not advisable.
contrast enhancement	Procedure in *image processing* that increases the difference between tones in an image.
contrast medium	A substance with a high attenuation for X rays, used to improve the X-ray visibility of vessels, cavities, intestines, and so on.
controlled clinical trial	A *clinical trial* consisting of a comparison of the outcomes of two different treatments (see Chapter 24, Section 5.1).
conversion	1. Changing internal computer data from one representation into another, e.g., from *integer* to *real number* format. 2. Changing an information system such that it can run on a computer system different from the one on which it originally was developed.
COPD	Chronic obstructive pulmonary disease, e.g., lung emphysema.
CORBA	Common Object Request Broker Architecture: specification of how objects can be distributed in a network and can be combined into services and applications.
coronary angiography	X-ray examination of the coronary arteries with the help of a contrast fluid applied through a *catheter* (see Chapter 12, Section 3.2).
correctness of data	Extent to which data are free of systematic and random errors (Chapter 3, Section 5).
correlation	The degree of the statistical relationship between two parameters.
correlation coefficient	Measure for the *correlation*.
cortex	The outer layer of the brain.
cost-benefit	The balance of costs and benefits of an (information) system, which is an important criterion for a go-no go decision of the management (see Chapter 32).

C

COSTAR	The Computer Stored Ambulatory Record System developed by the Massachusetts General Hospital in the 1970s.
Cox's regression	*Regression analysis* used in studies of *risk factors*, named after Cox. (see Chapter 24, Section 4).
CPR	See *computer-based patient record*.
CPT	Current Procedural Terminology: coding system scheme for diagnostic and therapeutic procedures for billing and reimbursement (see Chapter 6, Section 5).
CPU	Central processing unit: part of a computer that fetches and executes instructions stored in central memory (see Chapter 3, Section 3.1).
create-use matrix	A method used to develop an information architecture by setting up a matrix that describes the relation between activities or processes in a business and its relevant objects (data *entities*). This matrix describes for all activities or processes (the rows of the matrix) the allowed operations, such as create, use, delete, and so on, on data entities (the columns) and is used to subdivide the information processes in an organization.
critical pathway	The path through a *network* of activities that determines the shortest possible time that a process (e.g., a *project* or a patient's treatment) can be completed.
critiquing system	Decision-support system that allows the user to make the decision first; the system then gives its advice when the user requests it or when the user's decision is out of the system's permissible range.
crosscorrelation	*Correlation* between values of different signals (see Panel 25.4). Ant: *autocorrelation*.
cryptographic	See *encryption*.
CT	Computed tomography: a means of obtaining a two-dimensional image of the real tissue distribution in a single slice by means of X rays (see Chapter 9, Section 3.3).
cursor	Special sign on the *screen* indicating locations, e.g., where the next alphanumeric keyboard input will be located or where the *mouse* is pointing. The form of the cursor may indicate which activity is going on or may influence the next command of the user.
cutoff	See *threshold*.
cybernetics	The study of automatic control systems, especially the comparison of the nervous system with mechanical-electronic communications systems.
cyclotron	Equipment to accelerate charged particles such as electrons.
cytometry	Measuring of objective geometric parameters in cells and tissue.

D

D-A conversion	Conversion of *digital* data into *analog* data. Ant: *A-D conversion*.
data	Representation of observations or concepts suitable for communication, interpretation, and processing by humans or machines. Interpreted data form *information*.
data acquisition	Identification, selection, and sampling of data for further computer processing.
data collection	The gathering of source data.
data communication	The movement of digitally encoded data by means of electrical or electromagnetic transmission systems.
data compression	See compression.
data conversion	Changing the form of the representation of the data.

data dictionary	A description of *files*, *fields*, and variables in a *database*, mostly maintained in a computer.
data entry	The process of entering data into a computer, mostly by human action.
data glove	A glove that senses the movements of a hand or fingers and transmits these data to a computer and also gives feedback to the fingers to evoke the sense of pressure. It is used in *virtual reality* (see Panel 12.1).
data logger	Device that stores data sequentially without any further processing.
data mining	The use of the set of basic tools to extract patterns from the data in a *data warehouse*. Often artificial intelligence methods are used (see Panel 22.3).
data model	A model for the data used in a domain. See also *external data model* and *conceptual data model*.
data processing	Operations performed on data to provide useful data and information.
data protection	See *data security*.
data reduction	Transformation of raw data into more condensed data without loosing significant *semantic* information.
data security	Encompasses confidentiality, integrity, and availability of data (see Chapter 4, Section 2.2 and Chapter 33).
data validation	The examination of data for correctness.
data warehouse	A central data storage facility of large capacity for data imported periodically from multiple systems (see Chapter 22, Section 5). The technique to extract patterns from the data is called *data mining*.
data-driven reasoning	See *forward reasoning*.
database	1. A collection of data. 2. A structured set of logically related data together with software to define the structure of the data and to obtain access to the data (see Chapter 4).
database server	A computer system in a *distributed system* that contains a *database* and a *DBMS*.
dBase	A software package used to store and retrieve data in a *database*.
DBMS	Database management system: a software *shell* that handles all operations on data in a *database* (see Chapter 4).
ddf	See *density distribution function*.
DDL	Data definition language: tool of a *DBMS* that enables a description of the data such that an automatic *conversion* from the *implementation model* into the *physical data model* is possible (see Chapter 4, Section 2.1).
De Dombal's system	One of the first *decision-support systems*, diagnosing abdominal pain.
De Morgan's Law	A rule for the expansion of the negation of a *logical summation* or a *logical product*. (see Panel 23.1).
decision	An intentional choice out of a number of possibilities that will result in effects.
decision analysis	A decision analysis aims to support the clinician and the patient by an explicit and quantitative consideration of relevant aspects of a decision problem (see Chapter 18, Section 3.2).
decision table	A table containing the values for all *logical expressions* pertaining to a certain problem (the conditions) and the corresponding logical outcome using logical rules that connect conditions with results (see Chapter 15, Section 4.2.1 and Chapter 23). All logical expressions are considered simultaneously. See also *truth table*.
decision tree	A decision tree consists of nodes where a logical decision has to be made and connecting branches that are chosen according to the result of this decision. The

D

	nodes and branches that are followed constitute a sequential path through a decision tree that reaches a final decision in the end.
decision-support system	1. System consisting of a **knowledge base** and an **inference engine** that is able to use entered data to generate advice.
decoding	The inverse process of **coding**.
deduction	Deriving a particular conclusion from general principles and premises by logical reasoning.
Delphi technique	A **feedback** method to reduce interobserver **variability** by confronting each member of a panel of experts with the independent judgments of the other members and giving each member the possibility to adapt his or her judgment.
deltacheck	Checking the results of a biochemical test against earlier test results of the same patient to detect possible errors.
demographics	A person's data for address, birth date, gender, etc.
dendrogram	A visualization of a clustering process that looks like the branches of a tree (see Figure 27.6).
density distribution function	A function describing the number of events within an interval of an independent variable.
departmental system	A system that fulfills specific tasks encountered only in certain clinical departments (see Chapter 12).
depolarization	Breakdown of a potential difference (polarization) between two objects, for instance, in a cell between a separating cell membrane. Ant: **repolarization**.
design set	See **learning population**.
desktop metaphor	An imitation on a **VDU** screen of the top of a desk with folders, calendars, papers that cover each other (**windows**), and so forth.
desktop publishing	Preparing a document for publishing by use of a computer.
detection	The decision whether an event (e.g., a signal component) has occurred.
detection theory	The theory of how to discriminate a meaningful signal from a noisy background.
detector	Equipment, program, or observer that identifies an event or a phenomenon.
determinant	A factor that influences **health**.
deterministic signal	Signal that shows a definite form and sometimes periodicity (see Chapter 8, Section 2).
diagnosis	Description of a **health** problem in terms of known diseases.
diagnosis-related group	See **DRG**.
diagnostic-therapeutic cycle	A cycle consisting of the following elements: collection of patient data, diagnosis, therapy that may be circled several times (see Chapter 1, Section 2).
dialysis	Purification of blood by flow past semipermeable membranes, performed in case of renal failure.
dichotomous outcome	An outcome that can have only one out of two results.
DICOM	Digital Imaging and Communications in Medicine: a communication standard to exchange text and images, developed by **ACR/NEMA**.
differential diagnosis	A list of possible **diagnoses** that explain the current signs, symptoms, and measurements.
digital signal	Signal consisting of a series of numbers. Generally it is obtained by **A-D conversion**. Syn: discrete signal, Ant: **analog signal**
digital signature	A means of **authenticating** the identity of the sender of a digital message and proving the integrity of the message by means of data appended to that message, for instance

D

	by the **RSA** algorithm (see Chapter 34).
digital subtraction angiography	(DSA) Procedure to visualize blood vessels with **contrast medium** in a bony environment by subtracting the pre-contrast image (the mask) from the image with **contrast medium**.
digital-to-analog conversion	See **D-A conversion**.
digitize	See **A-D conversion**.
digitizing tablet	An input device that registers precisely the position of a pen. It is used to enter the **digitized** coordinates into a computer.
Diogene HIS	A hospital information system developed and used in Geneva, Switzerland (see Chapter 21, Section 5.1).
dipole	A pair of opposite electric charges or magnetic poles of the same strength, usually on a small distance.
direct access	See **random access**.
directory	See **folder**.
discrete number	Countable data; **integer**.
discrete signal	See **digital signal**.
discretization	See **A-D conversion**.
discrimination	Distinguishing a like object from another by discerning differences in **features** derived from the objects.
disk	See **hard disk** and **floppy disk**.
diskette	See floppy disk.
dispersion	See **standard deviation**.
display terminal	See **visual display unit**.
distributed database	A **database** located on several computers in a network.
distributed system	A set of computer systems interacting via a network and using data communications standards in which the various computers collaborate in common tasks.
distributive law	An algebraic rule that states that the same result is produced when an operation is applied on a whole as when operating on each apart and collecting the results, e.g., $a \bullet (b + c) = a \bullet b + a \bullet c$.
DM	See **data mining**.
DML	Data manipulation language: language used to store and retrieve data from a **database**.
DNA	Deoxyribonucleic acid: the substance within the chromosomes that carries the genetic attributes of a cell.
document management	Digital storage and retrieval of documents that in most cases are handled as images and not as **alphanumeric** data.
domain	1. The set of elements to which a variable or function is limited. 2. Any area of interest that might be modeled, e.g., to create an information system.
Doppler effect	The effect that the frequency of a reflected sound wave depends on the velocity of the target on which it reflects. This effect can be used to detect the target's velocities (see Chapter 9, Section 2.5).
DOS	Disk Operating System: an **operating system** residing on a **hard disk**. Examples for **personal computers** are MS-DOS (Microsoft) and the functionally identical PC-DOS (IBM)
dot matrix image	An image, mostly a character, formed by a number of dots selected out of a

D

	rectangular array of dots.
double blind	A clinical trial that is performed in such a way that neither the patients nor their physicians are aware of which patients have been assigned to receive the experimental intervention.
DRG	Diagnosis-Related Groups: a grouping of *ICD* codes based on costs of treatment, to be used for budgeting and hospital reimbursement (see Chapter 6, Section 5.11).
drug interaction	Interaction between two drugs administered at almost the same time causing a decrease or an increase of the effects of the drugs.
DSA	See *digital subtraction angiography*.
DSM	Diagnostic and Statistical Manual for Mental Disorders: a *nomenclature* system for mental disorders (see Chapter 6, Section 5.3).
DSS	Decision-support system: an active knowledge-based system that uses patient data to generate case-specific advice (see Chapter 16, Section 1.1).
DTP	Desktop publishing: a method to prepare a document with a computer that is ready to print.
dumb terminal	A computer terminal without its own processing capabilities.
duplicate records	The occurrence of two records for the same patient, usually with overlapping data (see Chapter 22, Section 2.3).
DW	See *data warehouse*.

E

e-mail	Mail in electronic form; the sender composes a message on his or her computer and transmits it via a communications network to the receiver's computer (see Chapter 5, Section 2.2).
EAN 128	Barcode specification that is able to encode all the characters that are on a conventional keyboard.
ECG	Electrocardiogram: recording of the body surface potential caused by the electrical activity of the heart muscle, giving information on the condition of the heart (see Chapter 13, Section 3).
echocardiography	Examination of the heart by means of *ultrasound* (see Chapter 9, Section 2).
echo scan	Imaging by means of the reflection of ultrasound on tissue boundaries (see Panel 9.11).
edge enhancement	Procedure in *image processing* that increases the visibility of an edge or a contour in an image.
EDI	Electronic Data Interchange: a form of e-mail to send and receive standard electronic messages, in which the *syntax* and the *semantics* are described (see Chapter 5, Section 2.3).
EDIFACT	Electronic Data Interchange for Administration, Commerce and Transport: *EDI* standard especially in use in commercial environments. EDIFACT is widely adopted in Europe (see Chapter 5, Section 2.3).
editor	A program that does additions or alterations in text-like files such as programs. Its functionality and user friendliness is usually less than that of *word processors*.
EDP	Electronic data processing: mostly electronic processing of administrative or registrative data.
EDP auditing	An examination by external experts of the functioning of the information-processing

	activities in an organization. This examination regards the contents of the procedures and the way they are obeyed.
EEG	Electroencephalogram: the recording of the electric activity of the brain.
efficacy	Effectiveness; the extent to which an activity reaches its goal.
EFMI	European Federation for Medical Informatics.
EIS	Executive information system: almost a synonym of *MIS*, but sometimes an EIS aggregates the data on a higher level than an MIS.
electrocardiography	The study of electrical phenomena in the heart by *ECG*, *VCG*, *His bundle* recording, and so forth (see Chapter 13, Section 3).
electrode	A conductor used to establish contact with nonmetallic objects .
electroencephalography	See *EEG*.
electromyography	See *EMG*.
electronic data interchange	See *EDI*.
electronic mail	See *e-mail*.
electronic signature	See *digital signature*.
electronic textbook	*Multimedia* document that permits different access paths, search strategies, and presentation facilities.
electrooculography	The examination of the electrophysiological part of the visual function.
ELIAS	Information system for primary care, widely used in the Netherlands.
EM radiation	Electromagnetic radiation: consisting of periodic variations of electric and magnetic fields. Examples are gamma waves, X rays, light, and radio waves.
EMG	Electromyography: recording of muscleaction potentials.
empirical variance	See *dispersion*.
EMR	Electronic medical record; see *computer-based patient record*.
emulation	The imitation of a hardware system by other hardware or by software such that the imitating system accepts the data and the instructions of the emulated system.
EMYCIN	*MYCIN's* backward chaining inference engine as a separately usable program.
encryption	The process of encoding (scrambling) data such that a specific key is needed to decode the data, mostly by means of methods that are based on the use of prime numbers.
endogenous determinant	An individual's personal possibilities and restrictions that influence his or hers *health* (see Panel 19.2).
endoscope	An instrument for visualizing the interior of a hollow organ.
engine	Software module that performs a certain task, for example a *database* engine or an *inference* engine.
entity	An object having meaning in a particular context.
entropy	1. A variable that describes the state of a thermodynamic system. It is a measure of the disorder of a closed system. 2. A measure of the amount of information in a message (see Chapter 2, Section 5).
epidemiology	A health science that (1) deals with the distribution and *incidence* of diseases in human populations; (2) identifies etiologic factors in the pathogenesis of diseases, and (3) prepares data for planning, implementation, and assessment of measures for the *prevention*, suppression and treatment of diseases.
epilepsy	Electrical disturbance in the central nervous system, giving rise to spasms and sometimes the loss of consciousness.
equivalency	A *logical operation* between two *logical expressions* that is then and only then TRUE

E

	when both expressions are TRUE (see Chapter 23, Section 2.2).
ERD	Entity Relation Diagram: method to describe a data structure by entities, i.e., the *object*s that are important for the user according to the *external data model* and by their relationships with other entities.
estimator	1. An estimation of a phenomenon (e.g., waveform) used to obtain a better *detection*, a better estimation, or a better numerical calculation. 2. A piece of equipment or a program that performs an estimation.
Ethernet	Communication protocol for linking computers and terminals in a *LAN*.
etiology	The causes of a disease or malcondition.
EU	European Union.
EUCLIDES	European Clinical Laboratory Information Data Exchange Standard: a European standard for the exchange of laboratory orders and reports.
eV	Electronvolt: a unit of energy used in particle physics and in radiation physics. It is the energy gained by an electron when it is accelerated by a potential difference of one volt.
evaluation	Measuring or describing something to assess its value with respect to a certain purpose. For the evaluation of clinical information systems, see chapter 30.
evidence-based medicine	Selection of diagnostic or therapeutic methods on the basis of scientifically based empirical evidence.
evoked response	See *evoked signal*.
evoked signal	Signal after stimulation of a signal source.
evoking strength	A measure used to express how strongly a finding suggests the presence of a disease.
Excel	Name of a *spreadsheet program*.
exclusive OR	See *XOR*.
exercise ECG	*ECG* recorded during physical exercise of the patient.
exogenous determinant	Factors coming from the outside world that influence somebody's *health* (see Panel 19.2).
expectation	The *mean* of a statistical function
EXPERT	A rule-based *shell*, used to create *DSS*s.
expert system	Older term for a *knowledge-based system*.
external data model	In the framework of a *DBMS*: data as seen from the viewpoint of the user (see Chapter 4, Section 2.1).
extrasystole	A premature ventricular contraction of the heart that may give rise to an arrhythmia. Syn: *PVC*.

F

false alarm	A *false-positive* alarm, a term especially used in patient *monitoring*.
false negative	A measure for the quality of a decision. The percentage of objects that have some attribute and for which a decision procedure incorrectly rejects this attribute (see Chapter 15, Section 4).
false positive	A measure for the quality of a decision. The percentage of objects that do not have some attribute but for which a decision procedure incorrectly detects this attribute (see Chapter 15, Section 4).
fast Fourier transform	(FFT) A method to quickly compute the *Fourier transform* (see Chapter 25, Section 2.1).
fax	Contraction from facsimile: equipment to send and receive documents via the public

	telephone network (see Chapter 5, Section 2.1).
FDA	Food and Drug Administration, the US government organization that certifies medical equipment and drugs.
feature	1. A measured or derived characteristic that is of importance for a decision or for a pattern-recognition problem. 2. The signs, symptoms, measurements, and results of tests.
feature extraction	see *feature selection*
feature selection	Selecting and extracting semantically or statistically relevant parameters for *classification* of, for instance, signals or images.
feature space	An abstract space of *n* dimensions in which the *n* *features* are the *axes*.
feature vector	A set of *features*.
feedback	The bringing back of part of the output of a system to the input.
FFT	See *fast Fourier transform*.
fibrillation	Disturbance in which the muscle cells contract chaotically and independently of each other, which makes a normal contraction impossible. In the heart, atrial fibrillation or ventricular fibrillation may occur.
fiducial marker	Marker point in a signal or an image that corresponds with a known or predefined position.
field	Part of a *record* containing one piece of data
file	A data-storage entity that has a name and that is divided into logical *records*. Mostly, a file contains related records (see Chapter 4, Section 1).
filter	Removes (equipment or software) or removing (activity) unwanted parts from the *frequency* spectrum of a signal or an image.
Fisher's test	Test to compare observed frequencies in populations.
floppy disk	Inexpensive lightweight removable disk with a limited storage capacity (storage capacity up to about 2 Mbytes [1996]) for a *personal computer* used to store and retrieve data . It consists of a flexible (floppy) disk coated with magnetic oxide surrounded by a hard plastic case.
flow cytometry	Assessing the DNA content in a flow of suspensions of cell contents by measuring the light intensity caused by fluorescent stains.
flowchart	1. A graphical representation of the definition, the analysis, or the solution of a problem, making use of symbols that represent processing, decisions, input/output, and so forth. 2. In *DSSs* a connection of decision units (microdecisions) that are traversed sequentially via a path that depends on the outcome of the microdecisions (see Chapter 15, Section 4.2.2). Compare *decision tree*.
fluid balance	The balance between fluid input and output of a patient within a fixed period.
flutter	In cardiology, a rapid and *quasi-periodic* atrial or ventricular excitation.
FN	See *false negative*
folder	A set of files that can be found under the name of the folder. Syn: *Dictionary*.
Food and Drug Administration	See *FDA*.
forms-driven data entry	Data entry by means of a form with a fixed layout which must be completed.
formulary	A collection of (allowed) medications.
forward chaining	See *forward reasoning*
forward reasoning	An *inference mechanism* that starts with case data and executes *production rules* that use these data (see Chapter 15, Section 4.2.3). Syn: data-driven reasoning. Ant:

F

	backward reasoning.
Fourier transformation	Mathematical transformation of a signal or an image from the time or spatial domain into the *frequency* domain, or vice versa (see Chapter 25, Section 2.1) (see also *FFT*).
fourth-generation programming languages	*Programming languages* that are sometimes considered successors to the *procedural languages*. They have a higher level of abstraction from the actual functioning of a computer. An example is *SQL*.
FP	See *false positive.*
frame	A form of knowledge representation in which concepts are associated explicitly with their defining *attributes*. *Instances* of a concept are created by assigning values to the attributes.
frame-based	A *DSS* in which the knowledge is condensed in coherent groups of decision rules.
frame-based inheritance	*Inheritance* of the values of attributes, that is, when concepts in a frame-based *knowledge-representation* system are organized hierarchically in a taxonomy, more specific concepts in the hierarchy automatically may assume the values for attributes of related concepts that are more general.
frame-based system	A *knowledge-based system* in which *frames* constitute the primary means for encoding knowledge.
free text	Natural language text without restrictions on format and word choice (see Chapter 2, Section 6.5). Syn: *natural language*. Ant: *structured* language.
free-form text	See *free text.*
frequency	The number of times that an event occurs in an interval.
frequency analysis	Analysis of the *frequency* components of a signal, mostly done by *bandpass filtering* or *Fourier transformation*.
frequency spectrum	The amplitude of the various frequencies in a signal or an image.
Friedman test	Test to compare data that are not *normally distributed* for multiple observations on same individuals.
FTP	File Transfer Protocol: an application under *TCP/IP* to retrieve a *file* from another computer over a *network* (see Panel 5.5).
function key	Special *keys* that may used to control the program flow (see Chapter 3, Section 3.3)
functional MRI	Use of magnetic resonance imaging to study metabolic processes in the brain (see Chapter 9, Section 4.7).
function laboratories	Departments that examine the dynamic (functional) properties of organs and organ systems.
fuzzy-set theory	An expansion of classical set theory, in which the membership of a set is not given by TRUE or FALSE, but rather by a distribution function.

G

g	See *Giga*.
GALEN	Reference model for medical concepts.
GAMES	A computer workbench supporting a methodology and containing tools to develop a *DSS*. Incorporates ideas from KAOS and *PROTÉGÉ*.
gamma camera	A device that transforms gamma radiation into a visual or electric image (see Chapter 9, Section 4).
gamma radiation	High-energy electromagnetic radiation used for imaging and radiotherapy.
gantry	Mechanical structure to support equipment.
gatekeeper	In health care: the function of a clinician who decides whether a patient should be

referred to the next higher level or to another type of health care or should be treated by the clinician himself or herself (see Chapter 11, Section 3.1).

gateway Special computer that resides on at least two **networks** to forward and translate data if the two networks run different communications protocols.

Gaussian distribution See **normal distribution**.

generic Relating to or characteristic for an entire class.

geographical information system (GIS) A system that manages, analyzes, and displays data with an explicit geographical component. It is based on a spatial database containing location data and a more or less integrated attribute database describing the application data (see Chapter 22, Section 2.5).

giga (G) Abbreviation for 1,000,000,000 (10^9).

GIS See **geographical information system**.

glass fiber Filament of glass used to optically transport digital signals with a large **bandwidth**.

glucose tolerance test Assessing glucose metabolism by administering glucose to a patient at fixed times and determining at intervals thereafter the blood glucose content.

goal-driven reasoning See **backward reasoning**.

gold standard The assessment of a **diagnosis** by independent clinical evidence for comparison with the results of a diagnostic method being **evaluated** (see Chapter 30, Section 2.3)

good laboratory practice (GLP) A formal quality control system for laboratories.

GP General practitioner: in some countries a primary care physician (see Chapter 11, Section 1).

GPS Global positioning system: accurate positioning system making use of earth-orbiting satellites.

gradient 1. Changes in the value of a quantity per unit of distance in a specified direction. 2. A quantity showing a gradual change.

graphic tablet Computer peripheral for interactive entry of image features.

graphical user interface A **user interface** that, besides keyboard characters, may contain windows, command buttons, and icons that the user can point at to issue a command (see Chapter 3, Section 2.3).

grey level Intensity grades of an image.

groupware Software used to prepare documents with many authors connected by an **Intranet**.

GUI See **graphical user interface**.

H

half-life Time in which an activity reduces to 50%. A measure especially useful for nonlinear decays, such as exponential radioactive decay.

handhold computer A small computer that can be held in one's hand so that it can be used at the **point of care**, also in **home care**.

hard copy Output on paper.

hard disk Auxiliary **random-access** magnetic memory. It contains one or more platters covered with magnetic material on which data can be written or read by means of read-write heads that can move in and out while the platters are spinning. Typical storage capacity for a **personal computer** is about 1 **G**byte (1997) (see Chapter 3, Section 3.3).

hardware Physical equipment. Ant: **software**.

harmonic A component of a periodic signal with a **frequency** that is an integer multiple of the

H

	basic *frequency* of the signal.
hashing	Part of the data of a *record* (the *key*) is entered into a formula that calculates from these data a number that is used as an *address* for the record.
HCI	See *human-computer interaction*.
health	A state of complete physical, mental, and social well-being, and not merely the absence of disease and infirmity (see Chapter 19, Section 2.1).
health information network	A network on a regional or a national scale to improve communications between health care centers.
health policy	The actions of governments and others aimed at maintaining and improving the population's *health* (see Panel 19.2).
health promotion	Measures directed to improving lifestyle *determinants* (see Panel 19.2).
health protection	Preventive measures that influence the physical and social environment to protect people's health (see Panel 19.2).
health status	A condition describing the health of an individual or a population by means of objective and measurable *indicators* (see Section Panel 19.1).
health surveillance	Monitoring the extent, trends and changes in disease occurrence.
HELP	*DSS* developed by the University of Utah to generate reminders.
help desk	Part of an information-processing department with the support of the user as its explicit task.
hemochromatosis	A congenital disease with an abnormality in iron metabolism. Excessive amounts of iron are deposited throughout the body.
heuristic classification	A *KBS* in which generalizations of the input features are heuristically associated with elements of the set of potential solutions by using rules of thumb (see Chapter 28, Section 4).
heuristic reasoning	Problem-solving method closely resembling human reasoning, in which a decision is reached after following paths of yes or no decisions using heuristics, that is, informal rules of thumb (see Chapter 15, Section 4.2).
heuristic system	*DSS* that uses *heuristic reasoning*.
hexadecimal	A number system with base 16: that is, numbers are represented with 16 different symbols, mostly 0 . . . 9, A . . . F. (see Chapter 23, Section 4).
hierarchical data model	*Database* model in which records are connected by *PCR* (parent-child relationships).
high-level language	A formal *programming language* that allows statements that are close to the problem description. A program written in a high-level language requires an *interpreter* or a *compiler* to execute it.
high-pass filter	*Filter* that reduces the low *frequencies* in a signal.
HIM	Hospital information model: a *reference model* for hospital organizations (see Chapter 19, Section 3.9).
HIN	Health information networks: computer networks for health information (see Chapter 22, Section 3.1).
HIR	Health information resources: information processing in the field of population-based health care (see Chapter 22).
HIS	Hospital information system: an information system used to collect, store, process, retrieve, and communicate patient care and administrative information for all hospital-affiliated activities and to satisfy the functional requirements of all authorized users.
HIS reference model	A model describing the functional components of a HIS and the data-flow

H

relationships among these components.

His-bundle electrogram | Registration of the activation of the His bundle. This bundle conducts the electrical signal in the heart from the *AV node* toward the bundle branches in the *ventricles*.

HISB | Health care Informatics Standards Board of *ANSI*.

Hiscom HIS | A hospital information system developed and widely used in The Netherlands (see Chapter 21, Section 5.1)

histogram | A graphical presentation of the number of events as a function of an independent variable. The values of the independent variable are generally divided in equal parts (bins), and the number of events in a bin is represented by the height of a block above that bin. It shows the distribution of a parameter (see Figure 27.2).

HIV | Human immunodeficiency virus, infection with which will likely cause AIDS.

HL-7 | Health Level 7: standard to define computer-computer messages.

HLA | Human leukocyte antigen: used in matching donor and receptor tissues in organ transplantation.

Holter ECG | Continuous ECG recording lasting many hours (typically 24 hours) (see Chapter 12, Section 3.1)

home care | A component of medical care in which patients who are unable to travel to a health-care provider receive evaluation and treatment in their homes.

HON | Health on the Net foundation: an organization that focuses on the appropriate and optimal use of health information on the *World Wide Web* (see Chapter 37, Section 4).

hospital information system | See *HIS*.

Hough transform | Originally a method to detect straight lines in digital images, later extended to more general digital curves.

HTML | *Hypertext* Mark-up Language: the language that describes *WWW*-documents and included links.

hub | See *gateway*.

human-computer interaction | (HCI) The design, *implementation*, and *evaluation* of interactive computer systems (see Chapter 31).

hyperlink | A link in a *hypertext* document to another set of data (text, images, sound) in the same or a different document.

hypermedium | Document that contains links to various media (see Chapter 31, Section 4.3).

hypertext | Text containing links to other texts, within or outside a document.

hypertext mark-up language | See HTML.

hypothesis testing | Testing the validity of a hypothesis by statistically analyzing the results of an experiment (see Chapter 24, Section 3.1).

Hz | Hertz: unit of *frequency*, equal to one cycle per second.

I

I/O | Input and output.

IARC | The *WHO* linked International Agency for Research on Cancer.

ICD | Intermittently connected device.

ICD | International Classification of Diseases: a coding system for disease terminology originally intended to be used to report mortality statistics but now also in use for patient record abstraction (see Chapter 6, Section 5.1)

ICD-O	International Classification of Diseases for Oncology: a *WHO* classification widely in use for cancer registrations (see Chapter 6, Section 5.5).
ICD-9-CM	Clinical modification (CM) of the ninth revision of *ICD*.
ICIDH	International Classification of Impairments, Disabilities, and Handicaps (*WHO*, 1980).
ICNP	International Classification for Nursing Practice: a lexicon describing nursing events and interventions (see Chapter 14, Section 7.4).
icon	A pictorial representation on the computer *screen* of a function to be performed by the computer.
ICPC	International Classification of Primary Care: classification for *diagnoses*, *reasons for encounter*, *therapies*, and laboratory tests (see Chapter 6, Section 5.2)
ICPM	International Classification of Procedures in Medicine. Though it never passed the trial phase, it has been a source for many procedural classifications (see Chapter 6, Section 5.7).
ICU	Intensive care unit: a nursing unit for patients who need intensive care (artificial respiration, monitoring of heart or brain functions, etc.).
ID	Identification (of a patient, a laboratory sample, and so forth).
identification	1. The unambiguous establishment that a set of data corresponds to a person. 2. A unique set of numbers and characters that is used to label a person in a computer.
IEC	International Electrotechnical Committee
IEEE	The Institute of Electrical and Electronical Engineers, which has proposed many standards for electrical equipment and their use.
ILIAD	A *DSS* for internal medicine developed at the University of Utah.
image analysis	The extraction of numerical information from images (see Chapter 10).
image processing	The enhancement of the quality of images (see Chapter 10).
image subtraction	Composing a new image that is the *pixel* by pixel difference of two images.
imaging	Generating images of organisms, organs, or parts of organisms or organs by means of radiation (see Chapter 9).
IMIA	International Medical Informatics Association: an association that unites national or regional *medical informatics* societies from around the world.
IMIA-LAC	Regional federation of health societies in Latin America.
implementation	The introduction of a developed information system in an organization by adapting (tuning) the application to the working practices of the users.
implementation model	Model derived from the *conceptual data model* to be used by a *DBMS* for implementation.
implication	A *logical operation* between two *logical expressions* that is then and only then FALSE when the left-hand variable is TRUE whereas the right-hand variable is FALSE (see Chapter 23, Section 2.2).
incidence	The relative frequency of an event.
inclusive OR	See OR.
index	A *key* of a *record* used for fast *retrieval* of that record.
index file	File connecting a *key* with an *address* or with another key (see Chapter 4, Section 4.4).
indicator	A variable for an abstract quantity such as *health*.
induction	*Inference* from particular to general (see also Chapter 1).
inference	Draw of conclusions from available knowledge and data.

inference mechanism	A procedure that operates on a *knowledge representation* to conclude new propositions.
informatics	The science that studies the use and processing of *data*, *information*, and *knowledge*.
information	Meaningful and useful facts extracted from *data*, or: interpreted data.
information analyst	A person who analyzes the current information flows in an organization.
information architecture	The existing or required framework of information processing.
information planning	An activity to describe the information needs in an organization and to propose technologies that will address those needs.
information processing system	Computer system that processes data to obtain information (Chapter 3, Section 2).
inheritance	In *object-oriented programming* and *frame-based DSS*: the fact that an descendant *object class* inherits characteristics of an ancestor (see Chapter 15, Section 4.2.4).
ink-jet printer	A printer that forms its output by directing selectively an ink jet to a place on paper.
instance	An *object* isolated from an *object class*.
instantiation	See *instance*
instruction	Command to the *CPU* to perform an action (see Chapter 3, Section 3.1)
integer	Zero, positive or negative natural number (. . . , -2, -1, 0, 1, 2, . . .).
integration	Data, presentation, or functions are available for the user in a consistent way (see Chapter 21, Section 3.4).
integrity control	Consistency control to safeguard the correctness of data (see Chapter 4, Section 2.2).
interface	1. A common boundary between two pieces of equipment or between a piece of equipment and a human being. 2. In programming, the outside view of a *procedure* or an *object*.
interference	1. Effect of one signal on another signal (e.g., light or electric signals). 2. Influence of one task on another task (see Chapter 31, Section 2.3).
International Agency for Cancer Research	See IARC.
interlingua	An artificial language used as an intermediate language for computer translation of a natural language into another one.
Internet	A worldwide *network* of computer networks. It provides exchange of information by *e-mail*, *bulletin boards*, *file* access and transfer, etc. (see Chapter 5, Section 6)
INTERNIST-I	A *DSS* covering the domain of internal medicine developed in the 1970s at the University of Pittsburgh.
INTERNIST-I/QMR	See *QMR*.
interoperability	The ability to approach data and functions from another *platform*.
interpolation	Estimation of values between known values.
interpreter	A program that processes high-level *program* statements, executing them immediately.
intersection	The intersection of two sets is the set that contains the objects that are in both original sets.
intersectoral health policy	Health-related policy that lies outside the official *public health* sphere, such as traffic safety or housing regulations (see Panel 19.2).
ionizing radiation	Radiation (high-energy *EM radiation*, " or $ particles from radioactive decay, and so forth) that causes ionization of atoms, which may result in cell damage in the body because of changes in molecular bonds.
IRD	Information requirement determination: methods used to obtain information about a

I

	domain, necessary to make a model of the information processes and their relationships (see Chapter 19, Section 6)
ischemic heart disease	Impaired flow of oxygen of parts of the heart muscle caused by obstructions in the coronary arteries.
ISDN	Integrated Services Digital Network: high-speed digital telephone network.
ISO	International Standards Organization: international organization that develops *standards*.
isodose curve	Curve that connects points that receive equal doses of radiation.
isotopes	Chemical elements that have almost the same chemical properties, but that show different physical behaviors, especially in their radioactivity.
ISPAHAN	An interactive system for *feature* evaluation, *supervised classification* and *clustering*.
IT	Information technology.

J

Java	An *object-oriented programming language* that has been designed specifically for running application programs on *World Wide Web* client systems (see Panel 5.5).
Java applet	Small *application program* written in a subset of *Java* and embedded in *HTML* pages.
joystick	A *pointing device* that translates two-dimensional movements of a stick to movements on a screen of a *VDU*. Its operation is generally faster than that of a *mouse* and it is therefore used in computer games and some medical applications.
junction	The junction of two sets contains the objects that are in one or both sets.

K

k	See *kilo*
K-means algorithm	Iterative *clustering* algorithm, assigning objects to K classes by using the distances to the class centers.
KADS	Knowledge Acquisition and Design Structuring: a methodology for the development of *DSSs*.
Karnaugh diagrams	Representation of all possible conditions expressed in a *truth table*.
karyogram	Visual representation of chromosomes after staining.
karyotyping	Classification of a *karyogram*.
KB	See *knowledge base*.
KBE	See *knowledge-based editor*.
KBS	Knowledge-based system: a system with a *knowledge base* and an *inferencing* mechanism operating on a patient *database*. (see Chapter 15, Section 4.2.8). Syn: DSS
kernel	A central or essential part.
key	1. Part of a *keyboard* used to enter symbols. 2. Part of a *record* that identifies that record. 3. Something to *encrypt* or decrypt a message.
keyboard	Input device consisting of a number of keys that have as a subset the standard typewriter keys (see Chapter 3, Section 3.3).
kilo	Abbreviation for 1000 (10^3)
kilobyte	1024 (2^{10}) bytes.
knowledge	Facts and relationships used or needed to obtain insight or to solve problems.
knowledge base	A systematically organized collection of *knowledge* stored in a *computer* to make decisions or to solve problems (see Chapter 15, Section 1).

J/K

knowledge engineer	A person who analyzes **knowledge** and represents it in the **knowledge base**. Now this person is more often simply called a **systems analyst**.
knowledge representation	A formal description of knowledge by means of, for instance, **decision trees**, **Bayesian** statistics, **production rules**, or **frames**.
knowledge-based editor	(KBE) A computer system used to enter **knowledge** directly into a **knowledge base**.
knowledge-based system	See **KBS**.
knowledge-driven data entry	A data entry system that contains a knowledge model that generates the most appropriate questions in response to the user's input (see Chapter 29, Section 3.4).
Kruskal-Wallis test	Test to compare not **normally distributed** observations for more than two groups.
kurtosis	Parameter that describes the steepness of a distribution.

L

LAN	Local area network: a high-bandwidth network within a restricted area, usually with a single network protocol (see Panel 5.3).
language	See **programming language**.
laparoscope	An instrument used to inspect or to act on the interior of the abdomen via a small incision.
laptop computer	A small and lightweight **personal computer** that is portable and that can be used comfortably on a person's lap.
laser printer	A printer that transfers images to paper by means of a light beam generated by a laser.
LCD	Liquid crystal display, see **screen**.
leaf	End node, that is, a node with input but no output branches in a **decision tree** or a **model**.
learning	In a **DSS** or **pattern recognition** system: the process in which such a system improves its performance by adapting its rules or methods.
learning population	A file of data to optimize **systems** and **models**, e.g., for classification. Syn: training set. Ant: **test population**
Leeds Abdominal Pain System	See **De Dombal's system**.
left bundle branch block	(LBBB) Electric conduction disturbance in the left-bundle branch of the heart, which is visible on the **ECG** by the occurrence of a widened **QRS** complex.
legacy system	Information system that is inherited from the past, but still in use.
library	Set of **programs** or **modules** organized in such a way that individual programs or modules can easily be retrieved.
license	The right to use a software package.
light pen	A handhold pen-like **pointing device** that can observe light when it is pointed to a **screen**. The moment that the pen senses the light caused by the writing beam, the position of the light is translated by the control program into the coordinates of the location on the screen.
linear accelerator	Equipment used to accelerate charged particles such as electrons. In a linear accelerator the particles travel in straight lines, not in orbits, as in cyclotrons.
linear regression analysis	Statistical analysis of the linear relationship of two variables.
linguistic pattern recognition	See **syntactic pattern recognition**.
Lissajous figure	Figure that is the result when the amplitudes of two signals at identical times are plotted along the x and y axes.

L

local area network	See *LAN*.
log file	A *file* documenting all changes to a file or database, usually since the time of the last *backup* (see also *roll forward*) (see Chapter 4, Section 2.2).
log in	*Procedure* to obtain access to a computer, usually consisting of identification by a user *identification* (e.g., name or number) and *authentication* by a *password*.
log on	See *log in*.
log-likelihood	The logarithm of the likelihood of the data given a model and a set of parameters.
log-normal distribution	A *normal distribution* obtained by performing a logarithmic transformation on the original data.
logging	To put transactions in a *log file*.
logical circuitry	Electronic circuitry consisting of components that can be in only one of two states.
logical deduction	*Deduction* using *logical reasoning*.
logical expression	1. An expression that has only two values, TRUE or FALSE, consisting of a *logical variable* or of *logical variables* connected by *logical operators*. Syn: *Boolean* expression. 2. A verbal statement that is TRUE or FALSE.
logical negation	See *NOT*.
logical operator	Operator on one or more *logical variables* or *expressions*, whose result is TRUE or FALSE.
logical product	Logical AND operation.
logical summation	Logical OR operation.
logical variable	A variable that has only two values, commonly denoted by TRUE or FALSE.
logistic regression	Multivariate regression of a logarithmically transformed dependent variable, frequently used in studies of *risk factors*. (see Chapter 24, Section 4)
logistics	The procurement, maintenance, and transportation of material, facilities, and personnel.
LOINC	Logical Observation Identifier Names and Codes: this database contains codes, names, and synonyms for more than 6,300 clinical chemistry test observations. It has been made available on the *Internet*.
longitudinal investigation	An investigation in which data for the same individuals are compared over time (see also *cohort study*).
longitudinal patient record	A patient record that contains data covering a period longer than one disease episode.
Lotus 123	Name of a *spreadsheet* program.
Lotus Notes	A *groupware* package from Lotus company (now part of IBM).
low-pass filter	*Filter* that reduces the high *frequencies* in a signal.

M

M	See *mega*.
M-mode	Motion mode: visualization of *ultrasound* reflections, in which the time interval between the pulse and the echo (corresponding to the distance between the *transducer* and the reflecting tissue) is plotted along one axis and the subsequent pulses are plotted along the other one. This enables the visualization of movements. The brightness of a point corresponds to the amplitude of the reflected signal (see Chapter 9, Section 2.2).
machine code	See *object code*.
machine language	See *object language*.
machine vision	Imitation of vision by means of sensing devices and *pattern recognition* programs.

magnetic card	Plastic card the size of a credit card that contains a magnetic strip for storing and reading data (see Chapter 3, Section 3.3)
magnetic disk	See **hard disk**.
magnetic resonance imaging	See **MRI**.
magnetic tape	A sequential storage device consisting of a long plastic tape, coated on one side with magnetic material on which data are stored (see Chapter 3, Section 3.3).
mailbox	A temporary storage location for **e-mail** messages to avert the necessity of keeping the receiving system on-line.
mainframe	A large, expensive computer, now gradually replaced by **distributed systems** or networks of **PCs**.
mammogram	Breast examination by X rays to detect breast cancer.
managed care	A system of health care in which providers do not receive reimbursement for specific services, but instead work for a fixed amount of money to pay for the care of each of patient. The system thus encourages conservation of resources, as health-care workers must provide care within a constrained budget.
management information	Information needed by managers to run an organization.
mark-sense form	Computer-readable paper form on which information can be placed by entering pencil marks in preprinted boxes.
mass storage device	A device used to supply a relatively inexpensive storage capability for a large amount of data, e.g., a **hard disk**.
mean	The average value of the data in a distribution.
MEANS	Modular **ECG** Analysis System: system for the interpretation of **ECGs** and **VCGs**.
median value	() Defined such that 50% of the observations have a value greater than.
medical informatics	Informatics applied to medicine, health care, and public health
medical logic module	See **MLM.**
medical record	An account of a patient's health and disease after he or she has sought medical help. Syn: patient record.
Medicare	Insurance coverage for hospital stay for elderly Americans.
MEDIX	Institute of Electrical Engineers/ medical data interchange.
MEDLINE	A large **database** of abstracts of articles in the international medical journals at the National Library of Medicine (**NLM**). The database is also accessible via the **Internet**.
mega	Abbreviation for 1,000,000 (10^6).
memory	Storage facilities of a computer, including both **volatile** central memory and background memory on **mass storage devices** such as **disks**.
menu	A list of options from which a user can choose.
menu-driven user interface	An interface in which the user selects an item from a menu or list on a display screen, which may produce a new list for further selection.
MeSH	Medical subject headings: a **classification** developed by **NLM** to index the world medical literature (see Chapter 6, Section 5.10).
meta-analysis	A critical review by statistically combining the results of previous research studies reported in the literature (see Chapter 17, Section 4.2).
meter	1. The **SI unit** for length. 2. A piece of equipment to show the value of a parameter. 3. An imitation of such a piece of equipment on a **VDU** screen.
MI	See **medical informatics**.
middleware	A **software shell** between the **operating system** and the **applications** or the user.

M

minicomputer	A computer, smaller than a *mainframe*, but larger than a *PC*. Nowadays minicomputers are mostly being replaced by *workstations* or *PCs*, which have increasing capacities.
Minnesota code	A code used for the formal description of *ECG* waveforms and arrhythmias, especially for population studies.
MIS	Management information system: an information system used to support the management of an organization by making available information about revenues, costs, and personnel.
missing data	Missing data in a record.
MLM	Medical logic module: encoding of a segment of medical knowledge (see Chapter 16, Section 4.2.2).
model	An abstraction of something in the real world into a verbal or pictorial description, a set of rules, a physical object, or a set of mathematical expressions. Important examples are the modeling of reality in *objects* or *entities*, e.g., to design a *database* or an *information processing system*, and the modeling of physiological processes or *pubic health* problems into mathematical computer models to run *simulations*.
modem	Equipment that modulates the digital computer signal into a signal acceptable for the analog telephone network and vice versa.
modular	A system that is divided into *modules*.
module	A rather independent component of a program package that, ideally, can be used as a building block to compose programs or systems.
MOLE	A knowledge-acquisition system for systems that perform fault diagnoses.
moment	1. A point of time. 2. A quantity describing the characteristics of a stochastic distribution, such as *mean*, *variance*, *skewness*, and *kurtosis*.
monitor	1. Equipment used to record the ongoing state of a patient, mostly patients in *ICUs*. 2. *visual display unit*.
monolithic system	A system's *architecture* whose structure is determined from the beginning and that incorporates in principle all hospital information functions (see Chapter 21, Section 2.3).
morphology	The study of form and structure of organs, cells, etc., without considering their function.
morphometry	Measuring the form and structure of objects, e.g., cells.
Morse alphabet	A *coding* system, invented by Morse, that transmits messages consisting of text by audible or visible signals (especially in telegraphy). The code consists of short and long signs denoting characters, digits, a few punctuation marks and pauses to separate characters and words.
mouse	A handheld device whose movements are read by the computer and converted into movements of a *cursor* on the *screen* (see Chapter 3, Section 3.3).
MPR	See *multimedia patient record*.
MRI	Magnetic resonance imaging: imaging of the interior of the body by means of magnetic resonance (see Chapter 9, Section 3.4).
MS-DOS	*Operating system* for *PCs*, manufactured by Microsoft.
MST	Minimal spanning tree: the graph with the minimal total length of the connections between all objects.
multicenter trial	A *clinical trial* in which more than one center participates.
multimedia	Interaction with a computer including graphics, sound, images, and movies.

M

multimedia patient record	Medical record with text, images, signals, and sounds (see Chapter 7, Section 7.2).
multiple regression	*Regression analysis* for more than one independent variable (see Chapter 24, Section 4). Syn: *multivariate regression*
multiprocessing	Simultaneous execution of two or more programs by a computer or a computer network (see Chapter 3, Section 3.1).
multiprogramming	Quasi simultaneous execution of two or more programs by a computer by switching quickly from one program to the other (see Chapter 3, Section 3.1).
multivariate analysis	Statistical analysis of data collected on several dimensions for the same individual.
multivariate regression	See *multiple regression.*
MUMPS	Programming language, also called M.
MYCIN	Early rule-based system *DSS* (Stanford) to determine possible causes of bacteremia and meningitis and assisting in therapy selection.

N

natural-language processing	(NLP) Accessing data in the form of narratic or *free text* and creating machine-understandable interpretations of those data (see Chapter 29, Section 2.4.1). See also *structured data entry.*
navigation	To find one's way through a large amount of data or text, also making jumps to other sets of data. Syn: *browse.*
NCID	National Center for Infectious Diseases (United States).
NCPDP	National Council of Prescriptions and Drug Programs.
nearest neighbor classification	Classification by determining for a new object the nearest neighbor or nearest neighbors of that object in feature space.
network	1. A set of nodes and connecting lines to describe intricate structures, e.g., the activities in *processes, conceptual models,* or *data models.* 2. In telecommunications, the technical facilities to permit voice and data transmission, e.g., the public switched telephone network. 3. A system of interconnected *computers* and *terminals* including their network protocols, e.g., *LAN* and the *World Wide Web.* 4. A computer representation of active or passive nodes and their connections, e.g., *artificial neural network* and models for *HIV* epidemiology. Syn: net.
network data model	A *database* model in which *records* may be accessed by arbitrary, predefined connections.
neural network	See *artificial neural network.*
neuron	1. A cell that is the basic functional unit of the nervous system. 2. A node in an *artificial neural network.*
NHS	National Health Service: governmental health organization of the United Kingdom.
NIS	Nursing information system.
NLM	National Library of Medicine (at the National Institutes of Health in the United States).
NLP	See *natural language processing.*
NMDS	Nursing minimum data set: a minimum set of nursing data elements with uniform definitions and categories, including nursing problems, diagnoses, interventions, and patient outcomes (see Chapter 14, Section 7.1).
nodal rhythm	A cardiac rhythm *paced* by the *AV-node.*
noise	Disturbance of a signal by unwanted extra sources, e.g., random noise or main line interference.
nomenclature system	A system that assigns codes to medical concepts and allows for the combination of

N

	these concepts (see Chapter 6, Section 2.2).
nonstationary signal	A *stochastic signal* whose statistical properties change over time (see Chapter 8, Section 3). Ant: *stationary signal*.
normal distribution	A distribution that can be described by a symmetric bell-shaped curve. Syn: Gaussian distribution.
nosology	The science of the *classification* of diagnostic terms (see Chapter 6, Section 2.5).
NOT	*Unary logical operator*, yielding the negation of its operand.
notebook computer	A portable *personal computer* that is about the size of a notebook and that is thus smaller than a *laptop computer*.
nuclear medicine	Diagnostic methods in which images of body parts are obtained by measuring the radiation of radioactive materials absorbed by parts of the body (see Chapter 9, Section 4).
null hypothesis	An assumption about the distributions of populations that is tested against *alternative hypotheses*. Mostly, the null hypothesis states that there is no difference between the populations (see Chapter 24, Section 3.1).
nursing informatics	Analyzing, formalizing, and modeling how nurses collect, manage, and process data (see Chapter 12).
nursing minimum data set	See NMDS.
Nyquist	See *Shannon-Nyquist theorem*.

O

object	1. In a *model*, a representation for a concept in the world; an entity. 2. In *object-oriented programming*, a software construct that encapsulates both a description of some entity and program fragments that affect the behaviors that that entity is capable of exhibiting.
object class	A set of *objects* that have common characteristics.
object code	Instructions in binary code that can be executed by a computer with no or with minimal translation. Syn: *machine code*; Ant: *source code*.
object language	The formal language for *object codes.* Ant: *object language*.
object oriented	Method in which an object is considered to be an instance of a more general type. The properties of an object are encapsulated (e.g., a record with its (encapsulated) data structure together with the operations allowed for this record forms an object). Descendants of an object *inherit* the properties of their ancestors, thus creating a taxonomy of objects. Object-oriented methods are applied in *object-oriented modeling*, in *object-oriented databases*, and in *object oriented programming*.
object-oriented database	Besides data storage, an object-oriented *DBMS* provides mechanisms for specifying data semantics and for implementing methods that perform database operations. A set of related records can be seen as one object; and associated with the object are methods for setting and updating *fields* contained in the object, for preserving its integrity, and for doing special computations (see Panel 4.4).
object-oriented modeling	Conceptual modeling that uses object-oriented means such as object classes and their relationships.
object-oriented programming	Type of *programming language* in which parts of the program are organized as objects; that is, functions and data structure are located within the object and are accessible only via a formal interface. This encapsulation prohibits undesired side effects when an object is used by different parts of the program. Object-oriented

0

	programming makes it possible that child objects *inherit* the properties of the parent object (see Panel 3.2).
occupational health care	See OHC.
OCIS	Oncology Clinical Information System: one of the first comprehensive *departmental information systems*, assisting both with information access and decision support developed at Johns Hopkins University Hospital in Baltimore, Md.
OCR	Optical character recognition: Computer reading of printed characters with a special OCR font.
odds ratio	The ratio of the number of events and the number of nonevents in two groups, differing in the exposition to a risk factor.
off-line	Not connected to a computer. Ant: *on-line*.
OHC	Occupational health care: services used to prevent work-related diseases, to promote and maintain employees' health and working ability, and to restore working ability to those with a diminished working ability (see Chapter 22, Section 3.3).
OLAP	On-line analytical processing: an OLAP application analyzes large on-line databases to extract statistical information.
OLE	Object linkage and embedding: a Microsoft method to link (make a connection) or embed (inserting information) *objects* from other applications into an application.
on-demand pacemaker	A *pacemaker* that starts triggering the heart only when an implanted device detects an irregular heart rate, or a heart rate that is too low, or an insufficient voltage.
on-line	1. For equipment, directly coupled to and under control of a central computer. 2. For a user, directly communicating with a computer.
ONCOCIN	Decision-support system for the treatment of cancer patients.
ontology	A *domain* of discourse for describing some reality. A set of concepts, the *attributes* of those concepts, and the relationships among concepts that characterize a given application area.
OPAL	An interactive, graphical knowledge acquisition system for *ONCOCIN* (see Panel 17.2).
open	A term denoting that a system not only is able to run programs developed for that system or to be connected with systems of the same type, but that intentionally has been designed to accept programs or connections from various origins. See also *UNIX* and *OSI*.
operand	Something on which an *operator* works.
operating system	The set of programs that control the computer. The main task are *I/O control*, starting and stopping of programs, and scheduling resources (see Chapter 3, Section 4.1).
operator	1. A person who is in charges of the daily operation of a computer system. 2. Indicator for some action, e.g., multiplication or AND, on variables or expressions.
OPS5	A rule-based *shell* developed at Carnegy-Mellon University in the 1970s.
optical card	Plastic card the size of a credit card on which data are stored like on a *CD-ROM* (see Chapter 3, Section 3.3).
optical storage	Storage of digital data by optical means (via laser beams) (see also *CD*).
OR	*Binary logical operator*, yielding only FALSE as result when both operands are FALSE.
order management	A system that handles physician's and nurse's orders for diagnostic and therapeutic actions. Input is done by the requesters themselves. Tracing of the order and data management of the reports are done by the system.
order-entry system	Part of an *HIS* that handles the orders of physicians and nurses to laboratories, the

0

	pharmacy department, etc.
order-management system	A system that processes requests for services, tracks the progress of that request, and handles the results of these actions.
ordinal data	A type of data that can be ordered according to a *code* derived from the data. (e.g., stages of an disease or a code for the quality of life).
orthogonal	Pairwise perpendicular.
OS/2	A *windows*-oriented *operating system* for *PCs* manufactured by IBM.
OSI	Open Systems Interconnection reference model developed by *ISO* that describes in a seven-layer stack, each needing its own standards, the functionality of the communications software and the interrelation of the tasks.
outlier	Observation with an extreme value.
outsourcing	Contracting out information systems handling to a third party.
oxytocin	Uterus-contracting hormone administered to accelerate parturition.

P

P-QRS-T	A complete complex of an *ECG*, starting with the *P-wave*, followed by the *QRS*-complex and the *T-wave*.
p-value	The value of the probability threshold for accepting or rejecting a hypothesis (see Chapter 24, Section 3.1).
P-wave	First part of the *ECG* waveform corresponding to the depolarization of the atria.
pacemaker	1. Region in the heart that sets the rate of the cardiac rhythm, in healthy hearts this is the *SA node*; 2. An electrical device performing the pacing function in case of a malfunctioning of the heart's own pacing (*artificial pacemaker*).
packet	Unit of datatransport in communications.
PACS	Picture archiving and communication system: a system for digital acquisition, storage and retrieval of images (see Chapter 13, Section 2).
paired *t*-test	A test for the comparison of *normally distributed* distributions of two observations for the same individuals.
paradigm	1. Example. 2. Pattern. 3. Fundamental concept.
parallel processing	Simultaneous processing of several programs or several parts of the same program.
parameter estimation	Estimation of the value of a population parameter and determination of the *confidence interval* (see Chapter 24, Section 3.2).
parasympathetic system	Part of the autonomic nervous system that increases secretion, the contractility of smooth muscles, and the dilatation of blood vessels. Ant: *sympathetic system*.
parse	To break input into smaller pieces, e.g., parsing a sentence to obtain the various words.
PASCAL	A *programming language* with a very well-defined structure.
password	A personal code word consisting of a series of symbols. It is used for user *authentication* when requiring access to a *network*, a *computer*, or a *program*.
patient identification	1. *Identification* of a patient. 2. A unique code that identifies the patient and that can be used as a *key* to his or her data records.
patient-driven data entry	Data entry, mostly concerning the *anamnesis*, performed by the patient before seeing the clinician.
pattern recognition	Techniques for *classifying* a set of objects into a number of distinct classes by considering similarities of objects belonging to the same class and the dissimilarities of objects belonging to different classes.

P

PC	See *personal computer*.
PC-DOS	*Operating system* for *PCs*.
PCL	Printer Control Language: a language used to control a printer.
PCR	Parent-child relationship: a hierarchical relationship between *records* in a *database*. Child records are dependent on the parent record. PCRs are used in the *hierarchical data model*
PDA	Personal digital assistant: a pocket-size computer used as organizer and for data entry.
PDF	*Portable* document format: a widely used *Adobe Acrobat* file format.
PDMS	Patient data management system: a computer system that manages patient data (acquisition, storage, data processing, and presentation) (see Chapter 12, Section 9).
PDQ	A base for oncology clinical trial protocols developed by the National Cancer Institute in the United States.
pen-based input	Input into a computer by means of a pen-like device whose movements are observed and interpreted by a computer.
perceptron	Early statistical method for the classification of objects that can be trained by a *learning population*. The perceptron is the predecessor of *artificial neural networks*.
periodic signal	A *deterministic signal* that is repeated with a fixed time interval (period) (see Chapter 8, Section 3).
peripheral device	Computer equipment not belonging to the central computer equipment (e.g., printers and terminals).
personal computer	(PC) Small computer intended to be used by one person at a time.
PET	Positron emission tomography: an imaging technique in nuclear medicine in which radiopharmaceuticals that emit positrons are used. The creation of a positron in the body is detected, and its location is reconstructed. In this way dynamic properties of biochemical and metabolic processes can be studied (see Chapter 9, Section 4.6).
pharmacokinetic model	*Model* of intake, transport through the body compartments, metabolism, and secretion of pharmaceuticals.
phonocardiogram	Recording of the sound produced by the beating heart.
photomultiplier	Equipment that multiplies the effect of an incoming photon by secondary emissions.
PHS	Public health surveillance: see *surveillance*.
physical data model	The organization of data in a *DBMS* as they are actually stored on the *mass storage device*.
pie chart	A graphical presentation in which the values of a variable are represented by segments of a circle, such that the result looks like a pie divided into unequal pieces.
piezo-electricity	Electrical change caused by pressure, especially in certain crystals.
pion	An unstable elementary particle, heavier than an electron, with positive, negative or no charge.
pixel	Contraction of 'picture element': the smallest part of a digital picture.
placebo effect	The effect caused by the suggestion of having received a possibly effective therapy.
platform	A characteristic combination of types of computer hardware and operating system, for example, a *UNIX* platform or a *Windows95* platform.
plethysmography	Method in lung physiology to determine the volume components of various respiratory gases.
plotter	A computer output device that draws images with ink pens.
PMS	See *postmarketing surveillance*
point process	A signal that is "0" most of the time, but when some event occurs it very briefly

P

	becomes a "1" (see Chapter 8, Section 3.1).
point-of-care system	A system that allows for the entry and retrieval of patient-specific data at the bedside.
point-to-point connection	Communication configuration in which each connection is a direct line (see Chapter 5, Section 4).
pointing device	A device whose movements are translated into the movement of a *cursor* on the computer *screen*.
population screening	Examination of a population to detect patients at risk or to find *risk factors* or diseases.
portability	The possibility of running a program on a machine different from the machine on which it has been developed.
posterior probability	Probability that an object belongs to a class given its *features* and *prior probabilities* of the classes.
postmarketing surveillance	Registering and monitoring of side effects and malfunctions of drugs, medical implants, and medical devices after their introduction to the market.
PostScript	A universal *command language* for printers.
Powerpoint	A presentation package from Microsoft used to prepare slide shows.
pragmatic	The effect of *information* on human actions (see Chapter 2, Section 4.3).
precision	Degree of exactness of a quantity (see Chapter 2, Section 6.3).
predictive value	The ratio between the correctly predicted outcome and the total of correctly and incorrectly predicted outcomes (positive predictive value for positive outcomes, negative predictive value for negative outcomes).
predictor	A *feature* of a disease process that can be used to predict a clinical outcome (see Chapter 18, Section 2).
prevalence	Fraction of the population with a certain *risk factor*, symptom, or disease.
prevention	Measures and activities to prevent health problems from occurring, to prevent the proliferation of diseases, and to prevent health deteriorating (see Panel 19.2).
primary care	The provision of integrated, accessible health care services by clinicians who are accountable for addressing a large majority of personal health care needs, developing a sustained partnership with patients, and practicing in the context of family and community (see Chapter 11).
primitive	In *pattern recognition*, an elementary component of an object.
printer	Computer device that can print characters or make drawings.
prior probability	The probability that an object belongs to a class without using the features of that object. It can be defined in the same way as *prevalence*.
privacy	The individual rights of a person to protect his or her personal life from the outside world, including the right to be left alone and to decide himself or herself how, what, and to what degree others may dispose of his or her data.
privacy regulation	The written policy of an organization with respect to privacy (see Chapter 33 , Section 3.3).
probabilistic reasoning	A *DSS* that uses statistical methods.
problem-oriented medical record	*Medical record* in which the notes are recorded for each problem assigned to the patient. Each problem is described according to the *SOAP* principle referred to Weed (see Chapter 7, Section 1).
problem-solving method	A generic strategy that can be abstracted from a class of *KBS*s (Chapter 28, Section 7).
procedural language	A high-level *programming language* (third-generation language). It contains statements that specify the steps that must be taken to perform a task.

P

procedure	1. A coherent set of actions that performs a certain task. 2. Part of a program that performs a subtask.
process	1. Something going on. 2. The systematic performing operations to produce a specified result. 3. The transformation of input data to output data that may be more suitable for further processing or interpretation.
process-control system	A computer system in which the decision-making process is part of the system, used to coordinate work processes such as manufacturing or assemby (see Chapter 3, Section 2).
production rule	Rule in a *DSS*-module that consists of a condition part and an action part. When the conditions are met, the action is executed.
program	Set of instructions or statements that let the computer perform a certain task.
programmer	A person who designs, writes, tests, and maintains *software*.
programming language	A formal language for the representation of a computer *program*. Syn: computer language.
project	A cluster of related activities that has a clear beginning and a clear ending in time. A project should deliver a specified product.
project leader	A person who has the day-to-day responsibility for a *project*.
prompt	A special sign on the device with which the user interacts (*VDU* or *printer-keyboard* combination), indicating that the computer expects a response.
propositional logic	See *Boolean algebra*.
prosthesis	An artificial device that replaces a part of the body.
PROTÉGÉ	A computer workbench supporting a formal methodology and containing tools used to develop a *DSS* from *domain ontologies* and reusable problem-solving methods (see Panel 17.3).
protocol	1. A standard means by which two devices can exchange data. It applies to the *syntax* or the *semantics*. 2. A standard *algorithm* that defines one precise manner in which certain classes of patients should be evaluated or treated.
prototype	A preliminary system that has part of the required properties of the intended system, such as the user interface.
provocative test	Signal issued by a biological system that is brought into a forced condition, e.g., by a stimulus, exercise, or *artificial pacing*.
pseudo-3D	Visualization of a three-dimensional image on a two-dimensional device by using techniques such as shadowing and hidden-line removal.
public domain software	Free software.
public health	Description of the health status of a population and the science and art of preventing disease, prolonging life, and promoting health through organized efforts of society.
PUFF	An *EMYCIN*-based *DSS* for the interpretation of pulmonary tests.
punched card	A now outdated storage and input medium that consists of a cardboard card in which the data were recorded by holes punched in the card.
PVC	Premature ventricular contraction: see *extrasystole*.

Q

Q wave	If the *QRS* complex of the *ECG* starts with a negative wave, then this wave is called the Q-wave. The presence of a Q-wave in some leads is an indication of a myocardial infarction.
QA	Quality assessment.

QC	Quality control.
QMR	Quick Medical Reference: a *DSS*, based on *INTERNIST-I* that assists in the diagnostic process in internal medicine (see Chapter 16, Section 4.2 and Panel 16.1). Syn: INTERNIST-I/QMR.
QMR-KAT	A *graphical KBE* used to support the creation and maintenance of *QMR* disease profiles.
QRS complex	Most prominent part of the *ECG* waveform. The first positive wave in the QRS complex is called the *R-wave*, a possibly preceding negative wave is called a *Q-wave*. The QRS-complex shows the electrical activity caused by the *depolarization* of the ventricles.
qualitative data	Data describing nominal categorical aspects (see Chapter 24, Section 2).
qualitative decision-support system	*DSS* that uses symbolic reasoning methods, e.g., logical deduction (see Chapter 15, Section 4.1)
qualitative model	A model in which relationships among concepts are defined in symbolic terms (e.g., *ontologies and knowledge bases*). Ant: *quantitative model*.
quality assessment	Measures used to determine the quality of medical care.
QUALY	Quality adjusted life years, a measure of the life expectancy corrected for loss of quality of that life caused by diseases and disabilities.
quantile	Division of a distribution such that a given percentage of the observations have values above that quantile. The 50% quantile is identical to the *median*.
quantitative data	Countable (*discrete*) or measurable (*continuous*) data (see Chapter 24, Section 2).
quantitative decision support	Decision support by statistical methods (see Chapter 15, Section 4.1).
quantitative model	A model in which relationships among concepts are defined in mathematical terms (e.g., compartment models and probabilistic models). Ant: *qualitative model*.
quasi-periodic signal	A *deterministic signal* that is repeated with almost the same time intervals and with almost the same waveshape (see Chapter 8, Section 3).
query language	A computer language to formulate orders for extractions from a *database*.
Quetelet index	Measure of the weight of a person corrected for his or her length. Syn: body-mass index.

R

R wave	The first positive wave in the *QRS complex*.
R&D	Research and development.
RAD	Rapid application development: a system development method that tries to speed up development, e.g., by using *prototyping*.
radio-opaque	Nontranslucent for certain *EM* radiation waves, such as *X rays*.
radio-pharmaceutical	A substance that is absorbed by the organ that is the subject of *nuclear medicine* examination, and that contains the radioactive *isotope* (see Chapter 9, Section 4).
radiotherapy	Treatment with localized high-energy radiation to destroy tumor tissue (see Chapter 12, Section 2.10).
RAM	Random access memory: the central memory of a computer.
random access	Access to data by reference to their storage location, independent of their storage sequence. Typical random access devices are central memory, disks (see Chapter 3, Section 3.3). Syn: direct access. Ant: *sequential access*
random noise	Noise with a random character, in many cases with a *normal distribution*.

randomization	Random division of a group of individuals into subgroups that, for instance, will each receive different treatments.
range	Difference between the largest and the smallest observation in a set of numeric data.
rank correlation test	Test used to analyze whether not *normally distributed* data are statistically linearly independent by means of a *rank score*.
rank score	A score derived from the ranks of the observed data that belong to a group.
RCC	Read Clinical Classification: a coding system, developed in the United Kingdom, that attempts to cover all terms that may be written in a patient record (see Chapter 6, Section 5.8).
Read codes	See *RCC*
real number	1. Mathematical: a number that can be approached with arbitrary accuracy by a quotient of two whole numbers 2. Informatics: a number that is internally represented in a computer memory by an exponent and a mantissa.
reason for encounter	(RfE) The reason why a patient contacts a clinician.
recognition	To perceive something to be previously known.
record	The smallest logical unit in a *file* or *database* system (see Chapter 4, Section 1).
record linkage	Combining data from different *databases* by linking personal records using direct or indirect identifications.
recovery	To restore the contents of a *database* after a disruption.
redundancy	The inclusion of more information than needed to derive *semantic* information.
reference model	A generic model for a class of organizations, such as hospitals or *primary care* that can be used for comparisons or as a reference for more detailed models. It describes both functionality and data (see Chapter 19, Section 3.6).
region growing	*Segmentation* performed by taking a *seed point* that is the starting point of a coherent region. Other points similar to the seed point are assigned to that region (see Chapter 10, Section 3.6).
region splitting	*Segmentation* by using discontinuities in the *gradient* of an image (see Chapter 10, Section 3.6).
region-of-interest	Part of an image that is selected for further *image processing*.
register	Part of a *CPU* for intermediate storage of instructions, addresses, and data.
registry	A collection of records containing health information for a population, such as specific diseases, transplants, congenital malfunctions, and immunization, in a region or country. Registries are usually established and enforced by legislation (see Chapter 22, Section 2.4).
regression analysis	Statistical analysis of the relationship between two sets of paired variables. *Linear regression analysis* is a special case in which the covariables have a linear relationship to a continuous outcome.
relational database	*Database* organization consisting of a series of tables, in which the rows are fixed-length *records* and the columns represent *fields*. Corresponding records in different tables are identified by means of *keys* (see Chapter 4, Section 4.1).
relative risk	The ratio of the *incidence* in two populations differing in the exposition to a *risk factor*.
relaxation	Returning back to an equilibrium state after being exposed to an external force.
reliability	Used to describe a measurement with low inter- and intraobserver *variabilities*.
remote sensing	Taking and analyzing measurements on the earth's surface or atmosphere by using aerial or satellite photography.

R

rendering methods	Methods in computer graphics to display three-dimensional structures.
repolarization	Restoration of the potential difference between objects such as in a cell between an isolating membrane after *depolarization*. Ant: *depolarization*.
repository	A consolidated or archival database that may combine records from a number of smaller databases and that is used in general for reference.
resolution	The density of *pixels* in a digital image.
retrieval	The act of retrieving earlier stored data.
reverse video	Part of a *screen* with colors for foreground and background complementary to the usual colors, intended to draw attention.
RGB	The red, green, and blue signal of a color television signal.
RICHE	Réseau d'Information et de Communication Hospitalier Européen: a *hospital information system* project founded by the European Union.
RIS	Radiology information system: a system that supports the medical and administrative functions of a radiology department (see Chapter 13, Section 2).
RISC	Reduced Instruction Set Computer: such a *computer* has a limited set of instructions that can be executed very fast. Complicated instructions are performed as a sequence of these elementary instructions. Ant: *CISC*.
risk factor	A *determinant* that has, in general, a negative influence on somebody's *health*.
RMIS	The Regenstrief Medical Information System: the system provides computer-based medical records and computer-generated reminders at the University of Indiana since the 1970s.
robot	A computer-controlled device that can physically manipulate its surroundings.
robotics	Creation and training of *robots*.
ROC	Receiver (or relative) operating characteristics: a curve of *false positive* and *false negative* results at various *threshold* values indicating the quality of a decision method (see Chapter 15, Section 4.1.2).
Roentgen radiation	See X ray
roll forward	Recovering the contents of a *database* from the last *backup* and the *log file*.
ROM	Read-only memory: a non-*volatile memory* that cannot be changed by the user. It often contains control programs, e.g., to *boot* the system.
RR interval	The distance in time between successive *R waves* in the *ECG*.
RSA	Rivest, Shamir, and Adelman: the initials of the inventors of an algorithm for a digital signature, using prime-number based *encryption* techniques.
rule-based reasoning	A *DSS* method based on *logical* (rule-based) reasoning (see Chapter 15, Section 4.2.3).
rule-based DSS	A *knowledge-based DSS* in which all the knowledge is encoded using *production rules*.

S

SA node	Sinoauricular node: the group of cells where the stimulation of the atrium starts.
sampling	Measuring the value of the output of a *process*.
sampling frame	A large population of *cases* from which samples for a *trial group* can be retrieved.
sampling frequency	*Frequency* at which samples are taken (see Chapter 8, Section 3). Syn: sampling rate.
sampling interval	Time interval over which the *sampling* of an *analog signal* takes places (see Chapter 8, Section 3).
sampling rate	See *sampling frequency*

sampling theorem	See **Shannon-Nyquist theorem**.
scanner	1. Equipment used to obtain images from a patient, e.g., **CT** or **MRI**. 2. Equipment used to enter information on documents or film into a computer.
scattergram	A presentation of bivariate data by plotting each variable as a point with (x,y) coordinates (e.g., Figure 27.5).
scintigram	In nuclear medicine, recording of detected scintillations caused by emission from an organ.
SCP	Standard communications protocol: a standard for the transmission of **ECGs** and their interpreted data.
screen	The surface of a display unit, consisting of phosphor that lightens up when hit by the electrode beam, or of liquid crystals that change their orientation when exposed to an electric field (see Chapter 3, Section 3.3).
SDE	See **structured data entry**.
SDI	Selective dissemination of information: a service that periodically runs user defined automatic **retrieval** searches on an **NLM database**.
searching	Selecting and retrieving data from a large data set, especially from a **database** or a **data warehouse**.
second opinion	Advice of another, independent clinician about a diagnosis or treatment.
sector	Part of a **track** of a **disk**. Syn: physical **block**.
security	See **data security**.
SEDAAR	Strategic Environmental Distributed Active Archive Resource: a **GIS** for environmental applications.
seed point	A starting point for **clustering** (see Chapter 27, Section 3.2).
segmentation	Decomposing a signal or an image into its constituent components (see Chapter 10, Section 3.6).
Seismed	A project within the European **AIM** program on security in medical information systems.
semantic	Relating to the meaning of a sign or a set of signs (see Chapter 2, Section 4.2).
semantic network	A representation of knowledge of a **domain** by means of a network of **concepts** (**object classes**) with **attributes** that provides **semantic** relationships among the **concepts**.
sensitivity	See **true positive**.
sensitivity analysis	Analysis of the change of an outcome of a calculation when input variables are changed.
sentinel GP	General practitioner belonging to a relatively small group of highly motivated, geographically distributed physicians who provide the data for epidemiological **monitoring**.
sequential access	A storage method in which the data must be read in the same order as they were written, such as for **magnetic tape** (see Chapter 3, Section 3.3). Ant: **random access**.
serial comparison	Comparison of **biosignals** (e.g., **ECGs**) over certain time intervals to detect intraperson changes.
SGML	Standard Generalized Markup Language: a formal standard for **hypertext** applications.
Shannon's formula	A formula that defines the information content of a message as the negative logarithm (base 2) of the probability of occurrence of that message (see Chapter 2, Section 4.4).
Shannon-Nyquist theorem	A theorem stating that a signal should be sampled at least at twice the highest-

S

	frequency component present in the signal to avoid the loss of information (see Chapter 8, Section 4.1).
shared care	Clinicians (general practitioners, specialists and nurses) jointly treating the same patient (see Chapter 11, Section 1).
shell	1. A software layer separating the user and the *operating system*. 2. A framework for a *DSS* without the domain knowledge.
shock	A state of severe disturbance of vital processes, associated with low blood volume and pressure.
SI units	Système Internationale d'unités: a system of internationally accepted units, whose use is mandatory in many countries. SI is based on the metric system with as basic units the meter, the kilogram, and the second, extended with units for current, temperature, and so forth. From the basic SI units other units can be derived, such as becquerel for the radioactivity of a substance and pascal for pressures.
signal analysis	Processing of signals to derive further information (see Chapter 8).
signal-to-noise ratio	(SNR) The ratio between the *variance* of the signal and the *variance* of the noise.
significance level	The maximal level for the probability of a *type-one error* in hypothesis testing.
significant digit	A digit in a number that has significance for the description of the result of a measurement or a calculation.
simulation	Use of a model of a physical or abstract system within another system (usually within a computer by means of a computer program) to study the behavior of the original system.
skewed data	Data that have a *bias*.
skewed distribution	A distribution that is not symmetric, that is, its *skewness* is not equal to 0.
skewness	Parameter that describes the asymmetry of a statistical distribution.
smart card	Plastic card the size of a credit card that is made intelligent by a small processor that is mounted in it (see Chapter 3, Section 3.3). Syn: *chip card*
SNOMED	Systematized Nomenclature of Human and Veterinary Medicine: a multiaxial *nomenclature system* for the coding of several aspects of a diagnosis (see Chapter 6, Section 5.4).
SNOP	Systematized Nomenclature of Pathology: a nomenclature system of the College of American Pathologists based on four coding axes: topography, morphology, etiology, and function. It is a predecessor to *SNOMED*.
SNR	See *signal-to-noise* ratio
SOAP	Acronym for the subjective (patient's complaints), objective (physician's findings), assessment (interpretations and conclusions), and plan (medical policy), ordering of the description of a problem in the *problem-oriented medical record*.
software	Computer programs and their documentation (see Chapter 3, Section 4). Ant: *hardware*.
software engineer	A person who does *software engineering*.
software engineering	The workmanship used to analyze, design, build, or maintain information systems.
solicited-advice DSS	A *DSS* that gives advice only on request of the user (see Chapter 16, Section 4).
sorting	Ordering groups of data in a sequence, according to given criteria.
source code	List of program statements (instructions) in the *language* in which that *program* was originally written. Ant: *object code* and *machine code*.
source-oriented medical record	*Medical record* in which the contents are ordered according to the method by which they were obtained. Within each section data typically have a chronological order

S

	(see Chapter 7, Section 2).
specificity	See *true negative*.
SPECT	Single-photon emission computed tomography: a method in *nuclear medicine* of obtaining three-dimensional reconstructions in a way similar to that used in *CT* (see Chapter 9, Section 4.6).
speech recognition	Computer transform of voice input into data (see Panel 7.5 and Chapter 31).
speech-based input	See *speech recognition.*
spirogram	Measurement of the lung volume, air pressures, and respiratory flows (see Chapter 13, Section 3).
spreadsheet	A computer program in which the *screen* is divided into cells. Data are entered and shown in the cells, and the cells may contain *algorithms* to perform operations with the contents of other cells.
SPSS	Statistical Package for the Social Sciences: a commonly used set of programs for performing statistical analyses of data.
SQL	Structured Query Language: a *database* language for *relational databases*. It contains a *DDL* to describe the data model and a *DML* to store and retrieve data (see Panel 4.2).
ST depression	Lowering of the signal in an *ECG* between *QRS complex* and *T-wave*, often indicating *ischemic heart disease*.
ST-T complex	Part of the *ECG* waveform immediately after the *QRS complex*, including the ST-segment and the *T-wave*. It describes the repolarization of the heart ventricular muscle.
standard	A document, established by consensus and approved by a recognized body, which provides rules, guidelines, or characteristics for activities (see Chapter 34).
standard deviation	Square root of the *variance* of a statistical variable, indicating the spread (or variability) of a distribution.
standardization	Activity of establishing a *standard.*
stat report	A report of a laboratory examination that has been declared urgent by the requester.
stationary signal	A *stochastic signal* whose statistical properties do not change over time see (see Chapter 8, Section 3). Ant: *nonstationary signal.*
statistical DSS	*DSS* based on statistical methods and making use of training populations; features are selected by using statistical methods as well. Ant: *symbolic DSS*.
statistical error	Variations between two measurements caused by natural fluctuations (see Chapter 2, Section 6.2). Ant: *Systematic error, bias*.
statistical pattern recognition	*Pattern* recognition in which objects are classified by numerical features.
statistical power	1. In hypothesis testing, a statistical parameter that gives the probability of a *false-negative* result (see Chapter 24, Section 3.1). 2. In stepwise selection, the probability that a *predictor* is selected if it indeed has a *predictive value* (see Chapter 18, Section 3.1).
statistical signal	See *stochastic signal.*
stepwise selection	A selection of features one by one starting with the feature explaining the highest (or lowest) amount of variance for a statistical or pattern recognition analysis (see Chapter 18, Section 3.2).
stochastic model	A model in which the results of an experiment are analyzed by statistical methods to obtain a conclusion valid within *confidence limits*.

S

stochastic signal	Signals that can only be described in statistical terms (see Chapter 8, Section 3). Ant: *deterministic signal;* Syn: statistical signal.
STOR	An early *CPR* developed at the University of California, San Francisco.
storage	1. A device of medium that can accept, hold and deliver *data*. 2. The act of storing data.
structured data entry	(SDE) Context-sensitive data entry in which the clinician completes part of a form presented on a *screen* by selecting from the screen a term that is related to the patient's problem or to the answer to a foregoing question (see Chapter 29, Section 2.4.2).
subroutine library	A *library* of *procedures*; in some *programming languages* procedures are called subroutines.
supervised classification	A technique in which an unclassified object is assigned to a class known beforehand.
surveillance	Routinely collecting data to examine the extent of a disease, to follow trends, and to detect changes in disease occurrence, e.g. infectious disease surveillance, *postmarketing surveillance.*
symbolic DSS	Decision-support model that uses *features* defined by experts or based on clinical studies. This type of decision-support methods uses logical reasoning. Ant: *statistical DSS.*
symbolic logic	See *Boolean logic.*
symbolic method	See *qualitative decision support.*
symbolic reasoning	Logical deduction.
sympathetic system	Part of the autonomic nervous system that decreases secretion, the contractility of smooth muscles, and the dilatation of blood vessels. Ant: *parasympathetic system.*
syndrome	A characteristic, concurrent combination of symptoms that cannot yet be connected to a disease causing the symptoms.
syntactic	Relating to the *syntax.*
syntactic pattern recognition	*Pattern recognition*, consisting of identification of the *primitives*, followed by identification of the *object class.*
syntax	The rules (the grammar) for the description, storage, and transmission of messages (see Chapter 2, Section 4.1) or for the composition of a program statement.
system	A combination of the people, procedures, programs, and machines used to perform a task.
systematic error	An error caused by an intrinsic difference in results between two measurement methods (see Chapter 2, Section 6.2). Syn: *bias*; Ant: *statistical error.*
systems analyst	A person who examines an activity to determine what should be accomplished and how the necessary operations should be performed by using computers.
systems designer	A person who analyzes the transformation of the information flows described by the *information analyst* into a *system.*

T

T	See *tera*
T wave	Last wave of the *ECG* waveform (see *ST-T complex*).
t-test	Statistical test used to compare the results of two *normally distributed* samples with identical *standard deviations*.
table	1. Collection of data in a form suitable for quick referencing. 2. Part of a relational database, consisting of records with identical structures.

tautology	A *logical operation* between two *logical expressions* that is always TRUE.
taxonomy	1. The study of classifications, including its bases, principles, procedures, and rules. 2. The resulting classification in related groups of a taxonomic process (see Chapter 6, Section 2.4).
TCP/IP	Transfer Control Protocol/Internet Protocol: a widely used protocol for communicating data over *networks*.
TEIRESIAS	A knowledge acquisition system for *MYCIN*.
telematics	Contraction of telecommunications and automatic information processing: the use of information technology over wide-area networks.
telemedicine	Diagnosis and therapy performed by somebody at a location remote from a patient, whose data are electronically transmitted.
teleoperation	Surgery in which the surgeon guides an operation or operates via *robotic* equipment on a patient at a distant location.
telepathology	Pathology in which the image of the specimen is *digitally transmitted* and examined by a pathologist at a remote location.
teleradiology	Radiology in which the radiological images and reports are electronically transmitted from one location to another.
Telnet	Protocol to enable logging into a remote computer via a network.
tera	Abbreviation for $1,000,000,000,000$ (10^{12}).
terminal	Computer *I/O* station.
terminal emulation	Imitating the functionality of a terminal by software.
test population	A set of *cases* independent of the *learning set*, to assess the performance of a *classification algorithm*. Ant: *Learning population*.
test set	1. A set of input data to validate a *program* or a *classification*. 2. A *test population*.
testing	Validation or *evaluation* of the performance of a computer system (*hardware* or *software*), *DSS*, or *pattern recognition* system by means of test procedures or a *test set*.
texture	Perceived structure of a surface.
therapy	Actions to treat a health problem.
thesaurus	Set of frequently used standard terms for a certain application area (see Chapter 6, Section 2.2).
threshold	1. In decision-support systems: a quantity for which a statement is false or true if the value of a feature is below or above that quantity, respectively. 2. In signal analysis: the level below which no signal is detected.
thresholding	*Segmentation* by cutting off all values above or below a *threshold*. Syn: *histogram segmentation* (see Chapter 10, Section 3.6).
time lag	Time interval between two not necessarily consecutive *samples* of the same or different signals.
time sharing	Use of a system by many users who may use the system in time slices in turn.
time-oriented medical record	*Medical record* with a chronological order of the data (see Chapter 7, Section 1).
TMR	A *CPR* for family medicine created at Duke University Medical Center.
TN	See *true negative*.
tomographic	See *CT*.
tomography	See *CT*.
toolkit	A set of *procedures* and stand-alone *programs* for the development or maintenance

T

	of a specific **application** or group of applications.
total performance	A measure for performance of a decision-support system expressed in one number (see Chapter 15, Section 4.1.3).
TOXNET	Information about toxic substances made electronically available by **NLM**.
TP	See **true positive**.
track	Circular part of a **disk** that can contain data. A track can be written or read without moving the read-write head after initial positioning.
tracking ball	A **pointing device** like a **mouse** consisting of a rotatable ball.
training set	See **learning population**.
transaction	A set of computer operations that performs a specific activity in the real world, e.g. the registration of a patient.
transaction processing	Processing of one **transaction** immediately after input of all necessary data (see Chapter 4, Section 2.2). Ant: **batch processing**.
transducer	A device that transforms an input signal into an output signal of a different type.
transfer function	Function that describes mathematically the transformation of the source signal by a system (e.g., a biological process) into the output signal.
transient signal	A signal caused by a sudden change in conditions that persists for a relatively short time after the change.
transmission channel	See **channel**.
transmitter	Transducer that transfers its signal by radio waves.
transmural	Care for an individual in a setting that is not limited to one health care organization.
trend analysis	Analysis of a variable over time to detect or investigate long-term changes.
trial group	A group of **cases** selected to perform a **clinical trial**.
trigger	1. The button on a **joystick**. 2. An event that causes a sequence of other events.
true negative	(TN) Measure of the quality of a decision. The percentage of objects that do not have some attribute and for which a decision procedure correctly rejects this attribute (see Chapter 15, Section 4).
true positive	(TP) Measure of the quality of a decision. The percentage of objects that have some attribute and for which a decision procedure correctly detects this attribute (see Chapter 15, Section 4).
truth table	1. A table containing the values of a **logical expression** for all possible combinations of its **logical variables**. 2. In **DSS**, making a **qualitative decision** by setting up a table to use all decision units (**logical expressions**) simultaneously (see also **decision table**).
turnkey	A ready-to-use system containing all the hardware, software, and training required to run an application.
twisted pair	Electrical connection consisting of a set of isolated wires that are twisted pairwise to reduce external noise influences.
type ahead	Entering data before the computer asks for it (see Chapter 3, Section 2.1).
type-one error	A false rejection of a **null hypothesis**.
type-two error	Falsely accepting the **null hypothesis**, although the **alternative hypothesis** is true.

U

ultrasound	Sound with a **frequency** far above the capability of human hearing (1-10 Mhz); it is used as a signal for patient imaging.
UMLS	Unified Medical Language System: contains a meta**thesaurus** with medical **concepts** and a **semantic network**. (see Chapter 6, Section 6).

UN/ECE	United Nations Economic Commission for Europe.
unary operator	An operator on one variable.
UNDP	United Nations Development Program.
unit dose system	A method in which drugs are packed and labeled individually for each patient and for each dose to prevent distribution errors.
UNIX	An *operating system* widely used in computers, from *main frames* to *personal computers*.
unsolicited advice DSS	A *DSS* that gives advice independently of a request of the user (see Chapter 16, Section 4).
unsupervised classification	See *clustering*.
URL	Universal Resource Locator: the *Internet* address system.
usability	The effectiveness and efficiency of a system and the user's attitude toward a system (see Chapter 31, Section 2.7).
user interface	The part of the computer system that communicates with the user (see Chapter 3, Section 2 and Chapter 31, Section 2.1).
utility	1. An assessment of the value of the expected result of a diagnostic and therapeutic treatment, expressed in units such as life expectancy or quality-adjusted life years (*QUALYs*). In general, the alternative with the highest utility will be preferred. 2. A software program that performs a task (e.g., *sorting* a *file*).

V

validity	Used to describe a measurement that reflects what is intended to be measured.
validity check	A check on the correctness of data by using their *semantics*.
variability	Variations in the results of a measurement, an observation, or an assessment. It is discerned in interobserver variability (differences between observers) and intraobserver variability (differences between repeated observations of the same observer).
variance	A measure for the spread of a distribution.
VCG	Vectorcardiogram: the representation of the *ECG* as a three-dimensional signal, visualized as three two-dimensional *Lissajous figures* in three *orthogonal* planes.
VDU	See *visual display unit*.
vectorcardiogram	See *VCG*.
Venn diagram	A graphical representation of all objects of a class (a set) by closed figures showing the relationships between subsets.
ventricle	1. Cavity in the body. 2. Heart chamber. 3. Cavity in the brain.
video teleconference	A conference with remotely located participants by telecommunication of sound and images.
videodisk	An *optical disk* with images or movies.
vigilance	Assessment and *prevention* of adverse drug reactions or *monitoring* of medical devices (see Chapter 22, Section 3.5).
virtual reality	Imitation of reality, usually with the help of a computer, which provides the user with a combination of visual, auditory, and possibly, tactile information reflecting the actions of the user, giving the user the impression of being present in some reality (see Panel 12.1).
Visible Humans Project	A project of *NLM* to make available detailed photographic, *MRI*, and *CT* data of normal humans by means of *data communication* for use in the study of anatomy,

V

	imaging research, and so on (see Chapter 26, Section 4.2 and Panel 26.1).
visual display unit	(VDU) A computer input/output device that allows presentation of characters and pictures on a screen.
vital signs	The most important parameters describing the condition of a patient, such as heart rate, blood pressures, respiration rate and volume, and blood gas levels.
voice input	See speech recognition.
voice recognition	See *speech recognition*.
volatile memory	Computer *memory* whose content is lost when the power is switched off.
voxel	A three-dimensional picture element (volume element) analogous to a *pixel*.
VR	See *virtual reality*.

W

WAN	Wide area network: a communications network that may span the whole world, but with a smaller bandwidth than a *LAN* (see Panel 5.3).
wavelet transform	Transformation of a signal into a linear composition of time-limited components (wavelets) (see Panel 25.3).
WBC	White blood cell.
WHO	World Health Organization: a United Nations organization having *public health* as its main concern.
WHOSIS	*WHO's* statistical information system.
Wilcoxon signed rank test	Test to compare two observations from the same sample that do not have a *normal distribution*.
Wilcoxon-Man-Whitney test	Test to compare two distributions that are not *normally distributed*.
window	Area on a computer *screen* that organizes data input and output and control data from a given program (see Chapter 3, Section 4.1).
Windows	A *windows*-oriented *operating system* for *PCs* manufactured by Microsoft.
windows-oriented interface	*Graphical user interface* that makes use of *windows*.
WORD	The name of a *word processor*.
word length	The number of *bits* in a *computer word*.
word processor	Program used to enter and manipulate texts.
WordPerfect	The name of a *word processor*.
workbench	A coherent set of computer programs used to support the design or development of information or knowledge systems.
World Bank	An international bank with activities for developing countries.
World Health Organization	See *WHO*.
World Wide Web	(WWW) An application on the *Internet* that facilitates access to information available at sites distributed throughout the world (see Panel 5.5).
WORM	Write once, read many times: a type of optical disk.
writing tablet	Computer input equipment that accepts human handwriting.
WWW	see World Wide Web.

X

X	A *windows-oriented* graphical user interface developed for *UNIX*.
X-Motif	A set of standardized high-level interaction components based on *X* (*graphical user interface* for *UNIX*).

W/X

X-ray	*EM radiation* of high energy (short wavelength). Its absorption by biological material depends on the kind of tissue.
X-ray image	Image obtained by means of *X rays*.
X-terminal	A terminal with the *graphical user interface X* (often used in *UNIX*) embedded in hardware.
X-Windows	A *graphical user interface* for *UNIX*.
X11	A *UNIX* standard for an *X*-type of *graphical user interface*.
XOR	A *logical operation* between two *logical expressions* that is then and only then TRUE when both expressions are TRUE (see Chapter 23, Section 2.2).

Z

Z score	A statistical test for normal distribution.

Key References

Van Bemmel JH, Willems JL, eds. *Handboek Medische Informatica*, Utrecht/ntwerpen: Bohn, Scheltema & Holkema, 1989 (in Dutch).

Webster's New World Dictionary of Computer Terms (4th ed.) New York: Prentice Hall, 1992.

Webster's Seventh New Collegiate Dictionary, Springfield, MA: Merriam Webster, Inc. 1965.

Seelos H-J, ed. *Wörterbuch der Medizinischen Informatik,* Berlin-New York: Walter de Gruyter, 1990 (in German).

Concise Oxford Dictionary (7th ed.) Oxford, UK: Oxford University Press, 1983.

Ball MJ, Hannah KJ, eds. *Using Computers in Nursing,* Reston, VA.: Reston Publishing Co., 1988.

Z

Keyword Index

Keyword Index

KI

KI

KI

KI

KI

KI

KI

KI

KI

KI

List of Authors

Dr. A.R. Bakker
Department of Medical Informatics
Faculty of Medicine,
University of Leiden
P.O. Box 2086
2301 CB Leiden
The Netherlands
Phone: +31 71 52 56 736
Fax: +31 71 521 6675
E-mail: abakker@hiscom.nl

Dr. M.J. Ball
First Consulting Group
2 Hamill Road, Quadrangle West 359
Baltimore, Maryland 21210-1999
United States
Phone: +1 410 433 0597
Fax: +1 410 433 0988
E-mail: mjb@fcgnet.com

Dr. P.J. Branger
Department of Medical Informatics
Faculty of Medicine and Health Sciences
Erasmus University
P.O. Box 1738
3000 DR Rotterdam
The Netherlands
Phone: +31 10 408 7050
Fax: +31 10 436 2882
E-mail: branger@mi.fgg.eur.nl

Dr. P.D. Clayton
Center for Medical Informatics
Columbia-Presbyterian Medical Center

Atchley Pavilion Rm 1301
161 Fort Washington Avenue
New York NY 10027
United States
Phone: +1 212 305 6896
Fax: +1 212 305 3302
E-mail: clayton@cucis.cis.columbia.edu

N.F. de Keizer, M.Sc.
Department of Medical Informatics, Division K
Amsterdam Medical Center, L0-062
Meibergdreef 15
1105 AZ Amsterdam
The Netherlands
Phone: +31 20-566 5205
Fax: +31 20-691 2432
E-mail: n.f.keizer@AMC.UvA.NL

Dr. G.J.E. De Moor
Department of Medical Informatics
State University Hospital
De Pintelaan 185
B-9000 Gent
Belgium
Phone: +32 9 240 3436
Fax: +32 9 240 3439
E-mail: gdemoor@allserv.rug.ac.be

Dr. P.F. de Vries Robbé
Department of Medical Informatics, Epidemiology &
Statistics
Catholic University of Nijmegen
P.O Box 9101
6500 HB Nijmegen

The Netherlands
Phone: +31 24 361 9158 / 3125
Fax: +31 24 361 3505
E-mail: p.robbe@mie.kun.nl

J.V. Douglas
First Consulting Group
2 Hamill Road, Quadrangle West 359
Baltimore, Maryland 21210-1999
United States
Phone: +1 410 433 0597
Fax: +1 410 433 0988
E-mail: jdouglas@fcgnet.com

J.S. Duisterhout, M.Sc.
Department of Medical Informatics
Faculty of Medicine and Health Sciences
Erasmus University
P.O. Box 1738
3000 DR Rotterdam
The Netherlands
Phone: +31 10 408 7049
Fax: +31 10 436 2882
E-mail: duisterhout@mi.fgg.eur.nl

C.J.W.A. Enning, M.Sc.
HISCOM
P.O. Box 901
2300 AX Leiden
The Netherlands
Phone: +31 71 52 56 789
Fax: +31 71 521 6675
E-mail: jenning@hiscom.nl

P.J.M.M. Epping, R.N., M.Sc., M.Ed.
Faculty of Nursing
Polytechnic Leiden
Endegeesterwatering 2
2333 CG Leiden
The Netherlands
Phone: +31 71 5171 121
Fax: +31 71 5154 041
E-mail: 75051.426@CompuServe.COM

dr. F.J. Flier
Department of Medical Informatics, Epidemiology &
Statistics
Catholic University of Nijmegen
P.O Box 9101
6500 HB Nijmegen
The Netherlands
Phone: +31 24 361 3125
Fax: +31 24 3613 505
E-mail: f.flier@MIE.KUN.NL

Dr. E.S. Gelsema
Department of Medical Informatics
Faculty of Medicine and Health Sciences
Erasmus University
P.O. Box 1738
3000 DR Rotterdam
The Netherlands
Phone: +31 10 408 7051 / 7050
Fax: +31 10 436 2882
E-mail: gelsema@mi.fgg.eur.nl

Dr. D.A. Giuse
Vanderbilt University Medical Center
Eskind Biomedical Library
2209 Garland Avenue
Nashville, TN 37232-8340
United States
Phone: +1 615 936 1556
Fax: +1 615 936 1427

Dr. N.B. Giuse
Vanderbilt University Medical Center
Eskind Biomedical Library
2209 Garland Avenue
Nashville, TN 37232-8340
United States
Phone: +1 615 936 1556
Fax: +1 615 936 1427

Dr. L. Gong
Department of Computer Science
Rutgers University
New Brunswick, NJ 08903
United States
Phone: +1 908 932 2006 / 2768
Fax: +1 908 932 0537

W. Goossen, R.N., B.S.N., Cert.Ed.
Nursing Sciences
Polytechnic Leeuwarden
P.O. Box 1080
8900 CB Leeuwarden
The Netherlands
Phone: +31 58 2934 365
Fax: +31 58 2934 335
E-mail: goossen@dns.nhl.nl

Dr. S.J. Grobe
LaQuinta Professor of Nursing
The University of Texas at Austin School of Nursing
1700 Red River
Austin, Texas 78701-1499
United States
Phone: +1 512 471 7311 ext. 355
Fax: +1 512 471 4910
E-mail: grobe@mail.utexas.edu

Dr. J.D.F. Habbema
Department of Public Health
Faculty of Medicine and Health Sciences
Erasmus University
P.O. Box 1738
3000 DR Rotterdam
The Netherlands
Phone: +31 10 408 7727 / 7712
Fax: +31 10 436 6831
E-mail: habbema@mgz.fgg.eur.nl

Dr. A. Hasman
Department of Medical Informatics
Faculty of Medicine and Health Sciences
University Maastricht
P.O. Box 616
6200 MD Maastricht
The Netherlands
Phone: +31 43 388 2240
Fax: +31 43 367 1052
E-mail: hasman@mi.unimaas.nl

Dr. R. Haux
Institute for Medical Biometry and Informatics
Department of Medical Informatics
University of Heidelberg

Im Neuenheimer Feld 400
D-69120 Heidelberg
Germany
Phone: +49 6221 56 7483
Fax: +49 6221 56 4997
E-mail: reinhold_haux@krzmail.krz.uni-heidelberg.de

Dr. J.C. Helder
Department of Medical Informatics
Faculty of Medicine and Health Sciences
Erasmus University
P.O. Box 1738
3000 DR Rotterdam
The Netherlands
Phone: +31 10 408 7050
Fax: +31 10 436 2882
E-mail: jchelder@knoware.nl

Dr. C.A. Kulikowski
Department of Computer Science
Rutgers University
New Brunswick, NJ 08903
United States
Phone: +1 908 932 2006 / 2768
Fax: +1 908 932 0537
E-mail: kulikows@cs.rutgers.edu

Dr. A.W. Kushniruk
Cognitive Studies in Science
Centre for Medical Education
McGill University
1110 Pine Avenue West
Montreal, Quebec
H3A 1A3 Canada
Phone: +1 514 398 4987 / 4988
Fax: +1 514 398 7246
E-mail: kushniruk@medcor.mcgill.ca

H.Y. Kwa, M.Sc.
SMS/Cendata
P.O. Box 1187
3430 BD Nieuwegein
The Netherlands
Phone: +31 30 6038 797
Fax: +31 30 6038 492
E-mail: ykwa@pi.net

Dr. F.J. Leven
Department of Medical Informatics
School of Technology Heilbronn
Max-Planckstr. 39
HD-74081 Heilbronn
Germany
Phone: +49 7131 504 396
Fax: +49 7131 52470
E-mail: leven@fh-heilbronn.de

Dr. J. Lindemans
Clinical Laboratory, L-154
University Hospital Dijkzigt
P.O. Box 2040
3000 CA Rotterdam
The Netherlands
Phone: +31 10 463 4509 / 3543
Fax: +31 10 436 7894
E-mail: lindemans@ckcl.azr.nl

H. Lodder, M.Sc.
Department of Medical Informatics
Faculty of Medicine,
University of Leiden
P.O. Box 2086
2301 CB Leiden
The Netherlands
Phone: +31 71 52 76 805
Fax: +31 71 52 76 799
E-mail: hlodder@informatics.medfac.leidenuniv.nl

Dr. A.T. McCray
Lister Hill Center,
National Library of Medicine
8600 Rockville Pike
Bethesda MD 20894
United States
Phone: +1 301 496 6280
Fax: +1 301 480 3035
E-mail: mccray@nlm.nih.gov

Dr. J. Michaelis
Institute for Medical Statistics and Documentation
University of Mainz
P.O. Box 3960
D91465 Mainz

Germany
Phone: +49 6131 173 252 / 177 369
Fax: +49 6131 172 968
E-mail: michael@imsd.uni-mainz.de

Dr. R.A. Miller
Vanderbilt University - Biomedical Informatics
Eskind Biomedical Library, room 436
2209 Garland Avenue
Nashville, TN 37232-8340
United States
Phone: +1 615 936 1556
Fax: +1 615 936 1427
E-mail: randy.miller@mcmail.vanderbilt.edu

Dr. P.W. Moorman
Department of Medical Informatics
Faculty of Medicine and Health Sciences
Erasmus University
P.O. Box 1738
3000 DR Rotterdam
The Netherlands
Phone: +31 10 408 8125 / 7050
Fax: +31 10 436 2882
E-mail: moorman@mi.fgg.eur.nl

Dr. M.A. Musen
Section on Medical Informatics
Stanford University School of Medicine
CA 94305-5479 Stanford
United States
Phone: +1 415 723 6979
Fax: +1 415 725 7944
E-mail: musen@smi.stanford.edu

Dr. V.L. Patel
Cognitive Studies in Medicine,
Centre for Medical Education
McGill University
1110 Pine Avenue West
Montreal, Quebec
H3A 1A3 Canada
Phone: +1 514 398 4987 / 4988
Fax: +1 514 398 7246
E-mail: patel@hebb.psych.mcgill.ca

Dr. L.A. Plugge
Department of Informatics
University Maastricht
P.O. Box 616
6200 MD Maastricht
The Netherlands
Phone: +31 43 388 3297 / 3504
Fax: +31 43 325 2392
E-mail: plugge@cs.unimaas.nl

Dr. P. Pop
Transmural and Diagnostic Center
University Hospital Maastricht
P.O. Box 1918
6201 BX Maastricht
The Netherlands
Phone: +31 43 387 5385
Fax: +31 43 387 7878

Dr. D.J. Protti
School of Health Information Science
University of Victoria
P.O. Box 3050
Victoria BC
V8W 3P5 Canada
Phone: +1 250 721 8814
Fax: +1 250 721 1457
E-mail: dprotti@hsd.uvic.ca

Dr. H.J. Rollema
Department of Urology
University Hospital Maastricht
P.O. Box 1918
6201 BX Maastricht
The Netherlands
Phone: +31 43 387 5259
Fax: +31 43 387 5255

R.J.A. Schijvenaars, M.Sc.
Department of Medical Informatics
Faculty of Medicine and Health Sciences
Erasmus University
P.O. Box 1738
3000 DR Rotterdam
The Netherlands
Phone: +31 10 408 7045 / 7050· ·

Fax: +31 10 436 2882
E-mail: schijvenaars@mi.fgg.eur.nl

Dr. E.W. Steyerberg
Department of Public Health
Faculty of Medicine and Health Sciences
Erasmus University
P.O. Box 1738
3000 DR Rotterdam
The Netherlands
Phone: +31 10 408 7053 / 7714
Fax: +31 10 436 6831
E-mail: steyerberg@ckb.fgg.eur.nl

Dr. J.L. Talmon
Department of Medical Informatics
University Maastricht
P.O. Box 616
6200 MD Maastricht
The Netherlands
Phone: +31 43 388 2243 / 2241
Fax: +31 43 367 1052
E-mail: talmon@mi.unimaas.nl

Dr. A.J. ten Hoopen
Department of Medical Informatics, Epidemiology &
Statistics
Catholic University of Nijmegen
P.O Box 9101
6500 HB Nijmegen
The Netherlands
Phone: +31 24 361 3125
Fax: +31 24 361 3505
E-mail: h.tenhoopen@mie.kun.nl

Dr. J.H. van Bemmel
Department of Medical Informatics
Faculty of Medicine and Health Sciences
Erasmus University
P.O. Box 1738
3000 DR Rotterdam
The Netherlands
Phone: +31 10 408 7050
Fax: +31 10 436 2882
E-mail: vanbemmel@mi.fgg.eur.nl

Dr. J. van der Lei
Department of Medical Informatics
Faculty of Medicine and Health Sciences
Erasmus University
P.O. Box 1738
3000 DR Rotterdam
The Netherlands
Phone: +31 10 408 8184 / 7050
Fax: +31 10 436 2882
E-mail: vanderlei@mi.fgg.eur.nl

A.A.F. van der Maas, M.D.
Department of Medical Informatics, Epidemiology &
Statistics
Catholic University of Nijmegen
P.O Box 9101
6500 HB Nijmegen
The Netherlands
Phone: +31 24 361 3125
Fax: +31 24 361 3505
E-mail: A.VanDerMaas@mie.kun.nl

Dr. A.M. van Ginneken
Department of Medical Informatics
Faculty of Medicine and Health Sciences
Erasmus University
P.O. Box 1738
3000 DR Rotterdam
The Netherlands
Phone: +31 10 408 7052 / 7050
Fax: +31 10 436 2882
E-mail: vanginneken@mi.fgg.eur.nl

Dr. E.M. van Mulligen
Department of Medical Informatics
Faculty of Medicine and Health Sciences
Erasmus University
P.O. Box 1738
3000 DR Rotterdam
The Netherlands
Phone: +31 10 408 7047 / 7050
Fax: +31 10 436 2882
E-mail: vanmulligen@mi.fgg.eur.nl

Dr. J.C. Wyatt
Biomedical Informatics Unit
Imperial Cancer Research Fund Laboratories
P.O. Box 123
London WC2A 3PX
United Kingdom
Phone: +44 171 242 0200 / 269 3637
Fax: +44 171 269 3067
E-mail: jeremy@biu.icnet.uk

C. Zeelenberg, M.Sc.
TNO Prevention and Health
Sector Medical Informatics
P.O. Box 2215
2301 CE Leiden
The Netherlands
Phone: +31 71 5181 789 / 181
Fax: +31 71 5181 906
E-mail: zeelenberg@pg.tno.nl

Dr. J.H.M. Zwetsloot-Schonk
Department of Medical Informatics
Amsterdam Medical Center
Meibergdreef 15
1105 AZ Amsterdam
The Netherlands
Phone: +31 20 566 5184 / 5200
Fax: +31 20 691 7233
E-mail: jschonk@amc.uva.nl